T0275468

Acupuncture for IVF and Assisted Reproduction

To my husband Alan and my children Daniel and Matthew. My life would not be complete without you!

Irina Szmelskyj

To my son Oliver Jacob Aquilina-Ford.

Also in the loving memory of my baby nephew Georgio Aquilina, and Indie.

Lianne Aquilina

For Elsevier
Content Strategists: Claire Wilson, Alison Taylor
Content Development Specialist: Sally Davies
Project Manager: Sukanthi Sukumar
Designer: Christian Bilbow
Illustration Manager: Richard Tibbitts
Illustrator: Antbits Ltd.

Acupuncture for IVF and Assisted Reproduction
An Integrated Approach to Treatment and Management

Irina Szmelskyj DipAc MSc MBAcC

Lead Clinician, True Health Clinics and Founder of The Fertility Foundation, Godmanchester, Huntingdon; Module Leader, Lecturer and MSc Supervisor, Northern College of Acupuncture, York; Guest Lecturer, University of Lincoln, Lincoln, UK

Lianne Aquilina DipAyuT APA BSc(Hons) MBAcC ATCM

Lead Clinician, Aquilia Acupuncture and Director of Aquilia Fertility, Stamford, Lincolnshire; BSc(Hons) Acupuncture Clinical Supervisor, University of Lincoln, Lincoln; Subject Specialist Guest Lecturer: Traditional Chinese Medicine in Fertility and IVF, University of Lincoln and Visiting Guest Lecturer, Northern College of Acupuncture, York, UK

Edited by
Alan O. Szmelskyj DO MSc AdvDipClinHyp FRSPH

Senior Clinician, True Health Clinics, Godmanchester, Huntingdon; Scientific Advisor, The Stress Management Foundation, Godmanchester, Huntingdon, UK

Foreword by
Giovanni Maciocia CAc (Nanjing)

Acupuncturist and Medical Herbalist
Visiting Professor, Nanjing University of Traditional Chinese Medicine, Nanjing, People's Republic of China

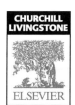

CHURCHILL LIVINGSTONE

ELSEVIER Edinburgh   London   New York   Oxford   Philadelphia   St Louis   Sydney   Toronto   2015

CHURCHILL
LIVINGSTONE
ELSEVIER

ISBN 978-0-7020-5010-7

British Library Cataloguing in Publication Data
A catalogue record for this book is available from the British Library

Library of Congress Cataloging in Publication Data
A catalog record for this book is available from the Library of Congress

Notices
Knowledge and best practice in this field are constantly changing. As new research and experience broaden our understanding, changes in research methods, professional practices, or medical treatment may become necessary.

Practitioners and researchers must always rely on their own experience and knowledge in evaluating and using any information, methods, compounds, or experiments described herein. In using such information or methods they should be mindful of their own safety and the safety of others, including parties for whom they have a professional responsibility.

With respect to any drug or pharmaceutical products identified, readers are advised to check the most current information provided (i) on procedures featured or (ii) by the manufacturer of each product to be administered, to verify the recommended dose or formula, the method and duration of administration, and contraindications. It is the responsibility of practitioners, relying on their own experience and knowledge of their patients, to make diagnoses, to determine dosages and the best treatment for each individual patient, and to take all appropriate safety precautions.

To the fullest extent of the law, neither the Publisher nor the authors, contributors, or editors, assume any liability for any injury and/or damage to persons or property as a matter of products liability, negligence or otherwise, or from any use or operation of any methods, products, instructions, or ideas contained in the material herein.

Printed in India

Contents

Contents

Biographies

IRINA SZMELSKYJ

Irina Szmelskyj is the co-director and lead clinician of True Health Clinics and is the founder of The Fertility Foundation.

With more than a decade of experience specializing in reproductive healthcare, including the healthcare needs of patients with infertility issues and the use of acupuncture in the clinical management of patients undergoing assisted reproductive treatments such as *In Vitro* Fertilization (IVF), Irina's method of managing subfertile patients is based on a thorough understanding of the value of combining the best of Traditional Chinese Medicine (TCM) and conventional medicine.

Her unique approach emphasizes the clinical utility of integrating both classically based traditional acupuncture treatment techniques and concepts with the practical clinical application of contemporary evidence-based advances, from the rapidly changing landscape of reproductive medicine research.

In addition to her clinical experience, Irina holds several academic posts at the Northern College of Acupuncture in York, including Module Leader for the MSc in Advanced Oriental Medicine and MSc in Advanced Complementary Medicine courses, as well as supervising Masters level acupuncture students. She also lectures undergraduate university students on the use of acupuncture treatment in the management of infertility and during IVF.

In 2006 she was the recipient of the British Acupuncture Council's nationally recognized Annual Research Excellence Award. She is a member of the Acupuncture Fertility Network (AFN), the National Network of Zita West Affiliated Fertility Acupuncturists, the British Fertility Society, the American Society for Reproductive Medicine (ASRM), and the European Society of Human Reproduction and Embryology (ESHRE).

LIANNE AQUILINA

Lianne Aquilina is from a family of nursing specialists and started her early career as a qualified dental nurse specializing in anxiety management and reduction – a skill that has proven invaluable in her fertility work. She went on to study complementary medicine with the specialization of Traditional Chinese Medical Acupuncture. In 2005 the Faculty of Health, Life and Social Sciences of the University of Lincoln awarded her the Dean's prize for Studies in Health. In 2008 Lianne was invited to join the University of Lincoln's teaching team as an acupuncture clinical supervisor.

Lianne was part of the first group of Traditional Chinese medical practitioners from England to complete further clinical training at the Guangdong Province Second Hospital of Traditional Chinese Medicine (TCM) in China. It was here that she observed the authentic combination of Traditional Chinese and orthodox medical strategies in treatment and management; she developed these insights for her patients undergoing *In Vitro* Fertilization (IVF) and other methods of Assisted Reproductive Medicine (ART).

Lianne's interests led to further study of Chinese medical classics as part of a Master of Arts programme, where she obtained a distinction from the College of Traditional Acupuncture, Warwick, UK, affiliated with Oxford Brookes University (2009).

Lianne Aquilina specializes in applied classical Chinese philosophy as the basis of Traditional Chinese Medicine reproductive health. She is an advocate of the importance of developing the therapeutic relationship and integrating acupuncture into mainstream medicine in response to the contemporary healthcare needs of subfertile patients.

Lianne's research project as part of her degree was published in order to demonstrate various approaches to qualitative research in healthcare.

For several years Lianne and Irina have teamed up to lecture undergraduate students on the use of Traditional Chinese Medicine and acupuncture treatment and the management of subfertility and IVF.

In 2012, Lianne was asked to join the British Acupuncture Accreditation Board (BAAB) as its accreditation observer for the accreditation of an MSc acupuncture course. Lianne is a member of the Association of Traditional Chinese Medicine (ATCM) and the British Acupuncture Council (MBAcC). She is an Associate Forum Member of Classical Chinese Medicine, an Associate member of the Ayurvedic Practitioners Association (APA), the American Society of Reproductive Medicine (ASRM), the British Fertility Society (BFS) and an Academic Associate of the British Medical Society (BMAS). She is the Founder, Director and Lead Clinician of Aquilia Acupuncture and Aquilia Fertility in Stamford, Lincolnshire.

ALAN SZMELSKYJ

For several years Alan Szmelskyj was an editorial board member of the *British Osteopathic Journal* before becoming chief editor of the peer-reviewed *Journal of Osteopathic Education and Clinical Practice*.

Alan has had articles and contributions published in several peer-reviewed medicine and healthcare journals including *Complementary Medical Research*, *Complementary Therapies in Medicine*, *Holistic Medicine*, *The Practitioner*, *Imaging* and the *BMJ* amongst others.

Previous appointments include preventative medicine roles in the Occupational Health Departments of both Hinchingbrooke NHS Trust and Papworth NHS Trust. As well as a Senior Research Fellowship, he has held lecturing roles at several osteopathic schools and lectured at international postgraduate conferences.

As well as being an enthusiastic supporter of preventative healthcare at both the individual patient level and in society in general, Alan has a longstanding interest in the role of bio-psychosocial aspects of health and medical care and the mediating role that psychosocial stress may play as an effector mechanism in the pathophysiology of ill health and disease morbidity.

Previously published work attests to Alan's fascination for trying to develop both novel theoretical hypotheses and clinical practical applications that can tap into some of the processes and techniques involved in the enhancement of the therapeutic value of the relaxation response. He was awarded his Masters degree in the Psychobiology of Stress at the University of Surrey and also completed an Advanced Diploma in Clinical Hypnosis and Stress Management at Staffordshire University.

In addition to his primary professional organizational memberships, he is also a member of The British Medical Acupuncture Society, the British Society of Clinical and Academic Hypnosis (BSCAH) and a Fellow of the Royal Society for Public Health. Alan is also trained in the Fertile Body Method. Alan is co-founder and lead clinician at True Health Clinics, Cambridgeshire, and founder of and scientific advisor to The Stress Management Foundation.

Foreword

Like all branches of Chinese medicine, traditional gynaecology has a long history. The earliest records of gynaecological medical writings date from the Shang dynasty (1600–100 BC): bones and tortoise shells from that period have been found with inscriptions dealing with childbirth problems. The text 'Book of Mountains and Seas' from the Warring States period (476–221 BC) describes medicinal plants to treat infertility.

The *Nei Jing – Su Wen* has many references to women's physiology and anatomy, as well as the diagnosis and treatment of gynaecological problems. It describes the function of the uterus and states its connection to the Heart and Kidneys via the *bao mai* (Uterus Vessel) and *bao luo* (Uterus Channel) respectively. For example, the 'Simple Questions' in Chapter 33 say: 'In amenorrhoea, the Uterus Vessel is shut. The Uterus Vessel pertains to the Heart and communicates with the Uterus; when Qi rebels upwards to press towards the Lungs, Heart-Qi cannot flow downwards and amenorrhoea results'.[1] In Chapter 47 it states: 'The Uterus Channel connects with the Kidneys; the Kidney channel reaches the root of the tongue'.[2]

That gynaecology already existed as a speciality during the Warring States period is recorded in the 'Historical Annals' (*Shi Ji*), which refer to the famous doctor Bian Que as one who 'treats diseases under the belt' (*Dai Xia Yi*), that is, a gynaecologist. Although Bian Que is not a historical figure, and the *Shi Ji* was compiled during the Han dynasty, it refers to events of the Warring States period.

During the Han dynasty (206 BC–AD 220), a gynaecologist was called a 'breast doctor' (*Ru Yi*) or 'women's doctor' (*Nu Yi*). The famous doctor Zhang Zhong Jing refers in his work 'Discussion on Cold-induced Diseases' (*Shang Han Lun*) to a previous book entitled 'Series of Herbs for Obstetrics' (*Tai Lu Yao Lu*), which proves that even before the Han dynasty there were books dealing exclusively with gynaecology, but all of these have been lost.

The 'Discussion of Prescriptions of the Golden Chest' (*Jin Gui Yao Lue Fang Lun*) by the same author has three chapters on gynaecology: 'On pregnancy', 'Post-partum diseases' and 'Women's miscellaneous diseases'. These chapters discuss disorders of menstruation, leucorrhoea, pregnancy, miscellaneous diseases, and post-partum problems. These three chapters on gynaecology represent one of the earliest gynaecological treatises, and they formed the model upon which subsequent books were based.

The 'Pulse Classic' (*Mai Jing*, AD 280) by Wang Shu He, a famous doctor of the Jin dynasty (AD 265–420), describes pulse pictures and differentiation of women's diseases in Volume 9. Wang Shu He also added a wealth of comments from his personal experience in the gynaecological field. For example, he says that 'The Kidneys govern the Uterus, and its condition is reflected at the Chi [Rear] position of the pulse. If the pulse at this region does not fade on pressure, it indicates pregnancy'.[3] In another passage he says that 'In pregnant women, a superficial pulse accompanied by

---

[1] 1979 The Yellow Emperor's Classic of Internal Medicine-Simple Questions (*Huang Ti Nei Jing Su Wen*), People's Health Publishing House, Beijing, first published c. 100 BC, p. 197.

[2] Ibid., p. 259.

[3] Wang Shu He 1988 A Revised Explanation of the 'Pulse Classic' (*Mai Jing Jiao Shi*), with commentary by the Fuzhou City People's Hospital, People's Health Publishing House, Beijing, p. 585. First published in AD 280.

abdominal pain referred to the midline of the lower back, indicates impending labour'.[4] The book also describes the qualities of the pulse before an imminent miscarriage, normal and abnormal pulses during the post-partum stage and pulses in women with abdominal masses in relation to prognosis.

All subsequent classic texts contain a wealth of knowledge and clinical information on gynaeco-logical and obstetric diseases. Especially of note are the 'General Treatise on the Symptomatology and Aetiology of Diseases' (*Zhu Bing Yuan Hou Zong Lun*, AD 610) by Chao Yuan Fang and the 'Thou-sand Golden Ducat Prescriptions' (*Qian Jin Yao Fang*, AD 652) written by Sun Si Miao. Sun Si Miao made the interesting observation that a metal knife should never be used to cut the umbilical cord: from a modern perspective, this was an important recommendation as, if dirty, a metal instrument can easily provoke a tetanus infection.

The 'Treasure of Obstetrics' (*Jing Xiao Chan Bao*), written during the Tang dynasty, is the earliest obstetrics book. The book contains twelve chapters on diseases of pregnancy, four chapters on dif-ficult labour and twenty-five chapters on post-partum diseases. Diseases of pregnancy discussed include morning sickness, bleeding, threatened miscarriage, miscarriage, urinary problems and oedema. The discussion on labour problems includes formulae for promoting labour, dealing with a dead foetus, prolonged labour and retention of the placenta. The discussion on post-partum dis-eases includes tetanus, puerperal infections, abdominal pain, persistent bleeding, retention of urine, lactation insufficiency and mastitis.

During the Song dynasty (960–1279) the imperial medical college was staffed by 300 people; there were nine departments, one of which was obstetrics and gynaecology. This was probably the earliest medical school department dedicated entirely to gynaecology and obstetrics. This led to the publica-tion of many books specializing in obstetrics and gynaecology, an important one being the 'Great Treatise of Useful Prescriptions for Women' (*Fu Ren Liang Fang Da Quan*, 1237) written by Chen Zi Ming during the Southern Song dynasty. The book comprises 24 volumes, including 20 chapters on menstrual diseases, 91 on miscellaneous diseases, 10 on infertility, 8 on 'foetal education', 9 on pregnancy problems, 70 on post-partum diseases and 10 on boils and ulcers. More than 260 diseases are discussed in all with various formulae for each. This book exerted a profound influence on the development of obstetrics and gynaecology in subsequent dynasties.

During the Yuan dynasty (1279–1368) many different medical schools of thought flourished, among which the main ones were those headed by Liu Wan Su, Li Dong Yuan, Zhu Dan Xi and Zhang Zi He. Liu Wan Su (1120–1200) maintained that Fire is the primary cause of disease, and he therefore advocated the use of cold herbs in gynaecological problems. For example, he attributed amenorrhoea to Heart-Fire.

Li Dong Yuan (1180–1251) was the founder of the 'School of Stomach and Spleen', which empha-sized a disharmony between these two organs as the main aetiology and pathology of diseases. He therefore advocated tonifying the Stomach and Spleen as the main method of treatment in gynaecol-ogy, too. In his book 'Secret Record of the Orchid Chamber' (*Lan Shi Mi Cang*), he says that prolonged deficiency of the Stomach and Spleen leads to amenorrhoea and that to treat this, one needs to clear Stomach-Heat, generate Stomach fluids and tonify Qi and Blood. He says that uterine bleeding is due to deficiency of the Stomach and Spleen, arousing Ministerial Fire of the Kidneys and causing Damp-Heat to infuse downwards: To treat this, he advocates tonifying the Stomach and Spleen and raising Qi.

Zhu Dan Xi (1281–1358) maintained that 'Yang is often in excess and Yin is often deficient' and therefore advocated nourishing Yin as one of the most important treatment principles. For example, for problems before childbirth he advised clearing Heat and nourishing Blood. He also indicated Huang Qin (*Radix Scutellariae baicalensis*) and Bai Zhu (*Rhizoma Atractylodis macrocephalae*) as two important herbs to prevent miscarriage. To this day, these are two important herbs used to prevent miscarriage.

The doctors of the Ming dynasty (1368–1644) consolidated and integrated the theories of these four great schools of medical thought. Many important gynaecological books were written during the Ming dynasty, such as 'Standards of Diagnosis and Treatment of Women's Diseases' (*Zheng Zhi Zhun Sheng - Nu Ke*, 1602) by Wang Ken Tang, 'Summary of Gynaecology and Obstetrics'

---

[4]Ibid., p. 588.

(*Nu Ke She Yao*, 1548) by Xue Ji and 'Summary of Fertility' (*Guang Si Ji Yao*) and 'Women's Secrets' (*Fu Ren Mi Ke*) by Wan Quan.

Interestingly, Wang Ken Tang said that, in order to conceive, the man should clear his Heart and control his sexual desire to nourish the *Jing*, while a woman should calm her Mind and settle Qi to nourish Blood.

The 'Complete Works of Jing Yue' (*Jing Yue Quan Shu*, 1624), by Zhang Jing Yue, has an extensive section on gynaecology and obstetrics that discusses the treatment of problems of pregnancy and labour, leucorrhoea, breast diseases, fertility, abdominal masses and menstruation. Zhang Jing Yue recommended paying particular attention to regulating menstruation in gynaecological diseases. He said that the key to regulate menstruation is to nourish Blood by tonifying the Stomach and Spleen and calming the chamber of Blood by tonifying the Kidneys. On the question of whether the Spleen or the Kidneys was the more important organ, he decided in favour of the latter.

During the Qing dynasty (1644–1911) many gynaecological treatises were written. The most notable one is 'Fu Qing Zhu's Gynaecology' (*Fu Qing Zhu Nu Ke*) by Fu Qing Zhu (1607–1684).

'Fu Qing Zhu's Gynaecology' is unlike any other gynaecology book in so far as the author proposes his own personal, and often unorthodox, ideas on the pathogenesis and treatment of gynaecological diseases and his formulae are unlike any of those from previous gynaecological books. One of the central theses of Fu Qing Zhu's book is that the Kidneys are the most important organ for the menstrual function as they are the origin of menstrual blood. According to him, menstrual blood is unlike normal Blood: it is a precious fluid derived from the Kidney-Jing. I personally completely agree with this view, and the importance of tonifying the Kidneys in gynaecological problems to me cannot be overemphasized.

Since 1949 the combination of Western and Chinese medicine has been emphasized, and many innovative treatments have been devised. For example, ectopic pregnancy is often treated with acupuncture and Chinese herbs without recourse to surgery; acupuncture is used in breech presentation of the foetus; Chinese herbs are used in the treatment of myomas and cervical carcinoma, and so on. Since the major colleges of Traditional Chinese Medicine were established in 1956, many modern gynaecology textbooks have been published and the ancient ones reprinted.

Of particular interest is the theory of the four phases of the menstrual cycle introduced by Dr. Xia Gui Cheng; this is a theory that cleverly integrates the Chinese view of Yin and Yang in the menstrual cycle with the Western view of oestrogen and progesterone and the follicular and luteal phases.

The treatment of female infertility has always occupied a major place in Chinese gynaecology. From a philosophical and social perspective, this could be attributed at least in part to the Confucian views on family and society. Confucian philosophy had a huge influence on Chinese medicine, an influence that in my opinion is not recognized. Most practitioners think that Chinese medicine is Daoist and that the *Nei Jing* is a Daoist text. In fact, the whole cultural background of the *Nei Jing* is completely Confucian and partly Legalist. For example, the view of the Internal Organs as 'ministers' and the Heart as 'ruler' is completely Confucian (Chapter 8 of the *Su Wen*). The Daoists would never make such a comparison because they disliked all political power and government structures. If we read Chapter 80 of the *Dao De Jing* we can see the description of the ideal Daoist society: a very small community where one hears cocks crow from a community next door, but the residents never feel the need to go there. Chapters 18, 19 and 38 of the *Dao De Jing* are stinging attacks on Confucian philosophy, even calling it the 'great hypocrisy'.

We should also remember that the *Nei Jing* was edited three times by Imperial Committees during the Song dynasty (960–1279), which saw the complete triumph of the Confucian ideology that remained the only accepted state ideology down to present times. I would even argue that many characteristics of the present regime are more Confucian than Marxist. Of course, that is not to say that there are no Daoist influences on the *Nei Jing*; there are. The very word *su* in the title *Su Wen* reflects the typical Daoist ideal of being 'unadorned' like raw silk, that is, 'simple'. Daoists advocated simplicity of lifestyle and shunning of political power.

Going back to women, fertility and children, Confucianists attached huge importance to children as a perpetuation of one's lineage and also as caretakers of the graves of their parents. Filial piety (*xiao*) is a fundamental cornerstone of Confucian philosophy. I think this is at least a partial explanation of the huge importance given to fertility in gynaecology books.

As we all know, Chinese medicine can be very effective in the treatment of infertility. However, with our patients, we are faced with new challenges that ancient Chinese doctors did not have, and that is the integration of our Chinese treatment with the modern techniques of ART. What would the ancient Chinese doctors think of freezing an embryo and keep it frozen for years?

Many questions arise when treating a patient who is undergoing or will soon undergo ART. Should we treat them according to the patterns seen in infertility, or should we do something different? If we do something different, how should we time it? All these questions and more are answered in depth in this book. Indeed, its title probably does not do it justice as the book does not deal only with the approach to a patient who is undergoing ART. It also gives an overview of the Chinese medicine view of the reproductive system and the Chinese patterns in subfertility.

I am delighted to introduce this book, the most comprehensive text on the integration of Traditional Chinese Medicine with modern ART techniques, which was written by practitioners with a great deal of experience and deep knowledge of the subject.

Giovanni Maciocia
Santa Barbara, 2014

Preface

Over the past decade or so, acupuncture treatment of patients undergoing Assisted Reproductive Technology (ART) treatments has gained in popularity. With this increased demand for acupuncture treatment, the role of fertility acupuncturists in the management of patients undergoing ART treatments has expanded. In contemporary fertility acupuncture practice, patients expect their acupuncturists to have a thorough understanding of not only Traditional Chinese Medicine (TCM), but also all Orthodox medical aspects that relate directly to the practice of fertility acupuncture. Patients expect their acupuncturists not only to treat them, but also to advise them about diagnoses, tests and investigations, clinic suitability, different treatment protocols, and stages of treatment and generally support them on many levels.

With these increased expectations, acupuncture practitioners find themselves looking for additional resources of information to supplement their often very limited training in this field of medicine. However, there is still a significant gap in the available literature on how to treat this patient group.

With this book, we aim to provide fertility acupuncturists with an 'all-in-one' resource on just about everything they are likely to need to know when managing patients undergoing ART treatments such as *In Vitro* Fertilization (IVF). This textbook is based on our combined 20 years of clinical experience, our experience of lecturing in this field and (whenever possible) on up-to-date evidence-based literature. This book draws its ethos and inspiration both from the technical complexities of the fast-moving and ever-developing field of conventional reproductive medicine and synthesizes this with traditional acupuncture practical approaches. The latter are derived from our interpretation of the classical acupuncture texts and supported with contemporary acupuncture research-based studies (where these are available). It attempts to simplify complex information into easily accessible and understandable material.

This book will take acupuncture students and practitioners, step by step, through every aspect of contemporary fertility and ART acupuncture practice. We believe it will cover just about everything that a novice or an experienced fertility acupuncturist is likely to need to know, including:

- Reproductive anatomy and physiology, both from Orthodox medical and TCM perspectives.
- Orthodox medical fertility tests and investigations, including information on how to interpret the results, what other tests may be suitable for patients, and when to refer them. Detailed reference ranges for the most commonly used tests are provided.
- The pathology and aetiology of TCM syndromes and their associated ART complications that are commonly seen in subfertile patients.
- Detailed information on how to take a fertility medical history and how to diagnose TCM syndromes. Case history templates are provided.
- Evidence-based information on how various lifestyle factors affect fertility and ART success rates. Ready-made factsheets are appended for acupuncturists to give to their patients.
- Guidelines on how to regulate the menstrual cycle in preparation for IVF treatment.
- How common fertility-related conditions such as endometriosis, Polycystic Ovary Syndrome, thyroid disease, and male factor infertility affect ART success rates and what can be done with acupuncture and lifestyle modifications to help patients succeed.

- Algorithmic acupuncture treatment pathways are provided for most conditions.
- How to adapt acupuncture treatment to different ART protocols including ovulation induction, Intra-Uterine Insemination and IVF, as well as for advanced treatment techniques such as Intra-Cytoplasmic Sperm Injection/Intra-Cytoplasmic Morphologically Selected Sperm Injection, assisted hatching, and third-party reproduction.
- How to support patients if their IVF is unsuccessful and how to treat patients during early pregnancy.
- How to manage patients with complex medical histories, including Recurrent Implantation Failure, reproductive immunology dysfunction, and recurrent miscarriages.
- How to build a therapeutic and trusting relationship with patients, which is critical in ART acupuncture practice.
- Ethical considerations relevant to fertility acupuncture practice.

We believe that infertility patients seeking out potential answers and solutions for their fertility issues may also benefit from this book by learning about how acupuncture may help them on their journey through the many ups and downs of fertility treatment.

Irina Szmelskyj
Lianne Aquilina
Huntingdon and Stamford 2014

Acknowledgements

Writing this book has been a long and in many ways challenging journey. It would not have been possible if not for the help and support of many people.

I would like to express my gratitude to Tom Williams, my MSc research module teacher, who believed in me; to my original research supervisor, Hugh MacPherson, who helped to steer me in the right direction; and to my research supervisor, Léonie Walker, for helping me achieve the highest possible standard of research. Without your input this book would not exist.

I would like to acknowledge my Northern College of Acupuncture colleagues, whose passion for research is an inspiration to me. I have learnt a lot from you and will carry on learning. A very special thanks to Lara McClure for helping me access the research material. I am humbled that the world-renowned acupuncture expert Giovanni Maciocia found the time in his busy schedule to review this book and write such a positive foreword – thank you! This book would not have been possible if it was not for help provided by Richard Blackwell, principal of the Northern College of Acupuncture. Richard, I am forever indebted to you.

My thanks to world expert on folliculogenesis, Alain Gougeon, for taking time to help me with my research on follicular development. This is a very important aspect of female reproductive physiology, which I believe acupuncture can directly influence. Thank you Raj Mathur and Stephen Harbottle of the Cambridge IVF, Amin Gorgy of the Fertility Academy and one other person who can not be named here (but I hope you know who you are) for your help with sourcing some of the laboratory images used in this book.

All my patients who agreed to be case studies for the book – thank you! Also all the patients I have treated over the years – I have learnt from treating each and every one of you and now I am sharing this knowledge with other acupuncturists.

Thank you to my colleagues at True Health Clinics for putting up with me while I was writing this book!

I would like to say an especially big thank you to Lisa Morton for creating some of the illustrations for this book. You are a very talented designer. Also the many night shifts of writing would have been much grimmer if it was not for your late-night support. You made me laugh so much that I cried. I will not miss the night shifts, but I will miss our laughs.

I am grateful for the support of all my wonderful friends, in particular Katarina and Oksana, who helped me to get through some difficult times.

This section would not be complete without expressing my sincere thanks to our publisher and our editors Claire Wilson, Sally Davies, Alison Taylor and our project manager, Sukanthi Sukumar. Thank you for being so patient with us and for allowing us the many extensions to the deadline that we so badly needed.

I would also like to acknowledge my co-author Lianne. Fate brought us together to work on this demanding project at possibly the most unsuitable times of our lives, when we had to juggle very young families and long hours of research and writing. Chinese medicine at times is not easy to understand and our combined efforts to take original TCM writings and to synthesize them into something more contemporary and appropriate for the nature of this book was quite challenging. We got through it, albeit somewhat battered and bruised!

Finally, my biggest thanks go to my family. To my husband Alan for suggesting that we write this book, for inspiring me and believing in me, for spending many hours painstakingly editing the manuscript and making it so much better, for making the countless cups of coffee to see me through the wee hours of the night, and for doing the household chores to give me the time to write.

To my mum Maria, my stepfather Peter, and to my brother Yura for always being there for me, even though I had very little time for you while writing this book.

And finally to Daniel and Matthew, my two very much loved and treasured children. Thank you for playing quietly while 'mummy was writing', for allowing me to have power naps while settling you and for ensuring that I stayed on schedule by checking the progress on my wall chart. You are my biggest inspiration. I hope that in turn this book will inspire you to achieve even greater things in your lives.

Irina Szmelskyj

I would like to acknowledge and thank all who have provided me with the opportunity to make this book a possibility. My special thanks go to Irina Szmelskyj, my co-author. As qualified acupuncturists with different backgrounds we each bring a range of different interests, skills, and experiences. Collaboration in the making and production of our book has been challenging, yet an invaluable personal and professional experience. I would also like to thank Alan Szmelskyj, our chief editor, for his time, expertise and advice. Thank you to our development editor, Sally Davies, and to Sukanthi Sukumar, our project manager, for their expertise and input in the making of our book. Thank you to Linda Husband, for securing me a place on the acupuncture course, and to Chris Low and Richard Bertschinger, my tutors, who willingly recommended a broad range of great Chinese medicine literature and shared their knowledge during my studies. Thanks also to Paul Franks and Martin Dean, my clinical supervisors, a great inspiration now and during my university days. Thank you to Venkat Kumarasamy for allowing us access to some of the difficult-to-obtain medical journal articles and for your help and advice.

Thank you, Gary Hares, 'Boss', for the position upon graduation as an acupuncturist in three of your busy clinics. Josephine Clegg of Sleaford Natural Health Centre, thank you for sharing your practice with me and for all your advice. You both gave me an opportunity and the start I needed (I am so grateful). Special thanks go to Fanyi Meng for inviting me back to the University of Lincoln (in my mid-twenties) to teach Chinese medicine and clinically supervise third-year acupuncture students. Working amongst a team of experts and eager students over so many years, in a vibrant, challenging and interactive learning environment has been a fundamental component in the continual development of my professional practice and fed my fascination of Chinese medical acupuncture. My experience of this is reflected wholeheartedly in this book.

I would like to extend my heartfelt thanks to my parents, whose work ethic has given me the aspiration to write. Both my mum, Karen Baza, and dad, Juzi Aquilina, have been ideal role models with regard to education, dedication and enrichment of my life. Thank you also Mr and Mrs Saleem. Oliver Aquilina-Ford, my gorgeous son, thank you for all that you teach me about life. Thank you, Aunty Susan, for looking after me so well. Big thanks, to Kelly Marie Bateson and Joel, Lou Congreve, Venkat and John Wheeler for their support when needed for aspects of this project. A special thanks, also, to Corinne Alexander, my associate acupuncturist for managing Aquilia Acupuncture marvellously.

Thank you to all my patients who consented to their case histories being used as a teaching tool. Thank you, Dawn, my first fertility and IVF patient of 2003, for stimulating my interest in and passion for fertility acupuncture.

I would like to thank those who helped me during my research for the TCM chapters and sections of this book. I am extremely grateful to: Elisabeth Rochat de la Vallée for her guidance and input on energies present at conception and Ming Men (Fire of Life); Dr Henry Lu for his response to my enquiries regarding his translation of the Nei-Jing and Nan-Jing; Alan Hext for discussions regarding the qi jing ba mai; Wainright Churchill for recommending the scholarly works of Russell Kirkland; Russell Kirkland for providing a range of his articles and collaborating with me; Tony Booker for reviewing the TCM energetics of food section; Care Fertility, Nottingham, for the images of eggs, sperm and embryos and for looking after my patients so well; and Davey Podmore, my neighbour, for the professional drawings of the TCM figures what a palaver that was!

The most exciting thought as I write now for the last time is the closure of this chapter of my life and in turn I hope that our book opens up new chapters in the life of subfertile patients.

Lianne Aquilina

Chapter 1

Subfertility overview

INTRODUCTION

'Now the girls are here it could be so easy to forget just how different things were when we first met. But I won't ever forget all of the advice and support you gave us, as well as your time (fitting us in around our [IVF] treatment even though it took some of your own valuable family time). You have made a real difference to us...'

'We can't thank you enough for all your help (with your magic needles) – without you we don't think we would have our beautiful daughter... We really believe you are... one of those who really make a difference in the world'.

'I just wanted to convey my warmest thanks for your support, advice and clinical expertise which has helped us to conceive. We are over the moon. I am absolutely sure that we couldn't have done it without your input. Not only the acupuncture itself, but [also] the additional advice'.

'I firmly believe that it was your knowledge, expertise and support that helped us conceive this much wanted baby and for this I thank you... I will never forget the impact you have made on my health, my grief and my ability to look to the future with positivity and happiness'.

'Please accept a huge thank you from us, we truly believe that our successful IVF treatment, which resulted in our gorgeous little boy, was down to not only the excellent and professional acupuncture treatment but also your support and positive attitude. We feel incredibly lucky to have him and are loving every moment with him'.

'A huge thank you for all the help and encouragement you have given me over the past year in the lead up to our IVF process. Your continued support during my pregnancy meant a lot and you gave me the added peace of mind... I am sure us now having our beautiful daughter is a result of your knowledge and care'.

'I truly believe that acupuncture was one amongst all the treatments I had that led to my conception'.

'We would like to just say a big thank you for all your help with the acupuncture and all the advice and support whilst I was going through my IVF...[for] going out of your way to always be available for our treatments. We will never forget your kindness and we will always be grateful we found such a good acupuncturist and also a lovely and caring person'.

'You've made our dreams come true!'

'We are pleased to announce the safe arrival of our baby boy. After five failed IVF cycles I am sure having acupuncture helped us to be successful on our sixth attempt. So thank you very, very much. Thank you once again and may all your good work continue to help others'.

Our treatment rooms' bookshelves are full of cards with messages such as these. They are from our past patients who were previously considered subfertile, people who experienced infertility first hand and conceived as a result of an integrated acupuncture approach to Assisted Reproductive Technology (ART) treatments.

Many patients believe that it was acupuncture alone that made all the difference. But as fertility acupuncturists, we know that the reality is more complex. Infertility is a multifactorial disease, with many causes and many approaches to treatment. What makes a difference is not a single solution, but a combined team effort on the part of patients, ART clinics, acupuncturists, and sometimes other professionals.

Being a reproductive medicine acupuncturist is both rewarding and challenging – rewarding because we make a real difference in other people's lives. We help them achieve their greatest dreams and become part of a team that helps to bring new life into the world. It is challenging because it takes a lot of dedication and determination to effectively help those suffering from infertility.

In this book, we hope to share with you the knowledge and experience that we have gained during our two decades of specializing in ART acupuncture. We begin by introducing you to infertility and explaining exactly what this disease is and what causes it.

DEFINITION OF INFERTILITY DISORDER

Most medical organizations agree that infertility should be defined as the inability to conceive after 1 year of regular unprotected intercourse (see Table 1.1). However, this definition can be confusing and open to varied interpretation.

Definition of pregnancy

Success in the field of reproductive medicine is defined as, for example, a 'clinical pregnancy', a 'successful pregnancy', and 'conception'. So what is meant by 'clinical' or 'successful'? The World Health Organization (WHO) defines a clinical pregnancy as 'a pregnancy diagnosed by ultrasonographic visualization of one or more gestational sacs or definitive clinical signs of pregnancy. It includes ectopic

Table 1.1 Definition of infertility

Organization	Infertility definition
WHO 2009[1]	Failure to achieve a clinical pregnancy after 12 months or more of regular unprotected sexual intercourse
ASRM 2013[2]	Failure to achieve a successful pregnancy after 12 months or more of appropriately, timed unprotected intercourse or therapeutic donor insemination
ESHRE 2010[3]	Failure to conceive after 12 months of regular unprotected sexual intercourse
National Institute for Health and Clinical Excellence (NICE) 2013[4]	Failure to conceive after frequent unprotected sexual intercourse for 1–2 years

pregnancy'.[1] The European Society of Human Reproduction and Embryology (ESHRE) definition is 'a pregnancy diagnosed by ultrasound or by definite signs of pregnancy'.[3] The American Society for Reproductive Medicine (ASRM) defines pregnancy as 'a clinical pregnancy documented by ultrasonography or histopathologic examination'.[2]

If a woman experiences 'pregnancy signs' such as delayed menstruation, nausea, swollen and tender breasts, yet a pregnancy test result is negative, should this be classed as 'clinical pregnancy'? Definite clinical signs of pregnancy can be evident within days of ovulation, yet up to 60% of pregnancies will fail even before they are confirmed by a pregnancy test.[5] Ultrasonographic evaluation is not usually utilized until 12 weeks gestation, by which time up to 70% of pregnancies fail.[5] So whilst WHO includes in its definition ectopic pregnancies, this may be inappropriate and more than just a tautological oxymoron. For example, if a woman loses both fallopian tubes as a result of ectopic pregnancies, she will be completely sterile. Yet by WHO's definition, she will be classed as fertile!

Definition of regular intercourse

The meaning of 'regular unprotected sexual intercourse' is another area for confusion. One couple may perceive that intercourse every 4–5 days is regular, whereas another couple may consider regular to be daily intercourse. What is probably more important is the timing of intercourse in relation to the menstrual cycle. Frequent intercourse during the fertile window (usually starting 5 days before and finishing on the day of ovulation) is most likely to result in conception.[6–12] Intercourse outside of the fertile window is almost certainly unlikely to lead to pregnancy.[11]

Length of time to achieve pregnancy

It is well known that older women take longer to conceive. Retrospective studies show that 75% of 30-year-old women will conceive within a year, whereas only 66% of 35-year-old women and 44% of 40-year-old women will conceive in this period.[13] Some would argue that 12 months is too long because prospective studies show that 80–90% of couples will conceive within 6 months.[9,10,14,15] Thus, the appropriateness of 12 months as a time frame within which to conceive remains debatable.

Implications

There have been calls for simplification and clarification of the definition of infertility and new definition and diagnosis models have been proposed.[16,17] The implications from the use of existing ambiguous definitions of infertility are widespread. In the clinical setting, couples may experience unnecessary distress as a result of being under- or overinvestigated or treated. Researchers may face difficulties in participant recruitment due to varying diagnostic interpretation criteria, or they may find it difficult to analyse and compare the results of research studies due to heterogeneous groups of patients.

Once a couple is diagnosed as infertile, they may experience significant psychological consequences. The term *infertility* is often associated with total sterility and implies a complete inability to conceive. Yet, in reality, the degree of infertility will vary, and the term *infertility* covers a spectrum from mild subfertility to complete sterility.

In acupuncture practice, patients often present with 'infertility', either medically or self-diagnosed. We would caution practitioners not to rely on such a diagnosis too rigidly. Taking a thorough medical history from which we can assess the appropriateness and the severity of the diagnosis is paramount.

In reproductive medicine, the terms *subfertility, subfecundity*, and even *sterility* are usually used synonymously with infertility. In this book, we use the terms *subfertility* and *infertility* interchangeably to refer to suboptimal fertility and to describe varying degrees and durations of involuntary childlessness in varying patient groups. We use the term *sterility* to indicate absolute inability to have a genetically related child.

PREVALENCE OF INFERTILITY

Infertility trends

It is estimated that between 5% and 15% of couples experience difficulty conceiving.[15,18–21] The prevalence of infertility is similar across the world:[19,22] 42% of women in the developed world seek medical advice, and 22.4% undergo infertility treatment, while it is estimated that 34.9% of women in less developed countries seek advice, and perhaps as many as 58% of these women receive treatment.[19]

Fecundability (that is, the probability of conceiving within a given menstrual cycle after unprotected sex) in a healthy fertile couple is estimated to be 0.25 or 25%.[23] This means that only one out of four couples will conceive in the first month of trying. Three percent of normal fertile couples will not get pregnant even after 12 months of trying because of bad luck.[23]

Some authors claim that infertility is on the increase.[24] However, there is very little good quality data to support this point of view. Most research points to the fact that the prevalence of infertility has remained stable in the developed world. A major survey, the results of which were published in 2012, analysed data from 277 demographic studies from 1999 to 2010. No evidence of changes in infertility patterns were found, except in the regions of sub-Saharan Africa and South Asia, where, although levels of infertility are still very high, they are declining.[19,22] One possible explanation for this decline is the reduction in Sexually Transmitted Infections (STIs) in less developed countries.

However, more couples in the developed world delay parenthood for economic and career reasons. As fertility declines with age, it is therefore likely that age-related infertility is likely to increase. However, a major 2012 survey did not find any evidence of this, except for secondary infertility (difficulty conceiving after successful live birth).[22]

One of the possible explanations for differences in opinions about infertility trends is that different research studies use different measures of fecundity. Historically, the time from marriage to pregnancy was used. Nowadays, especially in developed countries, couples delay parenthood until they are more economically secure. Therefore, time from marriage to pregnancy is no longer a relevant measure. Time to pregnancy is now used as a measure of fecundity. te Velde *et al.* argue that time to pregnancy in 'carefully selected populations' is a feasible option' to find out if the level of fecundity is declining.[25]

There are also reports that male fertility, measured by sperm counts, has decreased significantly.[26] However, because of heterogeneous measurement methodology, such as comparing data from different populations and using different methods of sperm analysis, this finding has been questioned by some.[27]

Different types of infertility vary between countries. For example, age-related infertility is becoming more prevalent in the more developed nations, secondary infertility is virtually nonexistent in China because of the one-child policy, and primary infertility is very low in Africa, where women are exposed to STIs only after they marry and have their first baby.[19]

Infertility treatment seeking

Less than 50% of subfertile couples seek medical advice.[15,19] However, this number is steadily increasing.[28] The increased willingness to seek medical help and the trend to delay parenthood[13] are likely to have social, economic, and medical implications.

Two out of three subfertile couples choose to use Complementary and Alternative Medicine (CAM) instead or alongside of Orthodox medical treatments. Forty-eight percent of these couples consult naturopaths, chiropractors, or acupuncturists.[29] Twenty-three percent of subfertile couples in the United States seek acupuncture to help them conceive.[30] Because the use of CAM in Europe is higher, it is conceivable that the percentage of couples consulting acupuncturists in European countries is also greater. The use of acupuncture is higher in older couples, those with higher education and income, and in couples undergoing *In Vitro* Fertilization (IVF).[30] With the increased willingness to seek medical advice and the likely increase in age-related infertility, it is reasonable to assume that over time there will be an increase in the demand for acupuncture treatment of subfertility.

MAJOR CAUSES OF SUBFERTILITY FROM AN ORTHODOX MEDICAL POINT OF VIEW

Estimates for medical causes of subfertility vary, but most fall within the following ranges: 20–30% of infertility is due to a male factor,[20,31,32] 20–35% is due to a female

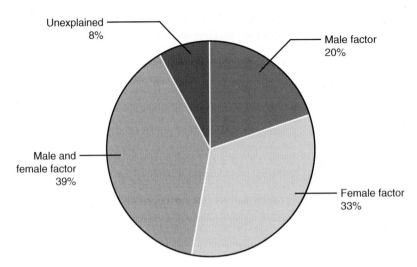

Figure 1.1 Estimated frequency of the causes of subfertility.[32]

factor,[20,32] 25–40% is due to both male and female factors,[20,21,32] and in 8–20% of cases no cause can be identified (Figure 1.1).[20,32]

The most common medical causes of female subfertility are ovulatory disorders (20–32%),[21,33] tubal disorders (14–26%),[21,33,34] and endometriosis (5–6%) (Figure 1.2).[21,33]

The most common medical causes of poor semen parameters in men include cryptorchidism (13%),[35] varicocele (10%),[35] congenital abnormality of the vas deferens (4%),[35] and endocrine abnormality (2%).[35] In 57% of men with severe oligospermia or azoospermia, no causes are found (Figure 1.3).[35]

Common medical causes of subfertility presenting in acupuncture practice

A 2010 survey of United Kingdom acupuncturists carried out by the British Acupuncture Council (BAcC) reported that the common symptoms and medical conditions acupuncturists frequently deal with in patients presenting with subfertility are irregular cycles, polycystic ovaries, and endometriosis (female factor); abnormal sperm (male factor); and unexplained infertility (both male and female factors).[36]

Tubal disease, which accounts for up to 26% of causes of female subfertility,[21] was not reported as a common presentation in acupuncture practice. Paradoxically and interestingly, a 2010 study found that acupuncture during embryo transfer resulted in a higher pregnancy rate in tubal-uterine or idiopathic cause cases.[37]

Importance of treating both male and female partners

The 2010 BAcC survey found that acupuncturists in the United Kingdom see 7.5 times more subfertile female patients than subfertile male patients.[36] In many cases, even where a cause of subfertility is confirmed to be due to a male

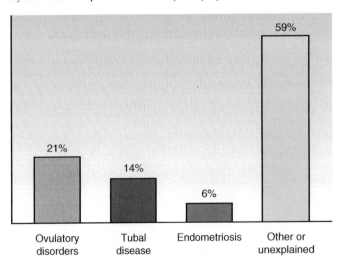

Figure 1.2 Common medical causes of female factor subfertility.[33]

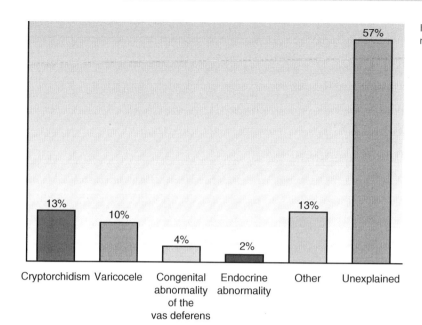

Figure 1.3 Common medical causes of male factor subfertility.[35]

factor, it is still the female partner who comes for acupuncture. As acupuncturists, we need to be aware that in two out of three couples we treat, there is likely to be a male-related subfertility cause, either alone or in combination with a female factor.

Conventional reproductive medicine practice is often guilty of ignoring the issue of male fertility. Most men have their semen analysed, but, in many cases, if the semen is found to be suboptimal, these couples are automatically referred for IVF, rather than the man undergoing further investigations to see if a cause of poor semen parameters can be found and corrected. There is a belief that IVF somehow magically overcomes male factor infertility. In part this is true, especially since the development of Intracytoplasmic Sperm Injection (ICSI). However, the success rates for IVF in male factor couples are only slightly higher than in couples with other causes of subfertility.

CONTRIBUTORY SUBFERTILITY FACTORS: THE ORTHODOX MEDICAL PERSPECTIVE

Many factors contribute to infertility, including cultural, social, economic, and environmental. Different factors may contribute to varying degrees in different populations and at an individual level at different stages of the reproductive cycle and reproductive development.

Socioeconomic factors

Delayed parenthood

Delayed parenthood is perhaps one of the biggest contributing factors to subfertility in more developed countries.

There is a well-documented trend that women in such countries are delaying motherhood until later in life. The mean age of a mother giving birth to her first child in England and Wales was 23.7 in 1970 and has steadily increased to 28.0 by 2011.[38] The data from the United States is comparable, 21.4 in 1970 to 25.0 in 2006.[39] Similar trends have been reported in other countries, including Switzerland, Japan, Netherlands, Sweden, Italy, Ireland, Greece, Denmark, Finland, Canada, France, Hungary, and Poland.[39]

Delaying parenthood until later in life can have a number of advantages. For example, commonly cited reasons are that the prospective parents are more financially and emotionally able to cope with bringing up a child and are in a more stable relationship.[40,41]

However, fertility declines with age in both men and women. Ovarian reserve declines rapidly after the age of 35.[42] Older men have lower sperm parameters and higher rates of sperm DNA damage.[43] Conception has a higher risk of complications in pregnancy and during delivery in reproductively older women. For example, one multicentre European study found that miscarriage rates were highest in couples where a woman was aged 35 or older and a man was 40 or older.[44] Pregnancies fathered by older fathers have been linked with higher rates of caesarean sections, preeclampsia, and preterm birth,[43] even after taking into account the age of their partners.

Children conceived by older parents are also at higher risk of health complications, including birth defects, childhood cancers, prostate and breast cancers, type I diabetes mellitus, multiple sclerosis, some forms of cerebral palsy, schizophrenia, bipolar disorder, autism, epilepsy, Alzheimer disease, and lower intelligence. However, some of these associations need to be researched further to confirm these findings.[43] Babies born to women aged 40 or more have a higher risk of being born prematurely, having a lower birth weight, and being admitted to intensive care units. Genetic abnormalities such as Down syndrome occur more often in children conceived by older mothers.

The trend to leave parenthood until later in life might have been influenced by the availability of ART treatments and the erroneous perception by many that IVF will 'fix' them should they have difficulties conceiving.[45] However, IVF is less successful in older women, with live birth rates 39% in women aged 34 or younger, going down to just 4% in women aged 43 or older.[46]

Education and financial status

Poor education and illiteracy result in women having limited or no access to family planning services and to contraception. This results in high rates of Sexually Transmitted Diseases (STDs), unwanted pregnancies, and septic abortions leading to subfertility. There is also some evidence that socially deprived people take longer to conceive.[47]

More educated couples are more likely to have access to knowledge about the menstrual cycle and how to optimally time their intercourse to conceive. This knowledge can lead to better coital practices, but, conversely, it can also put pressure on partners to 'perform' on demand and, therefore, negatively affect their fertility psychology.

Political policies

In an attempt to control population growth or decline, some governments put in place population-control policies. For example, for many years, China has maintained strict control of population growth through a one-child policy.

Opposite trends can be observed in other countries. Many developed countries see a decline in overall numbers of births while in the general population life expectancy is increasing. The trends in couples in these countries to delay having children until later in life can lead to an increase in the number of cases of age-related subfertility. Thus, some governments encourage couples to have more children through financial and employment incentives.

Healthcare spending

In third-world countries, spending on healthcare is low, and, consequently, medical care is poor. This can affect fertility in a number of ways. Poor family planning services lead to many unwanted pregnancies, which often results in many illegal abortions. Badly done, these can lead to infections and scarring. Limited services mean that STDs are not diagnosed early enough and, thus cause tubal and ejaculatory duct damage. Reconstructive surgeries for this type of damage are often unsuccessful. Preventative measures, such as better sex education, improved diagnosis and treatment of STDs, and better family planning services (including availability of contraception) could all help to reduce the rate of STDs and unwanted pregnancies.[48]

Limited healthcare budgets also affect the availability and access to subfertility treatments, such as assisted reproductive technologies. Poorly educated people may not be aware of reproductive treatments, or they might not be able to pay for them if these are not funded by the state. Also, there may be stigma attached to using reproductive treatment services.

Traditions, culture, and family values

There are many reasons why people choose to have children. Different cultures place different values on family life and parenthood. In some cultures, the only purpose people have in life is to reproduce and have as many children as they can. For some, it is insurance for when they are older, perhaps to have workers to help with domestic chores. For others, it is to ensure longevity of their family name. Often people choose to have children because it is what is expected of them by their family or society.

Some traditions in some parts of the world are blamed for adding to subfertility rates. For example, female circumcision is still widely practised and affects 80 million women, mostly in Africa.[48] Female circumcision is often performed by people without knowledge of hygiene or anatomy and in many cases leads to haemorrhage, infections, and subfertility. Even if these circumcised women get pregnant, there are often complications during labour, resulting in haemorrhage, shock, and perinatal maternal deaths.[48]

Environmental factors

Pollution can affect fertility and reproduction at different stages and in different ways. Exposure to environmental contaminants can happen in utero, during the developmental years when the reproductive organs grow and mature, and also in adulthood. Certain environmental hazards are linked to sperm issues, menstrual cycle irregularities, hormonal changes, miscarriages, foetal loss, early menopause, malformations of the reproductive tract, endometriosis, fibroids, altered puberty, and other reproductive changes.[49]

Men are possibly affected by exposure to environmental oestrogens, both at puberty and continually through their lives. This oestrogen may have an effect on the hypothalamic pituitary axis and spermatogenesis.[18]

More detailed information on which environmental pollutants and chemicals have been linked with subfertility can be found in Chapter 7.

Occupational factors

Certain occupations are associated with reduced fertility. Primarily this is through contact with environmental hazards.

Sedentary occupations have increased over the last century and are associated with an increase in intra-scrotal temperatures. Raised intra-scrotal temperature damages sperm DNA in animals. There is some evidence that a similar effect can be seen in human sperm.[50]

The level of evidence for occupational hazards varies, and more research is required to definitely determine causality. More detailed information on which occupations have been linked with subfertility can be found in Chapter 7.

Overview of other factors

Increased stress levels

Stress may be linked to reduced fertility. However, opinions vary about this. Chapter 7 reviews the evidence on the effects of stress on fertility in greater depth.

Nutrition, weight, and exercise

Being over- or underweight has been linked to subfertility and obstetric complications.[18]

Moderating exercise levels and keeping weight appropriately controlled may help to reduce the risk of ovulatory disorders.[51,52]

A nutritionally rich diet helps to improve fertility in both men and women.[51]

The roles of stress, nutrition, weight, and exercise are reviewed in much greater depth in Chapter 7.

Early puberty

An increased caloric intake and possible exposure to environmental oestrogens may be responsible for some causes of early female puberty and may potentially result in a shorter reproductive lifespan.[18] Girls who reach puberty early are more likely to be overweight, have Polycystic Ovarian Syndrome, fibroids, or endometriosis, all of which are linked to subfertility. Early puberty may also lead to early sexual activity with associated unwanted pregnancies and abortions or STDs, all of which can lead to infertility.

Sexual intercourse

It is estimated that 15% of couples will not conceive through any method other than ART. For the remaining 85%, conception should be possible through regular sexual intercourse.[53] Their chances of conception will be greatly affected by the frequency and timing of their intercourse.[54]

The use of water-based lubricants such as KY Jelly, olive oil, and even saliva is not advisable because sperm can be damaged by their presence. Mineral oils (such as canola oil) and hydroxyethylcellulose-based lubricants (such as Pre-Seed®) do not appear to have detrimental effects on sperm.[55] Chapter 7 provides more detail about the fertile window, intercourse, and coital practices.

Reproductive tract infections

The presence of microorganisms in the reproductive tract can cause it to become infected. Microorganisms can also be introduced during sexual intercourse, usually referred to as STIs or STDs, or through a medical procedure.[56]

WHO estimates that in 1999 there were over 340 million new cases of the four curable STIs (gonorrhoea, chlamydia, syphilis, and trichomoniasis). Viral STIs such as human papilloma virus, herpes simplex virus, and human immunodeficiency virus were not included in the estimate. If these were included, the number of STI cases might be three times higher.[56]

STIs are one of the biggest causes of subfertility in men and women. WHO estimates that the risk of infertility after one episode of pelvic inflammatory disease (a common complication of STIs) is increased by 15–25%, and it rises to 50–60% after a third episode.[56] STIs can also cause maternal deaths, miscarriages, stillbirth, preterm birth, and congenital infections.[56]

Delaying sexual activity, reducing the number of sex partners, correct and consistent use of condoms, and better hygiene practices in medical settings, particularly in poor countries, are some ways to prevent STIs.[56]

Negative lifestyle habits

Negative lifestyle habits, such as smoking, drinking excessive amounts of alcohol, and using recreational drugs are linked with increased time to conception. Chapter 7 discusses this in more detail.

CAUSES OF SUBFERTILITY FROM THE TCM POINT OF VIEW

In Traditional Chinese Medicine (TCM), health is achieved by maintaining a delicate balance between Qi (life force or energy) and the body, mind, and spirit. This delicate balance can be affected by numerous factors categorized into Internal, External, and Miscellaneous causes.[57] Once health is affected by these factors, according to TCM, it will begin to deteriorate and, if left untreated, will eventually cause a disease.

Internal causes of disease/injury through emotion

An Internal cause of a disease arises as a result of excessive emotions.[58] Experiencing emotions is necessary and healthy. However, excessively strong emotions can cause an imbalance of Qi, Qi Deficiency,[59] impaired Blood circulation,[58,60,61] and dysfunction of the Zangfu organs[62]; it can also affect the balance of Yin and Yang.[60]

Reproductive energy is the source of new life.[62] Suffering from infertility has an emotional impact on a couple. This emotional imbalance can damage the Zangfu organ system, depleting and reducing reproductive potential.[62] A combination and a range of emotions may impact the person in various ways. TCM recognizes that many emotions (for example, excessive joy or unexpected joy or anger)[63] can be pathological[64] but generally views pathological emotions as:

- Anger[65]
- Contemplation or worry[62]
- Sadness and grief[64]
- Fear[64]
- Shock[66]

Women are particularly prone to internal injury by emotion,[67] which is why women often require a great deal of support when dealing with subfertility:

- Women's Qi and Blood physiology make them susceptible to injury by emotion.
- Particular constitutional tendencies and pre-existing syndromes may predispose women to experience particular emotions (for example, women who are Wood/Liver type may feel angry, moody and irritable).
- Women may respond to subfertility in a reactive manner. This may be considered a normal reaction, but how they feel about the situation and cope with it may eventually lead to major ill health.
- Women are extra sensitive to the emotional upheaval of ART, and this can be further exacerbated by hormonal medication.
- Damage to Zangfu organs by excessive emotions causes Yin Deficiency[62] and a loss of reproductive energy.

Anger

Anger includes feelings of frustration and irritation. These feelings have a tendency to directly increase Liver Qi,[65] causing Liver Qi Stagnation, Liver Fire, Liver Blood Stasis, or Blood-Heat.[68] Anger makes energy rise upwards, which further damages the Liver.[69] An imbalanced Liver can negatively affect the regulation of the menstrual cycle and the Spleen's function of transportation and transformation of food and fluids,[61] leading to Qi Deficiency.

Feelings of frustration and resentment can present in a woman suffering with infertility and failed ART. Being aware and hypervigilant to the presence of pregnant women, babies, and celebrities with big 'bumps' can make subfertile women feel frustration, anger, jealousy, and resentment.

Contemplation or worry

Worry damages the Heart[65] and stagnates or blocks Qi,[62] especially the Qi of the Lungs, Spleen,[68] and Heart,

adversely effecting fertility. Spleen Qi Deficiency can lead to Internal Dampness, especially in the lower Jiao. Dampness from Spleen Qi Deficiency can cause Phlegm. Substantial accumulation of Damp-Phlegm clogs and blocks the Uterus, causing subfertility by hindering the vital flow of energy necessary for fertilization, conception, and pregnancy.[58] Fear combined with worry can injure the Heart.[70]

Fertility and IVF can be a source of worry for couples, especially for those who have experienced prior difficulties with ART. Such couples worry about producing enough eggs or sperm, eggs being fertilized, the number of or whether embryos will be available for transfer, whether the embryo(s) develop(s) to the blastocyst stage, the pregnancy test, and possible miscarriages.

Anxiety

Anxiety impairs the Spleen, the Kidney, and the Heart. By weakening the Spleen, anxiety can cause Blood Deficiency,[61] thus impacting upon fertility.

Fear

Fear affects the Kidneys, often leading to Kidney Yin Deficiency.[68] Fear or being fearful is like a stimulant, depleting Kidney reserves. Fear disperses and weakens Shen (Spirit).[62] A Deficiency of Liver Qi can cause Fear.[62]

Sudden fright can descend Kidney Qi,[61] and chronic fearfulness can make Qi ascend, causing a deficiency of Blood or Yin.[68]

Some patients, even before they start trying for a baby, fear they may not be successful. ART patients may fear the medical procedures involving numerous injections or be frightened of taking a pregnancy test. The effects of prolonged suffering from fear negatively impact the reproductive system.[62]

Sadness and grief

Sadness affects the Lungs,[61] the Liver,[62] and the Heart and may influence the functional relationship between these organs.[68] Sadness and grief induces Heart and/or Liver Blood Deficiency and may also impact the functions of the Uterus.[68] Deficiency of Heart Qi can cause sadness.[62] Sadness exhausts the meridians linked to the womb and causes infertility. Excessive sadness may injure the entire internal organ system, leading to an overall deficiency of energy.

Feeling disappointed and sad is common in subfertile patients. They grieve for what could have been and what they do not have. Each time a pregnancy test is negative, they may go through periods of grief, sadness, and sorrow.

Guilt

Guilt affects the Heart and Kidneys and creates Stagnation or induces the Sinking of Qi.[68]

Women who had an abortion when they were younger may feel guilty, incorrectly associating their infertility with the abortion. They feel like they are being punished for what they have previously done.

Both male and female partners can also experience guilt individually if they are the ones 'at fault'. They can also feel guilty for failing their other half or failing their parents by not providing a child or grandchild.

Interrelationship between the emotions, the body, and the Spirit

The relationship between the emotions, the body, and the Spirit is complex:

- Emotions can cause the disease and/or injure the Spirit.
- Zangfu organs produce Qi responsible for emotions.[64]
- Physical pathology can cause an emotional imbalance.
- A compromised Shen (Spirit) can affect the emotional balance and/or cause a disease.
- The Zangfu organs store Jing (Essence); when they are injured through emotion, reproductive Qi is lost.[62]

With subfertile patients undergoing ART, determining the cause and effect is even more difficult. ART treatment is often referred to as an emotional rollercoaster, forcing patients to experience short-term immense joy and hope, followed by despair soon after, followed by more emotional ups and downs. The acupuncturist's task in such situations is to identify primary causes of disease caused by emotion and acknowledge and prevent additional pathological emotions, which could cause a new disease or exacerbate pre-existing imbalances.

'Examine the syndromes to find the cause' serves as a good guide when determining primary or secondary causes of subfertility.[66,71] Examining the state of Shen (Spirit) of a person provides a useful example of this process.

The Zangfu organs encompass physical, spiritual, and emotional aspects of each person. They are referred to as storerooms because Spirits reside in and are stored there. The Heart stores Shen (Spirit), and the Lung stores strength. The Liver stores mental consciousness, the soul and the Spleen stores intention and sentiment. The Kidneys store Jing (Essence) and will (Table 1.2).[72]

Fright, fear, nervousness, deliberation, and worry cause injury to the Shen (Spirit).[62] All these emotions are very common in subfertile patients.

A compromised Shen (Spirit) can also cause an emotional imbalance and ill health. For example, a weak Spirit can cause fear, which can induce seminal emission, affecting the reproductive system in men.

In order to identify the syndrome(s) and derive appropriate treatment principles, acupuncturists should try to correlate the sound of a person with their colour, odour, the relationship with Spirit, emotions, and the Zangfu organ system because these interact with each other (see Chapter 5).

External causes of disease

External Pathogenic Factors (EPFs) are the beginning stages of disease.[76] A disharmony arises as a result of External causes when the body is invaded by EPFs or Six Evil Qi. EPFs tend to invade the body when it is weak,[77] not well protected, or exposed.

Fertility could be particularly compromised when the EPFs invade the Uterus. EPFs enter the Uterus directly or invade the space between the skin and muscles.[68] There are various traditional concepts regarding EPFs' transmission of disease. One example is where EPFs enter deeper into the body, finally ending up in the meridians, the five Zang organs, and then the Stomach.[78]

The EPFs Wind-Cold, Cold-Damp, and Damp-Heat can cause Girdle vessel (vaginal) discharges.[58] Vaginal discharges influence Bodily Fluids that exit[58] and reproductive energies that enter the vagina. Girdle vessel discharges are not dissimilar to the Orthodox medical concept of vaginal discharges caused by bacterial and viral infections.[58] Vaginal discharges can induce complexity of disease and reduce fertility further by transferring to the Chong Mai (Penetrating Vessel) and Du Mai (Governing Vessel) and then entering the rest of the body.[58]

Table 1.2 Summary of Zangfu organs and their associated characteristics[72]			
Zangfu organ	**Associated emotion**	**Store**	**How excessive emotions affect Zangfu**
Liver	Anger	Mental consciousness[62] and Soul[73]	Anger injures the Liver
Heart	Joy	Shen (Spirit)[73]	Joy or sadness injures the Heart, Liver,[74] Lungs[74]
Spleen	Deliberation	Intention, sentiment[73,75]	Deliberation, worry[74] weakens the Spleen, Heart[70]
Kidney	Fear	Jing (Essence),[73] Will	Fear injures the Kidneys
Lung	Sadness and grief	Strength[73]	Sadness and grief injure the Lungs

A woman is thought to be more prone to an EPF invasion during menstruation[61,68] or following childbirth.[61] EPFs are:

- Wind[65]
- Coolness/Cold[65]
- Heat/Fire[65]
- Dampness[65]
- Summer-Heat[65]
- Dryness[59]

Temperature and climatic factors[71] directly influence Blood. A Cold climate may congeal and stagnate Blood, while Hot climates may stir up Blood. A Windy climate can deregulate the menstrual cycle.[58] EPF Wind harms the Liver.[79]

Invasion by Cold, Heat/Fire, or Dampness EPFs is a common cause of subfertility.[61,68]

Cold EPF

Cold EPF enters the body from the surface of the body into the interior of the body.[80] Cold invasion can occur from being in a cold environment for a long period or wearing inadequate footwear or clothing. If a woman sits on a cold or damp surface for long periods, she may also suffer Cold-Damp invasion. Coolness is harmful to the lower Jiao.[65] Cold medical instruments can also introduce Cold inside the Uterus.

Cold is harmful to Blood.[64] Cold contracts and coagulates Qi and Blood, leading to Qi or Blood Stagnation. Stagnation can damage the Extraordinary Vessels, particularly the Chong Mai (Penetrating Vessel) and Ren Mai (Conception Vessel).[61] Both these Vessels are essential for fertility and pregnancy.

In men, Cold can cause seminal Essence-Cold, affecting men's fertility.[58] This Cold semen can then enter the Uterus during intercourse, creating difficulty in retaining semen[58] or inducing a Cold Uterus.

A Cold Uterus (whether arising from Cold EPF or from internal dysfunction) destroys 'things', including semen entering the Uterus, and, if conception progresses to this stage, the foetus.[58] A Cold Uterus is also unable to regulate Jing (Essence), causing conception difficulties.[58] This presentation is evident in some women with fertilization and embryo development issues, Repeated Implantation Failure, and reproductive immunology issues.

Heat/Fire EPF

Heat/Fire EPF can occur through climatic changes or hot environments. Heat or Fire is harmful to Qi.[64] Heat/Fire can consume Qi and Bodily Fluids and damage the Extraordinary Vessels. In particular, it can affect the functions of the Chong Mai (Penetrating Vessel) and Ren Mai (Conception Vessel).

Heat tends to affect the flow of Blood by speeding it up and making it 'reckless'. Once Heat has entered the body, it can move into the Blood-level, causing Blood-Heat,[68] thus adversely affecting fertility. Heat can be retained at a low level for long periods, causing subfertility. Heat can affect male fertility by negatively affecting sperm production.

Damp EPF

Damp living environments or being in a wet damp climate for prolonged periods can give rise to Damp invasion.[81] Dampness can invade the lower part of the body directly[68,80] or descend to the lower part of the body.[80] Dampness damages the Lower Jiao,[65] blocking the flow of Qi and Blood to the reproductive organs.

Miscellaneous causes of disease

In TCM, a disease can also arise as a result of miscellaneous causes. Miscellaneous causes include:

- Weak constitution
- Unhealthy lifestyle habits
- Poor diet and nutrition
- Surgery
- Physical overexertion
- Too much work and not enough rest
- Previous fertility treatment
- Miscarriage
- Coitus and inappropriate family planning
- Contraception

However, Sivin argues that mental overstimulation, unregulated diet, and overexhaustion are all External causes of disease.[71]

Constitution

The patient's state of health varies, depending on the constitution passed on to the patient by his or her parents.[61] The constitution of a child can be weaker if its parents were older or ill at the time they conceived that child. A weak constitution can affect most bodily systems, including the reproductive system.

Different constitutions and the influence of lifestyle generate various physiques that determine susceptibility to invasion by EPFs.[61]

Various imbalances in the constitution of individuals can be strengthened with acupuncture with appropriate needling technique, the use of herbal medicine, and improvements in lifestyle, diet, and exercises[61] such as qigong and tai chi.

Constitutional Deficiencies of the Kidney (for example, Kidney Yang Deficiency in the male and Kidney Yin Deficiency in the female) affect the transformation of vital energies essential for fertilization and conception. Poorly transformed vital energies may cause infertility because the foetus is unable to take form.[58] Conceptionally, this may be similar to poor fertilization rates or failure of embryos to implant.

Inappropriate diet

Irregular eating and excessive fatigue damage the Spleen and may cause extreme Deficiency[82] in several Zangfu organs, thus reducing reproductive potential.

The temperature of foods and fluids can influence the body in a way that causes pathology. Foods that are too hot or too cold in temperature can produce the same phenomena inside the body, i.e. hot foods generating Heat, and cold foods generating Cold.

Although TCM literature states that 'improper diet' is caused by excessive consumption of hot, cold, and raw foods or overeating,[61,68] even mild consumption of Cool or Hot foods over a period can have subtle implications on a patient's ability to conceive. However, eating and drinking hot and cold foods in moderation[83] and on a regular basis maintains harmony between the body and Shen (Spirit).[84,85] Dieting can cause Deficiency of the Stomach Qi, Deficiency of Jing (Essence), and low Shen (Spirit).[60]

From a TCM perspective, dieting or vegetarianism leads to Blood Deficiency.[68] Although vegetarians may still get a range of nutrition from a well-balanced vegetarian diet, a diet without TCM Blood-nourishing properties can produce Blood Deficiency.

Consumption of greasy foods will impact the bodily systems, especially in patients with pre-existing conditions such as Spleen Qi Deficiency, Dampness, or Phlegm. Greasy foods tend to create Dampness in the Lower Burner. A high intake of cheese, butter, cream, bananas, sweets, and sugar causes Dampness in the body.[68,71] These turbid energies of food damage the Middle Jiao.[80]

Surgery

Some women may have undergone surgery prior to ART. Surgery can create Qi or Blood Stagnation in the Lower Jiao. Stagnation can affect several Meridians and Extraordinary Vessels and the Uterus, as well as alter the physiological dynamics of Zangfu interrelationships.

Surgery can have an emotional element attached to it, affecting how women feel, and this connects with the Lower Jiao, potentially causing Heart–Uterus imbalance.

Social, recreational, and physical overexertion

Physical overwork can induce Stagnation or Deficiency. This is especially so if it occurred during puberty, for example, in young dancers[68] or young athletes. Such overexertion can have long-lasting effects. In adults, excessive exercise injures the Spleen, Liver, and Kidneys.[68] This is a common occurrence and delays conception in runners or people active in sports through the formation Qi Deficiency.

Work and rest

Overwork can consume Qi[61] and disperse Yang Qi.[79] Too much rest can Stagnate Qi.[61] Working long hours and not getting enough rest can cause Kidney Yin Deficiency[68] and affect the Liver and Heart, particularly if the work is perceived as stressful and is combined with a busy personal lifestyle.

A physically demanding job can cause Kidney Deficiency, impacting reproductive health. Sitting for long periods can cause Lung and Spleen Qi Deficiency. The psychosocial dynamics of the work environment can impact the well-being of a person, especially when exposed to mistreatment, intimidation, and pressure to perform. This often produces Spleen Qi Deficiency and Liver Qi Stagnation.

Physical overexertion can cause infertility and reduce reproductive potential. This is especially so for a certain subgroup of patients, for example, patients with Yin Deficiency who are undergoing ART and have very busy work and personal lifestyles. A balance between activity and rest helps preserve Kidney Jing (Essence)[83] and Yin and therefore fertility.

Couples may delay starting a family because of career pressures. This reduces fertility purely because of an age-related natural decline in fertility as, by the age of 40, Kidney Yin is significantly reduced.[64]

For some people, being overworked and needing to have constant communication (such as emails, mobile phones) combined with inadequate rest and sleep, uses up more Blood from the Liver and Heart. This decreases Blood and Jing (Essence) and the amount of nourishment available to the body.[86]

Previous fertility treatment

Previous fertility treatment can weaken Yin, Yang, Qi, and Blood. It can also lead to Heat and Stagnation. The Shen (Spirit) is easily disturbed by these factors, and it can be affected by the emotional consequences of failed ART treatment.

Miscarriages

Miscarriages are believed to be as draining to Qi and Blood as childbirths.[68] They affect the Kidney, Heart, and Liver and lead to Kidney Qi Deficiency, Blood Deficiency, or Stagnation.

Early miscarriages damage the Kidney, consume Qi, and weaken the Blood.[61]

Miscarriages usually happen in the background of pre-existing maternal Deficiency of Qi and/or Blood. The emotional impact for some women suffering from a miscarriage can create Heart Blood Deficiency, contributing to further subfertility and further miscarriage.

Coitus and family planning

Both excessive and infrequent sexual intercourse can deplete Kidney Jing (Essence) in men and, to a lesser extent, Kidney Jing (Essence) in women.[68] Sex in teenage-hood may damage Jing (Essence) in men and Qi and Blood in women.[87] In adulthood, both excessive and infrequent sexual intercourse can affect health.[88]

Anxiety about a possible lack of sexual satisfaction or inability to experience an orgasm may produce sexual frustration that consumes Yin. Zhu Dan Xi, a famous physician from the Jin and Yuan Dynasties, implies that, to avoid this, intercourse should occur at the right time and in a calm and mutually considered way in order to preserve Jing (Essence).[89] Reproduction relies on a good relationship between a male and a female partner, and coitus for the purpose of reproduction ought to occur at a time when Qi and Blood are strong.[89] Yet, when a couple try to conceive, they have very frequent intercourse, even if they do not feel like it or if they are tired or ill. A too-rigid approach to family planning can lead to Liver Qi Stagnation,[90] which can impair sexual enjoyment,[58] affecting the energies required for optimal conception.

Lack of education on natural family planning techniques, a delay in investigations, along with advanced maternal age and the 'biological clock ticking' phenomenon can create emotional upset in women. This adversely influences fertility by affecting the Heart, Liver, Spleen, and Kidney, creating Heat/Fire, Qi, Blood, and Yin or Yang Deficiency.

Many couples who are unsuccessful even after few months of trying to conceive may experience apprehension. After the initial subfertility investigations, many couples are advised to relax and continue trying. This can further exacerbate their emotional state. By the time a couple is referred for ART, emotional distress may already have been experienced; this potentially impacts negatively on their chance of a successful ART procedure.

Contraception

Long-term prior use of hormonal contraception can induce Blood Deficiency, Blood Stasis,[68] or Dampness. Sometimes the contraceptive pill is administered for a short duration prior to IVF. This can exacerbate pre-existing patterns of disharmony.

Summary of the causes of diseases in subfertility

Although invasion by EPFs causes subfertility, in contemporary acupuncture practice, Internal causes (e.g., excessive emotions) and Miscellaneous causes (e.g., inappropriate diet, overwork, weak constitution, unhealthy lifestyle habits, physical overexertion, excessive work and inadequate rest, coital issues, and inappropriate family planning) are more frequently observed in the authors' practice.

REPRODUCTIVE HISTORY AND DEVELOPMENT FROM AN ORTHODOX MEDICAL PERSPECTIVE

The first recorded successful birth following assisted conception happened in 1785 in London. Doctor John Hunter performed artificial insemination in a couple where the husband had hypospadias. It was not until the 1940s when further reports of intrauterine insemination (IUI) were recorded. IUI is still widely used today.[91]

In 1967, clomiphene citrate (clomid) was licensed for clinical use in the United States.[92] This medication is used to produce superovulation by stimulating follicular growth. In contemporary clinical practice, it is often used as a first-line subfertility treatment, especially in couples with known ovulatory problems.[91,92]

Between 1878 and 1953, many attempts were made to fertilize mammalian eggs *in vitro*. Some reported success. However, Bavister suggests most of these reports were unjustified.[93] One of the reasons was that 'capacitation' was not discovered until the 1950s by Chang and Austin.[93] *Capacitation* is the term used to describe the changes that happen to the sperm inside the female reproductive tract that allow the sperm to become capable of fertilizing the egg.

This discovery led to successful fertilization of a human egg. In 1969, Robert Edwards and his colleagues reported successful *in vitro* maturation and fertilization of human oocytes. Edwards attributed this success to the capacitation research done by Chang and Austin.[94]

Edwards believed this development would be useful in 'certain clinical and scientific uses for human eggs fertilized by this procedure'. However, the significance of this development was far greater than originally predicted.[93] In 1978, the first 'test tube' baby was born as a result of the pioneering work done by Patrick Steptoe and Robert Edwards, who developed the IVF technique. Initially, this technique involved no stimulation of the ovaries, and the egg was retrieved using laparoscopic surgery.

IVF has since been refined, but, along with several treatment derivatives, it remains the most frequently used ART procedure. To improve success rates, the ovaries are artificially stimulated by medication to produce more than one egg, and the eggs are retrieved transvaginally.[91,95]

In 1984, Gamete Intrafallopian Transfer was developed. In this procedure, both gametes (eggs and sperm) are placed inside the fallopian tubes, not inside the uterus as is done in IVF.[91,95] In 1983, the first pregnancy following frozen embryo transfer was reported.[96]

In 1991, a technique that revolutionized the treatment of certain male factor problems, called ICSI, was developed. In this procedure, the egg is injected with a single sperm in the hope that it will become fertilized. This has allowed men with very serious subfertility to father children.[95] Intracytoplasmic Morphologically Selected Sperm Injection is an even more refined sperm injection technique that

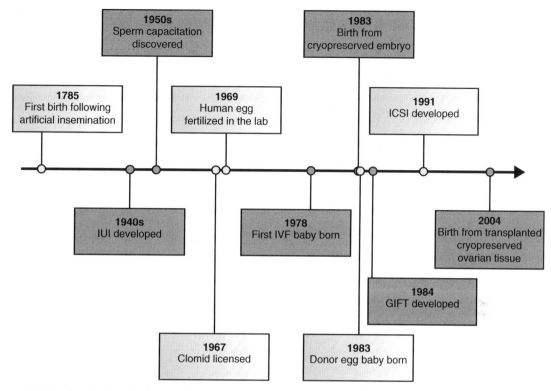

Figure 1.4 Timeline of major developments in ART.

promises even better results than ICSI.[97] Morphologically optimal sperm are identified using microscopy and injected into the egg, theoretically reducing the possibility of poorer quality sperm being used.

In 2004, the first birth from transplanted cryopreserved ovarian tissue was reported.[95]

ARTs are evolving rapidly, and many other techniques have been and are in the process of being developed. Figure 1.4 highlights major milestones in the development of ART.

Currently, researchers are focusing on fertility preservation, genetic diagnosis, improvement of ART success rates, and stem cell treatment of major diseases.

In 2010, ESHRE estimated that since the birth of the first test tube baby, over 3.75 million babies have been born as a result of IVF.[20]

REPRODUCTIVE HISTORY AND DEVELOPMENT FROM A TCM PERSPECTIVE

View and worship of fertility

Chinese fertility worship is derived from Chinese cultural perceptions. In Chinese culture, there are prolific illustrations of plants and animals that nonverbally articulate the aspiration to reproduce. The ability to reproduce is viewed as a form of power in society. In pre-industrial Chinese society, birth rates and death rates were high, and the growth rate of the population was therefore low.[98]

The notion of Yin and Yang represents the zenith of fertility. Yin and Yang exemplify male and female sexual organs. Yin is female, and Yang is male.[98] Yin Yang philosophy extends throughout the treatment and management of infertility.

When advising men and women on how to optimize their fertility in order to reproduce, the concept of Yin Yang philosophy is an integral part of fertility treatment. The male's fertility is thought to 'fluctuate on a daily basis corresponding with the rising Yang energies, particularly in morning'.[99]

The male is responsible for providing the 'Essence for conception' while the female takes charge of 'gathering the Essences'.[58]

Works of classical Chinese medicine physicians

Contemporary traditional Chinese reproductive and gynaecology Medicine is based on the classical work of TCM physicians, who provided insights and contemporaneous innovation to the practice of gynaecology. Some of the earliest records relating to gynaecology go back to the Shang Dynasty (1500–1000 BCE), where tortoise shells had details of childbirth-related complications scribbled on them.[100] As the knowledge base expanded, this was reflected in the writing of key texts (see Table 1.3).

Table 1.3 Summary of key TCM physicians and texts relating to gynaecology

Time periods	Physician	Knowledge development[101]	Texts
The Qin and Han Dynasties	–	• Natural patterns of female growth, development, and sexual maturation and decline • Female reproductive ability • Menstrual physiology • Diagnosis of pregnancy • Aetiology and pathology of gynaecological diseases (metrorrhagia, leucorrhoea, amenorrhoea, infertility, ovarian cyst) • Prescription for amenorrhoea and menorrhagia • Describes the physiology and functions of the Uterus	Huang Di Nei Jing Su Wen (The Yellow Emperor's Classic of Internal Medicine – Simple Questions)[100]
ca. 0–200 CE The Eastern Han Dynasty[102]	–	Anatomical term Zigong (Uterus) was introduced	Shen Nong Ben Cao Jing (Classic of Shen Nong's Materia Medica)[101]
150–219 CE The Eastern Han Dynasty[101]	Zhang Zhongjing (Zhang Zhong Jing)	Established principles of syndrome differentiation and treatment of: • Pregnancy diseases, nurturing the foetus, and damage to the foetus • Postpartum disease (e.g., convulsions, vertigo, postpartum abdominal pain) • Miscellaneous gynaecological diseases (including Heat invading the Blood Chamber, menstrual disease, leucorrhoea)	Jin Gui Yao Lue Fang Lun (Discussion of Prescriptions of the Golden Chest)[100]
ca. 280 CE Western Jin Dynasty[103]	Wang Shuhe (Wang Xi)	• Menstrual cycle rhythms classified into monthly, bimonthly, trimonthly, or annually • Prognosis of metrorrhagia, metrostaxis, impending labour or miscarriage by ascertaining pulse changes • Expertise in diagnosing pregnancy through Chinese pulse taking	Mai Jing (Canon of Pulses)[103]
ca. 610 CE The Sui Dynasty[101]	Chao Yuanfang	• Treatise on gynaecological diseases • Gynaecological diseases stemmed from injury to the Chong and Ren Mai (Penetrating and Conception Vessels)	Zhu Bing Yuan Hou Lun (Treatise on Causes and Symptoms of Diseases)[104]
581–682 CE The Tang Dynasty[103,105]	Sun Simiao	Presented a collection of medical essays and prescriptions (e.g., discussions on multifactorial contributions to infertility, early pregnancy support, nurturing of the foetus, cleansing the endometrium for implantation, prevention of recurrent miscarriage, positive reinforcement to the patients)	Bei Ji Qian Jin Yao Fang (Golden Prescriptions for Emergencies)[101]
ca. 852 CE The Sui and Tang Dynasties[106]	Zan Yin	52 chapters and 317 formulas to treat gynaecological and obstetric conditions	Jing Xiao Chan Bao (Treasured Knowledge of Obstetrics)[106]

Table 1.3 Summary of key TCM physicians and texts relating to gynaecology—cont'd

Time periods	Physician	Knowledge development[101]	Texts
ca. 1078 CE The Song Dynasty[107]	Yang Zijian	Practical manipulation of vaginal delivery	Shi Chan Lun (Treatise on Ten Obstetric Problems)[107]
ca. 1220 CE The Song Dynasty[99]	Qi Zhongfu	The term Bao Gong (Uterus) was introduced	Nu Ke Bai Wen (A Hundred Questions on Women's Diseases)[101]
1190–1270 CE The Song Dynasty[99]	Chen Ziming	• Systematic presentation on common gynaecological diseases • Recognized that treatment of gynaecological and obstetric conditions is complex • Stipulated that the most important factor in treating women is to regulate menses	Furen Da Quan Liang Fang (All-inclusive Good Prescriptions for Women)[99]
The Southern Song Dynasty[101]	Zhu Duanzhang	Symptoms and treatments for complex obstetric syndromes	Wei Sheng Jia Bao Chan Ke Bei Yao (A Precious Manual of Obstetrics for Home Use)[101]
ca. 1120–1200 CE The Jin and Yuan Dynasties[103]	Liu Wansu	Stipulated that treatment methods for women of different ages should be different: • Reinforce the Kidney in the treatment of girls at puberty • Regulate the Liver in the treatment of middle-aged women • Activate the Spleen in the treatment of the elderly	Su Wen Bing Ji Qi Yi Bao Ming Ji – Fu Ren Tai Chan Lun (Collected Writings on the Preservation of Life and Conditions of Qi According to Patho-Mechanisms of the Plain Questions – on Pregnancy and Birth)[101]
1281–1358 CE The Yuan Dynasty[103]	Zhu Danxi (Zhu Zhenheng)	• Postpartum treatment principles: clearing Heat and nourishing Blood, supplementing Qi • Herbal treatment to secure the foetus	Ge Zhi Yu Lun (Supplementary Treatise on Knowledge from Practice)[101]
ca. 1624 CE The Ming Dynasty[108]	Zhang Jiebin (Zhang Jingyue)	Divided gynaecological diseases into categories: • Channels and Vessels • Pregnancy and foetus • Pregnancy and delivery • Postpartum • Leucorrhoea • Breasts • Male offspring • Abdominal masses • Diseases of the genitalia Emphasized the Chong and Ren Mai Vessels, the Spleen, the Kidney, Yin and Blood, physiology between Yang Qi and Yin Essence	Jin Yue Quan Shu (Complete Works of Zhang Jingyue)[108]
The Ming Dynasty[109]	Wan Quan (Wan Mi-zhai)	• Five physiological defects that caused sterility: spiral stria of the vulva, stricture of the vagina, imperforate hymen, elongated clitoris, amenorrhoea	Guang Si Ji Yao – Ze Pei Pian (Summary of How to Have Many Children)[101]

Continued

Table 1.3   Summary of key TCM physicians and texts relating to gynaecology—cont'd

Time periods	Physician	Knowledge development[101]	Texts
		• Male lifestyle advice: Nourish semen by keeping a peaceful mind and limiting desires • Female lifestyle advice: Nourish Blood through a determined and calm mind	
The Qing Dynasty[101]	Fu Shan	Differentiated syndromes and treatment methods: • The Liver • The Spleen • The Kidney	Fu Qing Zhu Nu Ke (Fu Qing Zhu's Gynecology)[101]
1768–1831 CE The Qing Dynasty[103]	Wang Qingren	Developed concept of activating Blood to resolve Stasis	Yi Lin Gao Cuo (Corrections of Errors in Medical Field)[103]
The Qing Dynasty[101]	Wu Qian	Textbook on gynaecology and obstetrics organized by the government	Fu Ke Xin Fa Yao Jue (A Heart Approach to Gynaecology)[101]
1862–1918 CE The Late Qing Dynasty[110]	Tang Rongchuan (Tang Zong Hai)	Emphasized Qi and Blood regulation	Xu Zheng Lun (On Blood Disorder)[101]

- Knowledge regarding TCM biology of the reproductive system expanded with the information about normal menstrual cycle rhythms.
- The prognoses of conditions became scrutinized through clinical signs such as pulse diagnosis.
- Treatment protocols were endorsed for different age ranges in women, such as regulating the Liver in the middle aged (which is still salient when promoting fertility for women of advanced reproductive age).
- Roles of the physiological processes of Qi and Blood as well as the pathogenesis of Blood Stasis and Heat in the Blood Chamber were noted in gynaecological conditions. Qi and Blood are still fundamental concepts in contemporary reproductive TCM practice.
- The role of the Extraordinary Vessels was explored along with identifying pathology of the Chong (Penetrating) and Ren (Conception) Mai, the Spleen and Kidney, and the Liver.
- Deeper understanding was gained of differentiated syndromes and treatments.
- The understanding of the causes of disease evolved.
- The nosology of TCM advanced as gynaecological diseases were further divided into categories.
- The treatment and prevention of miscarriages and health in pregnancy and postpartum show enhanced understanding of the complexity of the subject.

Recognition by Chinese medicine of some of the fundamental concepts of fertility

TCM physicians observed and meticulously recorded some of the key concepts of fertility that are now accepted by both TCM and conventional Orthodox medical models.

Fertile window and intercourse timing

As in Orthodox medicine, the existence of the fertile window and the need for optimal timing of the intercourse was recognized. The best time for coitus was advised to be just after the end of menstruation[99] when old Blood has been eliminated and new Blood is generating.[58]

Chapter 3 reviews research on the fertile window and coitus in greater detail.

The effect of age on fertility

The classical TCM concept of the seven reproductive cycles (yearly cycles) in women and eight early cycles in men underpins TCM reproductive biology, recognizing age-related changes in the reproductive system (see Chapter 2 for more details).

The promptness for reproducing was associated with reproductive health, which was thought to be at its best

10 years after puberty in women.[99] Men were encouraged to marry at 30 years of age because that is when their fertility was believed to be in its prime.[99]

Importance of optimizing natural fertility

Classical TCM teachings recognized the importance of preservation and optimization of natural fertility.[99] The female was assigned procreative potential.[58]

Integrated approach

Since 1949 in China, TCM has been well integrated into Orthodox medicine. Acupuncture is often administered in hospitals. Doctors decide on the treatment plan, often combining the best of the Orthodox and TCM medical approaches. In the West, integrative approaches are extremely underused. This is especially so in ART medicine, where the potential for success may well be improved by the integration of TCM and Orthodox medical approaches.

SUMMARY

Rates of infertility appear to be static, yet increasingly more couples require ART treatments. This is in part caused by the fact that people delay having children until later in life.

As the numbers of people requiring ART has increased, so have the numbers of patients presenting for supportive acupuncture treatment during ART. Research suggests that these numbers are likely to rise further. This demand is in part fuelled by reports of several studies showing that acupuncture has a positive effect on IVF success rates.

TCM understanding of gynaecology and fertility goes back several millennia. TCM provides a different and alternative perspective on subfertility that has much to offer the subfertile couple on their journey toward conception. However, as with Orthodox medicine, the knowledge about how to manage patients during ART is a relatively modern concept, one that is rapidly evolving.

Infertility and ART is a challenging field of medicine. Neither Orthodox medical nor TCM medical paradigms have all the answers. An integrated approach, where acupuncturists have a thorough understanding of both concepts of reproductive health, may prove to be the most clinically useful approach. For example, when taking an initial medical history, acupuncturists must enquire into nonmedical causes of subfertility using both health models. A combined Orthodox medical and TCM approach to the assessment and management of subfertility enhances patient care by providing a holistic integrated approach and promoting optimal health, fertility, and well-being.

REFERENCES

1. Zegers-Hochschild F, Adamson GD, de Mouzon J, et al. The International Committee for Monitoring Assisted Reproductive Technology (ICMART) and the World Health Organization (WHO) revised glossary on ART terminology, 2009. Hum Reprod 2009;24:2683–7.

2. Practice Committee of the American Society for Reproductive Medicine. Definitions of infertility and recurrent pregnancy loss: a committee opinion. Fertil Steril 2013;99:63.

3. Assisted Reproductive Technology (ART) – glossary. Available from: http://www.eshre.eu/ESHRE/English/Guidelines-Legal/ART-glossary/page.aspx/1062 [accessed 26 January 2013].

4. National Collaborating Centre for Women's and Children's Health, Commissioned by the National Institute for Health and Clinical Excellence. Investigation of fertility problems and management strategies. In: Fertility: assessment and treatment for people with fertility problems. NICE clinical guideline. 2nd ed. London: The Royal College of Obstetricians and Gynaecologists; 2013. p. 80–132 [chapter 6].

5. Macklon NS, Geraedts JP, Fauser BC. Conception to ongoing pregnancy: the 'black box' of early pregnancy loss. Hum Reprod Update 2002;8:333–43.

6. Louis GM, Cooney MA, Lynch CD, et al. Periconception window: advising the pregnancy-planning couple. Fertil Steril 2008;89:e119–21.

7. Lynch CD, Jackson LW, Buck Louis GM. Estimation of the day-specific probabilities of conception: current state of the knowledge and the relevance for epidemiological research. Paediatr Perinat Epidemiol 2006;20:3–12.

8. Bigelow JL, Dunson DB, Stanford JB, et al. Mucus observations in the fertile window: a better predictor of conception than timing of intercourse. Hum Reprod 2004;19:889–92.

9. Brosens I, Gordts S, Valkenburg M, et al. Investigation of the infertile couple: when is the appropriate time to explore female infertility? Hum Reprod 2004;19:1689–92.

10. Stanford JB, White GL, Hatasaka H. Timing intercourse to achieve pregnancy: current evidence. Obstet Gynecol 2002;100:1333–41.

11. Dunson DB, Sinai I, Colombo B. The relationship between cervical secretions and the daily probabilities of pregnancy: effectiveness of the two day algorithm. Hum Reprod 2001;16:2278–82.

12. Dunson DB, Baird DD, Wilcox AJ, et al. Day-specific probabilities of clinical pregnancy based on two

studies with imperfect measures of ovulation. Hum Reprod 1999;14:1835–9.

13. Baird DT, Collins J, Egozcue J, et al. Fertility and ageing. Hum Reprod Update 2005;11:261–76.

14. Gnoth C, Godehardt E, Frank-Herrmann P, et al. Definition and prevalence of subfertility and infertility. Hum Reprod 2005;20:1144–7.

15. Hays B. Infertility: a functional medicine approach. Integr Med 2010;8:20–7.

16. Gurunath S, Pandian Z, Anderson RA, et al. Defining infertility – a systematic review of prevalence studies. Hum Reprod Update 2011;17:575–88.

17. Habbema JD, Collins J, Leridon H, et al. Towards less confusing terminology in reproductive medicine: a proposal. Fertil Steril 2004;82:36–40.

18. Barnhart KT. Epidemiology of male and female reproductive disorders and impact on fertility regulation and population growth. Fertil Steril 2011;95:2200–3.

19. Boivin J, Bunting L, Collins JA, et al. International estimates of infertility prevalence and treatment-seeking: potential need and demand for infertility medical care. Hum Reprod 2007;22:1506–12.

20. ESHRE ART fact sheet. Available from: http://www.eshre.eu/ESHRE/English/Guidelines-Legal/ART-fact-sheet/page.aspx/1061 [accessed 13 December 2012].

21. Wilkes S, Chinn DJ, Murdoch A, et al. Epidemiology and management of infertility: a population-based study in UK primary care. Fam Pract 2009;26:269–74.

22. Mascarenhas MN, Flaxman SR, Boerma T, et al. National, regional, and global trends in infertility prevalence since 1990: a systematic analysis of 277 health surveys. PLoS Med 2012;9:e1001356.

23. Olsen J, Zhu JL, Ramlau-Hansen CH. Has fertility declined in recent decades? Acta Obstet Gynecol Scand 2011;90:129–35.

24. Stephen EH, Chandra A. Declining estimates of infertility in the United States: 1982–2002. Fertil Steril 2006;86:516–23.

25. te Velde E, Burdorf A, Nieschlag E, et al. Is human fecundity declining in Western countries? Hum Reprod 2010;25:1348–53.

26. Carlsen E, Giwercman A, Keiding N, et al. Evidence for decreasing quality of semen during past 50 years. BMJ 1992;305:609–13.

27. Merzenich H, Zeeb H, Blettner M. Decreasing sperm quality: a global problem? BMC Public Health 2010;10:24.

28. Oakley L, Doyle P, Maconochie N. Lifetime prevalence of infertility and infertility treatment in the UK: results from a population-based survey of reproduction. Hum Reprod 2008;23:447–50.

29. Stankiewicz M, Smith C, Alvino H, et al. The use of complementary medicine and therapies by patients attending a reproductive medicine unit in South Australia: a prospective survey. Aust N Z J Obstet Gynaecol 2007;47:145–9.

30. Smith JF, Eisenberg ML, Millstein SG, et al. The use of complementary and alternative fertility treatment in couples seeking fertility care: data from a prospective cohort in the United States. Fertil Steril 2010;93:2169–74.

31. Practice Committee of American Society for Reproductive Medicine. Diagnostic evaluation of the infertile male: a committee opinion. Fertil Steril 2012;98:294–301.

32. Thonneau P, Marchand S, Tallec A, et al. Incidence and main causes of infertility in a resident population (1 850 000) of three French regions (1988–1989). Hum Reprod 1991;6:811–6.

33. Hull MG, Glazener CM, Kelly NJ, et al. Population study of causes, treatment, and outcome of infertility. Br Med J (Clin Res Ed) 1985;291:1693–7.

34. National Collaborating Centre for Women's and Children's Health, Commissioned by the National Institute for Health and Clinical Excellence. Introduction. In: Fertility: assessment and treatment for people with fertility problems. NICE clinical guideline. 2nd ed. London: The Royal College of Obstetricians and Gynaecologists; 2013. p. 47–9 [chapter 2].

35. ESHRE Capri Workshop Group. Diagnosis and management of the infertile couple: missing information. Hum Reprod Update 2004;10:295–307.

36. Bovey M, Lorenc A, Robinson N. Extent of acupuncture practice for infertility in the United Kingdom: experiences and perceptions of the practitioners. Fertil Steril 2010;94:2569–73.

37. Madaschi C, Braga DPAF, de Figueira RCS, et al. Effect of acupuncture on assisted reproduction treatment outcomes. Acupunct Med 2010;28:180–4.

38. Office for National Statistics. Live births in England and Wales by characteristics of mother 1. Report of the Office for National Statistics; 2011.

39. US Department of Health and Human Services, Centers for Disease Control and Prevention, National Center for Health Statistics. Delayed childbearing: more women are having their first child later in life. Report of the US Department of Health and Human Services, Centers for Disease Control and Prevention, National Center for Health Statistics; 2009.

40. Mac Dougall K, Beyene Y, Nachtigall RD. 'Inconvenient biology:' advantages and disadvantages of first-time parenting after age 40 using in vitro fertilization. Hum Reprod 2012;27:1058–65.

41. Skoog Svanberg A, Lampic C, Karlström PO, et al. Attitudes toward parenthood and awareness of fertility among postgraduate students in Sweden. Gend Med 2006;3:187–95.

42. Wallace WH, Kelsey TW. Human ovarian reserve from conception to the menopause. PLoS One 2010;5:e8772.

43. Sartorius GA, Nieschlag E. Paternal age and reproduction. Hum Reprod Update 2010;16:65–79.

44. de la Rochebrochard E, Thonneau P. Paternal age and maternal age are risk factors for miscarriage; results of a multicentre European study. Hum Reprod 2002;17:1649–56.

45. Maheshwari A, Porter M, Shetty A, et al. Women's awareness and perceptions of delay in

childbearing. Fertil Steril 2008;90:1036–42.

46. Centers for Disease Control and Prevention. Assisted Reproductive Technology success rates 2006. National summary and fertility clinic reports. Report of the Centers for Disease Control and Prevention, Birmingham, Alabama; 2008.

47. Hassan MA, Killick SR. Negative lifestyle is associated with a significant reduction in fecundity. Fertil Steril 2004;81:384–92.

48. Leke RJ, Oduma JA, Bassol-Mayagoitia S, et al. Regional and geographical variations in infertility: effects of environmental, cultural, and socioeconomic factors. Environ Health Perspect 1993;101:73–80.

49. Woodruff TJ, Carlson A, Schwartz JM, et al. Proceedings of the summit on environmental challenges to reproductive health and fertility: executive summary. Fertil Steril 2008;89:281–300.

50. Joffe M. What has happened to human fertility? Hum Reprod 2010;25:295–307.

51. Anderson K, Nisenblat V, Norman R. Lifestyle factors in people seeking infertility treatment – a review. Aust N Z J Obstet Gynaecol 2010;50:8–20.

52. Homan GF, Davies M, Norman R. The impact of lifestyle factors on reproductive performance in the general population and those undergoing infertility treatment: a review. Hum Reprod Update 2007;13:209–23.

53. Broekmans F. The initial fertility assessment: a medical check-up of the couple experiencing difficulties conceiving. In: de Haan N, Spelt M, Gobel R, editors. Reproductive medicine: a textbook for paramedics. Amsterdam: Elsevier Gezondheidszorg; 2010. p. 21–39 [chapter 1].

54. Gianotten W, Schade A. Sexuality and fertility issues. In: de Haan N, Spelt M, Gobel R, editors. Reproductive medicine: a textbook for paramedics. Amsterdam: Elsevier Gezondheidszorg; 2010. p. 167–78 [chapter 13].

55. Practice Committee of American Society for Reproductive Medicine in collaboration with Society for Reproductive Endocrinology and Infertility. Optimizing natural fertility. Fertil Steril 2008;90:S1–6.

56. WHO. Sexually transmitted and other reproductive tract infections: a guide to essential practice. Report of the WHO; 2005.

57. Wiseman N. Ellis. Disease and its causes. In: Zhong Yi Xue Ji Chu, editor. Fundamentals of Chinese medicine. 2nd ed. Massachusetts: Paradigm Publications; 1996. p. 77–87 [chapter 5].

58. Wu YL. Function and structure in the female body. In: Reproducing women: medicine, metaphor, and childbirth in late imperial China. Berkeley: University of California Press; 2010. p. 84–119 [chapter 3].

59. Lu HC. On pure and subtle energies. In: A complete translation of the Yellow Emperor's classics of internal medicine and the difficult classic (Nei-Jing and Nan-Jing). Vancouver: International College of Traditional Chinese Medicine; 2004. p. 367–71, Section two: Essential questions [Su Wen] [chapter 81].

60. Lu HC. Verbal questions. In: A complete translation of the Yellow Emperor's classics of internal medicine and the difficult classic (Nei-Jing and Nan-Jing). Vancouver: International College of Traditional Chinese Medicine; 2004. p. 481–7, Section three: Spiritual pivot [Ling Shu] [chapter 28].

61. Tan Y, Qi C, Zhang Q, et al. Etiology and pathogenesis of gynecological diseases. In: Gynecology of Traditional Chinese Medicine, Chinese-English bilingual textbooks for international students of Chinese TCM institutions. China: People's Medical Publishing House; 2007. p. 174–82 [chapter 3].

62. Lu HC. Spirit as the fundamental of needling. In: A complete translation of the Yellow Emperor's classics of internal medicine and the difficult classic (Nei-Jing and Nan-Jing). Vancouver: International College of Traditional Chinese Medicine; 2004. p. 402–4, Section three: Spiritual pivot [Ling Shu] [Chapter 8].

63. Lu HC. Inscriptions on bamboo sticks. In: A complete translation of the Yellow Emperor's classics of internal medicine and the difficult classic (Nei-Jing and Nan-Jing).

Vancouver: International College of Traditional Chinese Medicine; 2004. p. 535–8, Section three: Spiritual pivot [Ling Shu] [chapter 60].

64. Lu HC. Great treatise on Yin Yang classifications of natural phenomena. In: A complete translation of the Yellow Emperor's classics of internal medicine and the difficult classic (Nei-Jing and Nan-Jing). Vancouver: International College of Traditional Chinese Medicine; 2004. p. 86–98, Section two: Essential questions [Su Wen] [chapter 5].

65. Lu HC. Original causes of a hundred diseases. In: A complete translation of the Yellow Emperor's classics of internal medicine and the difficult classic (Nei-Jing and Nan-Jing). Vancouver: International College of Traditional Chinese Medicine; 2004. p. 549–51, Section three: Spiritual pivot [Ling Shu] [chapter 66].

66. Maciocia G. The causes of disease. In: The foundations of Chinese medicine: a comprehensive text for acupuncturists and herbalists. Edinburgh, NY: Churchill Livingstone; 1989. p. 127–42 [chapter 15].

67. Rochat de la Vallee E. Blood and Qi. In: Root C, editor. The essential women, female health and fertility in Chinese classical texts. Norfolk: Monkey Press; 2007. p. 1–7.

68. Maciocia G. Aetiology. In: Obstetrics and gynecology in Chinese medicine. New York: Churchill Livingstone; 1998. p. 53–68 [chapter 4].

69. Lu HC. Diseases (questions 48–61). In: A complete translation of the Yellow Emperor's classics of internal medicine and the difficult classic (Nei-Jing and Nan-Jing). Vancouver: International College of Traditional Chinese Medicine; 2004. p. 611–7, Section four: Difficult classic [Nan Jing] [chapter 4].

70. Lu HC. Symptoms of disease of viscera and bowels by pathogens. In: A complete translation of the Yellow Emperor's classics of internal medicine and the difficult classic (Nei-Jing and Nan-Jing). Vancouver: International College of Traditional Chinese Medicine; 2004. p. 384–91, Section three: Spiritual pivot [Ling Shu] [chapter 4].

71. Sivin N. Causes of medical disorders. In: Traditional medicine in contemporary China, science, medicine and technology in East Asia, vol. 2. USA: Center for Chinese Studies, University of Michigan; 1987. p. 273–90, Contents of translation [chapter 5].

72. Lu HC. Five pathogenic disorders. In: A complete translation of the Yellow Emperor's classics of internal medicine and the difficult classic (Nei-Jing and Nan-Jing). Vancouver: International College of Traditional Chinese Medicine; 2004. p. 494–5, Section three: Spiritual pivot [Ling Shu] [chapter 34].

73. Lu HC. On nine needles. In: A complete translation of the Yellow Emperor's classics of internal medicine and the difficult classic (Nei-Jing and Nan-Jing). Vancouver: International College of Traditional Chinese Medicine; 2004. p. 577–83, Section three: Spiritual pivot [Ling Shu] [chapter 78].

74. Lu HC. From beginning to end. In: A complete translation of the Yellow Emperor's classics of internal medicine and the difficult classic (Nei-Jing and Nan-Jing). Vancouver: International College of Traditional Chinese Medicine; 2004. p. 405–10, Section three: Spiritual pivot [Ling Shu] [chapter 9].

75. Lu HC. Viscera and bowels (questions 30–47). In: A complete translation of the Yellow Emperor's classics of internal medicine and the difficult classic (Nei-Jing and Nan-Jing). Vancouver: International College of Traditional Chinese Medicine; 2004. p. 606–12, Section four: Difficult classic [Nan Jing] [chapter 3].

76. Lu HC. Five disorders. In: A complete translation of the Yellow Emperor's classics of internal medicine and the difficult classic (Nei-Jing and Nan-Jing). Vancouver: International College of Traditional Chinese Medicine; 2004. p. 511–3, Section three: Spiritual pivot [Ling Shu] [chapter 46].

77. Lu HC. A separate treatise on meridian pulses. In: A complete translation of the Yellow Emperor's classics of internal medicine and the difficult classic (Nei-Jing and Nan-Jing). Vancouver: International College of Traditional Chinese Medicine;

2004. p. 141–3, Section two: Essential questions [Su Wen] [chapter 21].

78. Unschuld PU, Tessenow H, Zheng J. Discourse on the division and unity of Yin and Yang. In: Huang Di Nei Jing Su Wen, vol. 1. Berkeley: University of California Press; 2011. p. 127–35 [chapter 6].

79. Lu HC. On the correspondence of life energy with energy of heaven. In: A complete translation of the Yellow Emperor's classics of internal medicine and the difficult classic (Nei-Jing and Nan-Jing). Vancouver: International College of Traditional Chinese Medicine; 2004. p. 77–82, Section two: Essential questions [Su Wen] [chapter 3].

80. Lu HC. Nine needles and twelve original points. In: A complete translation of the Yellow Emperor's classics of internal medicine and the difficult classic (Nei-Jing and Nan-Jing). Vancouver: International College of Traditional Chinese Medicine; 2004. p. 372–6, Section three: Spiritual pivot [Ling Shu] [chapter 1].

81. Liu G, Hyodo A. Etiology and pathology of TCM. In: Fundamentals of acupuncture and moxibustion. Beijing: Huaxia Publishing House; 2006. p. 126–72 [chapter 4].

82. Lu HC. Separate duties of various officials. In: A complete translation of the Yellow Emperor's classics of internal medicine and the difficult classic (Nei-Jing and Nan-Jing). Vancouver: International College of Traditional Chinese Medicine; 2004. p. 560–3, Section three: Spiritual pivot [Ling Shu] [chapter 73].

83. Unschuld PU, Tessenow H, Jinsheng Z. Discourse on the true [Qi endowed by] Heaven in high antiquity. In: Huang Di Nei Jing Su Wen, vol. 1. Berkeley: University of California Press; 2011. p. 29–44 [chapter 1].

84. Lu HC. Nutritive energy. In: A complete translation of the Yellow Emperor's classics of internal medicine and the difficult classic (Nei-Jing and Nan-Jing). Vancouver: International College of Traditional Chinese Medicine; 2004. p. 456–7, Section three: Spiritual pivot [Ling Shu] [chapter 16].

85. Lu HC. On the heavenly truth. In: A complete translation of the Yellow Emperor's classics of internal

medicine and the difficult classic (Nei-Jing and Nan-Jing). Vancouver: International College of Traditional Chinese Medicine; 2004. p. 65–72, Section two: Essential questions [Su Wen] [chapter 1].

86. Larre C, Rochat de la Vallee E. Xue Blood. In: Root C, editor. Essence Spirit Blood and Qi. Norfolk: Monkey Press; 1999. p. 68–75 [chapter 4].

87. Liu Z, Ma L. Common methods used in health preservation of TCM. In: Health preservation of Traditional Chinese Medicine. Beijing: People's Medical Publishing House; 2007. p. 294–442 [chapter 2].

88. Maciocia online: sexual life in Chinese medicine. Available from: http://maciociaonline.blogspot.co.uk/2011/07/sexual-life-in-chinese-medicine.html [accessed 26 September 2012].

89. Zhu Dan-Xi. Admonitions on sexual desire. In: Yang S and Duan W, editors. Extra treatises based on investigation and inquiry: a translation of Zhu Dan-Xi's Ge Zhi Yu Lun. Boulder, CO: Blue Poppy Press; 1994. p. 3–4.

90. Unschuld PU, Tessenow H, Jinsheng Z. Discourse on the hidden canons in the numinous orchid [chambers]. In: Huang Di Nei Jing Su Wen, vol. 1. Berkeley: University of California Press; 2011. p. 155–62 [chapter 8].

91. Wilkes S. Management of infertility in primary care. Br J Healthc Manag 2009;15:543–8.

92. Feinberg EC, Bromer JG, Catherino WH. The evolution of in vitro fertilization: integration of pharmacology, technology, and clinical care. J Pharmacol Exp Ther 2005;313:935–42.

93. Bavister BD. Early history of in vitro fertilization. Reproduction 2002;124:181.

94. Edwards RG. An astonishing journey into reproductive genetics since the 1950's. Reprod Nutr Dev 2005;45:299–306.

95. Wang J, Sauer MV. In vitro fertilization (IVF): a review of 3 decades of clinical innovation and technological advancement. Ther Clin Risk Manag 2006;2:355–64.

96. Ghobara T, Vandekerckhove P. Cycle regimens for frozen-thawed embryo transfer. Cochrane

Database Syst Rev 2008;23: CD003414.

97. Souza Setti A, Ferreira RC, Paes de Almeida Ferreira Braga D, et al. Intracytoplasmic sperm injection outcome versus intracytoplasmic morphologically selected sperm injection outcome: a meta-analysis. Reprod Biomed Online 2010;21:450–5.

98. Wang X. Cultural origin of TCM. In: A guide to Traditional Chinese Medicine culture, National planned university textbook for international Traditional Chinese Medicine education. Beijing: Gao Deng Jiao Yu Chu Ban She; 2007. p. 157–84 [chapter 1].

99. Furth C. The development of Fuke in the Song Dynasties. In: A Flourishing Yin: gender in China's medical history, 960–1665. California and Los Angeles: University of California Press; 1999. p. 59–93 [chapter 2].

100. Maciocia G. History of gynecology in Chinese medicine. In: Obstetrics and gynecology in Chinese medicine. New York: Churchill Livingstone; 1998. p. 3–6 [chapter 1].

101. Tan Y, Qi C, Zhang Q, et al. Introduction. In: Gynecology of Traditional Chinese Medicine. China: People's Medical Publishing House; 2007. p. 153–9 [chapter 1].

102. Shen nong ben cao Jing (Shennong's herbal), the earliest pharmacopoeia of China. Available from: http://en.tcm-china.info/ science/zt1/zq2/80934.shtml [accessed 23 January 2013].

103. Liao Y. Stories about famous doctors in history. In: Traditional Chinese Medicine. 3rd ed. Cambridge: Cambridge University Press; 2011. p. 93–110.

104. Earliest discovery of infectious diseases. Available from: http://en. tcm-china.info/science/zt1/zq4/ 80946.shtml [accessed 22 January 2013].

105. Discovery of *Ashi* points and catheterization. Available from: http://en.tcm-china.info/science/ zt1/zq4/Science4.15.1.html [accessed 22 January 2013].

106. Wang Z, Chen P, Xie P. The full development of Chinese medicine and pharmacology (from Jin, Northern and Southern Dynasties to Sui, Tang and Five Dynasties, 265A.D.–960A.D.). In: Chen P, editor. History and development in Traditional Chinese Medicine. Ohmsha, Beijing: Science Press, IOS Press; 1999. p. 94–155.

107. Wang Z, Chen P, Xie P. Medical systematization, improvement and learned debates (Song and Ming Dynasties, 960–1368 A.D.). In: Chen P, editor. History and development in Traditional Chinese Medicine. Ohmsha, Beijing: Science Press, IOS Press; 1999. p. 158–99.

108. Wang Z, Chen P, Xie P. New developments in medical theory and practice (covering the entire Ming Dynasty and Qing Dynasty before the opium war, 1368–1840 A.D.). In: Chen P, editor. History and development in Traditional Chinese Medicine. Ohmsha, Beijing: Science Press, IOS Press; 1999. p. 200–57.

109. Flaws B. Introduction. In: A handbook of TCM pediatrics: a practitioner's guide to the care and treatment of common childhood diseases. 2nd ed. Boulder, CO: Blue Poppy Press; 2006. p. 3–6.

110. West Z. Foreword to first edition. In: Acupuncture in pregnancy and childbirth. Edinburgh: Churchill Livingstone/Elsevier; 2001. p. viii.

Chapter | 2 |

Anatomy and physiology of the reproductive system: Prerequirements for conception

Many patients with fertility issues like to know precisely what is happening in their body and how this is related to their ability to conceive. In this chapter, we will explain the key elements of human reproductive anatomy and physiology, which are essential for fertility acupuncturists to understand. Orthodox medical and Traditional Chinese Medicine (TCM) concepts in relation to reproductive structure and function will be explained.

FUNCTIONAL ANATOMY OF THE REPRODUCTIVE SYSTEM FROM AN ORTHODOX MEDICAL PERSPECTIVE

Female reproductive anatomy

The main functions of the female reproductive system are:

- Production of eggs (oocytes)
- Fertilization of an egg by a spermatozoa
- Providing an environment for nourishment, growth, and development of an embryo and foetus
- Childbirth

The female reproductive system is split into genitalia and internal organs. The external genitalia are commonly referred to as the **vulva** and consist of:

- Labia majora
- Labia minora
- Clitoris
- Vestibule
- Hymen
- Greater vestibular glands

The internal organs consist of (Figure 2.1):

- Two Ovaries
- Two fallopian tubes (oviducts)
- Uterus (womb)
- Vagina

The ovaries and follicles

The **ovaries** are two glands. The male equivalent is the testicles. Each ovary lies on the lateral side of the pelvis. The ovaries were first described by Soranus, a gynaecologist living in the Roman Empire in the second century CE.[1] The ovaries are approximately 2.5–3.5 cm long, 2 cm wide, and 1 cm thick[2] or the size of an unshelled almond.[3] The ovaries are attached to the uterus by the ovarian ligaments and by the suspensory ligament to the pelvic wall. The uterus and the ovary are attached by the broad ligament.[3]

The main function of the ovaries is to develop and mature **eggs** (oocytes), which are then released, usually one egg at a time, during a process called *ovulation*. Each ovary contains two main types of tissue: the *medulla* and the *cortex*. The medulla is the central part of the ovary and contains fibrous tissue, blood vessels, and nerves. The cortex surrounds the medulla and contains **ovarian follicles** (*folliculus* = little bag),[3] all at various stages of development and maturation.[2] Each follicle contains an egg (oocyte), and the surrounding cells are called follicular cells. As the egg within these cells grows and matures, the follicular cells form more layers, called *granulosa cells*. As the follicle grows bigger, these cells secrete oestrogen.[3]

The fallopian tubes

The **fallopian tubes** (oviducts) are approximately 10 cm (4 in.) long and extend laterally from the uterus.[3] The tubes consist of two parts: the *isthmus* (short, narrow, thick-walled portion nearer the uterus) and *ampulla* (wider, longer portion of the tube, nearer the ovaries).[3] From the ampulla of

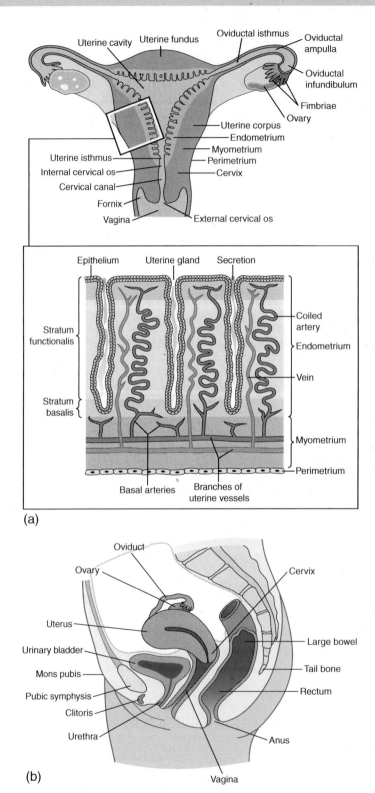

Figure 2.1 Female reproductive anatomy: (a) coronal plane; (b) sagital plane.

Reprinted from Jones R, Lopez K. The female reproductive system. In: Human Reproductive Biology, 3rd ed.; 2006. p. 31–72 [chapter 2]; with permission from Elsevier.

each ovary, there are finger-like projections called *fimbriae*, one of which (the biggest one) is attached to the ovary.

The main function of the fallopian tubes is to facilitate the transportation of the sperm to the egg and afterward to actively facilitate the passage of a fertilized egg into the uterus. The fallopian tube achieves this through a peristaltic and ciliary movement.[2] The fallopian tubes also secrete mucus, thereby aiding the transportation of both sperm and egg. The fertilization of the egg usually happens in the ampulla part of the fallopian tube.

Uterus

The **uterus** (womb) is a pear-shaped organ, which lies antero-posteriorly in the pelvis between the urinary bladder and the rectum. The existence of the uterus was acknowledged by the ancient Egyptians in the papyrus writings from 2500 BCE.[4]

The uterus is hollow and is approximately 7.5 cm (3 in.) long and 5 cm (2 in.) wide, with walls 2.5 cm thick. The uterus has three parts:[2]

- The *fundus*: the upper part above the opening to the fallopian tubes, with two *horns*, one on each side of fundus
- The *body*: the middle part
- The *cervix*: the lowest and narrowest point of the uterus, connecting the uterus and the vagina

The uterine walls have three layers: *perimetrium, myometrium*, and *endometrium*. The thickness of the endometrium depends on the stage of the menstrual cycle. It is at its thinnest just after the menstrual bleed (around 7 mm on day 4),[5] and it then gradually thickens to allow an embryo to implant (around 11 mm on ovulation day).[5]

After implantation, the main function of the uterus is to provide the environment that nourishes and protects the embryo.[2]

If an egg is fertilized, it travels through the fallopian tubes into the uterus, where it then attempts to implant into the uterine wall. If it succeeds, the foetus grows in the uterus until approximately 40 weeks' gestation, at which point the baby will be born and the placenta expelled.

During labour, the upper part of the uterus contracts intermittently, while the cervix relaxes and dilates. As labour progresses, the contractions become more frequent, and the cervix keeps gradually dilating. Once it is fully dilated (10 cm), the second stage of labour begins. This is when a woman helps to push her baby out.

The cervix also produces mucus, which can act as a barrier to ascending infections. During the fertile window (around 5–6 days before ovulation), rising oestrogen levels make the cervical mucus less viscous. A thinner, less tenacious mucus allows the sperm to enter the uterus more easily.

Vagina

The **vagina** is a tube that connects the vulva and the uterus. It runs obliquely upward and backward at a 45° angle, with the bladder in front and the anus behind the vagina. Its anterior wall is 7.5 cm (3 in.) long, and the posterior wall is 9 cm (3.5 in.) long. This is because the cervix (lower part of the uterus) protrudes onto the anterior side of the vagina.[2]

A main function of the vagina is to act as a barrier to stop microorganisms from entering the uterus. *Lactobacillus acidophilus* microbes are normally present in the vagina of women of reproductive age. These microbes secrete lactic acid, which helps to maintain an acidic environment in the vagina (pH 4.9–3.5). This acidic environment reduces the chance of microorganisms surviving and entering the uterus.[2]

Abnormalities of the female reproductive anatomy

Ovarian factors

The ovarian follicles may fail to grow and release an egg. This may be either temporary (for example, in women with certain conditions such as Polycystic Ovary Syndrome or thyroid disease) or permanent (for example, in women with Premature Ovarian Failure). Sometimes when an egg is released, it may be of poor quality. The collapsed follicle (known as the *corpus luteum*) that released the egg may not function properly and may fail to produce adequate amounts of progesterone. The number of ovarian follicles still available for ovulation (ovarian reserve) may be affected by previous ovarian surgery, for example, where healthy ovarian tissue is removed along with diseased tissue.

Tubal factors

The fallopian tubal factor is another common cause of subfertility.[6] The fallopian tubes may be partially or completely blocked and unable to allow the passage of sperm and egg. This is usually caused by a previous history of Pelvic Inflammatory Disease, infections, or endometriosis. Some women with a history of ectopic pregnancy may have had their tube(s) removed. For women with both tubes missing or blocked, Assisted Reproduction Technology (ART) treatment is the only way for them to conceive.

Sometimes the fallopian tubes may be filled with fluid. This is called *hydrosalpinx*. Fluid is believed to leak into the uterus and be toxic to an embryo.[6] In some women, hydrosalpinx necessitates the complete removal of the affected tubes.[7]

Uterine factors

Congenital uterine abnormalities are found in 5.5% of the female population, increasing to 8% of infertile women, 13.3% of women with a history of miscarriages, and 24.5% of women with a combined history of infertility and miscarriages (Figure 2.2).[8]

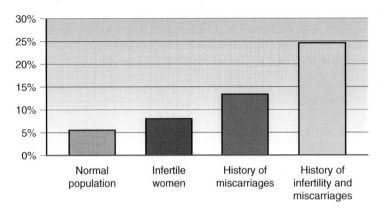

Figure 2.2 Incidence of uterine factors in different female population groups.[8]

Several categories of congenital uterine anomalies have been classified by the American Fertility Society (Figure 2.3).[9]

The most common congenital uterine abnormalities that may affect reproduction are:[8]

- *Arcuate* uterus (a uterus with concave fundus protruding into the uterine cavity, possibly more common in patients with a history of miscarriages but not significantly so)
- Canalization defect: *septate* and *subseptate* uterus (a wedge-like septum partially or completely partitions the uterus longitudinally; compared to the normal population, this is significantly more common in patients with miscarriages and a combined history of infertility and miscarriages, 2.3% versus 5.3% versus 15.4%, respectively).

- Unification defects:
  - *Bicornuate* uterus (a 'heart-shaped' uterus, compared to the normal population, has a significant association with infertility, miscarriages, and combined infertility and miscarriages, with a frequency of 0.4% versus 1.1% versus 2.1% versus 4.7% in the respective patient groups)
  - *Unicornuate* uterus (where only one uterine horn is present; compared to the normal population, this is significantly associated with infertility, miscarriages, and combined infertility and miscarriages, 0.1% versus 0.5% versus 0.5% versus 3.1% respective frequency)
  - *Uterus didelphys* (duplication of corpus and cervix, significantly more common in women with mixed

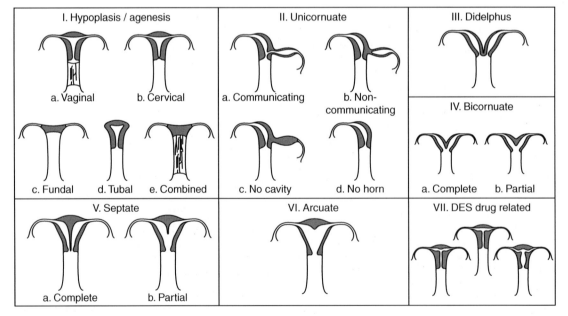

Figure 2.3 American Fertility Society classification of congenital uterine anomalies.
Reprinted from Taylor E, Gomel V. The uterus and fertility. Fertil Steril 2008; 89(1): 1–16; with permission from American Society for Reproductive Medicine; published by Elsevier Inc.

infertility/miscarriage history when compared to normal population: 2.1% versus 0.3%, respectively).

Other uterine abnormalities include problems with the endometrial lining not developing properly or certain other uterine abnormalities that may impede implantation (for example, scarring from previous surgeries, fibroids, polyps, or endometritis).

Cervical problems include issues with the quality and quantity of cervical mucus production. However, it is a rare cause of subfertility.[6]

Male reproductive anatomy

The main functions of the male reproductive system are production and transportation of sperm. The male reproductive system consists of (Figure 2.4):

- Two testes
- Two epididymides
- Two vas deferens (deferent or sperm ducts)
- Two seminal vesicles
- Two ejaculatory ducts
- A prostate gland
- A urethra
- A penis

Testes

The **testes** (testicles) are two oval glands measuring 5 cm (2 in.) in length and 2.5 cm (1 in.) in diameter.[2] They

are contained inside the *scrotum* and suspended outside the body in front of the upper thighs and behind the penis. This ensures that the temperature inside the testes is 2–3°C lower than the normal body temperature of 37°C. This lower temperature is necessary for optimal sperm production (spermatogenesis). Curiously, the left testis is often suspended lower than the right one. If the temperature gets too cold, the muscles in the testes can contract, and the testes will ascend inside the body as very cold temperature is also not ideal for spermatogenesis.[10]

The main function of the testicles is the production of sperm and testosterone. Spermatozoa and nutrient fluid are produced by *germ cells*, which line the *seminiferous tubules* inside the testicles, and testosterone is produced by the *Leydig cells*, which are located between the seminiferous tubules. There are hundreds of seminiferous tubules inside each testis, each measuring 80 cm (31 in.) long.[10]

Epididymides

The seminiferous tubules merge into the **epididymides**, where spermatozoa mature and are stored. This maturation process takes 6 weeks. In the head of the epididymis, there are 5–10 separate tubules, which merge into one tubule. This tubule is twisted and condensed, 5 cm (2 in.) in its compressed form, and approximately 6 m (19 ft) long if extended.[10]

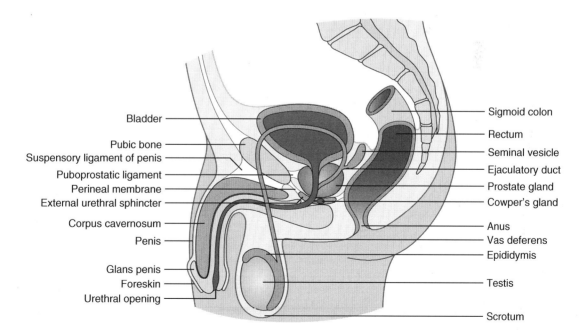

Bladder
Pubic bone
Suspensory ligament of penis
Puboprostatic ligament
Perineal membrane
External urethral sphincter
Corpus cavernosum
Penis
Glans penis
Foreskin
Urethral opening

Sigmoid colon
Rectum
Seminal vesicle
Ejaculatory duct
Prostate gland
Cowper's gland
Anus
Vas deferens
Epididymis
Testis
Scrotum

Figure 2.4 Male reproductive anatomy.
Reproduced with permission from © Elf Sternberg elf@halcyon.com.

Vas deferens

The epididymis continues into the **vas deferens** (also called the sperm duct). There are two vas deferens, one on each side, each measuring 45 cm (17 in.) long. They ascend into the abdomen next to the bladder.[10] When a man is sterilized, the vas deferens are severed and each end is then sealed. This stops sperm from being ejaculated. Although this procedure can be reversed, the reversal is not always successful. In such cases, if a man wants to have a baby, he and his partner would almost certainly need to undergo ART treatment in order to conceive.

Seminal vesicles

Each vas deferens transitions into *ejaculatory ducts*. Where the transition happens, there are two **seminal vesicles**, one on each side. Seminal vesicles are sac-like structures that produce 50% of semen plasma. Seminal fluid contains fructose, which provides energy to sperm. It is also highly viscous and chemically basic (pH 7.2).[11] The vagina has high acidity (pH 4.9–3.5),[2] which is harmful to sperm. The low acidity in semen helps to neutralize the high acidity of the vagina.[10]

Ejaculatory ducts, prostate gland, and prostatic urethra

The **ejaculatory ducts** each measure 2 cm in length.[2] They pass through the **prostate gland** and join the **prostatic urethra**. The prostate gland surrounds the ejaculatory ducts at the base of the urethra. It produces lubricating fluid, which forms part of semen.[10]

Urethra

The **Urethra** is approximately 19–20 cm (8 in.) long, and it extends from the bladder to the tip of the penis.[2] Its main function is transportation of urine and semen.

Penis

The **Penis** contains the urethra and erectile tissue. When it is sexually stimulated, it fills with a large volume of blood, and the penis becomes erect.

During ejaculation, the sperm is propelled by the peristaltic action of the vas deferens, seminal vesicles, ejaculatory ducts, and prostate gland into the urethra and then out of the penis. Sometimes a small amount of semen comes out before an ejaculation, and sometimes men have nocturnal ejaculation when asleep.[3] If they are not ejaculated, spermatozoa can survive for several months and eventually get reabsorbed by the seminiferous tubules.[2]

Abnormalities of the male reproductive anatomy

Many things can go wrong with the male reproductive system. The testicles may fail to produce sperm or may produce only a limited amount or abnormal sperm. In some men, the testicles fail to descend (known as *cryptorchidism*), only one testicle may be present, or the testicles may be too small or undeveloped. The vas deferens may be missing on one or both sides (for example, in men with cystic fibrosis). There may be partial or full obstruction of the ejaculatory ducts. There may be congestion of the veins in the scrotum (known as *varicocele*). A varicocele may lead to inflammation and affect sperm production. Erectile dysfunction of the penis can result from physical and psychological reasons.

SPERM AND EGG PRODUCTION

Spermatogenesis and spermiogenesis

Spermatogenesis is the process of spermatozoa (sperm) formation.[12] Spermatogenesis starts at puberty, when the Leydig cells in the testes start to produce androgens under the influence of the Follicle-Stimulating Hormone (FSH) and the Luteinizing Hormone (LH), which are in turn controlled by the Gonadotrophin-Releasing Hormone (GnRH) produced by the hypothalamus.[3] In the absence of LH and FSH, androgen levels drop, and spermatogenesis stops.[12]

Spermatogenesis begins with *spermatogonia* (the diploid (*2n*) immature sperm cells derived from embryonic germ cells) dividing by *mitosis*.[3] During their prolonged meiotic phase, the spermatocytes are sensitive to damage.[13] Some of the spermatogonia develop into *primary spermatocytes*.

At puberty, there is an increase in testosterone levels; this initiates *meiosis I*. During this stage, a primary spermatocyte generates two *secondary spermatocytes*, which then undergo *meiosis II*. Two haploid *spermatids* (haploid cells) are generated by each secondary spermatocyte, resulting in a total of four spermatids. **Spermiogenesis** is the final stage of spermatogenesis, and, during this phase, spermatids mature into spermatozoa (sperm cells) (Figure 2.5).[3]

The spermiogenesis phase is completed with maturation of a spermatozoon.[12] Spermatogenesis takes 65–75 days[3] and takes place simultaneously at different times in different regions of the testis for an even production and availability of mature sperm.

Structure of sperm

Spermatids change their round shape to become elongated spermatids. A *tail* develops to help with forward movement, a *midpiece* forms that contains the mitochondria, and *centrioles* link the midpiece to the *head* of the spermatozoon.

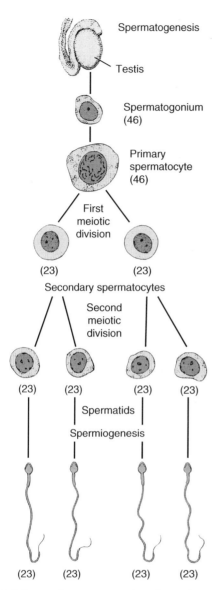

Spermatogenesis

Testis

Spermatogonium
(46)

Primary
spermatocyte
(46)

First
meiotic
division

(23)   (23)
Secondary spermatocytes

Second
meiotic
division

(23)   (23)   (23)   (23)

Spermatids

Spermiogenesis

(23)   (23)   (23)   (23)

Figure 2.5 Stages of spermatogenesis and spermiogenesis.
Reprinted from Jones R, Lopez K. The male reproductive system. In: Human Reproductive Biology, 3rd ed.; 2006. p. 97–124 [chapter 4]; with permission from Elsevier.

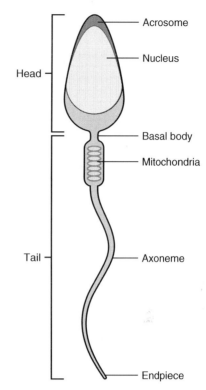

Head

Acrosome

Nucleus

Basal body

Mitochondria

Tail

Axoneme

Endpiece

Figure 2.6 Structure of a spermatozoon.
Reprinted from Jones R, Lopez K. Gamete transport and fertilization. In: Human Reproductive Biology, 3rd ed.; 2006. p. 231–52 [chapter 9]; with permission from Elsevier.

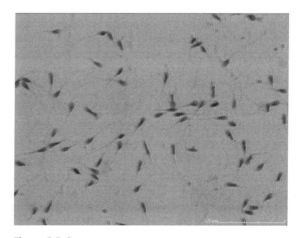

Figure 2.7 Sperm.
Courtesy of Care Fertility, Nottingham, UK.

Aspects that are important for sperm–oocyte fertilization start developing. For example, the *acrosome* becomes able to penetrate an oocyte (this is discussed in more detail in Chapter 3). The nucleus in the head of the sperm contains the chromosomes (DNA).[12] Figure 2.6 shows the structure of a mature spermatozoon, and Figure 2.7 is a photograph of mature sperm.

Oogenesis

Oogenesis is the creation of an egg (also known as an ovum or oocyte) in the female foetus. Oogenesis starts in the foetus at around 7 weeks' gestation, when *primordial germ cells* colonize the newly formed ovary. They are now referred to as *oogonia*.[16]

Oogonia undergo *mitosis* or rapid proliferation (multiplication). The number of oogonia is estimated to increase rapidly from 43,740 at 7 weeks' gestation to 148,785 at 9 weeks' gestation to 5.5 million at 14–15 weeks' gestation (Figure 2.8).[17]

At around 20 weeks' gestation, oogonia become *primary oocytes*, and their development is arrested in *prophase I* of *meiosis*.[19]

The oocytes' development remains in this arrested state until the onset of ovulatory cycles at puberty.[2] At around 28 weeks' gestation, mitosis ends, and a rapid rate of follicular atresia (degeneration) begins although reasons for this are not known.[16] Only about 1 million oocytes survive to the birth of the baby girl.[18]

Oocyte atresia continues throughout the adult reproductive lifespan. By puberty, only 300,000–400,000 oocytes remain,[18] and they are reduced to 158,900 at 18–24 years of age and 62,100 at 25–31 years of age. The number of oocytes remains relatively stable at about 63,000 at 32–38 years of age, dropping noticeably to 9600 at 40–44 years of age and 6100 at 46–50 years of age (Figure 2.9).[20] Over a woman's reproductive lifespan, only around 300–400 oocytes will reach the ovulatory state; the rest undergo atresia.[16]

The eggs remain dormant until nearer ovulation time when the rise in the levels of LH triggers continuation of the *first meiotic division* of the egg (oocyte).[21] When *meiosis I* is completed, the oocyte will have two cells: a bigger one (the secondary oocyte), which has most of the cytoplasm, and a smaller one (the polar body), consisting of a nucleus. *Meiosis II* of the secondary oocyte follows immediately after meiosis I is completed but arrests in the *metaphase* and will remain in this phase until fertilization.[21] The follicle ruptures, and the egg is released. If and when the egg is penetrated by a spermatozoon, this activates the egg, and meiosis II is completed (approximately 3 h later).[14]

Structure of the egg

A mature egg (ovum, oocyte) is the biggest cell in the body at 0.1 mm.[21] It contains a large *nucleus* and within it the DNA material of the egg. The egg is surrounded by the *corona radiata* and the *zona pellucida*. They are protective layers of the egg, which a spermatozoon needs to penetrate during fertilization. The *cytoplasm* contains yolk granules that nourish the embryo early in development until it is nourished by its mother (Figure 2.10).[3]

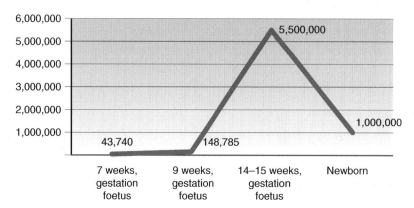

Figure 2.8 Estimated number of egg cells in the ovaries of a female foetus and newborn.[17,18]

Figure 2.9 Estimated mean number of egg cells in adult human ovaries.[20]

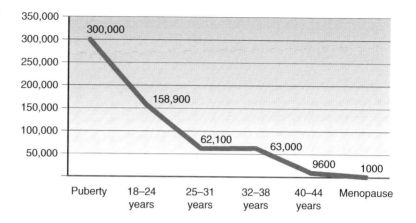

Figure 2.10 Human egg: (a) a photograph; (b) human egg structure.
(a) Courtesy of Care Fertility, Nottingham, UK.

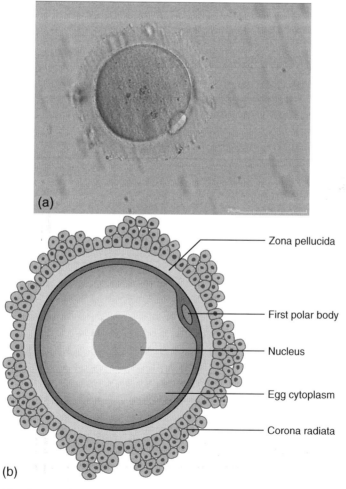

Folliculogenesis

The eggs (oocytes) develop within ovarian follicles (*folliculus* = little bag).[3] The development of *primordial* (resting) follicles into *preovulatory* follicles is known as *folliculogenesis*.

As follicles grow and develop within the foetus, they acquire certain characteristics and are classified according to these characteristics (Figure 2.11):[24]

- Primordial
- Primary
- Secondary
- Preantral (class 1)
- Early antral (class 2, 3, and 4)
- Antral (class 5 and 6)
- Early ovulatory (class 7)
- Preovulatory or Graafian (class 8)

Primordial follicles are seen on the foetal ovaries as early as 15 weeks' gestation.[16] They surround the oocytes, which have completed the first stage of meiosis.[1] The development of primordial follicles continues until all oocytes are surrounded; this takes place between 6 and 9 months' gestation.[27]

Initial recruitment and development of primordial follicles up to class 5 antral follicles

The folliculogenesis process begins when primordial follicles are recruited to resume their development.[1,27] The number of recruited follicles depends on factors such as the woman's age and ovarian reserve. Until this point, the primordial follicles remain dormant.[16] What initiates the resumption of primordial follicular development is largely unknown.[28–30]

It is not known precisely how long it takes for a follicle to develop from the primordial to the preovulatory stage. It has been suggested it takes about a year.[24] The development of primordial follicles into small class 2 follicles is estimated to take around 300 days, and this stage of development is largely independent of gonadotrophic hormone influence.[26] When secondary follicles reach 0.08 mm in diameter, they acquire one or two arterioles, suggestive of hormonal and nutritional environmental influences affecting follicular development.[25] Class 2–5 follicles depend on gonadotrophins (in particular, FSH)[26] for their further development; this stage takes 55 days.[24]

Cyclical recruitment (selection) and development of antral into preovulatory follicles

At any point in a woman's reproductive lifespan, the ovaries contain a number of follicles, all at different stages of development.[27] Beginning in puberty, when the hypothalamus starts to secrete large amounts of gonadotrophins, important

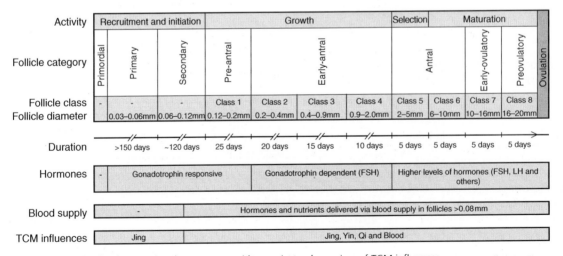

Figure 2.11 Follicular development in a human ovary with a conjectural overview of TCM influences. *Data from Gougeon 1986,[24] Gougeon 1996,[25] and Zeleznik 2004.[26]*

changes occur in the ovaries. At the end of the luteal phase of every menstrual cycle (days 23–28), several antral follicles are selected to continue developing. This is known as *selection* or *recruitment* of antral follicles (not to be confused with recruitment of primordial follicles). Class 5 antral follicles take around 20 days to develop to preovulatory class 8 follicles,[24] and this phase is dependent on high levels of gonadotrophins, in particular, FSH and LH.[26]

Early in the follicular phase, one follicle is selected from a pool of class 5 follicles (2–5 mm in diameter) to become a dominant follicle.[25] The dominant follicle grows very rapidly, reaching 6.9 mm on day 2, 13.3 mm on day 7, and 18.8 mm on day 12.[31]

The rest of the follicles undergo atresia during both preantral and antral phases, although follicles that are bigger than 2 mm in diameter are more commonly destined for atresia and do not normally develop beyond medium stage class 6 follicles (maximum 10 mm in diameter).[27] The development of follicles beginning during the early antral phase depends on FSH secretions. If FSH is absent, the follicles will stop developing.[27]

During the downregulation phase of IVF, the levels of FSH are pharmacologically depleted, which temporarily stops the development of antral follicles, allowing a more homogeneous group of follicles to be available during the ovarian stimulation phase. During this phase, a woman injects a large dose of FSH (usually into the abdomen), which helps to rescue some of the class 5–6 antral follicles that otherwise would be destined for atresia.

Figure 2.11 summarizes all stages of follicular development and suggests where TCM concepts and influences may be most usefully applied.

TCM integrated perspective on follicular and egg development

Understanding Orthodox medical physiology of follicular and egg development aids in understanding TCM influences.

Influence of acupuncture on primordial, primary, and early secondary follicles (approximately 360 and 190 days before ovulation)

The transition of primordial follicles to early secondary follicles (around 360 to 190 days before ovulation) is independent from gonadotrophin and blood supply. The follicles largely control their own growth and development during this period. Therefore, it is likely that primarily Pre-Natal Jing (Essence) influences this phase because a woman is born with her complete ovarian reserve. It might be possible to influence this phase with acupuncture by nourishing Pre-Natal Jing (Essence). Acupuncture points REN4,[32] KID3,[33] BL23,[34] BL52,[34] GB39,[35] and DU4[36] tonify Jing (Essence).

Influence of acupuncture on late secondary to preovulatory follicles (approximately 190–0 days before ovulation)

Follicles bigger than 0.08 mm in diameter (secondary follicles, around 190 days before ovulation) begin to respond to their environment by acquiring arterioles. This allows the delivery of reproductive hormones and nutrition to the follicles via these arterioles. Therefore, in addition to Jing [Essence] and Yin, Blood and Qi influence the development of follicles from this point on.

It is hypothesized that acupuncture may improve the quality of the follicles and the eggs within them by improving the blood flow to the ovary.[37] But the outcome depends on the duration of acupuncture treatment[38] because it takes about 1 year for the follicles to develop.[24] The last 190 days are particularly important because that is when the follicles begin to respond to their environment[25] and therefore become even more likely to be influenced by acupuncture. During this phase of follicular development, acupuncture treatment should be aimed at tonifying Pre- and Post-Natal Jing (Essence), Yin, Blood, and Qi. In addition to the Jing (Essence) points listed above, use acupuncture points such as BL17,[34] ST36,[39] SP6,[40] KID6,[33] LIV3,[41] LIV8,[41] and REN6.[32]

INTERESTING FACTS

FOLLICLES AND FOLLICULOGENESIS

- The process of primordial follicle recruitment is continuous. It starts in the foetus, continues after birth, and runs until the ovarian reserve is depleted.[16]
- Follicles up to 5 mm in size (class 5) are always present in ovaries, from infancy to menopause. This is because these follicles require only small amounts of gonadotrophins. However, class 5 or bigger follicles are dependent on larger quantities of hormones during the 20 days preceding ovulation.[25]
- In a small number of cycles, two follicles become dominant, which may result in dizygotic (nonidentical) twins.

REPRODUCTIVE PHYSIOLOGY FROM AN ORTHODOX MEDICAL PERSPECTIVE

The Hypothalamic–Pituitary–Gonadal Axis

The activity of the *gonads* (ovaries and testes) is controlled by the *hypothalamus* and the *pituitary glands*.[42] This is referred to as the *Hypothalamic–Pituitary–Gonadal Axis* (*HPGA*), also known as the *Hypothalamic–Pituitary–Ovarian Axis* in women and the *Hypothalamic–Pituitary–*

Testicular Axis in men. The HPGA is where reproductive hormones from the ovaries or testes, hypothalamus, and anterior pituitary gland exert control over circulating levels of one another (Figure 2.12). The HPGA matures at puberty, activating the cyclical development of antral follicles and eggs, as well as the onset of ovulation and the menstrual cycle.[30] In men, HPGA maturation starts the onset of sperm production.

The hypothalamus is situated between the midbrain and the forebrain.[43] It connects to the pituitary gland through the neural and vascular links by receiving neurohumoral signals from other parts of the brain and the central nervous system and hormonally derived messages from the ovaries and the testes.[43] The hypothalamus has many roles in controlling reproductive functions, such as the onset of puberty, reproduction, pregnancy, and lactation.[42,43]

The hypothalamus releases GnRH in a pulsatile manner (at about 90–120 min intervals).[43] GnRH is transmitted through the portal vessels to the anterior pituitary.[43] Here GnRH binds to receptors of gonadotrophic cells in the pituitary to affect the rate of the production and release of gonadotrophin hormones (FSH and LH)[43] and prolactin.[42] The anterior pituitary also secretes Growth Hormone (GH) and Thyroid-Stimulating Hormone.[42,43]

In women, FSH and LH stimulate the ovaries to grow and mature follicles and eggs. The largest dominant follicle starts to produce oestrogens and inhibins during the mid-follicular phase.[44] Oestrogens and inhibins suppress FSH production by the pituitary, which stops the development of nondominant antral follicles, which then undergo atresia.[44] In men, FSH and LH stimulate the testes to produce sperm, testosterone, and inhibin.

Oestrogens, testosterone, and inhibins suppress the production of FSH, LH, and GnRH by the pituitary and the hypothalamus.

INTERESTING FACTS

HYPOTHALAMUS IN REPRODUCTION

The emotional environment has a profound effect on the reproductive process.[42] The hypothalamus' function is influenced by signals it receives from other parts of the brain, for example, the amygdala and hippocampus.[43]

Key reproductive hormones

Gonadotrophin-Releasing Hormone

GnRH is released by the hypothalamus.[3] It controls the secretion of FSH and LH both in the male and the female.[3,42]

Follicle-Stimulating Hormone

In females, FSH stimulates the growth and maturation of ovarian follicles.[3]

In males, FSH stimulates sperm production.[3]

Luteinizing Hormone

In females, rising oestrogen levels cause LH to rise exponentially (peaking approximately 36 h before ovulation). This surge of LH triggers final maturation and the release of the egg (ovulation). After the egg is released, the remainder of the follicle becomes luteinized under the influence of LH,

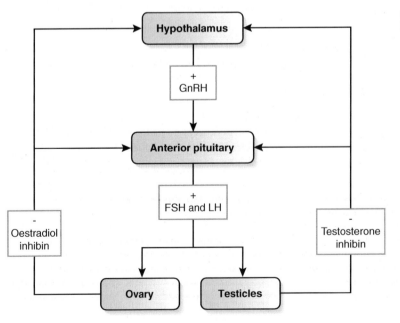

Figure 2.12 The Hypothalamic–Pituitary–Gonadal Axis.

which stimulates the formation of progesterone in the follicular granulosa and theca cells.[43] LH also stimulates ovarian androgen production by the ovarian theca cells.[45]

In males, LH stimulates testes to produce testosterone and inhibin.[43]

Oestrogens

In women, increasingly higher levels of oestrogens are secreted by the dominant follicle, resulting in increased GnRH secretions by the hypothalamus. This causes the anterior pituitary gland to secrete higher levels of FSH and LH.[3] This leads to the preovulatory LH surge, which triggers the dominant follicle to release its egg during ovulation[45]; this occurs approximately 36 h later. In the beginning of the menstrual cycle, oestrogen levels are low, thereby keeping the GnRH, FSH, and LH levels relatively low.[45]

In men, oestrogens are also secreted but in smaller quantities.[46] Oestrogen has an inhibitory effect on GnRH release.[47]

Progesterone

In women, after ovulation, the corpus luteum (collapsed follicle) begins to secrete high levels of progesterone.[45] The levels of progesterone peak midway through the luteal phase of the menstrual cycle. Progesterone, synergistically with oestrogens, helps to prepare the endometrium for implantation. High levels of progesterone also inhibit production of GnRH and LH.[3] Progesterone supports embryonic development until the placenta takes over at approximately 10–12 weeks' gestation.

In men, progesterone regulates sperm capacitation and motility and affects the receptors on the sperm's acrosomal membrane.[48]

Human Chorionic Gonadotrophin

In women, if implantation occurs and pregnancy follows, the trophoblast (implanting embryo) produces the Human Chorionic Gonadotrophin (hCG) hormone, which keeps the corpus luteum producing progesterone and oestrogen until 10–12 weeks' gestation, by which stage the placenta makes enough oestrogen and progesterone to support itself.[45]

In men, hCG stimulates testosterone production in the testes.[49]

Testosterone

In men, the Leydig cells in the testes produce testosterone. Testosterone controls spermatogenesis,[43] whereby high testosterone levels inhibit GnRH secretion by the hypothalamus. This causes the anterior pituitary gland to release less LH. Lower levels of LH lead to lower testosterone levels produced by the Leydig cells in the testes. During puberty, testosterone controls male sexual development.[3]

Women also produce testosterone, but its reproductive role is not well understood although it is accepted that testosterone plays a role in sexual arousal.[50] Low testosterone levels are associated with low ovarian reserve.[51]

Inhibin

In the male, inhibin is secreted by Sertoli cells in the testes. It inhibits spermatogenesis by inhibiting FSH secretions by the anterior pituitary gland.[3]

In the female, inhibin is secreted by granulosa cells in a growing follicle and by the corpus luteum.[3] It controls FSH secretions[43] and, to a lesser degree, LH secretions.[3]

Relaxin

In women, a small amount of relaxin is secreted by the corpus luteum to help with implantation by relaxing the uterus.[3] During pregnancy, more relaxin is produced by the placenta.[3]

The role of relaxin in men is less clear. It is secreted by prostate and is found in semen. It increases sperm motility and sperm fertilizing capacity.[52]

Other hormones

There are other hormones that are involved in reproduction. These will be referred to and explained in this book where relevant.

Menstrual cycle

The cycles of physiological changes that occur in women of reproductive age are known as the *menstrual cycles*. Menstrual cycles are regulated through feedback of ovarian hormones, GnRH, LH, and FSH.[28]

Typically the menstrual cycle length averages 28[53–55] or 29 days.[56] It can range from 22[56] or 23 days[55] up to 35[55] or 36[56] days in women from their early 20s to mid-30s.

Cycle lengths change with age. A large study involving the measurement of thousands of cycles reported mean cycle lengths to be 29 days in 18- to 20-year-old women, gradually reduced to 27 days by the age of 44, and then increased to 28 days in 45- to 47-year-olds, 32 days in 48- to 50-year-olds, and 39 days in 51- to 53-year-olds. There was very little cycle variability in the younger women, but in women 45 years or older cycle lengths varied considerably.[57]

Factors such as weight,[58] physical activity,[59] smoking,[60] and psychosocial stress[60] can affect cycle length.

Long, irregular cycles with intermenstrual bleeding are associated with infertility.[58] Long cycles double the risk of foetal loss.[58]

Menstrual cycles are split into two main phases: the follicular phase and the luteal phase. The follicular phase varies in length (for example, 14 days in a 28-day cycle, 7 days in 21-day cycle, and 19 days in a 33-day cycle), and the luteal phase is usually fixed at around 14 days (Figure 2.13). Ovulation marks the end of the follicular phase and the beginning of the luteal phase.

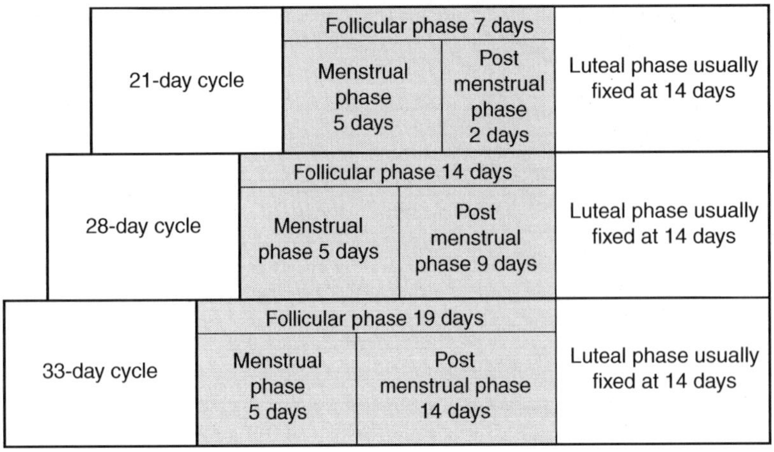

21-day cycle	Follicular phase 7 days		Luteal phase usually fixed at 14 days
	Menstrual phase 5 days	Post menstrual phase 2 days	

28-day cycle	Follicular phase 14 days		Luteal phase usually fixed at 14 days
	Menstrual phase 5 days	Post menstrual phase 9 days	

33-day cycle	Follicular phase 19 days		Luteal phase usually fixed at 14 days
	Menstrual phase 5 days	Post menstrual phase 14 days	

Figure 2.13 Variations in length of menstrual cycles: The luteal phase is usually fixed at 14 days, whereas the follicular phase is variable.

Follicular phase

Events in the uterus

The declining levels of progesterone in the last few days of the previous menstrual cycle trigger the release of prostaglandins. These prostaglandins cause the uterine spiral arterioles to constrict and the endometrial cells to become starved of oxygen and die. The dead endometrial tissue is then shed through the vagina during menstruation. Around 50–150 mL of blood is lost during menstruation.[3]

The first day of menstruation is day 1 of the menstrual cycle and is also day 1 of the follicular phase (also known as the proliferation phase).

Following menstruation, the endometrium is at its thinnest, approximately 4 mm[3] to 7 mm[5]. The rising oestrogen levels secreted by a growing follicle initiate uterine endometrial proliferation (thickening). Just before ovulation the endometrium thickens to about 10 mm[3] to 11 mm[5].

Events in the ovaries

At the end of the previous menstrual cycle, a cohort of antral follicles is selected (recruited) to continue developing under the influence of FSH. The exact number of selected follicles depends on a woman's age, ranging from around 20[3] in younger women to only 1 or 2 in older women. By about day 6,[3] one follicle dominates. The dominant follicle is more advanced and larger than the rest of the follicles. It undergoes rapid growth, and the egg within it matures. As it grows, it secretes oestrogens and inhibin, which suppress the growth of other follicles, causing them to undergo atresia. When the dominant follicle is 18 mm[61] to 25 mm[28] in diameter, it is ready for ovulation.

Ovulation

Ovulation is when the mature egg is released. This happens at the end of follicular phase. Increasing levels of oestrogen secreted by the dominant follicle trigger the hypothalamus to release more GnRH. This, in turn, triggers the anterior pituitary gland to release even more FSH and LH.[3] The LH levels peak at around 36 h before ovulation, which causes the dominant follicle to grow further and the egg within it to mature.

A protuberance appears from the ovarian surface because of the enlargement of the follicle. With the final increase in follicular size, the enlarged protuberance ruptures and the egg is released through the ruptured follicle.[28] Follicular fluid flows out onto the surface of the ovary, transporting with it the egg and a mass of surrounding cumulus cells.[28] Cumulus cells help to protect and nourish the egg and help with egg and sperm interactions. Chapter 3 describes the sequence of what happens to the egg after ovulation.

Unique images of spontaneous ovulation have been recently captured by Jacques Donnez while performing laparoscopic observation. These images are shown in Figure 2.14.[62]

Luteal phase

The luteal phase (also known as the secretory phase) begins just after ovulation, when the empty follicle collapses and becomes fully vascularized in a process called luteinization. The collapsed empty follicle is subsequently referred to as a *corpus luteum*.[28] The corpus luteum produces up to 40 mg of progestogens a day.[63] It also produces some oestrogens,[3] inhibin, and oxytocin.[28]

Events in the ovary

If no pregnancy occurs, the corpus luteum remains functional for about 14 days.[3] It then regresses in size and function, resulting in a reduction of progesterone, oestrogen, and inhibin levels.[3] This initiates increased GnRH, FSH, and LH secretion,[3] a new cohort of follicles is selected, and the cycle is repeated.

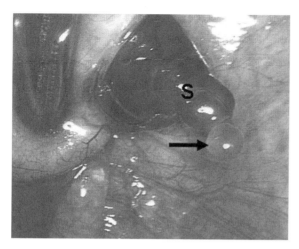

Figure 2.14 Images of ovulation (arrow points to the egg and S points to the follicle).
From Lousse J-C, Donnez J. Laparoscopic observation of spontaneous human ovulation. Fertil Steril September 2008; 90(3): 833–34. Reproduced with kind permission of Jacques Donnez and Elsevier Ltd.

If implantation occurs, the trophoblastic cells of the implanting embryo start to secrete hCG, which 'rescues' the corpus luteum. The corpus luteum then continues producing progesterone beyond the usual 2-week time frame. In doing so, it supports early pregnancy.[63]

Events in the uterus

Progesterone and oestrogens secreted by the corpus luteum stimulate endometrial gland secretions.[3] Stromal proliferation increases, the endometrial cells become 'larger' and 'plumper', and spiral arteries fully develop[64] to support implantation. The endometrium thickens to 12–18 mm.[3]

If no implantation occurs, the levels of progesterone decline. The epithelium of the uterus breaks down and is shed as menstruation.[28]

REPRODUCTIVE PHYSIOLOGY FROM A TCM PERSPECTIVE

TCM and Orthodox medical paradigms

It would be easy to assume that ART can solve all fertility problems. However, the reality is that overall ART success rates are low. ART can successfully bypass certain fertility issues by extracting eggs, fertilizing them in the laboratory, and then replacing the embryos inside the uterus. But Orthodox medical procedures have limited control over factors such as egg and sperm quality, the environment inside the uterus, and a woman's ability to carry the pregnancy successfully to full term.

TCM thinking and concepts in reproductive physiology are very different from the Orthodox medical model. TCM may offer an additional approach to achieving conception, especially in those cases where, despite the very best efforts on the part of fertility clinics, patients still fail to conceive.

TCM view of the human body

TCM originated several thousand years ago. Subsequently, over time it has evolved a rich repertoire of concepts, resulting in different perspectives of health and illness compared to Orthodox medical thought.[65] TCM's understanding of human anatomy and physiology is based on historical record or anecdotally based detailed observations of the functions of the human body and much less on the detailed anatomical structures and locations used in Orthodox medicine. Instead of blood vessels and nerve pathways, TCM recognizes energy meridians, which carry Qi and Blood. Instead of hormonal balance, TCM has the concept of Yin and Yang balance.

However, anatomy is also relevant in classical Chinese medical literature. The anatomy of Zangfu organs was mentioned in the Nan Jing and Ling Shu.[66,67] In the seventh century, the anatomical shape of the Uterus was used as a diagnostic method in treating subfertility,[68] presumably via some form of internal examination.

In classical Chinese medicine, there are three unified concepts: Heaven, the Body, and Earth.

The Body is influenced by Heaven and Earth. This is a reciprocal arrangement; one cannot exist without the other.

There are three aspects of the Body. These are Shen, Ti, and Xing.[69] Shen is the individual, Ti is holistic unity, and Xing is the visible and tangible aspect of the body in corporeal form.[69,70] These three aspects combine to form the Body.

In TCM, the main components of human body physiology are Jing (Essence), Shen (Spirit), Blood, Qi, the Zangfu organs, Meridians, Extraordinary Vessels, and Extraordinary Fu.

The reproductive lifespan in TCM: The yearly cycles

As in Orthodox medicine, TCM recognizes that women and, to lesser degree, men have limited reproductive lifespans. In TCM, physiological changes occur during eight yearly cycles in the male and seven yearly cycles in the female (Figure 2.15).[71]

The onset of reproductive life is when Tian Gui arrives.[72] Tian means Heaven,[70] and Gui pertains to Water.[73] Tian Gui (Heavenly Gui) represents the sperm[73,74] and more recently has been referred to as the egg.[73] Tian Gui (Heavenly Gui) also represents Yin, Heavenly Water, or Menses.[71]

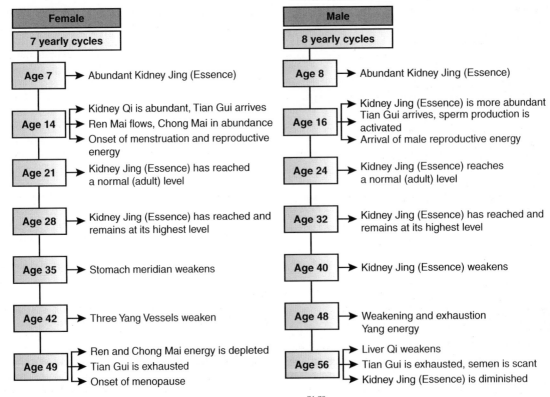

Figure 2.15 Male and female yearly cycles in relation to reproduction.[71,72]

Tian Gui initiates menarche and reproductive potential in the female. At the age of 14, Tian Gui arrives.[72] The Ren Mai (Conception Vessel) is activated and flows, and the Chong Mai (Penetrating Vessel) is abundant and menses occurs harmoniously. This is the onset of reproductive potential in a female.

A woman is most fertile in her 20s. Blood is the precursor to reproductive decline in the female. At the age of 35, a woman's Blood decreases and fertility declines. At the age of 42 to 49, the Ren Mai (Conception Vessel) and the Chong Mai (Penetrating Vessel) begin to weaken and eventually become Deficient, Tian Gui is drained,[72] and a woman is almost infertile.

In the male, at the age of 16, Kidney Qi thrives and Tian Gui arrives, which indicates the beginning of his reproductive potential.[72] The Kidney is the precursor to reproductive decline in the male.[71] At 40 years of age, male reproductive ability declines, marked by a weakening of Kidney Jing (Essence). At 48 to 56 years of age, a man's Kidney Yang becomes exhausted, Tian Gui is depleted, sperm is scant, and the Kidneys become weak.[72] Figure 2.15 summarizes reproductive ageing from the TCM point of view.

Qi, Blood, and Jing (Essence)

Qi

There is no word in the English language that translates and encompasses the meaning of Qi. Qi is described as breath that occurs through transformation, 'an exhalation and releasing movement'.[75] Taoism provided the conceptual framework for TCM. Concepts of Qi are therefore strongly related to Taoism. Qi is everywhere; Qi gives life to all things. In a human being, Qi is 'profoundly interactive in the body',[76] and it interacts with vital substances (for example, Jing (Essence) and Blood) and the external environment[77] (for example, the seasons).[76]

As with other aspects of TCM, Qi is not a physical matter that can be measured or investigated in the laboratory setting.

In traditional and contemporary TCM practice, Qi is understood through its context, type, and function and by the assessment of health and illness. For example, one of the functions of Qi is to facilitate circulation. If this function fails, Qi is said to be Stagnant.

The main functions of Qi are:

- **Powering function**:[78] Qi stimulates and completes growth, development, activity, circulation, and distribution.[79] For example, Qi aids in the creation and the development of an embryo.
- **Warming function**:[78] Qi, in particular Yang Qi, produces heat to keep the body warm. In reproduction, Qi helps to warm the Uterus and maintain an appropriate environment for the embryo.
- **Protecting function**:[78] Qi acts as a defensive boundary and protects the body from the external environment. Wei (Defensive) Qi helps to prevent EPFs from entering the body.[80] For example, it prevents External Wind-Cold from invading the body.
- **Holding function**:[78] Qi holds and supports a form, shape, and position. For example, Qi helps to hold the foetus in the Uterus and the Blood in the Vessels.
- **Transforming function**:[78] Qi facilitates transformation from one form to another. For example, in the menstrual cycle Qi facilitates transformation from Yin into Yang and vice versa. Transformation creates the embryo. The transformation of Qi generates the five emotions: Joy, Anger, Sadness, Anxiety, and Fear.[81]

Qi is categorized according to its functions in the body. The main types of Qi are:

- **Zheng (Right or Correct) Qi**: facilitates harmony in the body by being 'present in the correct place at the correct time'. It rectifies incorrect functions of Qi to prevent illness.[82] Zheng Qi is opposite to disease-causing or pathogenic Qi.
- **Zong (Gathering or Chest) Qi**: combination of different types of Qi,[82] stored in the chest.[79] It is a familial hereditary Qi, which is responsible for producing, consuming, and the circulation of Qi and Blood.[82,83]
- **Yuan (Original) Qi**: Qi potential, which is Qi before it is expressed in 'specific forms'.[82] The original supply of Yang and Yin[83] provided by parents. Jing (Essence) assists in the functions of Yuan (Original) Qi[83] and acts as a catalyst in the formation of Zhen Qi and Blood.
- **Zhen (True) Qi**: represents the laws of nature.[83,84]
- **Gu (Food or Grain) Qi**: produces Jing (Essence) and Blood; together, they nourish the body.[81]
- **Wei (Defensive) Qi**: circulates, defends,[80] protects, and nourishes the body.[79,85]
- **Ying (Nutritive) Qi**: nourishes, rebuilds, and maintains the whole body, including channels and Zangfu organs; activated by acupuncture.[82,85]

Blood

Although TCM and Orthodox medicine use the word *blood*, the meaning of Blood in TCM is very different to that of Orthodox medicine. In TCM, Blood is defined by its main purpose, which is the distribution and expression of energy in the body,[83,86] rather than just the contents of the circulatory system. Blood is a material form of Qi.[85] Blood and Qi represent a Yin Yang pair, Blood being more Yin and Qi being more Yang.[87] In TCM, Blood is essential for life and is central to reproductive health. It delivers nutrients to the body.[79,87] Blood and Qi determine initiation and function of menstruation and conception.[88,89]

The Stomach transforms food and drink into Gu (Food) Qi, which is referred to as [Post-Natal] Jing (Essence).[83] The Stomach transforms and distributes Unclear Gu (Food) Qi to the Heart.[90,91] After Blood has passed through the Heart,[86] it turns red.[92] The Spleen sends Clear Gu (Food) Qi to the Lung where it combines with [Air] Qi.[86,90,91] The Lung propels it to the Heart.[85] Zong (Chest) Qi assists the circulation of Qi and Blood.[82] The Stomach also distributes Gu (Food) Qi [Essence] directly to the Liver, and this form of Jing (Essence) is stored as [Liver] Blood.[90,91] Figure 2.16 summarizes the main steps in Qi and Blood production.

Interestingly, Maciocia states that Yuan (Original) Qi and Bone Marrow, which is generated by Kidney Jing (Essence), are involved in the production of Blood and that Blood is produced by Bone Marrow.[85] Other authors state that Bone Marrow does not produce Blood, but instead Kidney Yin nourishes Liver Blood,[94,95] which, according to other authors, is why Liver Blood is synergistic in presentation and ability with Kidney Jing (Essence).[86] The relationship of mutual engenderment and balance between the Kidney and Liver is where the saying that the Liver and Kidney share the same source comes from.[96]

The functions of Blood include:

- Circulating around the body[83]
- Nourishing and moistening the tissues[79,83]
- Being the basis for mental activity[79] and clarity[83] of Shen (Mind)
- Governing the woman. Blood is a sign of procreative and generative power[97]
- Creating and nourishing life, including the embryo and the foetus

Blood is influenced by the environment, for example, the waxing and waning of the moon.[98] EPFs and internal dysfunction also influence Blood.[68,97] Lifestyle and diet affect Blood quality and quantity.[68] In ill health, Blood can become Deficient and/or Stagnant, Hot or Cold, and this can contribute to subfertility.[68]

Blood is closely related to Qi, Jing (Essence), and Body Fluids; these relationships are outlined in Figure 2.17.

Jing (Essence)

Jing (Essence) is a substance that is able to create, produce, organize, rebuild, and maintain life. It is the basis of the body[99] and reproduction. Jing (Essence) ensures the quality and vitality of a human being.[87,100] It has been described as 'Vital essence, one's innate reservoir of Qi'.[77]

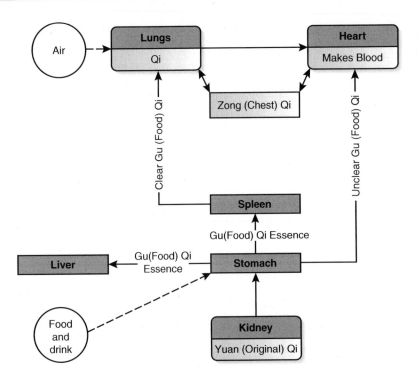

Figure 2.16 Conjectural overview of Qi and Blood production based on synthesis of several classical and contemporary authors' hypotheses.[82,83,85,86,90,91,93]

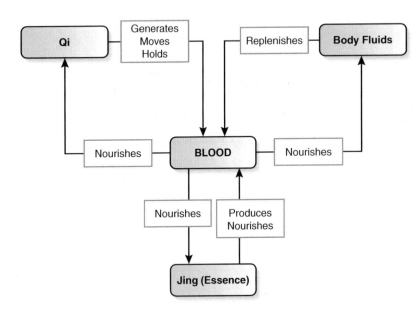

Figure 2.17 The relationships among Blood, Qi, Jing (Essence), and Body Fluids.[79,85,86]

There are two types of Jing (Essence): Pre-Natal and Post-Natal.[79,101] Pre-Natal Jing (Essence) is the energy passed to an embryo by its parents. The Kidney stores and releases Pre-Natal Jing (Essence),[102,103] and this function is governed by Yuan (Original) Qi.[101] Yuan (Original) Qi is responsible for the flourishing of Pre-Natal Jing (Essence). Yuan Qi is the functional manifestation of Pre-Natal Jing (Essence).[101]

Food and water transform into Post-Natal Jing (Essence) and nourish Pre-Natal Jing (Essence).[85,100,101,104]

Jing (Essence) characteristics include:[81]

- Being a source of life[74]
- Transforming Qi[81] and transforming into Qi
- Determining life cycles: growth, reproduction, and development[85]
- Circulating around the body[79]
- Determining an individual's constitution[85]
- Controlling sexual desire[101]
- Manifesting as Heavenly Water (menstruation),[101] sperm,[100] and eggs
- Controlling the health[101] and development of the embryo
- Pre- and Post-Natal Jing (Essences) and Qi are the material basis for Shen (Spirit)[105]

For conception, both Kidney Jing (Essence) and Yuan (Original) Qi need to be healthy.[101] Weak Jing (Essence), Blood, Qi,[68] and Bodily Fluids cause infertility, poor egg and sperm quality and quantity, or difficulty in forming the embryo.[101]

Egg

In classical TCM literature, an embryo was thought to be formed from male Kidney Jing (Essence) and female Blood.[106] In contemporary TCM literature, very few references exist that explain what eggs are. Some authors suggest that eggs are Jing (Essence)[107,108] or Tian Gui.[73]

In our opinion, it is too simplistic to say that eggs are Jing (Essence) or Tian Gui. In our understanding and interpretation of classical TCM female physiology, we hypothesize that eggs are made and influenced by several additional key components:

- We know that a female foetus has all the eggs she is going to have for her entire reproductive lifespan. So we can confidently suggest that this supply of eggs is equivalent to **Pre-Natal Jing (Essence)** that is passed to the female foetus by her parents.
- At the age of 14, when the Kidney Jing (Essence) is abundant, **Tian Gui** arrives (as described earlier in this chapter), and the woman's reproductive life commences. We can equate this to the activation of the Hypothalamic–Pituitary–Ovarian Axis (HPOA), which regulates reproductive function in women. Thus, eggs will not continue developing unless there is a correct hormonal balance, which is provided by activation of the HPOA. (This equates to additional influences from a TCM perspective.)
- From the Orthodox medical point of view, it is well documented that follicles require a good blood supply in order to continue developing. Therefore, we hypothesize that from TCM point of view, a woman's eggs depend on good supply and circulation of **Blood, Yin, Qi,** and **Post-Natal Jing (Essence)**.

There may also be other important influences. We hypothesize that the ones listed above are the most significant ones.

If this hypothesis is correct, then in women with ovarian reserve issues or history of poor follicular development, acupuncturists need to examine which of these key components are suboptimal and address this in their treatment plan. For example, if present, Blood Deficiency may be associated with the Liver, the Heart, or both. Yin Deficiency may involve the Kidney and/or the Liver and/or the Stomach. Pathogenic Factors may be blocking Jing (Essence), Blood, Qi, or Yin or may damage Yin or Qi. Pre-Natal Jing (Essence) may be linked to women with a lower-than-expected ovarian reserve for their age. Where women have good ovarian reserve but produce low numbers of or low-quality eggs, Post-Natal Jing (Essence) and/or Qi may be implicated.

Figure 2.18 summarizes our interpretation of the mature egg from a contemporary integrated TCM point of view.

Sperm

In the classical TCM literature, semen is associated with Jing (Essence).[68,106,109] In contemporary TCM literature, sperm is said to be Kidney Jing (Essence)[110] or Tian Gui.[73]

With the current medical knowledge of male reproductive physiology, the explanation of what sperm is can be developed further:

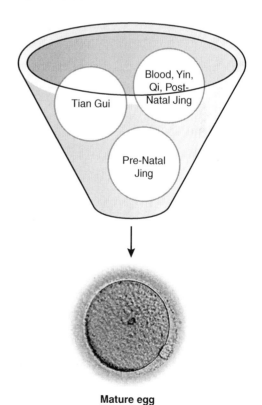

Mature egg

Figure 2.18 Integrated interpretation of what a mature egg is.

- Men produce sperm continually. But this production would be impossible without testicular tissue, which develops in the male foetus and therefore is dependent on **Pre-Natal Jing (Essence)** that is passed to the male foetus by his parents.
- At the age of 16, when the Kidney Jing (Essence) is abundant, **Tian Gui** arrives, and the man produces sperm. We can equate this to the activation of the Hypothalamic–Pituitary–Testicular Axis, which regulates reproductive function in men.
- The continual production of sperm also depends on a good state and supply of **Yang, Yin, Qi**, and **Post-Natal Jing (Essence)**.

Figure 2.19 summarizes our interpretation of the mature sperm from a contemporary integrated TCM point of view.

The menstrual cycle

Menarche

In TCM, the onset of menstruation is considered to be healthy if it occurs at 14 years of age.[72] Earlier or later than this is a sign of pathology (see Chapter 5 for further details).

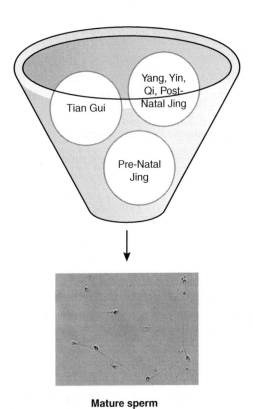

Mature sperm

Figure 2.19 Integrated interpretation of what mature sperm is.

Menstrual discharge

Menses in TCM is considered to be Heavenly Water.[72] Liu Yi-ren, a physician from the Qing dynasty, stated that menstruation is not Blood but 'menstrual water', which is Yin-Blood and relies on Qi for its movement.[111] Figure 2.20 summarizes what menses is from the TCM perspective.

Menstruation occurs when Blood (Heavenly Water) surges, increases, and spreads beyond its limit, flowing out of the Uterus in a monthly flow.[97]

'When the Qi of the Kidney is complete and abundant, the thoroughfare and the controlling vessel are passed by a flow. The menstrual Blood gradually accumulates and moves down when its time comes'.[72]

Heavenly Water (menses) is red, similar to the redness of Blood after it passes through the Heart. Red colour illustrates a harmonious interrelationship between the Heart, Kidney, Liver, the Extraordinary Vessels, and the Uterus. Heavenly Water (menses) is a reflection of the state of a woman's Mind and her Pre- and Post-Natal Jing (Essences), Blood, and Qi circulation.

Menstrual cycle

The menstrual cycle (metaphorically referred to in TCM literature as the 'monthly affair') is considered regular if it occurs every 28–30 days.[72] In medieval times, Sun Simiao acknowledged the role of the menstrual cycle in female health and fertility.[68,112] Sun Simiao described irregular menstruation as menses that did not occur monthly.[68,112] In the classical TCM literature, menses was considered irregular if it occurred early or was delayed.[68,88,112]

The assessment of menses included the flow, consistency, and the amount of Blood lost.[88,113] The flow of menses is central to fertility. For example, stop–starting or spotting is considered abnormal[68,112] because this illustrates pathology of Blood, Qi, and Bodily Fluids.

Examination of the colour of menses (according to the five-phase system of correspondence) was also relevant.[68,112]

Broader manifestations in relation to the menstrual cycle included the role of emotions in female health and tiredness.[68,112]

Fu Qing-zhu and Sun Simiao described manifestations of abnormal menstruation to include symptoms such as menstrual pain.[68,88,112] Pain could occur in the abdomen or legs.[68,112]

The menstrual cycle is regulated by Kidney Jing (Essence), Tian Gui (Heavenly Water), Yin and Yang, Blood, Qi, the Zangfu organs, the Extraordinary Vessels, and Fu.

Fu Shan stated that menstrual flow originates from the Kidneys and that 'freeing Essence' is one among several ways to regulate the menstrual cycle.[88] He discussed how Liver Qi Stagnation blocks the flow of Kidney Qi and thus

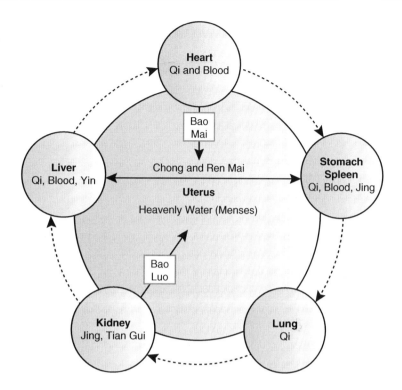

Figure 2.20 Conjectural composition of menstrual blood from TCM point of view.

affects the time of arrival of the menses, with irregular cycles leading to difficulty conceiving.[88]

More recently, Liu Feng Wu (1976) described menstrual irregularities as 'a manifestation of dysfunction of the integrated function of the body'.[114] He related nonstandard variations of a menstrual cycle to dysfunction of the Zangfu organs, particularly the Kidney, Liver, and Spleen. Liu Feng Wu stated that menstrual disease results from loss of regulation of the Kidneys, Qi, Blood, and Extraordinary Vessels, in particular, the Chong (Penetrating) and Ren (Conception) Mai. He concluded that the treatment of Blood disharmony should be the primary method of regulating menstrual cycles. Liu Feng Wu drew an analogy between the regulation of the menstrual cycle and the regulation of hormones.[114]

The four phases of the menstrual cycle and Yin Yang

Chinese philosophers view the world in terms of natural laws that govern life. These principles include Yin Yang theory.[115] In the 1960s, Xia Guicheng developed the four-phase menstrual cycle model based on Yin Yang principles:[116]

'The four phases of the menstrual cycle illustrates physiology and pathology corresponding to the ebb and flow of Yin and Yang. During the first half of the cycle Yin increases and Yang decreases, while in the second half Yang increases and Yin decreases. Ovulation marks a rapid change from Yin to Yang (i.e. Yang increases and Yin decreases), while menstruation marks a rapid change from Yang to Yin (i.e., Yang decreases and Yin starts to increase)'.[116]

However, Guicheng did not make any attempts to equate Yin Yang with a typical pattern of reproductive hormone level.[116] The functions of Yin and Yang in the menstrual cycle allow us to draw some comparisons between the hormones and Yin Yang. FSH, oestrogen, and LH dominate the first half of the cycle (follicular phase),[117] and they are at their highest just before ovulation,[117] which according to Guicheng is when Yin peaks. Progesterone is highest in the second half of the cycle (luteal phase),[117] and this phase is under the influence of Yang. Oestrogen peaks at ovulation time, then rapidly declines and rises again a few days later.[117] Therefore, oestrogen is under the influence of both Yin and, to a lesser degree, Yang.

Table 2.1 summarizes the complex interactions between the key reproductive hormones, Yin Yang, and follicular and endometrial development; it also provides a summary of key events from Orthodox medical and TCM points of view. Chapter 8 discusses menstrual cycle regulation with acupuncture.

Yin and Yang are closely related[121] to the menstrual cycle. The harmonious relationship of Yin and Yang is essential for a healthy menstrual cycle:

Table 2.1 The menstrual cycle: Key reproductive hormones, Yin Yang, follicular and endometrial development, TCM and Orthodox medical menstrual cycle activity (day 0 = ovulation day)[116,117]

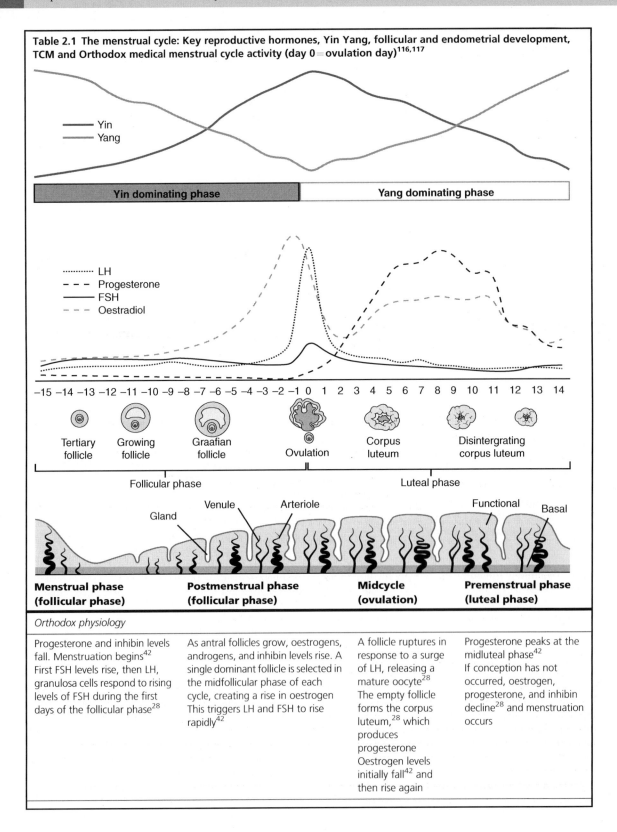

Menstrual phase (follicular phase)	Postmenstrual phase (follicular phase)	Midcycle (ovulation)	Premenstrual phase (luteal phase)
Orthodox physiology			
Progesterone and inhibin levels fall. Menstruation begins[42] First FSH levels rise, then LH, granulosa cells respond to rising levels of FSH during the first days of the follicular phase[28]	As antral follicles grow, oestrogens, androgens, and inhibin levels rise. A single dominant follicle is selected in the midfollicular phase of each cycle, creating a rise in oestrogen This triggers LH and FSH to rise rapidly[42]	A follicle ruptures in response to a surge of LH, releasing a mature oocyte[28] The empty follicle forms the corpus luteum,[28] which produces progesterone Oestrogen levels initially fall[42] and then rise again	Progesterone peaks at the midluteal phase[42] If conception has not occurred, oestrogen, progesterone, and inhibin decline[28] and menstruation occurs

Table 2.1 The menstrual cycle: Key reproductive hormones, Yin Yang, follicular and endometrial development, TCM and Orthodox medical menstrual cycle activity (day 0 = ovulation day)—cont'd

TCM physiology

Yang at its peak begins to decline. Yin is born. Chong Mai empties. Blood develops[118] Free flow of Liver Qi aids Blood movement[119]	Blood and Yin are relatively empty, the Ren and Chong Mai are depleted[119] Kidney Yin starts to grow[120] Before ovulation, Yin peaks, the Chong Mai is full of Blood[118]	Blood and Yin gradually fill the Chong, Ren, and Du Mai[119] The action of the Heart via Bao Mai facilitates ovulation[118] As ovulation occurs, Kidney Yin transforms into Kidney Yang[120]	Yang rises and Liver Qi moves in preparation for the period[119] If a woman is not pregnant, 1[118] to 3[120] days before menstruation, Yin and Yang become insufficient

- **The opposition of Yin Yang**: occurs during the menstrual cycle, for example, when comparing the Yin phase to the Yang phase and vice versa. Also, there is always an element of Yin in Yang and Yang in Yin.
- **The interdependence of Yin and Yang**: one phase of the menstrual cycle does not exist without the other; the Yin phase is caused by the Yang phase, and the Yang phase is dependent on the Yin phase.
- **Mutual consumption of Yin and Yang**: the Yang phase is a product of Yin (for example, the luteal (Yang) phase is only possible if the ovarian follicle grows during the follicular (Yin) phase).
- **The intertransformation of Yin and Yang**: ovulation marks the intratransformation of Yin into Yang, and, if no pregnancy occurs, mutual consumption generates another menstrual cycle, and Yang transforms back into Yin with the onset of menses.

Assessing the menstrual cycle according to the natural affinity of Yin and Yang provides key information about a patient's reproductive physiology and well-being. Figure 2.21 summarizes the key Yin Yang relationships in a menstrual cycle.

Key Zangfu organs in fertility and early pregnancy

Zang are solid organs, and they are Yin. Fu are hollow organs, and they are Yang.[99] The Fu organs process liquids and food and spread Body Fluids.[122,123] The Zang organs combine with Fu organs, and all organs are linked to corresponding meridians.[124] Shen (Spirit), Jing (Essence), Qi, and Blood circulate through the body to nourish and maintain life.[122,123] The five Zang organs are reservoirs of these.[124] The key Zangfu organs for fertility are the Kidney, Liver, Heart, Stomach, Spleen, and Lung.

Zangfu organs are interconnected and interrelated with each other in physiology and pathology. The Zang organ system is discussed in this chapter with an emphasis on fertility and early pregnancy. Where possible, links are drawn between the essential functions of Zang organs and key aspects of reproductive physiology related to the treatment and management of subfertile patients and patients undergoing ART.

The Kidney

Achieving a pregnancy and live birth is strongly linked, though not limited to, healthy functioning Kidneys. The Kidney influences the functions of all the other Zangfu organs. The Kidney's reproductive functions are closely related to Mingmen (the Gate of Life).[125,126]

There are several records regarding the location of Mingmen (the Gate of Life).[126] One view is that the space between the Kidneys is Mingmen (the Gate of Life).[81,125,126] Another view is that the right Kidney is Mingmen (the Gate of Life).[66,125–127] Thus, the term Mingmen (Gate of Life) either signifies the Fire existing between the Kidneys[125] or refers to the right side where there is Mingmen (Gate of Life).

Nanjing 36 states, 'The Gate of Life is where Essence-Spirit (Jing-Shen) is stored and Yuan (Original) Qi is enclosed'.[127] In a male, the Gate of Life is connected to the Chamber of Semen, which stores sperm. In a female, the Gate of Life is connected to the Uterus (Figure 2.22).[66]

The basic functions of the Kidney are:

- The Kidney stores[128,129] and provides Pre-Natal Jing (Essence) and Yuan (Original) Qi[81,127] for reproduction, development, and growth.[89]
- Kidney Jing (Essence) is the origin for the formation of Tian Gui (Heavenly Water), which influences reproduction.[119] It is formed under the influence and abundance of Kidney Qi.[119]
- The Kidney governs sperm, menstruation (including the opening and closing function[101] of the genitals),

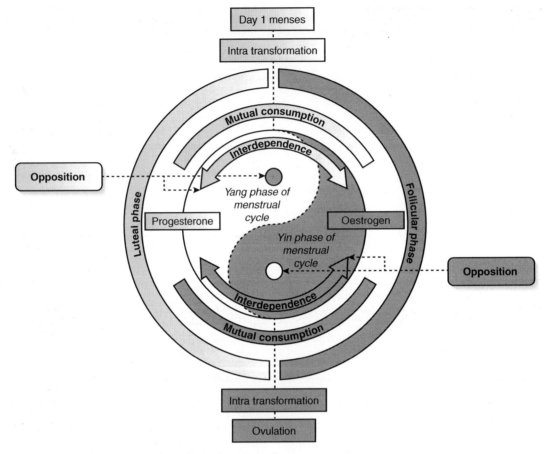

Figure 2.21 Taiji symbol: Yin Yang relationship in the menstrual cycle.

conception, and the embryo and foetus through Pre-Natal Jing (Essence), Qi, and Blood.

- The Kidney connects to the Uterus[89] through the Bao Luo (Uterine Channel), providing the Uterus with Jing (Essence) to nourish follicles and eggs, for menstruation, conception, and nurturing the embryo and foetus.[89]
- The Kidney sustains the quality and function of all other Zangfu organs.[128]
- It fills the bones with Pre-Natal Jing (Essence), generates Marrow,[95,124,130] and fills the Brain with Jing (Essence).
- It enriches and nourishes the Liver by providing it with Kidney Yin.[94]
- The Kidney supports the flow of Yin in the Ren Mai (Conception Vessel) and supplements Blood in the Chong Mai (Penetrating Vessel).[131]

Female fertility depends on the abundance of Blood, Qi, and Jing (Essence).[132] The Kidney provides Jing (Essence); therefore, it can be thought of as the fundamental basis of fertility. It provides the foundation for Pre-Natal Jing

(Essence) and affects the quality and firmness of it, an important function implicated in the quality of an embryo.

Kidney Qi is responsible for governing menstruation and pregnancy through its opening, releasing, and closing functions. Kidney Qi ensures that Pre-Natal Jing (Essence), Blood, and Fluids are released properly as menses.[101]

The Kidney is equally important for male fertility. Pre-Natal Jing (Essence), also referred to as Tian Gui, is a source of sperm.[73] The sperm duct and semen are governed and controlled by Kidney Jing (Essence) and Kidney Qi through the storing, releasing, and closing functions.[133] Semen is strongly allied with Pre-Natal Jing (Essence) and Qi.[74] A reduction in Kidney Jing (Essence), Yin Yang, or anything blocking or preventing it (for example, Stagnation, Dampness, or Phlegm) can lead to male subfertility.

The Kidney is also responsible for the viability and proper development of an embryo. The foetus's survival depends on maternal and paternal Jing (Essence) from the Kidney.[84,134] The mother nurtures her embryo through all its stages of growth and development.[134]

Figure 2.22 Gate of Life and connections with reproductive organs.

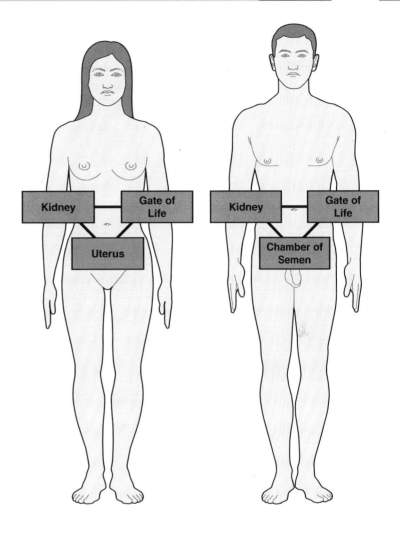

Reproductive failure is strongly linked with Kidney Jing (Essence) Deficiency.[72] Eggs and sperm are related to Pre-Natal Jing (Essence) and Kidney Yin and Yang. Any problems with eggs and sperm can be a direct result of any Kidney pathology.

Kidney Deficiency is associated with reduced ovarian reserve. The ovarian reserve is often lower in older women or in women with Kidney Jing (Essence) Deficiency. During IVF, even if several eggs are collected, their quality and the quality of any resulting embryos may be compromised. This is why IVF pregnancy rates are lower in older women.

The quality of the egg is also strongly linked with the quality of Yin and/or Blood. There is a strong relationship between the Kidney and Zangfu organs involved with Blood. For example, a Deficiency of Kidney Yin may lead to Deficiency of Liver Blood and, therefore, poor quality eggs and embryos. Or Stomach and Spleen Qi Deficiency may reduce Post-Natal Jing (Essence), and this, in turn, may influence Blood and Pre-Natal Jing (Essence).

In extreme cases, Kidney Jing (Essence) Deficiency may lead to complete sterility, where no eggs or sperm are produced and donor eggs or sperm are required in order to conceive. Kidney pathology is associated with infertility issues such as age-related decline in fertility, poor follicular response to IVF medication, cancelled IVF cycles, repeated IVF failures, and miscarriage(s).

Figure 2.23 summarizes the complex interactions and reproductive functions of the Kidney and all key Zangfu organs.

The Liver

Although the Kidney is the basis for reproduction, the Liver allows conception to occur.

'It is due to her Liver that Blood is able to make life'.[132]

The basic functions of the Liver are:

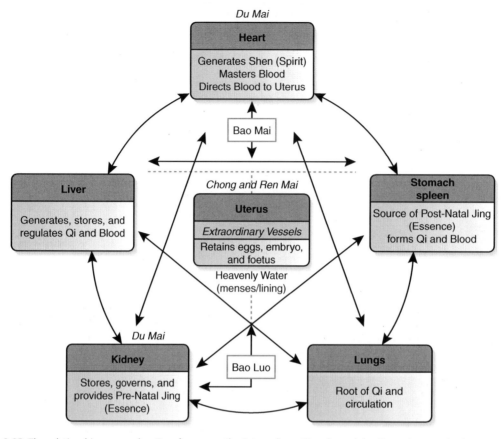

Figure 2.23 The relationships among key Zangfu organs, the Extraordinary Vessels, and the Uterus in reproduction.

- Storing, generating, and regulating Blood[128] and Qi.[128,129,135]
- Releasing Blood for menses.[89,132]
- Taking charge of the eyes.[66,95]

The Liver generates the energy of Blood and stores Blood; this is responsible for correct movement and circulation of Blood in the body[132] and the regulation of menses.

> *'It is the movement of the Liver on the Yin side storing the Blood, and on the Yang side giving the impulse for all circulation, sending forth and spreading out, Yin is the basis for Yang'.*[132]

The Liver regulates the menstrual cycle by moving Qi and Blood.[132] A healthy menstrual cycle promotes fertility and optimizes a woman's response to IVF treatment.

The Liver and Kidney both help to facilitate implantation and pregnancy, particularly in the early stages. The first month of pregnancy is when Jing (Essences) concentrate, Blood coagulates, and the embryo 'knots'.[84]

In our opinion, pathology of the Liver is strongly linked to menstrual cycle irregularities, infertility, implantation and IVF failure, and early miscarriages.

In our experience, issues with ovarian reserve can result from Kidney Jing (Essence) Deficiency and/or Liver Blood Deficiency. A history of problems with the endometrium during IVF can result from Kidney Jing (Essence) and Yin and Liver Blood Deficiency. Follicular recruitment and development is connected to the Liver's function of generating and regulating Blood as well as the Liver's, Kidney's, and Heart's interrelationship with each other and the Uterus.

Figure 2.23 summarizes the complex interactions and reproductive functions of the Liver and all key Zangfu organs.

The Heart

The Heart is the centre of fertility. It promotes Blood circulation to the Uterus. The basic functions of the Heart are:

- Generating[92,128] and controlling changing[128] of Shen (Spirit)

- Connecting to the Uterus through the Bao Mai (Uterine Vessel)
- Mastering Blood,[66] promoting Blood circulation,[66,95] directing Blood to the Uterus,[89] and filling up Blood vessels[136] in the Uterus
- Enabling menstruation, conception, and pregnancy[89]
- Manifesting in the complexion[137]

The Heart and the Mind of a woman should be harmonized throughout menstruation, fertility, conception, and pregnancy.[84]

'Human life is brought about in the Essences and both Essences are drawn together in Spirit'.[128]

The Heart generates and stores Spirit. The terms *Shen* and *Spirit* are often used synonymously.[138] Shen (Spirit) is acquired when the Body, Heart, and Mind are settled, calm, and 'properly aligned'.[139] Shen (Spirit) promotes movement and vitality of Jing (Essence), Qi, and Blood by invigorating and circulating them around the body.

'Suppression of menstruation is due to a blockage of meridian within the womb, which belongs to the Heart and is linked with the internal region of the womb'.[140]

Follicular growth and egg maturation depend on Blood circulation and the Heart's function of directing Blood to the Uterus. Weakness of this function will compromise fertility, follicular development during IVF, and conception. Figure 2.23 summarizes the complex interactions and reproductive functions of all key Zangfu organs.

The Stomach

The basic functions of the Stomach are:

- Generating Qi and Blood[119,129,136] and Post-Natal Jing (Essence)
- Transforming and distributing Gu (Food) Qi[141] to the Heart and the Spleen, which in turn transforms and distributes[128] Gu (Food) Qi and Post-Natal Jing (Essence)[86] into Qi and Blood for reproductive purposes
- Supporting, and facilitating the Chong Mai's (Penetrating Vessel) role of regulating menstruation by supplementing Blood and Jing (Essence)[131]

Jing (Essence) consists of Pre- and Post-Natal components. The Stomach (together with the Spleen) supports fertility as it is the source of Post-Natal Jing (Essence), Qi, and Blood. Post-Natal Jing (Essence) nourishes, rebuilds, and maintains the body.[83] Diet is important in the reproductive field because the Stomach's ability to produce Post-Natal Jing (Essence) depends on good dietary habits. Post-Natal Jing (Essence) nourishes Pre-Natal Jing (Essence).

The Stomach links with the Chong (Penetrating) Vessel, strengthening the Sea of Blood by providing Jing (Essence) and Qi[131] for menstruation. The Stomach also enriches Yin, thus helping the Ren Mai (Conception Vessel).[142]

Figure 2.23 summarizes the complex interactions and reproductive functions of the Stomach and all key Zangfu organs.

The Spleen

The basic functions of the Spleen are:

- Forming Blood[86]
- Keeping Blood in the correct place[89]
- Supporting the Chong (Penetrating) Mai in regulating menstruation by supplementing Blood and Jing [Essence][131] through Qi
- Enriching Kidney Yin and Yang through Qi and Blood[143]
- Nourishing the body and aiding regeneration of Bodily Fluids (together with Stomach and Kidney)[144,145]
- Lifting and securing the Uterus[89]
- Nurturing the embryo[132,134]

Yin, Blood, and Qi support fertility and conception. Copious Blood is essential for conception.[119] The Spleen supports fertility by forming Qi and Blood, while the Heart masters Blood. Qi and Blood can transform into Post-Natal Jing (Essence), and Jing [Essence], in turn, can transform into Blood.

The Spleen is affiliated with the Uterus via the Chong (Penetrating) and the Ren (Conception) Mai.[89] The abundance of Stomach and Spleen Blood and Qi ensures nutritional enrichment and renewal of Blood to support the Chong Mai.[142]

By delivering Qi, Blood, and Jing (Essence) to the embryo via the Chong and Ren Mai, the Spleen (together with the Stomach) provides essential nutrients to the embryo in order for it to survive.[132,134]

During IVF, if Spleen Qi and/or Blood is Deficient, the embryo may fail to implant, or, if it implants, it may stop developing, and the pregnancy will fail.

Figure 2.23 summarizes the complex interactions and reproductive functions of the Spleen and all key Zangfu organs.

The Lung

The basic functions of the Lung are:

- Generating Qi,[136] Blood,[83] Jing (Essence), and Bodily Fluids, which are all essential for menstruation, conception, and pregnancy[146]
- Governing Qi[66] and regulating rhythms of the Zangfu[146]
- Filling up the skin with Lung energy[130] and defending the body from EPF invasion[66]

The Lung is situated near the Heart. Its physiological and anatomical connection closely assists the Heart in its reproductive functions.

The Lung is the root of Qi. It provides a balance of Qi[146] and supports the functions of Qi within the body and the Zangfu organ system. It governs breathing and regulates essential rhythms of the Zangfu organs, which assists fertility.

The Lung assists fertility by circulating Qi, Jing (Essence),[101] Blood, and Bodily Fluids around the body.[101] These substances are also the foundation for menstruation and nourishment of the embryo.[89]

Weakness of the Lung leads to poor generation of Qi, along with poor circulation of Qi and Blood, which compromises fertility.

Figure 2.23 summarizes the complex interactions and reproductive functions of the Lung and all key Zangfu organs.

The Uterus

The basic functions of the Uterus are:

- Regulating menstruation,[147] conception, and pregnancy[147]
- Gathering Blood and Qi from all Zang organs[148]
- Receiving Pre-Natal Jing (Essence) from the Kidney and Post-Natal Jing (Essence) from the Stomach and Spleen[149] via the Chong Mai (Penetrating Vessel)
- Storing Jing (Essence) and Blood for menstruation[149]
- Retaining and releasing the egg(s)
- Retaining sperm after intercourse or artificial insemination
- Accepting, holding, and protecting the embryo and foetus[148] and facilitating the embryo's health, nutrition, and development

Influenced by the Extraordinary Vessels and Zangfu organs, the Uterus allows the entire TCM reproductive physiology system to interact and bring new life into the world.

The Uterus is an Extraordinary Fu organ[150] because it transforms, transmits,[151] and releases Heavenly Water (menses).

As discussed earlier, the TCM term *Uterus* encompasses the ovaries. Thus, the Uterus acts as an Extraordinary Fu organ, by storing and retaining[151] eggs, storing the Heavenly Water (menses), and releasing Pre-Natal Jing (Essence) (the egg) at ovulation and menses at menstruation. The Uterus also stores the embryo and facilitates its development.

The Uterus, with the aid of the Zangfu organs and Extraordinary Vessels (and the Brain), facilitates the completion of the whole embryological process and the formation of the embryo and foetus.[151]

The Extraordinary Vessels, in particular the Ren (Conception), Du (Governing), and Chong (Penetrating), occupy the centre of the Uterus.[149] (The Section 'The key Extraordinary Vessels in reproduction' later in this chapter discusses this in more detail.)

The Uterus receives Pre-Natal Jing (Essence) from the Kidney and Qi and Blood from the Heart. The Uterus is connected to the Heart 'as if it was its own viscera'[149]

and is joined also to the Kidney. The Bao Mai (Uterine Vessel) links the Uterus and Heart. The Bao Mai is an important connection that links the Shen (Spirit/Mind) of the female to the Uterus. The Bao Mai enables circulation and regulates the distribution of Blood to the ovaries and Uterus. During conception and pregnancy, this network nourishes and protects the embryo.[148] The Bao Luo (Uterine Channel) links the Uterus and Kidney in order to provide Pre-Natal Jing (Essence).[148]

Figure 2.23 summarizes the complex interactions and reproductive functions of the Uterus and all key Zangfu organs.

Zangfu organ interactions and IVF

During the stimulation phase of an IVF treatment cycle, the Heart, Kidney, and Liver (and Extraordinary Vessels) regulate the ovaries, thus facilitating follicular growth, egg maturation, and the endometrial lining. The Uterus also receives Qi, Blood, and Jing (Essence) from other Zangfu organs, in particular, the Stomach and Spleen.

In IVF, the embryo is transferred into the Uterus. The embryo continues to develop and grow in the Uterus with the aid of the Extraordinary Vessels and Zangfu and under the influence of Jing (Essence), Shen (Spirit), Qi, and Blood. The embryo also develops through its own embryonic Qi (see Chapter 3).

The key Extraordinary Vessels in reproduction

The Zangfu organs and Extraordinary Vessels regulate the menstrual cycle. They are referred to as reservoirs because they regulate the amount and flow of Qi, Blood, and Jing (Essence) during the menstrual cycle. The Extraordinary Vessels strengthen meridians by circulating and distributing Yin, Yang, Blood, Qi, and Jing (Essence).

There are eight Extraordinary Vessels:[152,153]

- Chong Mai (Penetrating Vessel)
- Ren Mai (Conception Vessel)
- Du Mai (Governing Vessel)
- Dai Mai (Girdling Vessel)
- Yinqiao Mai (Yin Motility Vessel)
- Yangqiao Mai (Yang Motility Vessel)
- Yinwei Mai (Yin Linking Vessel)
- Yangwei Mai (Yang Linking Vessel)

This section focuses on the Chong, Ren, Du, and Dai Mai (Penetrating, Conception, Governing, and Girdling Vessels) because they play a critical role in fertility. The Chong, Ren, and Du Mai (Penetrating, Conception, and Governing Vessels) connect to the Uterus and are affiliated with the Stomach, Kidney, Liver, and Spleen. The Du Mai (Governing Vessel) enters the Brain and connects to the Kidney and Heart.

The Extraordinary Vessel pathways are discussed in this section because they illustrate interrelationships that have fundamental roles in women's reproductive physiology.

The Chong Mai (Penetrating Vessel)

The Chong Mai (Penetrating Vessel) originates in the area between the Kidneys, travels through the Uterus to REN1, then to ST30 (the meeting point of the Chong Mai), where it emerges.[73]

It then travels with the Stomach[153,154] or Kidney[155,156] meridian alongside the umbilicus, reaches the chest, and disperses.[153–156]

Ling Shu 38 describes a branch of the Chong Mai that travels down the leg and nourishes the Liver, Spleen, and Kidney meridian.[157,158]

The main functions of the Chong Mai (Penetrating Vessel) are:

- Connecting Pre- and Post-Natal Jing (Essence) and Qi[159]
- Mastering all circulation[158–161] and regulating Qi and Blood,[158–161] the Uterus,[73] and the menstrual cycle to benefit fertility and conception[162]
- Providing Yang with Jing (Essence) and Blood[159]
- Warming Mingmen (Fire of Life)[163]
- Receiving Jing (Essence) and assistance from the Kidney meridian[79,89]
- Nourishing the Kidney, Liver, and Spleen and warming collaterals[157,164]

The Chong Mai (Penetrating Vessel) is used to improve and ensure a good and appropriate amount and flow of Qi and Blood in the Uterus. The Chong Mai (Penetrating Vessel) connects with Pre- and Post-Natal Jing (Essence), the Kidney, and the Stomach. It improves reproductive health and fertility by nourishing the Kidney and warming Mingmen. The Chong Mai (Penetrating Vessel) also nourishes the Liver and the Spleen[164] and provides the Uterus with Jing (Essence) and Blood for healthy menses. For this reason, it is called the Sea of Blood.

The Du Mai (Governing Vessel)

The Du Mai (Governing Vessel) originates in the area between the Kidneys, travels to the Uterus, and emerges at REN1.[73,153]

It then travels to its primary point DU1, ascends inside the spine up to DU16, and enters the Brain.[153,154]

Su Wen 60 describes in detail the importance of the Du Mai (Governing Vessel) in reproductive anatomy and physiology and how the Du Mai (Governing Vessel) tracks the female genitalia and, in the male, travels along the penis.[156]

Su Wen 60 also describes how the Du Mai (Governing Vessel) merges with the Kidney meridian, enters the spine, and connects with the Kidneys.[156]

Su Wen 60 states that the Du Mai (Governing Vessel) penetrates the umbilicus, ascends and enters the Heart, travels through the throat to the lower cheek, moves around the lips, and travels to below the centre of the eyes.[156]

The main functions of the Du Mai (Governing Vessel) are:

- Mastering Yang Qi[165] and connecting Yang meridians[89]
- Entering the Kidney, Heart, and Brain[156]
- Governing fertility and conception[165] by influencing male and female genitals[165]
- Together with the Ren Mai (Conception Vessel), maintaining a balance of Yin and Yang[89]

The Du Mai's (Governing Vessel's) affiliation with the Kidney, Heart, Brain, and Liver creates a supportive environment for fertilization, conception, implantation, and pregnancy. For example, DU20 is the meeting point of the Du Mai (Governing Vessel) with the Liver.[166] It raises and stabilizes Yang, interrelates the body with Heaven, and provides a calming effect on Shen (Spirit). This point can be used before an embryo transfer and for early pregnancy support. Acupuncture and moxibustion on DU4 is often used to tonify the Kidney for fertility and conception purposes.

The Ren Mai (Conception Vessel) and the Du Mai (Governing Vessel) arise together,[142] sustaining an essential balance and maintaining Yin and Yang function.[32] However, Unschuld, Tessenow and Jinsheng state that the Du Mai (Governing Vessel) is assigned a more important role[80] in reproductive health than the Ren Mai (Conception Vessel) because it enters the Kidney, Heart, and Brain. According to TCM concepts, it is through these connections that fundamental physiological changes in fertility, conception, and early pregnancy happen.

Thus, with so many connections with male and female genitalia, disorders in the Kidney, Heart, and Brain in both classical TCM literature and contemporary TCM infertility practice are believed to be caused by disorders of the Du Mai (Governing Vessel).[155]

The Ren Mai (Conception Vessel)

The Ren Mai (Conception Vessel) originates in the area between the Kidneys, travels to the Uterus, and emerges at REN1.[73] It then ascends inside the abdomen through the acupuncture point REN4 toward the throat.[153,154]

The Ren Mai (Conception Vessel) meets with the Liver meridian at REN2, the Spleen meridian at REN3, and the Kidney meridian at REN4.[32]

The main functions of the Ren Mai (Conception Vessel) are:

- Facilitating menarche and fertility[142] by receiving nourishment from Pre- and Post-Natal Jing (Essence)[89,131]
- Controlling and nourishing Yin through governing Jing (Essence),[142] Bodily Fluids, and Blood[89]
- Enabling conception by governing the Uterus and menses[89]

Table 2.2 Key differences between Chong, Du, and Ren Mai (Penetrating, Governing, and Conception Vessels)

Extraordinary Vessel	Vital substances and Yin Yang	Zangfu connections	Extraordinary Fu connections	Main function	TCM terminology
Chong Mai (Penetrating Vessel)	Jing (Essence), Qi[73] and Blood	Stomach Kidney Liver Spleen	Uterus	Regulates, controls, and supplements Qi and Blood	Sea of Blood Sea of 12 Channels
Du Mai (Governing Vessel)	Jing (Essence), Blood, Yang	Kidney Heart Liver	Uterus Brain	Controls Yang	Represents the Gate of Life (Mingmen)[73]
Ren Mai (Conception Vessel)	Jing (Essence), Body Fluids, Yin[73]	Kidney Liver Spleen	Uterus	Activates, controls, nourishes, and supplements Yin	Sea of Yin Channels

- Controlling the embryo[163] and foetus[79,89,142]

The Ren Mai (Conception Vessel), and to some extent the Du Mai (Governing Vessel), ensure good quality, timely, and plentiful cervical mucus by regulating the circulation of nourishing Blood, Yin, and vaginal fluids.

The Ren Mai (Conception Vessel) helps to improve egg quality by nourishing and enriching Jing (Essence), Yin, and Blood. REN12 is a Front Mu point of the Stomach, which provides Post-Natal Jing (Essence) and supports Qi and Blood. REN4 is a meeting point of the Kidney, Liver, and Spleen and can be used to tonify Pre-Natal Jing (Essence).

Disorders of the Ren Mai (Conception Vessel), such as Deficiency of Jing (Essence), Yin, Blood, or Stagnation, can manifest in the Liver, Spleen, and Kidney.[131]

Table 2.2 summarizes key differences between the Chong, Ren, and Du Mai.

The Dai Mai (Girdling Vessel)

The Dai Mai (Girdling Vessel) arises from the tenth rib and completes a full circle around the waist[153,154] like a belt. As it circles the waist, it passes through GB26, GB27, and GB28.[73]

The Kidney Divergent Channel[167] is associated with the Dai Mai (Girdling Vessel),[168] thus demonstrating a key relationship between the Kidney and the Dai Mai (Girdling Vessel). Other sources describe an association of the Dai Mai (Girdling Vessel) with the Spleen and, therefore, with 'liquids'.[89,169]

The main functions of the Dai Mai are:

- Uniting with[169] and restraining the Chong (Penetrating), Ren (Conception), and Du Mai (Governing) Vessels, thus linking with the Uterus[89]
- Harmonizing, regulating, and balancing Qi and Blood[169]
- Supporting the functions of the Uterus[89]

SUMMARY

Reproductive anatomy and physiology

- From a conventional Orthodox medical point of view, both female and male reproductive anatomy is important for fertility. Abnormalities of the uterus, ovaries, fallopian tubes, testicles, or penis could lead to subfertility or sterility.
- TCM places less importance on physical anatomical structures and more on the functions of each organ. However, references to the anatomical observation of the Uterus (corporeal form of the Body) date as far back as medieval times in the classical TCM literature.[68] In contemporary acupuncture practice, practitioners have access to more detailed observations of the anatomy, such as scans of the fallopian tubes, the ovaries, and the uterine lining. This information can help to refine and enhance the TCM diagnosis. (Chapter 4 discusses interpretation of diagnostic tests in greater detail.)

Reproductive ageing

- Women are born with an ovarian reserve of about 300,000 follicles, which decreases to 1,000 follicles by menopause. Thus, women's reproductive lifespan is very limited. Men begin to produce sperm at puberty and continue to do so until they die. However, the quality of sperm declines with advancing age.
- Classical TCM acknowledges reproductive decline through a concept of 'yearly cycles'. Women are most fertile in their 20s. In their mid-30s, their meridian energy weakens, and, by the age of 49, their fertility is depleted. TCM views male fertility similarly, with fertility being in its prime in the 20s and declining in the 40s.

Egg maturation

- Eggs take over a year to develop from their dormant state to ovulatory phase. Once the follicles reach 0.08 mm in diameter, they gain a blood supply (estimated to be between 120 and 190 days before ovulation). A good blood supply, and, therefore, hormone and nutrient delivery to the follicles, improves egg quality. Acupuncture has been shown to improve the blood supply to the ovaries. Therefore acupuncture may also have the potential to help follicular growth during this last phase of follicular development.

Reproductive system physiology

- Both TCM and Orthodox medicine recognize the importance of the menstrual cycle although its physiology and the emphasis on what is important or pathological differ.

- From the Orthodox medicine point of view, reproductive physiology is regulated by the Hypothalamic–Pituitary–Gonadal Axis and reproductive hormones, in particular, FSH, LH, oestrogen, progesterone, inhibin, and testosterone.

- From the TCM point of view, the female reproductive physiology is complex and dynamic. Good fertility depends on a rich supply and free-flowing circulation of Jing (Essence), Tian Gui (menses), copious amounts of Blood and Qi, a good state of Shen (Spirit/Mind) and emotion, Yin Yang balance, good functioning of the Zangfu, the Uterus, and the Extraordinary Vessels (in particular, the Chong (Penetrating) and Ren (Conception) Mai).

- Male reproductive physiology is less complex and is mainly associated with a good amount of Kidney Jing (Essence), Tian Gui, Yin Yang, and good functioning of Qi.

REFERENCES

1. Speroff L, Fritz MA. The ovary-embryology and development. In: Clinical gynecologic endocrinology and infertility. 7th ed. Philadelphia: Lippincott Williams & Wilkins; 2005. p. 97–113 [chapter 3].

2. Wilson KJW, Waugh A, Ross JS. The reproductive systems. In: Ross and Wilson anatomy and physiology in health and illness. 8th ed. New York: Churchill Livingstone; 1996. p. 421–41 [chapter 18].

3. Tortora GJ, Grabowski SR. The reproductive systems. In: Principles of anatomy and physiology. 9th ed. New York; Chichester: John Wiley & Sons Inc.; 2000. p. 974–1021 [chapter 28].

4. Speroff L, Fritz MA. The Uterus. In: Clinical gynecologic endocrinology and infertility. 7th ed. Philadelphia: Lippincott Williams & Wilkins; 2005. p. 113–45 [chapter 4].

5. Sangeetha M, Shobha N, Thavamani D. A prospective study for the assessment of follicular growth, endometrial thickness and serum estradiol levels in spontaneous and clomiphene citrate induced cycles in unexplained infertility patients. Int J Biol Med Res 2012;3:1345–7.

6. Harris-Glocker M, McLaren JF. Role of female pelvic anatomy in infertility. Clin Anat 2013;26:89–96.

7. ASRM patient fact sheet. Hydrosalpinx. Available from: http://www.asrm.org/Hydrosalpinx_factsheet/ [accessed 9 February 2013].

8. Chan YY, Jayaprakasan K, Zamora J, et al. The prevalence of congenital uterine anomalies in unselected and high-risk populations: a systematic review. Hum Reprod Update 2011;17:761–71.

9. Taylor E, Gomel V. The Uterus and fertility. Fertil Steril 2008;89:1–16.

10. Kastrop P. Laboratory aspects of male infertility. In: de Haan N, Spelt M, Gobel R, editors. Reproductive medicine: a textbook for paramedics. Gezondheidszorg, Amsterdam: Elsevier; 2010. p. 57–72 [chapter 3].

11. WHO. Reference values and semen nomenclature. In: Cooper TG, editor-in-chief. WHO laboratory manual for the examination and processing of human Semen. 5th ed. Geneva: World Health Organization; 2010. p. 223–6 Appendix 1.

12. Johnson MH, Everitt BJ. Testicular function. In: Essential reproduction. 5th ed. Oxford: Blackwell Science; 2000. p. 53–68 [chapter 4].

13. Bungum M. Sperm DNA, integrity assessment: a new tool in diagnosis and treatment of fertility. Obstet Gynecol Int 2012;2012:531042.

14. Speroff L, Fritz MA. Sperm and egg transport, fertilization, and implantation. In: Clinical gynecologic endocrinology and infertility. 7th ed. Philadelphia: Lippincott Williams & Wilkins; 2005. p. 187–231 [chapter 7].

15. Johnson MH. Making sperm. In: Essential reproduction. 7th ed. Chichester, West Sussex: John Wiley & Sons; 2012. p. 105–21 [chapter 6].

16. Oktem O, Urman B. Understanding follicle growth in vivo. Hum Reprod 2010;25:2944–54.

17. Mamsen LS, Lutterodt MC, Andersen EW, et al. Germ cell numbers in human embryonic and fetal gonads during the first two trimesters of pregnancy: analysis of six published studies. Hum Reprod 2011;26:2140–5.

18. Oktem O, Oktay K. The ovary: Anatomy and function throughout human life. Ann N Y Acad Sci 2008;1127:1–9.

19. Skinner MK. Regulation of primordial follicle assembly and development. Hum Reprod Update 2005;11:461–71.

20. Bukovsky A, Caudle MR, Svetlikova M, et al. Origin of germ cells and formation of new primary follicles in adult human ovaries. Reprod Biol Endocrinol 2004;2:1–30.

21. Vergouw C. Egg cells. In: de Haan N, Spelt M, Gobel R, editors. Reproductive medicine: a textbook for paramedics. Amsterdam: Elsevier Gezondheidszorg; 2010. p. 73–8 [chapter 4].

22. Weima S. Embryology. In: de Haan N, Spelt M, Gobel R, editors. Reproductive medicine: a textbook for paramedics. Amsterdam: Elsevier Gezondheidszorg; 2010. p. 79–92 [chapter 5].

23. Rienzi L, Balaban B, Ebner T, et al. The oocyte. Hum Reprod 2012;27 (Suppl. 1):i2–i21.

24. Gougeon A. Dynamics of follicular growth in the human: a model from preliminary results. Hum Reprod 1986;1:81–7.

25. Gougeon A. Regulation of ovarian follicular development in primates: facts and hypotheses. Endocr Rev 1996;17:121–55.

26. Zeleznik AJ. The physiology of follicle selection. Reprod Biol Endocrinol 2004;2:31.

27. Erickson GF. Gynecology and obstetrics. Available from: http://www.glowm.com/resources/glowm/cd/pages/v5/v5c012.html?SESSID=4o2r5knl4qtpq11cpqc5ssfd02#r2.

28. Johnson MH, Everitt BJ. Adult ovarian function. In: Essential reproduction. 5th ed. Oxford: Blackwell Science; 2000. p. 69–87 [chapter 5].

29. Elder K, Dale B. Gametes and gametogenesis. 3rd ed. In-vitro fertilization, Cambridge: Cambridge University Press; 2011. p. 28–49 [chapter 3].

30. Baerwald AR, Adams GP, Pierson RA. Ovarian antral folliculogenesis during the human menstrual cycle: a review. Hum Reprod Update 2012;18:73–91.

31. Gougeon A, Lefèvre B. Evolution of the diameters of the largest healthy and atretic follicles during the human menstrual cycle. J Reprod Fertil 1983;69:497–502.

32. Deadman P, Al-Khafaji M, Baker K. The conception vessel. In: A manual of acupuncture. England: Journal of Chinese Medicine Publications; 1998. p. 493–526.

33. Hecker H-U, Steveling A, Peuker E, et al. The Kidney channel. In: Color atlas of acupuncture: body points, ear points, trigger points. 2nd ed. Stuttgart: Thieme; 2008. p. 57–60.

34. Deadman P, Al-Khafaji M, Baker K. The Bladder channel. In: A manual of acupuncture. England: Journal of Chinese Medicine Publications; 1998. p. 249–328.

35. Hecker H-U, Steveling A, Peuker E, et al. The Gallbladder channel. In: Color atlas of acupuncture: body points, ear points, trigger points. 2nd ed. Stuttgart: Thieme; 2008. p. 73–84.

36. Hecker H-U, Steveling A, Peuker E, et al. The Governor Vessel (GV) (Du Mai). In: Practice of acupuncture: point location, treatment options, TCM basics. Stuttgart: Thieme; 2005. p. 338–56.

37. Anderson BJ, Haimovici F, Ginsburg ES, et al. In vitro fertilization and acupuncture: clinical efficacy and mechanistic basis. Altern Ther Health Med 2007;13:38–48.

38. Anderson B, Rosenthal L. Acupuncture and in vitro fertilization: critique of the evidence and application to clinical practice. Complement Ther Clin Pract 2013;19:1–5.

39. Deadman P, Al-Khafaji M, Baker K. The Stomach channel. In: A manual of acupuncture. England: Journal of Chinese Medicine Publications; 1998. p. 123–74.

40. Deadman P, Al-Khafaji M, Baker K. The Spleen channel. In: A manual of acupuncture. England: Journal of Chinese Medicine Publications; 1998. p. 175–206.

41. Deadman P, Al-Khafaji M, Baker K. The Liver channel. In: A manual of acupuncture. England: Journal of Chinese Medicine Publications; 1998. p. 467–92.

42. Johnson MH, Everitt BJ. The regulation of gonadal function. In: Essential reproduction. 5th ed. Oxford: Blackwell Science; 2000. p. 88–118 [chapter 6].

43. Elder K, Dale B. Endocrine control of reproduction: controlled ovarian hyperstimulation for ART. In: In-vitro fertilization. 3rd ed. Cambridge: Cambridge University Press; 2011. p. 19–27 [chapter 2].

44. McGee EA, Hsueh AJ. Initial and cyclic recruitment of ovarian follicles. Endocr Rev 2000;21:200–14.

45. Yaqoob M. Endocrine disease. In: Kumar P, Clark M, editors. Kumar and Clark's clinical medicine [ebook]. 7th ed. Saunders Ltd.; 2012 [chapter 19]. Available from: http://www.amazon.co.uk/Kumar-Clarks-Clinical-Medicine-ebook/dp/B008IZKYGY/ref=sr_1_1?s=books&ie=UTF8&qid=1375020189&sr=1-1.

46. Hess RA, Bunick D, Lee KH, et al. A role for oestrogens in the male reproductive system. Nature 1997;390:509–12.

47. De Ronde W, Pols HA, Van Leeuwen JP, et al. The importance of oestrogens in males. Clin Endocrinol (Oxf) 2003;58:529–42.

48. Sabeur K, Edwards DP, Meizel S. Human sperm plasma membrane progesterone receptor(s) and the acrosome reaction. Biol Reprod 1996;54:993–1001.

49. Nieschlag E, Swerdloff R, Behre HM, et al. Investigation, treatment and monitoring of late-onset hypogonadism in males. Aging Male 2005;8:56–8.

50. Drillich A, Davis SR. Androgen therapy in women: what we think we know. Exp Gerontol 2007;42:457–62.

51. Gleicher N, Kim A, Weghofer A, et al. Hypoandrogenism in association with diminished functional ovarian reserve. Hum Reprod 2013;28(4):1084–91.

52. Weiss G. Relaxin in the male. Biol Reprod 1989;40:197–200.

53. Chiazze L, Brayer FT, Macisco JJ, et al. The length and variability of the human menstrual cycle. JAMA 1968;203:377–80.

54. Cole LA, Ladner DG, Byrn FW. The normal variabilities of the menstrual cycle. Fertil Steril 2009;91:522–7.

55. Alliende ME. Mean versus individual hormonal profiles in the menstrual cycle. Fertil Steril 2002;78:90–5.

56. Fehring RJ, Schneider M, Raviele K. Variability in the phases of the menstrual cycle. J Obstet Gynecol Neonatal Nurs 2006;35:376–84.

57. Harlow SD, Lin X, Ho MJ. Analysis of menstrual diary data across the reproductive life span applicability of the bipartite model approach and the importance of within-woman

variance. J Clin Epidemiol 2000;53:722–33.

58. Rowland AS, Baird DD, Long S, et al. Influence of medical conditions and lifestyle factors on the menstrual cycle. Epidemiology 2002;13:668–74.

59. Liu Y, Gold EB, Lasley BL, et al. Factors affecting menstrual cycle characteristics. Am J Epidemiol 2004;160:131–40.

60. Fenster L, Waller K, Chen J, et al. Psychological stress in the workplace and menstrual function. Am J Epidemiol 1999;149:127–34.

61. Diagnostic Products Corporation. Hormonal levels during the early follicular phase of the menstrual cycle. Report of the Diagnostic Products Corporation. Los Angeles; 1999.

62. Lousse JC, Donnez J. Laparoscopic observation of spontaneous human ovulation. Fertil Steril 2008;90:833–4.

63. Devoto L, Fuentes A, Kohen P, et al. The human corpus luteum: life cycle and function in natural cycles. Fertil Steril 2009;92:1067–79.

64. Johnson MH, Everitt BJ. Actions of steroid hormones in the adult. In: Essential reproduction. 5th ed. Oxford: Blackwell Science; 2000. p. 133–52 [chapter 8].

65. Kuriyama S. Visual knowledge in classical Chinese medicine. In: Bates D, editor. Knowledge and the scholarly medical traditions, illustrated ed. Cambridge; New York, USA: Cambridge University Press; 1995. p. 205–31, Part 2. [chapter 10].

66. Lu HC. Viscera and bowels (questions 30–47). In: A complete translation of the Yellow Emperor's classics of internal medicine and the difficult classic (Nei-Jing and Nan-Jing). Vancouver: International College of Traditional Chinese Medicine; 2004. p. 606–12 Section four: Difficult classic [Nan Jing]. [chapter 3].

67. Lu HC. Five observations and five effects of viscera. In: A complete translation of the Yellow Emperor's classics of internal medicine and the difficult classic (Nei-Jing and Nan-Jing). Vancouver: International College of Traditional Chinese Medicine; 2004. p. 499–500 Section three: Spiritual pivot [Ling Shu]. [chapter 37].

68. Sun Si-Miao. Prolegomena. In: Wilms S, translator. Bèi Jí Qian Jin Yào Fang. Essential prescriptions worth a thousand in gold for every emergency. Portland: The Chinese Medicine Database; 2007. p. 4–50 [chapter 1: 3 Volumes on Gynecology.

69. Larre C, Schatz J, Rochat de la Vallée E, et al. The body. In: Survey of Traditional Chinese Medicine. 1st ed. Columbia Maryland: Institut Ricci; 1986. p. 107–10, Part 2 [chapter 2].

70. Wiseman N, Feng Y. Grammar. In: Chinese medical Chinese: grammar and vocabulary. Brookline: Paradigm Publications; 2002. p. 1–70 [chapter 1].

71. Lu HC. Natural span of life. In: A complete translation of the Yellow Emperor's classics of internal medicine and the difficult classic (Nei-Jing and Nan-Jing). Vancouver: International College of Traditional Chinese Medicine; 2004. p. 526–9 Section three: Spiritual pivot [Ling Shu] [chapter 54].

72. Unschuld PU, Tessenow H, Jinsheng Z. Discourse on the true [Qi endowed by] Heaven in high antiquity. In: Huang Di Nei Jing Su Wen, vol. 1. Berkeley: University of California Press; 2011. p. 29–44 [chapter 1].

73. Maciocia G. Women's physiology. In: Obstetrics and gynecology in Chinese medicine. 2nd ed. Edinburgh: Elsevier Health Sciences; 2011. p. 7–49 [chapter 2].

74. Larre C, Rochat de la Vallée E. Life cycles. In: Root C, editor. The Kidney. 2nd ed. Norfolk: Biddles; 1989. p. 37–46 Su Wen [chapter 1].

75. Larre C, Schatz J, Rochat de la Vallée E, et al. The breaths. In: Survey of Traditional Chinese Medicine. 1st ed. Columbia Maryland: Institut Ricci; 1986. p. 49–52, Part 1. [chapter 8].

76. Kirkland R. Chinese religion: Taoism. In: Rumbold BD, Puchalski CM, Cobb M, editors. Oxford textbook of spirituality in healthcare. Oxford. Oxford University Press; 2012. p. 19–24 [chapter 3].

77. Kirkland R. Neiye "inner cultivation". In: Pregadio F, editor. The encyclopedia of Taoism. Richmond: Curzon; 2000. p. 771–3.

78. Larre C, Rochat de la Vallee E. Qi. In: Root C, editor. Essence, Spirit, Blood and Qi. Norfolk: Monkey Press; 1999. p. 41-56 [chapter 2].

79. Liu G, Hyodo A. Morphology and function of TCM. In: Fundamentals of acupuncture and moxibustion. Beijing: Huaxia Publishing House; 2006. p. 35–125 [chapter 3].

80. Unschuld PU, Tessenow H, Jinsheng Z. Prolegomena. In: Huang Di Nei Jing Su Wen, vol. 1. Berkeley: University of California Press; 2011. p. 9–25.

81. Unschuld PU, translator and annotator. Transportation holes, the sixty sixth difficult issue. In: Janzen JM, Leslie C, editors. Nan-ching, the classic of difficult issues, medicine in China. London: University of California; 1986. p. 626–9 [chapter 5].

82. Rochat de la Vallee E. Qi in classical texts. In: Root C, editor. A study of Qi. Kings Lynn: Monkey Press; 2006. p. 55–118.

83. Larre C, Schatz J, Rochat de la Vallée E, et al. The differential energies. In: Survey of Traditional Chinese Medicine. 1st ed. Columbia Maryland: Institut Ricci; 1986 Part 2. [chapter 3].

84. Rochat de la Vallee E. The Zhubing Yuanhou Lun. In: Root C, editor. Pregnancy and gestation, in Chinese classical texts. Norfolk: Monkey Press; 2007. p. 28–108.

85. Maciocia G. The vital substances. In: The foundations of Chinese medicine: a comprehensive text for acupuncturists and herbalists. New York: Churchill Livingstone, Edinburgh; 1989. p. 35–57 [chapter 3].

86. Larre C, Rochat de la Vallee E. Xue Blood. In: Root C, editor. Essence, Spirit, Blood and Qi. Norfolk: Monkey Press; 1999. p. 68–75 [chapter 4].

87. Sivin N. Chi, Blood, Ching, and dispersed Bodily Fluids. Traditional medicine in contemporary China, science, medicine and technology in East Asia 2. USA: Center for Chinese Studies, University of Michigan; 1987 Contents of translation. p. 237-47. [chapter 3].

88. Fu Qing-Zhu. Tiao Jing regulating the menses. In: Flaws B, editor. Yang S, Liu D, translators. Fu Qing-Zhu's

gynecology. 2nd ed. Chelsea: Blue Poppy Press; 1992. p. 29–54, Part 1 [chapter 3].

89. Tan Y, Qi C, Zhang Q, et al. Characteristics of female anatomy and physiology. In: Gynecology of Traditional Chinese Medicine, Chinese-English bilingual textbooks for international students of Chinese TCM institutions. China: People's Medical Publishing House; 2007. p. 160–73 [chapter 2].

90. Lu HC. A separate treatise on meridian pulses. In: A complete translation of the Yellow Emperor's classics of internal medicine and the difficult classic (Nei-Jing and Nan-Jing). Vancouver: International College of Traditional Chinese Medicine; 2004. p. 141–3 Section two: Essential questions [Su Wen] [chapter 21].

91. Unschuld PU, Tessenow H, Jinsheng Z. Further discourse on the conduit vessels. In: Huang Di Nei Jing Su Wen, vol. 1. Berkeley: University of California Press; 2011. p. 369–81 [chapter 21].

92. Larre C, Schatz J, Rochat de la Vallée E, et al. The Zang and the Fu. In: Survey of Traditional Chinese Medicine. 1st ed. Columbia Maryland: Institut Ricci; 1986. p. 157–224, Part 2 [chapter 5].

93. Larre C, Rochat de la Vallee E. The origins of Blood and Qi. In: Root C, editor. Essence, Spirit, Blood and Qi. Norfolk: Monkey Press; 1999. p. 109–21 [chapter 8].

94. Liu F. Medical essays. In: The essence of Liu Feng-Wu's gynecology. 1st ed. Boulder: Blue Poppy Press; 1998. p. 21–33 Section 3. Why is it said the Liver is the thief of the Five Viscera and Six Bowels, [chapter 1].

95. Lu HC. Great treatise on Yin Yang classifications of natural phenomena. In: A complete translation of the Yellow Emperor's classics of internal medicine and the difficult classic (Nei-Jing and Nan-Jing). Vancouver: International College of Traditional Chinese Medicine; 2004. p. 86–98 Section two: Essential questions [Su Wen] [chapter 5].

96. Wiseman N, Feng Y. B. A practical dictionary of Chinese medicine. 2nd ed. Brookline, Mass: Paradigm Publications; 1998. p. 14–52.

97. Wu YL. Function and structure in the female body. In: Reproducing women: medicine, metaphor, and childbirth in late Imperial China. Berkeley: University of California Press; 2010. p. 84–119 [chapter 3].

98. Furth C. The development of Fuke in the Song Dynasties. In: A flourishing Yin: gender in China's medical history, 960–1665. California and Los Angeles: University of California Press; 1999. p. 59–93 [chapter 2].

99. Unschuld PU, Tessenow H, Jinsheng Z. Discourse on the true words in the golden chest. In: Huang Di Nei Jing Su Wen, vol. 1. Berkeley: University of California Press; 2011. p. 83–94 [chapter 4].

100. Larre C, Rochat de la Vallee E. Jing. In: Root C, editor. Essence, Spirit, Blood and Qi. Norfolk: Monkey Press; 1999. p. 21–40 [chapter 1].

101. Liu F. Medical essays. In: The Essence of Liu Feng-Wu's gynecology. 1st ed. Boulder: Blue Poppy Press; 1998. p. 13–9 Section 2. A talk on the Kidneys [chapter 1].

102. Larre C, Rochat de la Vallee E. The power to arouse. In: Root C, editor. The kidney. 2nd ed. Norfolk: Biddles; 1989. p. 47–9 Su Wen [chapter 8].

103. Larre C, Rochat de la Vallee E. Su Wen. In: Root C, editor. The Kidney. 2nd ed. Norfolk: Biddles; 1989. p. 51–4 [chapter 9].

104. Unschuld PU, Tessenow H, Jinsheng Z. Comprehensive discourse on phenomena corresponding to Yin Yang. In: Huang Di Nei Jing Su Wen, vol 1. Berkeley: University of California Press; 2011. p. 95–126 [chapter 5].

105. Larre C, Rochat de la Vallee E. Blood and Qi, Spirit and Qi. In: Root C, editor. Essence, Spirit, Blood and Qi. Norfolk: Monkey Press; 1999. p. 121–30 [chapter 9].

106. Sun Si-Miao. Translation. In: Wilms S, translator. Bèi Jí Qian Jin Yào Fang. Essential prescriptions worth a thousand in gold for every emergency, vol. 2. Portland: The Chinese Medicine Database; 2007. p. 52–216 3 Volumes on Gynecology [chapter 2].

107. Lyttleton J. A tale of two clinics – the treatment of infertility with Chinese medicine or Western medicine. In: Treatment of infertility with Chinese medicine. London:

Churchill Livingstone; 2004. p. 1–6 [chapter 1].

108. Maughan TA, Zhai X. The acupuncture treatment of female infertility – with particular reference to egg quality and endometrial receptiveness. The Journal of Chinese Medicine 2012;98:13–21.

109. Larre C, Rochat de la Vallee E. Nan Jing difficulty 36. In: Root C, editor. The Kidney. 2nd ed. Norfolk: Biddles; 1989. p. 9–13.

110. Deadman P. The treatment of male subfertility with acupuncture. J Chin Med 2008;88:5–16.

111. Liu Y. Women's menstrual irregularities are all ascribed to Qi counter flow. In: The Heart transmission of medicine. Boulder: Blue Poppy Press; 1997. p. 168–9 [chapter 69].

112. Sun Si-Miao. Translation. In: Wilms S, translator. Bèi Jí Qian Jin Yào Fang. Essential prescriptions worth a thousand in gold for every emergency, vol. 4. Portland: The Chinese Medicine Database; 2007. p. 404–540 3 Volumes on Gynecology [chapter 4].

113. Furth C. Nourishing life: Ming bodies of generation and longevity. In: A flourishing Yin: gender in China's medical history, 960–1665. California and Los Angeles: University of California Press; 1999. p. 187–223 [chapter 6].

114. Liu F. Medical essays. In: The Essence of Liu Feng-Wu's gynecology. 1st ed. Boulder: Blue Poppy Press; 1998. p. 121–30 Section 10. A preliminary exploration of the treatment of menstrual irregulatory based on Chinese medical pattern discrimination [chapter 1].

115. Unschuld PU, Tessenow H, Jinsheng Z. The generation and completion of the Five depots. In: Huang Di Nei Jing Su Wen, vol. 1. Berkeley: University of California Press; 2011. p. 185–201 [chapter 10].

116. Guicheng X, Zhiwen F. Discussion of the menstrual cycle. The cycle-regulating treatment. The Journal of Chinese Medicine 2001;67:30–3.

117. Stricker R, Eberhart R, Chevailler MC, et al. Establishment of detailed reference values for luteinizing hormone, follicle stimulating hormone, estradiol,

and progesterone during different phases of the menstrual cycle on the abbott ARCHITECT analyzer. Clin Chem Lab Med 2006;44:883–7.

118. Lyttleton J. The menstrual cycle. In: Treatment of infertility with Chinese medicine. London: Churchill Livingstone; 2004. p. 7–46 [chapter 2].

119. Maciocia G. Women's physiology. In: Obstetrics and gynecology in Chinese medicine. New York: Churchill Livingstone; 1998. p. 7–29 [chapter 2].

120. Lian F. TCM treatment of luteal phase defect – an analysis of 60 cases. J Tradit Chin Med 1991;11:115–20.

121. Maciocia G. Yin and Yang. In: The foundations of Chinese medicine: a comprehensive text for acupuncturists and herbalists. Edinburgh, New York: Churchill Livingstone; 1989. p. 1–14 [chapter 1].

122. Sunu K, Lee Y. Original aspects of the Tsang. In: The canon of acupuncture: Huangti Nei Ching chapter 41–50, vol. 2. Korea: Yon Un Publishing; 1985. p. 35–46 [chapter 7].

123. Lu HC. Internal organs as roots and causes. In: A complete translation of the Yellow Emperor's classics of internal medicine and the difficult classic (Nei-Jing and Nan-Jing). Vancouver: International College of Traditional Chinese Medicine; 2004. p. 513–6 Section three: Spiritual pivot [Ling Shu] [chapter 47].

124. Lu HC. On the ultimate truth in the Emperor's golden bookcase. In: A complete translation of the Yellow Emperor's Classics of internal medicine and the difficult classic (Nei-Jing and Nan-Jing). Vancouver: International College of Traditional Chinese Medicine; 2004. p. 82–6 Section two: Essential questions [Su Wen] [chapter 4].

125. Larre C, Rochat de la Vallee E. Nan Jing difficulty 39. In: Root C, editor. The Kidney. 2nd ed. Norfolk: Biddles; 1989. p. 14–7.

126. Unschuld PU. Medical thought during the Ming and Ch'ing Epochs: The individual search for reality. In: Medicine in China: a history of ideas. Berkeley: University of California Press; 1985. p. 189–228 [chapter 8].

127. Unschuld PU, translator and annotator. The depots and the palaces, questions 30–47. In: Janzen JM, Leslie C, editors. Nan-Ching. Medicine in China. The classic of difficult issues. The Chinese medical classics. Berkeley: University of California Press; 1986. p. 341–445 [chapter 3].

128. Bertschinger R. Zang imagery. In: The single idea in the mind of the Yellow Emperor, a primer of Chinese medical texts from the Huangdi Nei Jing. Montacute, Somerset: Tao Booklets; 2008. p. 130–78 [chapter 5].

129. Unschuld PU, Tessenow H, Jinsheng Z. Discourse on the six terms [of a year] and on phenomena [associated with the condition] of the depots. In: Huang Di Nei Jing Su Wen, vol 1. Berkeley: University of California Press; 2011. p. 163–84 [chapter 9].

130. Lu HC. On nine needles. In: A complete translation of the Yellow Emperor's classics of internal medicine and the difficult classic (Nei-Jing and Nan-Jing). Vancouver: International College of Traditional Chinese Medicine; 2004. p. 577–83 Section three: Spiritual pivot [Ling Shu] [chapter 78].

131. Liu F. Medical essays. In: The Essence of Liu Feng-Wu's gynecology. 1st ed. Boulder: Blue Poppy Press; 1998. p. 35–44 Section 4. A discussion of the [saying] Chong and Ren cannot move by themselves [chapter 1].

132. Rochat de la Vallee E. Zang and Fu. In: Root C, editor. The essential women, female health and fertility in Chinese classical texts. Norfolk: Monkey Press; 2007. p. 26–46.

133. Maciocia G. The functions of the Kidney. In: The foundations of Chinese medicine: a comprehensive text for acupuncturists and herbalists. Edinburgh, New York: Churchill Livingstone; 1989. p. 95–101 [chapter 10].

134. Hsu Ta-Ch'un. On [the] fetus and birth. In: Unschuld PU, translator. Forgotten traditions of ancient Chinese medicine: a Chinese view from the eighteenth century: the I-hsüeh Yüan Liu Lun of 1757. Brookline: Paradigm Publications; 1998. p. 140–2 [chapter 15].

135. Larre C, Rochat de la Vallee E. Liver functions and related symptomatology. In: Root C, editor. The Liver. 1st ed. Norfolk: Monkey Press; 1994. p. 106–15.

136. Lu HC. Spirit as the fundamental of needling. In: A complete translation of the Yellow Emperor's Classics of internal medicine and the difficult classic (Nei-Jing and Nan-Jing). Vancouver: International College of Traditional Chinese Medicine; 2004. p. 402–4 Section three: Spiritual pivot [Ling Shu] [chapter 8].

137. Maciocia G. The functions of the Heart. In: The foundations of Chinese medicine: a comprehensive text for acupuncturists and herbalists. Edinburgh, New York: Churchill Livingstone; 1989. p. 71–87 [chapter 6].

138. Kirkland R. Taoism and early Chinese thought. In: Pregadio F, editor. The encyclopedia of Taoism. Richmond: Curzon; 2000. p. 132–4.

139. Kirkland R. Varieties of Taoism in ancient China: a preliminary comparison of themes in the Nei Yeh and other Taoist classics. Available from: http://www. optim.ee/mati/Taoism/ VARIETIES.pdf.

140. Lu HC. Comments on hot diseases. In: A complete translation of the Yellow Emperor's classics of internal medicine and the difficult classic (Nei-Jing and Nan-Jing). Vancouver: International College of Traditional Chinese Medicine; 2004. p. 172–4 Section two: Essential questions [Su Wen] [chapter 33].

141. Li Dong-Yuan. Treaties on the transmutation of vacuity and repletion of the Stomach and Spleen. In: Yang S, Li J, translators. Li Dong-Yuan's treatise on the Spleen and Stomach: a translation of the Pi Wei Lun. Boulder, CO: Blue Poppy Press; 1993. p. 3–9 Section 1 [chapter 1].

142. Larre C, Rochat de la Vallée E. Ren Mai. In: Hill S, editor. The Eight Extraordinary Meridians. Norfolk: Monkey Press; 1997. p. 85–106.

143. Liu F. Book one. Medical essays. The clinical significance of the Spleen and Stomach's upbearing and down bearing. In: The Essence of Liu Feng-Wu's gynecology. 1st ed. Boulder: Blue Poppy Press; 1998. p. 3–12.

144. Lu HC. Five separate channels of the Body Fluids and their blockage. In: A complete translation of the Yellow Emperor's classics of internal medicine and the difficult classic (Nei-Jing and Nan-Jing). Vancouver: International College of Traditional Chinese Medicine; 2004. p. 498 Section three: Spiritual pivot [Ling Shu] [chapter 36].

145. Unschuld PU, Tessenow H, Jinsheng Z. Discourse on how the Qi in depots follow the pattern of the seasons. In: Huang Di Nei Jing Su Wen, vol. 1. Berkeley: University of California Press; 2011. p. 384–400 [chapter 22].

146. Larre L, Rochat de la Valle E. In: Root C, editor. The Lung, revised ed. Norfolk: Monkey Press; 2001. p. 1–85.

147. Maciocia G. The functions of the six Extraordinary Yang organs. In: The foundations of Chinese medicine: a comprehensive text for acupuncturists and herbalists. Edinburgh; New York: Churchill Livingstone; 1989. p. 123–5 [chapter 14].

148. Rochat de la Vallee E. Bao Luo. In: Root C, editor. The essential women, female health and fertility in Chinese classical texts. Norfolk: Monkey Press; 2007. p. 18–25.

149. Larre C, Rochat de la Vallée E. The Bao. In: Root C, editor. The Extraordinary Fu. London: Monkey Press; 2003. p. 159–94.

150. Lu HC. A discerning treatise on five viscera. In: A complete translation of the Yellow Emperor's classics of internal medicine and the difficult classic (Nei-Jing and Nan-Jing). Vancouver: International College of Traditional Chinese Medicine; 2004. p. 111–2 Section two: Essential questions [Su Wen] [chapter 11].

151. Unschuld PU, Tessenow H, Jinsheng Z. Further discourse on the Five depots. In: Huang Di Nei Jing Su Wen, vol. 1. Berkeley: University of California Press; 2011. p. 203–10 [chapter 11].

152. Larre C, Rochat de la Vallée E. Introduction. In: Hill S, editor. The Eight Extraordinary Meridians. Norfolk: Monkey Press; 1997. p. 1–22 [chapter 1].

153. Lu HC. Meridians (questions 23–29). In: A complete translation of the Yellow Emperor's classics of internal medicine and the difficult classic (Nei-Jing and Nan-Jing). Vancouver: International College of Traditional Chinese Medicine; 2004. p. 601–6 Section four: Difficult classic [Nan Jing] [chapter 2].

154. Unschuld PU, translator and annotator. The conduits and vessels. Difficult questions 23–29. In: Janzen JM, Leslie C, editors. Nan-Ching. Medicine in China. The Classic of Difficult Issues, The Chinese Medical Classics. Berkeley: University of California Press; 1986. p. 285–332 [chapter 2].

155. Lu HC. On joint cavities. In: A complete translation of the Yellow Emperor's classics of internal medicine and the difficult classic (Nei-Jing and Nan-Jing). Vancouver: International College of Traditional Chinese Medicine; 2004. p. 231–4 Section two: Essential questions [Su Wen] [chapter 60].

156. Unschuld PU, Tessenow H, Jinsheng Z. Discourse on bone hollows. In: Huang Di Nei Jing Su Wen, vol. 2. Berkeley: University of California Press; 2011. p. 73–88 [chapter 60].

157. Lu HC. Techniques of acupuncture as applied on normal and abnormal energy flow and on flat and thin pulses. In: A complete translation of the Yellow Emperor's classics of internal medicine and the difficult classic (Nei-Jing and Nan-Jing). Vancouver: International College of Traditional Chinese Medicine; 2004. p. 500–2 Section three: Spiritual pivot [Ling Shu] [chapter 38].

158. Lu HC. Pulsating spots and transmission of energy. In: A complete translation of the Yellow Emperor's classics of internal medicine and the difficult classic (Nei-Jing and Nan-Jing). Vancouver: International College of Traditional Chinese Medicine; 2004. p. 539–40 Section three: Spiritual pivot [Ling Shu] [chapter 62].

159. Larre C, Rochat de la Vallée E. Chong Mai. In: Hill S, editor. The Eight Extraordinary Meridians. Norfolk: Monkey Press; 1997. p. 107–32.

160. Lu HC. On the four seas of the human body. In: A complete translation of the Yellow Emperor's classics of internal medicine and the difficult classic (Nei-Jing and Nan-Jing). Vancouver: International College of Traditional Chinese Medicine; 2004. p. 492–4 Section three: Spiritual pivot [Ling Shu] [chapter 33].

161. Lu HC. On paralysis. In: A complete translation of the Yellow Emperor's classics of internal medicine and the difficult classic (Nei-Jing and Nan-Jing). Vancouver: International College of Traditional Chinese Medicine; 2004. p. 196–8 Section two: Essential questions [Su Wen] [chapter 44].

162. Maciocia G. The Eight Extraordinary Vessels (part 2). J Chin Med 1989;30:3–8.

163. Rochat de la Vallee E. The Extraordinary Meridians. In: Root C, editor. The essential women, female health and fertility in Chinese classical texts. Norfolk: Monkey Press; 2007. p. 47–53.

164. Jianghan M. The Extraordinary Channel Chong Mai and its clinical applications. J Chin Med 1993;43:27–31.

165. Larre C, Rochat de la Vallée E. Du Mai. In: Hill S, editor. The Eight Extraordinary Meridians. Norfolk: Monkey Press; 1997. p. 23–84.

166. Deadman P, Al-Khafaji M, Baker K. The Governing Vessel. In: A manual of acupuncture. England: Journal of Chinese Medicine Publications; 1998. p. 527–62.

167. Deadman P, Al-Khafaji M, Baker K. The Kidney channel. In: A manual of acupuncture. England: Journal of Chinese Medicine Publications; 1998. p. 329–64.

168. Lu HC. Separate master meridians. In: A complete translation of the Yellow Emperor's classics of internal medicine and the difficult classic (Nei-Jing and Nan-Jing). Vancouver: International College of Traditional Chinese Medicine; 2004. p. 438–42 Section three: Spiritual pivot [Ling Shu] [chapter 11].

169. Larre C, Rochat de la Vallée E. Dai Mai. In: Hill S, editor. The Eight Extraordinary Meridians. Norfolk: Monkey Press; 1997. p. 133–57.

Chapter | 3 |

The magic of conception

For many of our patients, conception is still possible, for example, while they are waiting for Assisted Reproductive Technology (ART) treatment to begin. They want to understand how to increase their chances of conception by understanding what happens in their body at different stages of conception. They may ask questions, such as what exactly happens during ovulation, when is the fertile window, and when does the embryo implant. This chapter will introduce the reader to key events that happen before, during, and after conception.

The ability to conceive naturally depends on several key components. A woman must ovulate and release a mature egg. Sperm must be ejaculated inside the female reproductive tract through sexual intercourse. Sperm needs to pass through the vagina and uterus and get into the fallopian tubes where it will remain until the egg is ovulated. The egg must then be fertilized by a single spermatozoon and, while dividing, travel down the fallopian tube and into the uterus where it must implant.

Other factors that affect the chances of conception are the maternal uterine environment, correct hormonal balance, and practical aspects, such as sexual intercourse. This chapter discusses each of these elements in greater detail.

It also examines what Traditional Chinese Medicine (TCM) views as key components of conception.

SEXUAL INTERCOURSE

Sexual intercourse (also known as coitus – a coming together) is required for unassisted conception to happen. Couples often refer to intercourse as 'baby dancing' or 'BD'. Sperm needs to be inseminated inside the vagina. From there it will travel through the uterus and into the fallopian tubes where it will fertilize the egg. Several models of human

sexual response exist, but most models describe four main stages:

- Desire, excitation, and arousal
- Plateau
- Orgasm
- Resolution

During the initial stage of desire, excitation, and arousal, genital tissues become engorged with blood, resulting in an erection of the penis in men and of the clitoris and labia in women.[1] Engorgement causes lubricating fluids (also known as *mucus*) to ooze through the skin, more so in women (partly from the vagina and partly from the cervix). Men also contribute a small amount of mucus. Inadequate amounts of these fluids will lead to painful intercourse, which may inhibit the potential for orgasm.

Sexual arousal is enhanced by direct physical contact, such as kissing and rubbing.[1] Some authors argue that higher levels of arousal are better for conception.[2] Anticipation of pain or discomfort, tension, or stress may reduce the level of sexual excitement and, therefore, affect sexual arousal. Although having frequent intercourse during the fertile window can help increase the odds of conception, both partners may find it too stressful to be able to 'perform on demand'. This may result in erection issues in men and lack of lubrication in women.[1]

The period of excitement and arousal can last just a few seconds or many minutes. During the late stages of arousal, the distal third of the vagina swells and grips the penis tightly. This helps to stimulate the penis more strongly and orgasm usually follows although not always and not necessarily simultaneously in both partners.[1]

Men usually ejaculate during orgasm. Both men and women usually experience several rhythmic muscular contractions during orgasm. Some experts[3,4] believe that these contractions in women may help to propel sperm quickly into the uterus and inside the fallopian tubes. However, as Levin has noted, this opinion is based on only three anecdotal cases.[2]

After an orgasm, a couple usually remain motionless. Leaving the penis inside the vagina until it becomes flaccid (between 5 and 10 min) helps with the painless withdrawal of the penis.[2]

SPERM TRANSPORTATION UP THE FEMALE REPRODUCTIVE TRACT

The journey sperm makes up the female reproductive tract is tough. Out of 300–500 million ejaculated spermatozoa, less than 1% reach the egg.[5] First, sperm has to survive the mechanical stress of the ejaculation process (estimated to happen at 28 miles/h)[6] and the biochemical hazard of oxidative stress as it passes through many defensive mechanisms in the female reproductive tract. After ejaculation, sperm pools in the anterior vagina near the cervical os (opening of the uterus). The physiological benefit of being deposited here is that it can quickly escape (within minutes) the tough environment of the vagina, which protects the reproductive tract from the outside influences, such as infection.[7]

Within a minute of being ejaculated, the semen forms a gel (coagulates). Coagulation serves to hold sperm by the cervical os and may have a protective function against the harsh environment of the vagina.[7] On average, only 65% of sperm enter the cervical mucus. In a study done by Baker and Bellis, they observed that 35% of sperm are lost through *flowback* into the vagina. This happens approximately 30 min after coitus. This flowback was observed in 94% of copulations. However, in 12% of copulations, almost 100% of sperm were lost. Female orgasm between 1 min before ejaculation and up to 45 min after increases sperm retention.[8]

Once in the cervix, sperm mixes with cervical mucus. Cervical mucus composition changes throughout the menstrual cycle. During the most fertile time of the cycle, the mucus is most hydrated and is more than 96% water. The structure of cervical mucus helps to filter out normal and abnormal sperm as well as assist sperm in transportation. The female immune system mounts an immune response to the presence of sperm, stimulating migration of leukocytes (mainly neutrophils and macrophages). However, these leukocytes take time to build up and do not form a significant barrier to sperm transportation unless the females become immunized against sperm and form anti-sperm antibodies. In these cases, neutrophils will bind to sperm and destroy it. Immunoglobulins (IgG and IgA) are also secreted in cervical mucus to fight bacteria.[7]

It is interesting to note that vaginal, cervical, and uterine contractions often present in the pre-orgasmic and orgasmic phases are not actually required for effective sperm transport although they may potentially assist it.[9] Spermatozoa are transported mostly via their own activity.[2,9]

From the cervix, sperm travels upward through the uterus toward the fallopian tubes. Sperm is estimated to swim through the uterus at a speed of 5 mm/min. As the uterus is only a few centimetres in length, it would take around 10 min for sperm to reach the fallopian tubes.[10] Uterine smooth muscle contractions aid sperm movement. In one study, sperm was found in the fallopian tubes just 5 min after insemination.[11] However, these findings are dismissed by most authors because the women in this study were anaesthetized, not sexually aroused, and the semen was pre-incubated and placed directly into the cervical os. Another study showed that it can take up to 1 h for sperm to reach the tubes.[12] The longer transit time in this study might have been caused by uterine abnormalities, such as fibroids, polyps, and endometriosis whilst shorter times in other studies do not necessarily mean fertilization is possible because the physical stress of going too quickly through the tubes may possibly cause damage to sperm.[7] Although some sperm have been found in the cervix 5 days after insemination, it is unlikely that many sperm would be able to reach the fallopian tubes 24 h after ejaculation.[7]

The entrance to the fallopian tubes at the uterotubal junction is narrow but fairly easy for sperm to pass through.[7] The fallopian tubes contain viscous mucus, but, unlike the vagina, cervix, and uterus, the fallopian tubes are fairly safe for sperm because the tubes do not mount an immunological defence. The fallopian tubes are believed to act as storage for sperm and help to maintain the potency of sperm until ovulation. When in the fallopian tubes, the sperm bind to the epithelium lining. This process has been shown to be disrupted in women with endometriosis.[13] The fallopian tube mucus and epithelial binding help to slow down sperm progression toward the ampulla part of the fallopian tubes, thus reducing the chance of polyspermic fertilization (where the egg is fertilized abnormally by more than one sperm).[7]

PREFERTILIZATION SPERM CHANGES

In order to fertilize the egg, sperm undergo two changes: *capacitation* and *hyperactivation* (hypermobility).[7,14] Capacitation, possibly the greatest discovery in ART, was discovered in 1951 by Chang and Austin; it is a process in which a sperm sheds its major protein coating. This protein facilitates a sperm's movement through the cervical mucus and helps it bind to the epithelium of the fallopian tubes.[14] In 1969, when Robert Edwards and his colleagues reported successful *in vitro* maturation and fertilization of human oocytes, they attributed their success to the capacitation research done by Chang and Austin.[15] Capacitation is believed to happen in the fallopian tubes.

Once the protein coat is shed, sperm unbind from the fallopian tube epithelium and move toward the egg. This stage is facilitated by sperm hyperactivation, the process where the velocity of sperm increases;[14] this process involves a change in the flagellar (tail) beating.[7] Capacitation and hyperactivation are believed to be triggered by chemical and hormonal signals released by the pre-ovulatory follicle. Hyperactivation is also thought to help sperm penetrate the zona pellucida.[7]

When sperm reach the egg, they undergo the acrosome reaction. This is where the spermatozoa plasma membrane and the outer acrosomal membrane breakdown and merge, the change that is required for the egg and sperm to fuse.[14] The acrosome reaction is triggered by sperm binding to the outer shell of the egg, the zona.[16]

In summary, after insemination in the vagina, sperm move as quickly as possible through the cervix and uterus and bind to the epithelial lining of the fallopian tubes. Out of 300–500 million ejaculated sperm, fewer than 1% reach the egg.[5] Here sperm wait for a signal that the egg is about to be ovulated (sometimes as long as 5 days), at which point spermatozoa unbind from the epithelium of the fallopian tubes, undergo chemical changes, and move toward the ampulla part of the fallopian tube where they attempt to fertilize the egg.

INTERESTING FACTS

TRANSPORTATION OF SPERM IN THE FEMALE REPRODUCTIVE TRACT

- Sperm is ejaculated at 28 miles/h.[6]
- Fewer than 1% of ejaculated sperm reach the egg.[5]
- Semen is made up of spermatozoa and seminal plasma. Plasma provides transport medium and nutrition to ejaculated spermatozoa.[17]

EGG MATURATION AND OVULATION

As already discussed in Chapter 2, approximately 36 h before ovulation (when the follicle is approximately 18 mm[18] in diameter), luteinizing hormone (LH) peaks. This happens as a result of raised oestrogen levels, which stimulate the hypothalamus to release more gonadotropic releasing hormone (GnRH) and the anterior pituitary gland to produce more LH. GnRH promotes the release of follicle-stimulating hormone (FSH) and more LH by the anterior pituitary.[1]

The majority of home ovulation detection kits detect raised LH levels in the urine; this is an indication that the woman is about to ovulate. If progesterone is present at the same time, the delicate hormonal balance necessary for ovulation will be disrupted;[1] this is how many hormonal contraceptive pills work.

The high levels of LH trigger continuation of the *first meiotic division* of the egg (oocyte).[19] When *meiosis I* is completed, the oocyte will have two cells: a bigger one (the secondary oocyte), which has most of the cytoplasm, and a smaller one (the polar body) consisting of a nucleus. Meiosis II of the secondary oocyte follows immediately after meiosis I is completed, but the oocyte arrests in the *metaphase* and will remain in this phase until fertilization.[19] At this stage, the egg is considered to be mature. The follicle then ruptures, and the egg is released. This is called ovulation, and, for many women, this occurs on day 14 in a 28-day cycle.[1] Meiosis II is completed once the egg is fertilized.

The remainder of the ruptured follicle collapses and, under the influence of LH, becomes luteinized. It is now referred to as the *corpus luteum*. The main function of corpus luteum is to produce progesterone, oestrogen, relaxin, and inhibin.[1] These hormones are necessary for the uterine lining to be maintained and, if fertilization occurs, to support the embryo. The lifespan of the corpus luteum is 2 weeks, at which point it degenerates into a *corpus albicans*.[1] However, if fertilization has occurred, the embryo will start to produce Human Chorionic Gonadotropin (hCG) hormone, and this rescues the corpus luteum, which in turn continues producing hCG until approximately 10 weeks' gestation when the placenta takes over hCG production.

EGG FERTILIZATION

It could be argued that the most important event in reproduction is when the egg and sperm fuse, the process referred to as fertilization. The first demonstration of fertilization was done in 1875 in Germany by Wilhelm August Oscar Hertwig, who demonstrated the fusion of a sea urchin's sperm and egg.[14] However, it was only following the development of *in vitro* fertilization that more was learned about what happens during fertilization.

The egg can be fertilized within 12–24 h after ovulation *in vivo* (in the body)[5,14] and up to 36 h *in vitro* (in the laboratory dish).[14] It is estimated that sperm maintains its capacity to fertilize the egg for 48–72 h after insemination.[14]

When an egg is ovulated, it is carried by the fluid currents toward the fimbriae part of the fallopian tube. The fimbriae move towards and sweep over the ovary in order to pick up the egg. The fimbriae initiate the movement of the egg into the tube. Once the egg enters the tube (approximately 15–20 min after ovulation), its movement toward the ampullary–isthmic junction of the tube is facilitated by the presence of many cilia in the ampulla part of the tube.[14] Once in the fallopian tube, the egg might be fertilized by sperm already waiting for it.

The egg is surrounded by the *zona pellucida* (a transparent shell). This shell has chemicals that are recognized by the spermatozoon of the same species, thus preventing cross species reproduction.[19] The spermatozoon binds to the zona pellucida for approximately 1 min and then penetrates it. The penetration involves a physical thrust of the tail and rapid lateral oscillations of the head. Fertilization takes place near the ampullary–isthmic junction.[20]

As already discussed in Chapter 2, when the egg is penetrated by a spermatozoon, the egg is activated, and meiosis II is completed (approximately 3 h later).[14] At the end of this stage, two further cells are formed: a bigger cell that has most of the cytoplasm and the second polar body. Now the egg cell and the sperm cell (each carrying 23 chromosomes) can fuse.[19] Fusion of the egg and sperm results in the formation of a *zygote*,[21] from Greek meaning *joined*. This is the earliest developmental stage of the embryo, and it contains the DNA of both parents. The zygote phase ends when the egg and sperm pronuclei merge together.[5,22] Once the egg is fertilized, the zona pellucida becomes impervious to other sperm.[5,14] Once meiosis II is completed, the second polar body is released, and the now fertilized egg contains 46 chromosomes, 23 from the sperm and 23 from the egg. The newly formed embryo has two cells, and it is now ready to migrate down the fallopian tube and continue dividing.

TRANSPORTATION OF THE EMBRYO DOWN THE FEMALE REPRODUCTIVE TRACT

After ovulation, the egg is inside the fallopian tube within 15–20 min[14] where it is fertilized; the fertilized egg takes approximately 3.5 days[23] or 80 h[14] to travel through the fallopian tube before it enters the uterus. It is aided by ciliary beating, smooth muscle contractions, and tubal mucus.[24] Ninety percent of this time is spent near the junction of the ampulla and the isthmus of the tube where fertilization is believed to take place.[14]

There is evidence that the embryo is able to slow down its transportation from 133 μm/s (prefertilization) to 46 μm/s (postfertilization). This helps the embryo start its communication with its mother. The characteristics of the fallopian tube containing a fertilized egg are different from the physiology of the tube on the opposite side of the body, suggesting that the embryo triggers a reaction in the tube that ensures the embryo's optimal microenvironment and nutrition during the first 24–48 h after fertilization.[23] A small proportion of embryos implant in the fallopian tube, resulting in an ectopic pregnancy. This type of pregnancy is not viable and is potentially life threatening, often resulting in surgical removal of the damaged tube (see Chapter 12 for more detailed information on ectopic pregnancies).

As the embryo moves down the tube, its cells (blastomeres) divide very rapidly, 18 h for each cell. This speed of division is only comparable to tumour cells or to regenerating somatic

tissue.[22] Blastomeres are totipotent, meaning that until the embryo has four to eight cells (usually 2–3 days after fertilization), blastomeres are not destined to grow into any particular tissue. Animal studies show that, during this phase, an embryo can be split into two, each part potentially capable of growing into a separate viable offspring.[22]

This is one of the methods of cloning that would result in monozygotic (identical) twins. Other methods of cloning exist, for example, where a nucleus is transferred from donor cell into an egg that has no nucleus, resulting in an identical genetic copy of the first cell. Any method of tissue cloning for the purpose of reproduction is highly controversial, and, so far, all cloned embryos have been destroyed before 14 days development.

COMPARISON OF NATURAL FERTILIZATION (*IN VIVO*) WITH ART FERTILIZATION (*IN VITRO*)

The main differences between a natural cycle and ART treatment cycle are outlined in Table 3.1.

EMBRYOGENESIS

Embryogenesis refers to the process of embryo development, starting from the moment the egg and sperm fuse (fertilization) to approximately 8 weeks after fertilization. From this point on, the embryo is referred to as a foetus.

When a sperm penetrates the egg, embryogenesis begins with the formation of a one cell **zygote** (Figure 3.1), which is defined as an embryo because it contains a full set of chromosomes. When the pronuclei of the egg and sperm merge, a two-celled embryo is created and is no longer called a zygote. This two-celled embryo continues dividing, a process called **cleavage**.

The first division of the zygote begins 24 h after fertilization and completes 30 h after fertilization.[5] By the end of the second day after fertilization, an embryo is expected to have four cells.[25] By the end of day 3, there will be around eight cells.[25] When the embryo has divided into 8 cells, it starts the process of **compaction** (where cells bind very tightly together), and the embryo enters the **morula** stage with 32 cells[22] approximately 4 days after fertilization.[5] Throughout this time, the embryo travels down the fallopian tube. Over the next 24 h, **cavitation** occurs, where an outer cell layer (**trophectoderm**) begins to pump fluid inside the embryo. This is the first time that the embryo not only keeps dividing into further cells (40–150 cells) but also starts to expand. This phase is called the **blastocyst** stage, and the embryo will have now reached the uterus. The blastocyst is made of a *trophoblast* (an outer layer of cells that becomes the placenta), an *inner cell mass* (most of which develops into the embryo), and a *blastocoele* (hollow space).[5]

Table 3.1 Comparison of natural and artificial ovulation and fertilization

Stage	Natural cycle (*in vivo*)	ART cycle (*in vitro*)
Follicular phase	Only enough FSH is secreted for 1 out of about 20 follicles to develop	A high dose of FSH is injected daily, allowing for more than one follicle to develop
Ovulation and fertilization	Ovulation is triggered by a raised LH level. An egg is picked up by the fallopian tube, and it travels into the ampulla part of the tube where it is fertilized by sperm deposited earlier	Ovulation is triggered by injecting hCG hormone (which is similar in action to LH). Eggs are retrieved surgically 36 h later In the meantime, sperm is provided by a male partner who masturbates and ejaculates into a container. Alternatively, previously frozen or donor sperm can be used The retrieved eggs are fertilized by one of the following two methods: • *In Vitro* Fertilization (IVF): Eggs are placed in a Petri dish with 50,000–100,000 sperm • Intracytoplasmic Sperm Insemination (ICSI): One spermatozoon is injected directly into the egg
Postfertilization stage	The fertilized egg travels down the fallopian tube while undergoing division; it enters the uterus approximately 3.5 days later and attempts to implant after day 5	Fertilized eggs are left in the laboratory to divide. Embryo(s) can be transferred into the uterus on days 2, 3 or 5 postfertilization where they may then implant

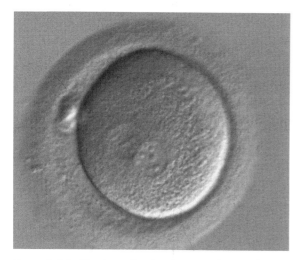

Figure 3.1 Fertilized egg showing two pronuclei.
Courtesy of Mr A. Gorgy at The Fertility and Gynaecology Academy and City Fertility, London, UK.

Eventually, the embryo can no longer expand within the zona pellucida (its shell) and it **hatches**, usually on day 6 or 7 postfertilization[22] or 72 h after the embryo enters the uterus.[26] The implantation stage begins. All of these stages are sometimes referred to as the **conceptus** stage.[21] Table 3.2 and Figures 3.2 and 3.3 summarize different stages of embryo development.

INTERESTING FACTS

OVULATION AND FERTILIZATION

♦ LH surge occurs at approximately 3 am, beginning between midnight and 8 am in two-thirds of women.[27]

♦ Ovulation happens mostly in the morning in spring (50% of women ovulate between midnight and 11 am) and in the evening during autumn and winter (90% of women will ovulate between 4 and 7 pm).[28]

♦ Ovulating from the right ovary is more frequent (55% of ovulations) and more likely to result in conception.[29]

♦ Younger women often ovulate from alternate ovaries. Women over the age of 30 ovulate more frequently from the same ovary. A contralateral pattern of ovulation is more likely to result in pregnancy.[30]

♦ A fallopian tube can pick up the egg released by the ovary on the contralateral side.[14]

♦ A woman is more likely to ovulate the more nights she spends sleeping next to a man. One study found that 92% of women who slept next to a man for more than one night in a 40-day period ovulated, compared to 56% of women who slept next to a man for a day or less in a 40-day period.[31] Perhaps this presents an example of the TCM theory on the interaction of Yin and Yang, where one depends on another (female being Yin and male being Yang).

Table 3.2 Summary of embryo development stages

Stage	Developmental term	Days/weeks postfertilization
Early embryo stage (sometimes referred to as conceptus stage)	Embryo-zygote (1 cell)[5]	Fertilization day
	Embryo (2–4 cells)[5,22]	Day 2
	Embryo (6–10 cells)[22]	Day 3
	Embryo-compaction/morula stage (up to 32 cells)[5]	Day 4
	Embryo-blastocyst stage (40–150 cells)[5]	Day 5
	Embryo-hatching blastocyst	Day 6
Embryo stage	Embryo	From day 1 postfertilization until week 8 postfertilization (10 weeks' gestation)
Foetal stage	Foetus	From 8 weeks postfertilization (10 weeks' gestation) until birth

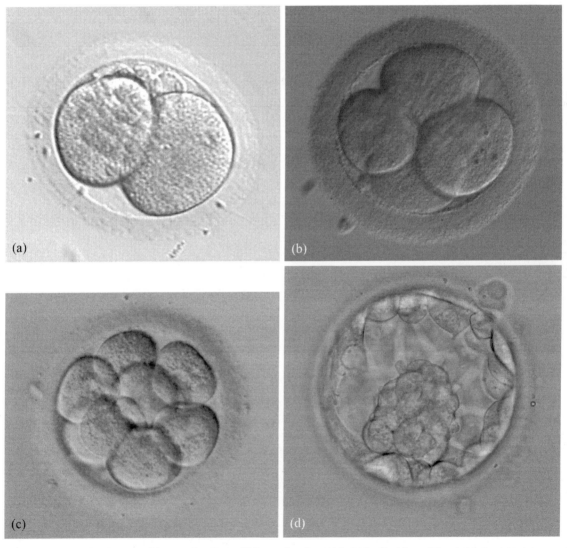

Figure 3.2 Embryo development: (a) two-cell embryo; (b) four-cell embryo; (c) eight-cell embryo; (d) early blastocyst;

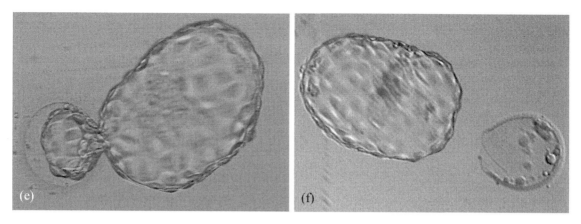

Figure 3.2—cont'd (e) hatching blastocyst; (f) hatched blastocyst.
Images (b) and (e) courtesy of Mr A. Gorgy at The Fertility and Gynaecology Academy and City Fertility, London, UK. Image (d) courtesy of Mr R. Mathur and Mr S. Harbottle at Cambridge IVF, Cambridge, UK.

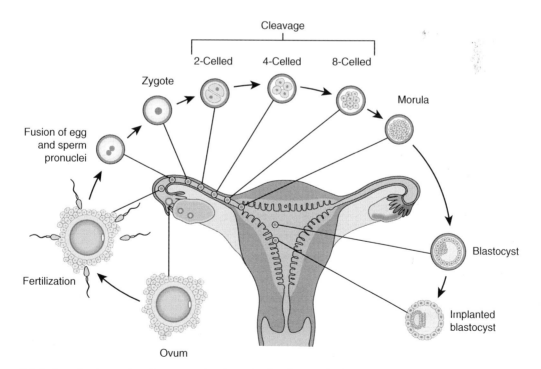

Figure 3.3 Embryo development and transportation down the female reproductive tract.

IMPLANTATION: THE FIRST COMMUNICATION BETWEEN THE MOTHER AND HER EMBRYO

Implantation is the process whereby the blastocyst attaches itself to the endometrium, and it also results in the formation of the placenta. This is an essential step in reproduction.

Implantation window

The blastocyst is only able to implant when the endometrial surface is receptive to the embryo. This phase is referred to as an 'implantation window'. The endometrium is receptive to the embryo for less than 48 h, but the exact cycle days vary in different women and in different cycle types, for example:[32]

- In natural cycles, 6–8 days post-LH surge (approximately 5–7 days postovulation)
- In controlled ovarian stimulation cycles (such as IVF), 4–8 days post-egg retrieval

Implantation is complete when the embryo begins to secrete hCG, usually on days 8, 9, or 10 after fertilization but can be as early as day 6 and as late as 12 days after fertilization.[33] Late implantation is linked to increased risk of pregnancy loss, with no clinical pregnancies recognized if implantation happens more than 12 days postovulation.[33] Pregnancy is more likely to succeed if implantation happens by day 9 postfertilization.[33]

Process of implantation

Implantation is a complicated process involving complex communication between the blastocyst and uterus, resulting in extensive biological changes.[34]

On entering the uterus, the embryo positions itself in either the posterior portion of the fundus or the body of the uterus[5] with its inner cell mass facing the endometrial lining. It then dissolves its zona pellucida (i.e., hatches).[5,35] Hatching is estimated to happen around 72 h after the embryo enters the uterus.[26] The embryo is now ready to implant.

Hoozemans et al. describe the basic steps of implantation as follows:[36]

- Apposition
- Attachment
- Invasion

Apposition is where the embryo begins to form a very loose and unstable connection with the uterine wall.[26]

Then the embryo begins to attach to the endometrium, and the connection becomes more stable.[26] Attachment creates changes in the endometrium, which initiates the development of the maternal component of the placenta.[37]

A brief period of stable attachment is followed by a longer phase where trophoblasts invade the uterus. By day 10 postconception, the blastocyst is completely covered by uterine epithelium.[26] With the formation and invasion of the decidua, the implantation process is complete. As a result, there is a physical hold and a nutritional source of decidual yolk, and the basis of placental development is established, thus enabling an initiation of adjacent circulations and exchange of nutrients.[37]

Figure 3.4 summarizes the steps involved in implantation.

Embryo–maternal interaction

The embryo starts to communicate with its mother as early as 2 days postfertilization by triggering Early Pregnancy Factor (EPF) secretions.[38] The embryo is made of maternal and paternal DNA. Immunomodulation is necessary in order for the maternal immune system not to reject the embryo.[36] EPF is one example of the many immunosuppressant agents involved in immunomodulation of implantation.[36]

Once implanted, in order to survive, the embryo needs to signal its presence to its mother[39] and change her reproductive status to pregnant. hCG is secreted by the embryo to extend the functioning of the corpus luteum. The extended secretion of progesterone by the corpus luteum is believed to be fundamental for sustaining pregnancy.[26,40]

The embryo engages with its mother through short-range and long-range interaction.[39] Short-range interaction is the physical and nutritional contact of the embryo with the endometrium. This ensures that the embryo receives the nutrition it requires in order to grow.[39]

Long-range interaction is where the embryo signals its existence to the Hypothalamic–Pituitary–Ovarian Axis. This signal ensures that the embryo is acknowledged and, thus, prevents luteal regression. The embryo's tasks are to alter the reproductive system and create and maintain a progesterone-predominant environment. Pregnancy is said to occur when the 'embryo has signalled its presence successfully' to its mother.[39]

Factors affecting implantation

Implantation in humans is poorly understood and remains a major challenge in ART treatment.[41] As many as 22–60%[42,43] of pregnancies fail between fertilization and the clinically recognizable pregnancy stage.

Any issues with egg maturation may result in impaired implantation or early pregnancy loss. Research shows that, among other factors, maternal age, uterine environment, and embryo quality may affect implantation.[44] In ART, a considerable proportion of implantation failures is ascribed to the embryo.[34] Therefore, in acupuncture practice, it is important to treat patients preconceptually to optimize egg and sperm quality. Chapter 12 provides more detailed information on implantation failure.

Figure 3.4 The process of implantation of an embryo: (a) the blastocyst moves close to the uterine lining; (b) the trophoblast penetrates the epithelium and begins to invade the stroma; (c) the blastocyst sinks further into the stroma; the amniotic cavity appears; (d) the uterine tissue grows over the implanted embryo (deciduoma response).
Reprinted from Jones R, Lopez K. Pregnancy. In: Human reproductive biology, 3rd ed., p. 253–96; 2006 [chapter 10], with permission from Elsevier.

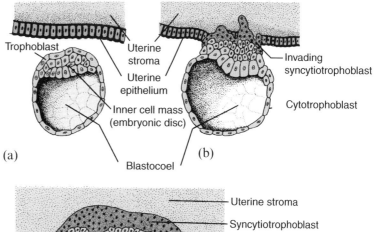

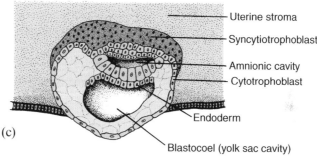

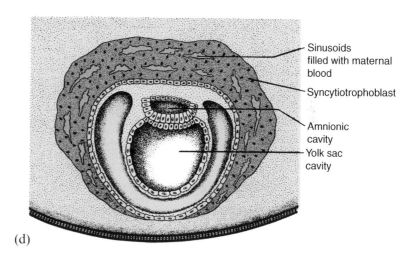

CONCEPTION FROM THE TCM POINT OF VIEW

Natural conception

Classical Chinese literature

In classical Chinese literature, Water is considered to be the source and power of life and conception. Water is everywhere. 'It collects in the Heavens and on Earth'[45] and is stored and gathered in all forms of life. Water is Jing (Essence), Blood, and Qi.

> *'When the vital Essence and vital force of male and female unite, Water passes between them and assumes form'.*[45]

Conception is described as.

> *'The Dao gives birth to the one, the one gives birth to two, two gives birth to three, three gives birth to the ten thousand things'.*[46]

'As both fine spirits are drawn to each other, they unite and fit together to complete the human form. This precedes the life of the physical body. This is the function of the Essences'.[47]

'When two spirits struggle against each other and meet together to form physical shape a fetus will come into existence. The energy responsible for this formation is called pure energy (Essence)'.[48]

Traditional Chinese Medicine

The creation of an embryo in TCM can be described as transformation. For example, Water assumes form and new life begins, or male and female Jing (Essences) unite and transform to create a human being.[45,47,48]

TCM also discusses Mingmen (the Fire of Life) as essential for conception (see Chapter 2). Mingmen (the Fire of Life) is created by Water[49] and is regulated by the Kidneys.[49] The embryo is created through Jing (Essence) of the Kidneys and Mingmen (the Fire of Life).[49]

Mingmen (the Fire of Life) is housed by the Gate of Life, which is housed by the Kidney (see Chapter 2). It is associated with the origin of life and is therefore essential for conception.

Conception in IVF or by ICSI from the TCM point of view

In IVF, fertilization occurs outside the body (in the laboratory dish), resulting from the combination of the sperm and egg Jing (Essences) (Figure 3.5).

As discussed in Chapter 2, the egg and sperm are Kidney Jing (Essence) and are influenced by Blood and Qi. Fertilization and the resulting embryo is a consequence of combining Kidney Jing (Essences).[47–51]

The physiology of fertilization, according to the Yin Yang classification of IVF, involves the male sperm (Yang) fertilizing the female egg (Yin). The egg (Yin) is the foundation for fertilization, and the sperm (Yang) is the instigator. This is not so dissimilar from a concept in classical Chinese medicine where life begins in Yin.

'At first the embryo is brought into being by a combination of two energies called Yin and Yang'.[51]

'The fetus is created by the interaction and mutual stimulation of Yin [female] and Yang [male]'.[52]

'Yin and Yang blend in harmony, the two qi respond to each other, and yang bestows and yin transforms'.[53]

The embryo's energy (Pre-Natal Qi)

Larre *et al.* discuss TCM physiology before birth, in other words, the physiology of the embryo and foetus.[54] The embryo is said to be made up of four Qi (Figure 3.6) although it is important to remember that the four aspects operate in unity and are not separate entities.

- Yuan (Original) Qi
- Kidney Jing (Essence)
- Zhen (True) Qi
- Shen (Spirit)

The prefertilization Qi of the male and the female combine to produce the Qi of the resulting embryo.[54] In other words, the embryo is a direct expression of its parents' Qi.

Yuan (Original) Qi

The sperm and egg at the time of fertilization transmit Yuan (Original) Qi. It is the original supply of Yang and Yin of the embryo. Yuan (Original) Qi initiates and facilitates

Figure 3.5 Conjectural overview of fertilization by IVF from the TCM point of view.

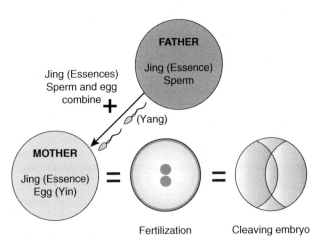

Jing (Essences) Sperm and egg combine

FATHER
Jing (Essence) Sperm

(Yang)

MOTHER
Jing (Essence) Egg (Yin)

Fertilization   Cleaving embryo

Figure 3.6 The embryo's Qi.

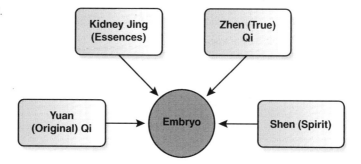

the development of the embryo and remains the source of life of the person,[54] from the embryonic state (*in vivo* or *in vitro*) and throughout adulthood.

Pre-Natal Jing (Essence)

Kidney Jing (Essence) creates and nourishes[55] the embryo. The embryo is derived from the parents' reproductive organs. Kidney Jing (Essence) of the parents unite to become the embryo. The father and mother pass on their Jing (Essence) at the time of fertilization. The grading of the embryo for the purposes of ART (see Chapter 6) and the way it divides depends on the parents' state of health and their Jing (Essence).

Zhen (True) Qi

The correspondence between Heaven and Earth[56,57] is Zhen (True) Qi. Zhen (True) Qi resembles and represents natural order,[57] the law of nature, and transformation of Qi.[58] Zhen (True) Qi initiates the possibility of conception[57] along with the parents.

Shen (Spirit)

Shen (Spirit) is responsible for the vitality of the embryo and lays the earliest foundation for the character of the newly conceived individual.[54]

SUMMARY

Both Orthodox and Chinese medicines recognize that natural conception is a complex process involving several key components. These components are:

- Sexual intercourse (coitus)
- A healthy sperm
- A healthy egg
- Ability of sperm to fertilize the egg
- Free passage of sperm and egg in the female reproductive tract
- Uterine environment receptive to the embryo
- Properly regulated hormonal balance and the menstrual cycle

The quality of the embryo greatly influences the chances of successful conception. Parental energy influences the quality and potential of embryonic development and, hence, greatly influences the success of IVF treatment. Therefore, in order to optimize their reproductive health, it is essential to assess and treat both parents' Kidney Yin and Yang, Blood, and Qi during the preconceptual phase.

ACKNOWLEDGEMENT

Energies discussed at the time of conception – the type, nature, and physiology – have been further developed via personal communications and courtesy of Elisabeth Rochat de la Vallée. This concept and adaptation is somewhat different to earlier works by the authors, which are stipulated in Survey of Traditional Chinese Medicine 1986.[54]

REFERENCES

1. Tortora GJ, Grabowski SR. The reproductive systems. In: Principles of anatomy and physiology. 9th ed. New York, Chichester: John Wiley & Sons Inc.; 2000. p. 974–1021 [chapter 28].

2. Levin RJ. Sexual arousal – its physiological roles in human reproduction. Annu Rev Sex Res 2005;16:154–89.

3. Fox CA, Wolff HS, Baker JA. Measurement of intra-vaginal and intra-uterine pressures during human coitus by radio-telemetry. J Reprod Fertil 1970;22:243–51.

4. Beck JR. How do the spermatozoa enter the uterus? Am J Obstet 1874;7:350–91.

5. Tortora GJ, Grabowski SR. Development and inheritance. In: Principles of anatomy and physiology. 9th ed. New York, Chichester: John Wiley & Sons Inc.; 2000. p. 974–1021 [chapter 29].

6. West Z. A man's fertility. In: Zita West's guide to fertility and assisted conception: essential advice on preparing your body for IVF and other fertility treatments. London: Vermilion; 2010. p. 55–72 [chapter 3].

7. Suarez SS, Pacey AA. Sperm transport in the female reproductive tract. Hum Reprod Update 2006;12:23–37.

8. Baker RR, Bellis MA. Human sperm competition: ejaculate manipulation by females and a function for the female orgasm. Anim Behav 1993;46:887–909.

9. Johnson MH. Sperm and eggs. In: Essential reproduction. 7th ed. Chichester, West Sussex: John Wiley & Sons; 2012. p. 176–88 [chapter 10].

10. Mortimer ST, Swan MA. Variable kinematics of capacitating human spermatozoa. Hum Reprod 1995;10:3178–82.

11. Settlage DS, Motoshima M, Tredway DR. Sperm transport from the external cervical os to the fallopian tubes in women: a time and quantitation study. Fertil Steril 1973;24:655–61.

12. Rybenstein BB, Strauss H, Lazarus ML, et al. Sperm survival in women; motile sperm in fundus and tubes of surgical cases. Fertil Steril 1951;2:15–9.

13. Reeve L, Lashen H, Pacey AA. Endometriosis affects sperm-endosalpingeal interactions. Hum Reprod 2005;20:448–51.

14. Speroff L, Fritz MA. Sperm and egg transport, fertilization, and implantation. In: Clinical gynecologic endocrinology and infertility. 7th ed. Philadelphia: Lippincott Williams & Wilkins; 2005. p. 159–233 [chapter 7].

15. Edwards RG. An astonishing journey into reproductive genetics since the 1950's. Reprod Nutr Dev 2005;45:299–306.

16. Natali A, Turek PJ. An assessment of new sperm tests for male infertility. Urology 2011;77:1027–34.

17. Johnson MH, Everitt BJ. Coitus and fertilisation. In: Essential reproduction. 5th ed. Oxford: Blackwell Science; 2000. p. 153–71 [chapter 9].

18. Diagnostic Products Corporation. Hormonal levels during the early follicular phase of the menstrual cycle. Report of the Diagnostic Products Corporation, Los Angeles; 1999.

19. Vergouw C. Egg cells. In: de Haan N, Spelt M, Gobel R, editors. Reproductive medicine: a textbook for paramedics. Amsterdam: Elsevier Gezondheidszorg; 2010. p. 73–8 [chapter 4].

20. Croxatto HB. Physiology of gamete and embryo transport through the fallopian tube. Reprod Biomed Online 2002;4:160–9.

21. Shenfield F, Pennings G, Sureau C, et al. The moral status of the pre-implantation embryo. Hum Reprod 2001;16:1046–8.

22. Weima S. Embryology. In: de Haan N, Spelt M, Gobel R, editors. Reproductive medicine: a textbook for paramedics. Amsterdam: Elsevier Gezondheidszorg; 2010. p. 79–92 [chapter 5].

23. Kölle S, Reese S, Kummer W. New aspects of gamete transport, fertilization, and embryonic development in the oviduct gained by means of live cell imaging. Theriogenology 2010;73:786–95.

24. Lyons RA, Djahanbakhch O, Mahmood T, et al. Fallopian tube ciliary beat frequency in relation to the stage of menstrual cycle and anatomical site. Hum Reprod 2002;17:584–8.

25. Alpha Scientists in Reproductive Medicine and ESHRE Special Interest Group of Embryology. The Istanbul consensus workshop on embryo assessment: proceedings of an expert meeting. Hum Reprod 2011;26:1270–83.

26. Norwitz ER, Schust DJ, Fisher SJ. Implantation and the survival of early pregnancy. N Engl J Med 2001;345:1400–8.

27. Cahill DJ, Wardle PG, Harlow CR, et al. Onset of the preovulatory luteinizing hormone surge: diurnal timing and critical follicular prerequisites. Fertil Steril 1998;70:56–9.

28. Testart J, Frydman R, Roger M. Seasonal influence of diurnal rhythms in the onset of the plasma luteinizing hormone surge in women. J Clin Endocrinol Metab 1982;55:374–7.

29. Fukuda M, Fukuda K, Andersen CY, et al. Right-sided ovulation favours pregnancy more than left-sided ovulation. Hum Reprod 2000;15:1921–6.

30. Fukuda M, Fukuda K, Andersen CY, et al. Characteristics of human ovulation in natural cycles correlated with age and achievement of pregnancy. Hum Reprod 2001;16:2501–7.

31. Veith JL, Buck M, Getzlaf S, et al. Exposure to men influences the occurrence of ovulation in women. Physiol Behav 1983;31:313–5.

32. Nikas G, Makrigiannakis A, Hovatta O, et al. Surface morphology of the human endometrium. Basic and clinical aspects. Ann N Y Acad Sci 2000;900:316–24.

33. Wilcox AJ, Baird DD, Weinberg CR. Time of implantation of the conceptus and loss of pregnancy. N Engl J Med 1999;340:1796–9.

34. Parks JC, McCallie BR, Janesch AM, et al. Blastocyst gene expression correlates with implantation potential. Fertil Steril 2011;95:1367–72.

35. Clancy KB. Reproductive ecology and the endometrium: physiology, variation, and new directions. Am J Phys Anthropol 2009;140:137–54.

36. Hoozemans DA, Schats R, Lambalk CB, et al. Human embryo implantation: current knowledge and clinical implications in assisted reproductive technology. Reprod Biomed Online 2004;9:692–715.

37. Johnson MH, Everitt BJ. Implantation and the establishment of the placenta. In: Essential reproduction. 5th ed. Oxford: Blackwell Science; 2000. p. 173–92 [chapter 10].

38. Fan XG, Zheng ZQ. A study of early pregnancy factor activity in preimplantation. Am J Reprod Immunol 1997;37:359–64.

39. Johnson MH, Everitt BJ. Maternal recognition and support of pregnancy. In: Essential

reproduction. 5th ed. Oxford: Blackwell Science; 2000. p. 194–202 [chapter 11].

40. Guzeloglu-Kayisli O, Basar M, Arici A. Basic aspects of implantation. Reprod Biomed Online 2007;15:728–39.

41. Edwards RG. Human implantation: the last barrier in assisted reproduction technologies? Reprod Biomed Online 2006;13:887–904.

42. Wilcox AJ, Weinberg CR, O'Connor JF, et al. Incidence of early loss of pregnancy. N Engl J Med 1988;319:189–94.

43. Chard T. Frequency of implantation and early pregnancy loss in natural cycles. Baillieres Clin Obstet Gynaecol 1991;5:179–89.

44. Roberts SA, Hirst WM, Brison DR, et al. Embryo and uterine influences on IVF outcomes: an analysis of a UK multi-centre cohort. Hum Reprod 2010;25:2792–802.

45. Rickett WA, translator. Shui Di Water and Earth. In: Guanzi. Political, economic, and philosophical essays from early China. Volume II, Chapters XII, 35-XXIV, 86. 2nd ed. New Jersey: Princeton University Press; 2001. p. 98–107.

46. Bertschinger R. The Dao transformed. In: The Daode Jing. The Dao and its energy. Montacute, Somerset UK: p. 44, Part 42.

47. Bertschinger R. Zang imagery. In: The single idea in the mind of the Yellow Emperor, a primer of Chinese medical texts from the Huangdi Nei Jing. Montacute, Somerset UK: Tao Booklets; 2008. p. 130–78 [chapter 5].

48. Lu HC. Various types of energy. In: A complete translation of the Yellow Emperor's classics of internal medicine and the difficult classic (Nei-Jing and Nan-Jing). Vancouver: International College of Traditional Chinese Medicine; 2004. p. 489–90, Section three: Spiritual pivot [Ling Shu] [chapter 30].

49. Unschuld PU. Medical thought during the Ming and Ch'ing Epochs: the individual search for reality. In: Janzen JM, Leslie C, editors. Medicine in China: a history of ideas. Berkeley: University of California Press; 1985. p. 189–228 [chapter 8].

50. Larre C, Rochat de la Vallee E. Nan Jing difficulty 39. In: Root C, editor. The Kidney. 2nd ed. Norfolk: Biddles; 1989. p. 14–7.

51. Lu HC. Meridians. In: A complete translation of the Yellow Emperor's classics of internal medicine and the difficult classic (Nei-Jing and Nan-Jing). Vancouver: International College of Traditional Chinese Medicine; 2004. p. 411–37, Section three: Spiritual pivot [Ling Shu] [chapter 10].

52. Sun Si-Miao. Prolegomena. In: Wilms S, translator. Bèi Jí Qian Jin Yào Fang. Essential prescriptions worth a thousand in gold for every emergency. 3 Volumes on gynecology. Portland: The Chinese Medicine Database; 2008. p. 4–50 [chapter 1].

53. Sun Si-Miao. Translation. In: Wilms S, translator. Bèi Jí Qian Jin Yào Fang. Essential prescriptions worth a thousand in gold for every emergency. 3 Volumes on gynecology, vol. 2. Portland: The Chinese Medicine Database; 2008. p. 52–216 [chapter 2].

54. Larre C, Schatz J, Rochat de la Vallée E, et al. The differential energies. In: Survey of Traditional Chinese Medicine. 1st ed. Columbia, MD: Institut Ricci; 1986. p. 111–39, Part 2 [chapter 3].

55. Maciocia G. The vital substances. In: The foundations of Chinese medicine: a comprehensive text for acupuncturists and herbalists. Edinburgh, NY: Churchill Livingstone; 1989. p. 35–57 [chapter 3].

56. Unschuld PU, Tessenow H, Jinsheng Z. The five periods, the five agents, and the ten stems. In: Huang Di Nei jing Su Wen: nature, knowledge, imagery in an ancient Chinese medical text, with an appendix, the doctrine of the five periods and six Qi in the Huang Di Nei Jing Su Wen. Berkeley: University of California Press; 2003. p. 399–414, The five periods. [Section 2].

57. Rochat de la Vallee E. The Zhubing Yuanhou Lun. In: Root C, editor. Pregnancy and gestation, in Chinese classical texts. Norfolk: Monkey Press; 2007. p. 28–108.

58. Soulie de Morant G, Grinnell L, Jeanmougin C, et al. Energy (Qi). In: Zmiewski P, editor. Chinese acupuncture, vol. 1. Brookline: Paradigm Publications; 1994. p. 46–56 [chapter 7].

Chapter 4

Orthodox medical tests and investigations: Optimizing patient care

Being able to interpret results of subfertility tests and investigations is of vital importance to fertility acupuncturists. The knowledge gained can provide information about a patient's medical diagnosis and prognosis; therefore, it can help the acupuncturist to better plan treatment. For example, if a patient's tests results show that her level of Follicle-Stimulating Hormone (FSH) is very high, this may be a sign of poor ovarian reserve. This patient may potentially need to be rapidly referred for *In Vitro* Fertilization (IVF). A consensus view of some of the world's leading acupuncturists who specialize in the treatment of subfertility is that 'biomedical information should inform decisions about (acupuncture) diagnosis and treatment'.[1]

This chapter explains what tests should ideally be done at various stages of subfertility treatment, how to interpret them, the implications, and the optimal timing and appropriateness of each test.

THE INITIAL CONSULTATION

After a certain period of unsuccessfully trying for a baby, a couple may realize that they need help and visit their doctor. What will happen to them then will depend on the experience and specialist knowledge of that doctor, the local regulations and policies, and, in many cases, the availability of funding for that couple's treatment.

A 2010 review by the world's top authoritative organizations in the field of reproduction, including the American College of Obstetricians and Gynecologists (ACOG), the American Society for Reproductive Medicine (ASRM), the Canadian Fertility and Andrology Society (CFAS), the European Society of Human Reproduction and Embryology (ESHRE), the Human Fertilisation and Embryology Authority (HFEA), the Royal College of Obstetricians and

Gynaecologists (RCOG), and the World Health Organization (WHO), proposed the following protocol for a primary care physician dealing with a subfertile couple.[2]

Medical history

One of the first things a doctor should do is take a detailed medical and fertility history. It is recommended that both partners should be interviewed not only together but separately as well because they may wish to disclose information when their partner is not present that they would otherwise not disclose.[2] A female partner may be asked questions about:[2]

- Present history
  - Age
  - Current problem/complaint
  - Occupation
  - Recent cervical smear findings
  - Breast changes (milk discharges)
  - Excessive hair growth with or without acne on the face and chest
  - Hot flashes
  - Eating disorders
  - Current associated medical illness (diabetes, hypertension)
  - Medication currently being taken
  - Sex steroid, cytotoxic or recreational drug intake
  - Smoking
  - Alcohol consumption
  - Caffeine consumption
- Menstrual history
  - Age of menarche
  - Cycle characteristics and associated symptoms (such as spotting or pain)
  - History of primary or secondary amenorrhoea

- Obstetric history
  - Previous pregnancies (in the current or previous relationships)
  - Previous pregnancy losses
  - Previous terminations
  - Posttermination infections or puerperal sepsis
- Contraception history
  - Previous use of contraceptive methods (including intrauterine devices) and any associated problems
- Sexual history
  - Intercourse frequency and timing
  - Lubricant use
  - Intercourse problems (difficult or painful coitus)
  - Vaginal douching
  - Loss of libido
  - History of previous relationships
- Past medical or surgical history
  - Pelvic infections
  - Tuberculosis
  - Bilharziasis
  - Ovarian cysts
  - Appendectomy
  - Laparotomy
  - Caesarean sections
  - Cervical conization
  - Rubella status
  - Sexually transmitted infections
- Family history
  - Consanguinity
  - Diabetes mellitus
  - Hypertension
  - Twin delivery
  - Breast cancer

A male partner may be asked questions about:[2]

- Present history
  - Age
  - Current problem/complaint
  - Occupation
  - Breast changes (enlargements)
  - Current associated medical illness (diabetes, hypertension)
  - Medication currently being taken
  - Sex steroid, cytotoxic or recreational drug intake
  - Smoking
  - Alcohol consumption
  - Caffeine consumption
  - Previous seminal analysis findings
- Obstetric history
  - Previous pregnancies (in the current or previous relationships)
  - Previous pregnancy losses
- Contraception history
  - Previous use of contraceptive methods (vasectomy in men) and any associated problems

- Sexual history
  - Intercourse frequency and timing
  - Lubricant use
  - Intercourse problems (erectile dysfunction or ejaculatory problems)
  - Loss of libido
  - History of previous relationships
- Past medical or surgical history
  - Tuberculosis
  - Bilharziasis
  - Appendectomy
  - Mumps
  - Sexually transmitted infections
  - Hydrocele
  - Varicocele
  - Undescended testis
  - Inguinal hernia repair
  - Bladder-neck suspension operations
- Family history
  - Consanguinity
  - Diabetes mellitus
  - Hypertension

Initial physical examination

After the interview, it is recommended that the doctor physically examine both partners.[2] However, in reality, very few patients are actually examined by their doctor. Physical examination of a female partner should include the following:[2]

- General examination
  - Vital signs (including blood pressure)
  - Body height, weight, and body mass index (BMI)
  - Secondary sexual characteristics
  - Excessive hair growths with/without acne on face or chest
  - Acanthosis nigricans
  - Abnormal skin depigmentation such as vitiligo
  - Thyroid glands
- Breast examination
  - Development check
  - Enlargements and other pathology
  - Presence of occult galactorrhoea (milky secretions)
- Chest examination
  - Lungs and heart
- Abdominal examination
  - Abdominal mass
  - Organomegaly (the abnormal enlargement of organs)
  - Ascites
  - Abdominal striae
  - Surgical scars
- Genital examination
  - Circumcision

- Size and shape of clitoris, hymen, vaginal introitus
- Site, size, shape, surface, consistency, mobility, and direction of uterus
- Palpable adnexal mass
- Vaginal discharge or tenderness
- Uterosacral ligament thickening
- Nodules in the cul-de-sac (possible sign of endometriosis or tuberculosis)

Physical examination of a male partner should include the following:[2]

- General examination
  - Vital signs (including blood pressure)
  - Body height, weight, and BMI
  - Secondary sexual characteristics
  - Thyroid glands
  - Arm span
- Breast examination
  - Gynaecomastia
- Abdominal examination
  - Abdominal mass
  - Organomegaly (the abnormal enlargement of organs)
  - Ascites
  - Undescended testis
  - Inguinal hernia
  - Genital examination
  - Shape and size of penis
  - Prepuce (foreskin)
  - Position of external urethral meatus
  - Testicular volume (by using Prader's orchidometer)
  - Palpation of epididymis and vas deferens
  - Check for varicocele or hydrocele
  - Perineal sensation
  - Rectal sphincter's tone
  - Prostate enlargement

Once a comprehensive medical history has been obtained and both partners have been thoroughly physically examined, there should be a preliminary diagnosis. The doctor can decide on further management, guided by local policies and guidelines.

TESTS AND INVESTIGATIONS OVERVIEW

The Practice Committee of ASRM recommends that the initial investigations

'. . . should be conducted in a systematic, expeditious, and cost-effective manner so as to identify all relevant factors, with initial emphasis on the least invasive methods for detection of the most common causes of infertility. . . . The pace and extent of evaluation should

take into account the couple's preferences, patient age, the duration of infertility, and unique features of the medical history and physical examination'.[3]

Both US and UK guidelines recommend that a couple who fails to conceive after 12 months or more of regular unprotected intercourse should be investigated.[4,5] Investigations after 6 months are justified in a couple if the female partner is more than 35 years old,[4,5] if there is a known medical cause of subfertility, or if there is a history of factors that may lead to subfertility,[5] for example, endometriosis or pelvic inflammatory disease. In couples with known infertility (for example, patients whose fertility is compromised by previous cancer treatment), then an early fertility specialist referral should be initiated.[5]

CLINICAL TIPS

INFERTILITY TESTS AND INVESTIGATIONS

- When were the most recent tests undertaken? Any tests that are over 6 months old may need to be repeated.
- Have the appropriate tests been performed correctly (for example, at the right time in the menstrual cycle)? If you find discrepancies, then refer your patient for retesting.
- Patients often say that all their tests results are 'normal'. Always request a copy of the test results and check that they are in the normal ranges.
- Treat low/high ends of normal ranges with caution because these may be early indications of abnormalities.
- Some tests may need to be repeated (for example, abnormal semen analysis). Check that this has been done.
- Familiarize yourself with local guidelines and policies and adapt your treatment plan according to these guidelines. Incorrectly timed or delayed referral for investigations can result in IVF not being funded.

 ### Case study

Tests and Investigations: Timely Referral

- Jo, an almost 40-year-old teacher, presented for acupuncture treatment to help her with fertility. Jo mentioned that her husband's semen analysis was abnormal and that he had had problems with fertility in a previous relationship. Jo also had a blockage in one of her fallopian tubes.
- It appeared very likely that this couple would need IVF because the chances of natural conception were low. The local policy was that IVF funding was available for women under the age of 40. Jo was advised that, if IVF

Continued

Case study—cont'd

was an option for her and her husband, then they should not wait and should proceed straight to IVF.

♦ Jo's referral was fast tracked and she started IVF stimulation 2 days before turning 40, just in time for funding to be available. She conceived and had a baby boy.

♦ Timely referral for IVF ensured that funding was available for this couple.

TESTS AND INVESTIGATIONS: FEMALE

Ovulation assessment

One of the first tests a doctor will do is check the level of progesterone to see if a woman is ovulating. Ovulation dysfunction is one of the most common causes of female infertility, identified in approximately 20–32% of infertile women.[6,7] A menstrual history of regular 25- to 35-day cycles is often enough to assume normal ovulation. However, in infertile women an objective measure of ovulation is necessary. As explained in Chapter 2, progesterone levels rise soon after ovulation and peak at the mid-luteal phase. Therefore, the test needs to be done 7 days before the expected start of the next period to coincide with the progesterone peak.

Serum progesterone levels of >3 ng/mL (>9.54 nmol/L) suggest ovulation has occurred.[3,8] However, progesterone levels of ≥10 ng/mL (≥31.8 nmol/L) may suggest a better quality luteal function,[3,9] which may create a better environment for implantation. However, progesterone levels in this higher reference range may not be a reliable finding as progesterone secretions are pulsatile, and the levels may vary up to sevenfold within a few hours.[3,10]

Thyroid disorders and/or hyperprolactinaemia are common causes of anovulation.[3] So, if a woman is not ovulating, serum thyroid-stimulating hormone (TSH) and prolactin levels should be checked. TSH is discussed in more detail in the section on thyroid disease in Chapter 8. Reference ranges for progesterone and prolactin hormones are provided in Table 4.1.

Red flag

Increased prolactin levels

Even mildly elevated prolactin may be a sign of central nervous system lesion (tumour). Therefore, a referral for an MRI scan is indicated.[12]

Women who are not having any periods should have their FSH and oestradiol (E2) levels investigated to distinguish between amenorrhoea due to ovarian failure (high FSH, low E2) and hypothalamic amenorrhoea (low FSH, low E2). For FSH and E2 reference ranges, see Table 4.2.

Table 4.1 Ovulation investigations: reference ranges for progesterone and prolactin

Hormones	Timing relative to menstrual cycle	Reference range[a]	Notes
Progesterone	7 days before expected start of next period In women with irregular cycles, the test may need to be repeated every 7 days until the next period starts[5]	>9.54 nmol/L (>3 ng/mL): ovulation has occurred[3] ≤3 ng/mL (≤9.54 nmol/L): ovulation has not occurred[3]	Some fertility clinics prefer to see higher levels, as levels ≥31.8 nmol/L (≥10 ng/mL) may be suggestive of better quality luteal function[9]
Prolactin	Any cycle day	Values depend on assay used by the laboratory, ranging from[11] 3.35–4.65 μg/L (71–98 mIU/L) (lower limit) to 16.4–23.2 μg/L (348–492 mIU/L) (upper limit)	Even mildly elevated prolactin may be a sign of a central nervous system lesion. Therefore, magnetic resonance imaging (MRI) is indicated in all cases of raised prolactin[12] Other causes of raised prolactin include physical and emotional stress, high protein diet, and intense breast stimulation,[13] kidney or thyroid disease, use of certain drugs and hypersensitive prolactin releasing cells in the pituitary[14]

[a] Reference values may vary among different laboratories and assays used. Therefore, laboratory reports should be checked for reference ranges applicable to the individual patient's results profile.

Table 4.2 Ovarian reserve reference ranges: FSH, LH, E2

Hormones	Timing relative to menstrual cycle	Reference ranges[a]	Notes
FSH[b]	Cycle days 2–5	ASRM:[3] <10 IU/L (<10 mIU/mL): normal ovarian reserve[a] 10–20 IU/L (10–20 mIU/mL): poor ovarian reserve >20 IU/L (>20 mIU/mL): may signify menopause National Institute for Health and Care Excellence (NICE):[5] <4 IU/L (<4 mIU/mL): likely high ovarian response[a] >8.9 IU/L (>8.9 mIU/mL): likely low ovarian response	An imperfect measure as FSH fluctuates from cycle to cycle
LH	Days 2–5 together with FSH	1.4–7.8 IU/L (1.4–7.8 mIU/mL): normal range[17]	High LH + normal FSH suggests Polycystic Ovarian Syndrome (PCOS)[18] although this is not a diagnostic test and specific PCOS tests need to be carried out (see Chapter 8 for further details on PCOS) High LH + high FSH suggest diminished ovarian reserve (DOR)
E2	Days 2–5 together with FSH	>188–210 pmol/L (51–57 pg/mL): high levels[17]	Helps to interpret FSH correctly. If FSH is within normal range, raised E2 may be artificially supressing FSH, thus giving a false normal FSH level. E2 levels during IVF may be much higher E2 also helps to distinguish between different types of amenorrhoea:[3] • High FSH + low E2 = ovarian failure requiring egg donation • Normal FSH + low E2 = hypothalamic amenorrhoea requiring exogenous gonadotrophin stimulation for ovulation induction

[a] Reference values may vary among different laboratories and assays used. Therefore, laboratory reports should be checked for reference ranges applicable to the individual patient's results profile.
[b] Should be tested and interpreted together with E2. High E2 may suppress FSH, resulting in false normal FSH reading.[15,16] This is usually seen in premenopausal women.

In Traditional Chinese Medicine (TCM), ovulatory disorders are associated with the following syndromes:

- Heart Shen (Spirit) impairment[19]
- Kidney Jing (Essence) Deficiency
- Qi and Blood Deficiency[20]
- Yin, Yang Deficiency[20]
- Blood-Stasis with Phlegm-Dampness[19]
- Qi Stagnation[19]
- Heat[19]
- Heart and/or Liver Qi Stagnation

Ovarian reserve screen

Diminished ovarian reserve (DOR) is defined as 'women of reproductive age having regular menses whose response to ovarian stimulation or fecundity is reduced compared to those women of comparable age'.[3] Reduced response to ovarian stimulation is defined as <2–3 follicles or ≤4 retrieved eggs.[16]

Ovarian reserve should be assessed in women at increased risk of DOR. This includes women who:[3]

- Are more than 35 years old
- Have a family history of early menopause
- Have a history of damage to the ovaries from chemotherapy, pelvic radiation therapy, or ovarian surgery or have only one ovary
- Have unexplained infertility
- Have a history of poor response to ovarian stimulation with gonadotrophins
- Are planning to undergo Assisted Reproductive Technology (ART) treatment

There are no perfect measures of ovarian reserve. Even if reduced ovarian reserve is established following investigations, this only has a predictive value in determining the likely response to ovarian stimulation and does not necessarily signify inability to conceive.[3] Women can conceive with even extremely low ovarian reserve markers, and age is a more accurate predictor of a future live birth.[21]

Ovarian reserve tests include hormonal blood tests, such as FSH, E2, Anti-Müllerian Hormone (AMH), Antral Follicle Count (AFC) ultrasound scan, and provocative tests, such as the Clomiphene Citrate Challenge Test (CCCT).

FSH, E2 (and LH)

As explained in Chapter 2, FSH is released by the anterior pituitary gland in order to stimulate ovarian follicles to grow and develop. In some women, the pituitary has to release much higher levels of FSH in order for the ovaries to respond. This commonly happens in women whose ovarian reserve is in decline.

The FSH test was, and to some extent still is, the most commonly used test to measure ovarian reserve. However, it is not as reliable as AMH[22] and AFC[21] (information on these tests is provided later in this section).

FSH should be tested on days 2–5 of the menstrual cycle, usually with tests for Luteinizing Hormone (LH) and also ideally E2. Reference values for FSH vary, but most laboratories use a cut-off point for FSH at <10 mIU/mL.[15,18] Values of >12 mIU/mL on the third day of the menstrual cycle (especially levels >20 mIU/mL) suggest very poor prognosis of pregnancy.[15]

Care should be taken to check E2 concentrations at the same time as those of FSH because high E2 levels can have a negative feedback on FSH values (by artificially suppressing FSH, thus giving false normal FSH values).[15,16]

However, E2 levels on their own should not be used to measure ovarian reserve.[3,5,16]

E2 levels can also help to distinguish between:[3]

- Amenorrhoea due to ovarian failure (high FSH, low E2), which requires egg donation, and
- Hypothalamic amenorrhoea (normal FSH, low E2), which requires exogenous gonadotrophin stimulation for ovulation induction.

FSH, LH, and E2 reference ranges are shown in Table 4.2.

From the TCM point of view, FSH, E2, and LH abnormalities are associated with impairment of the Heart and Kidney axis. Syndromes to look for are:

- Empty syndromes
  - Kidney Jing (Essence) Deficiency
  - Kidney Yin Deficiency[20,23]
  - Empty-Heat from Yin[24–26] or Blood Deficiency[23]
  - Spleen Qi and Blood Deficiency[25]
  - Liver Blood Deficiency
- Mixed syndromes
  - Heart and/or Liver Qi Stagnation[26] with Blood Deficiency and Heat
  - Blood-Stasis[24,25]

AMH

AMH is the hormone produced by the granulosa cells of primary, preantral, and antral follicles.[16] The higher the number of these early follicles, the higher AMH levels are. AMH is relatively constant and therefore can be tested on any day of the menstrual cycle.[3,27] AMH is a better predictor of response to ovarian stimulation than FSH but not as good as AFC.[21]

Low values (<1.5–5.0 pmol/L or <0.2–0.7 ng/mL DSL Enzyme-linked Immunosorbent Assay (ELISA)) have been shown to be highly predictable of poor ovarian response (<3 follicles or ≤2–4 retrieved eggs).[16] However, women with low or undetectable AMH values can still respond well to ovarian stimulation and become pregnant.[16]

Ovarian surgery, for example, endometrioma[28–30] or cyst[29] surgery, may damage healthy ovarian and follicular tissue and, therefore, reduce AMH and ovarian reserve. One study showed that the AMH levels slightly recover 3 months postsurgery.[29] Another recent study, however, demonstrated that ovarian reserve is lower in patients with endometriomas even before they undergo ovarian surgery.[31]

High AMH values (>48 pmol/L or >6.7 ng/mL) are associated with PCOS.[32]

As discussed in Chapter 2, the follicular pool reduces naturally as women age. Therefore, AMH level naturally declines with age. Assessing AMH values relative to a woman's age may be a more useful tool when deciding if a woman's ovarian follicular pool is declining with her age or prematurely.

Table 4.3 summarizes how to interpret AMH values.

Table 4.3 Ovarian reserve reference ranges: AMH

Hormones	Timing relative to menstrual cycle	Reference ranges[a]			Notes
AMH	Any cycle day	ASRM:[16]			Very good predictive value of ovarian response[16]
		<1.4–5 pmol/L (<0.2–0.7 ng/mL DSL ELISA): likely low ovarian response, poor embryo quality, and low chance of achieving pregnancy			
		NICE:[5]			
		≤5.3 pmol/L (≤0.7 ng/mL): likely low ovarian response			
		≥25.0 pmol/L (≥3.5 ng/mL): likely high ovarian response			
		>48 pmol/L (>6.7 ng/mL): likely PCOS[32]			
		Age	pmol/L	ng/mL[33]	Age-specific AMH values may be better for assessing ovarian reserve on an individual basis[34]
		24	29.3	4.1	
		25	29.3	4.1	
		26	30.0	4.2	
		27	26.4	3.7	
		28	27.1	3.8	
		29	25.0	3.5	
		30	22.8	3.2	
		31	22.1	3.1	
		32	17.9	2.5	
		33	18.6	2.6	
		34	16.4	2.3	
		35	15.0	2.1	
		36	12.9	1.8	
		37	11.4	1.6	
		38	10.0	1.4	
		39	9.3	1.3	
		40	7.9	1.1	
		41	7.1	1.0	
		42	6.4	0.9	
		43	5.0	0.7	
		44	4.3	0.6	
		45	3.6	0.5	
		46	2.9	0.4	
		47	2.9	0.4	
		48	1.4	0.2	
		49	0.7	0.1	
		50	0	0	

[a] Reference values may vary among different laboratories and assays used. Therefore, laboratory reports should be checked for reference ranges applicable to the individual patient's results profile.

From the TCM point of view, low AMH levels are associated with:

- Kidney Jing (Essence) Deficiency
- Kidney Yin[23] Deficiency with or without Empty-Heat
- Liver Qi Stagnation with Blood Deficiency[26]
- Heart and/or Spleen Qi Deficiency

AFC

AFC is a transvaginal ultrasound scan during which antral follicles on both ovaries are counted.[16] It is usually performed during the early follicular phase,[16] but it can be performed at any point in a cycle.[27] Different clinics define antral in different ways. For example, some count follicles measuring 2–10 mm in diameter, others 3–8 mm.[16]

AFC is the most direct measure of ovarian reserve and corresponds to how many eggs are likely to be retrieved during IVF.[21] A meta-analysis of 11 studies showed that the AFC scan is currently as accurate in predicting ovarian response to stimulation as using several different markers.[35] In one study, AFC was the only measure of ovarian reserve that predicted ovarian response to IVF stimulation when compared to AMH and FSH.[21]

Table 4.4 summarizes how to interpret the results of AFC.

CCCT

CCCT involves administering 100 mg of Clomiphene Citrate (sometimes referred to as Clomid) daily on days 5–9 of the cycle. FSH is measured before (day 3) and after (day 10). Elevated FSH on day 10 (10–22 IU/L or 10–22 mIU/mL) suggests diminished ovarian reserve.[3] This test is not as sensitive as AMH or AFC.[16] In the UK, it is not widely used and is not recommended because of lack of evidence of its ability to predict response to IVF.[5]

Inhibin B

The use of Inhibin B hormone level tests is no longer recommended in ovarian reserve testing because it is not a reliable measure.[5,16] AMH and AFC are the gold standard measures of ovarian reserve.

Other blood tests

Rubella status, full blood count, ferritin levels, hepatitis B and C, and Human Immunodeficiency Virus serology are usually also carried out as part of the initial investigations.[18]

Cervical assessment

Cervical factors, such as abnormalities of cervical mucus or interaction of sperm and cervical mucus, are rarely primary causes of infertility. Examination of cervical mucus is the only cervical assessment recommended by ASRM.[3] The postcoital test is no longer recommended because it lacks accuracy and usefulness.[3]

Uterine anomalies, tubal patency, and other peritoneal factors

Tubal disorders contribute to between 14% and 26% of infertility cases.[6,7,37] Uterine causes are relatively rare. However, both need to be excluded when evaluating the female partner.

From the TCM perspective, anatomic abnormalities of the Uterus may involve Kidney Jing (Essence) Deficiency. Tubal pathology is discussed in greater detail in Chapter 8.

Ultrasound

Transvaginal ultrasonography (ultrasound scan) can be used to prove ovulation by observing a collapsed follicle

Table 4.4 Ovarian reserve reference ranges: AFC			
Scan	Timing relative to menstrual cycle	Reference ranges	Notes
AFC	Usually performed during the early follicular phase (but can be done at any point)[27]	ASRM:[3,16]	Very good predictive value of ovarian response[16]
		>10 total antral follicles: good ovarian reserve	
		3–10 total antral follicles: poor ovarian reserve, likely to have poor response to stimulation and low chance of achieving pregnancy	
		NICE:[5]	
		≤4 total antral follicles: likely low ovarian response	
		>16 total antral follicles: likely high ovarian response	
		≥12 follicles on each ovary measuring 2–9 mm indicates PCO[36]	

although, if possible, cheaper investigative methods such as a progesterone test should be used first to detect ovulation.[3]

Ultrasound can also be used to diagnose uterine pathology, for example, myomas.[3] However, uterine pathology is better detected by hysteroscopy (see later in this chapter).[3]

Ultrasound can also be used to assess the ovaries, for example, for the presence of endometriomas.[3]

Ultrasound can be used to assess the fallopian tubes for the presence of hydrosalpinges (see the tubal pathology section about hydrosalpinges in Chapter 8). Ultrasound is not useful for identifying other tubal pathology.[38]

Transvaginal ultrasonography is used during ART treatment to monitor follicular and endometrial growth during ovarian stimulation or ovulation induction.[38]

Hysterosalpingography

Hysterosalpingography (HSG) is a procedure where oil- or water-based contrast media is injected via a catheter into the uterus and into the fallopian tubes. As this contrast media fills the uterine cavity and the fallopian tubes, X-ray images are periodically taken to record the filling of the uterus and fallopian tubes. Various degrees of pelvic pain may be experienced during and after the procedure, and light spotting may last for up to 24 h following the procedure.[38] During HSG, patients are exposed to radiation; therefore, HSG cannot be done during pregnancy.[38] HSG also cannot be used during active pelvic infection.[38] HSG is usually performed between cycle days 6 and 11 when the chances of pregnancy are lowest and the endometrium is at its thinnest.[38] Prophylactic antibiotics may be given after the procedure.[38]

HSG is used as first-line investigation of tubal pathology in women with no known comorbidities (such as pelvic inflammatory disease, endometriosis, history of ectopic pregnancy).[5] For these women, laparoscopic investigations with dye may be more suitable (see later in this chapter).[5]

HSG is effective for documenting proximal and distal tubal blockage and other tubal abnormalities.[3] However, some authors argue that better and safer alternatives exist (for example, hysterosalpingo-contrast-ultrasonography (Hy-Co-Sy) or Chlamydia Antibody Test (CAT), which are discussed later in this section) and that these should be used instead of HSG.[39]

HSG can also be used to examine the uterine cavity for anomalies such as abnormal uterine development (unicornuate, septate, bicornuate uterus), acquired abnormalities (endometrial polyps, submucous myomas, synechiae), but HSG is not useful for detecting endometrial polyps and submucous myomas.[3] HSG is not as sensitive at detecting intrauterine abnormalities. Other methods, such as hysteroscopy, may be more effective for intrauterine investigations.[40]

Hysterosalpingo-contrast-ultrasonography

Hy-Co-Sy is a procedure where a small amount of effervescent fluid is introduced into the uterus and through it to the fallopian tubes. A concomitant ultrasound scan is carried out to assess the uterus and the patency of the fallopian tubes.

As with HSG, following the procedure, women may experience some discomfort, vaginal bleeding, and referred shoulder pain.[38] The procedure needs to be done during the early follicular phase.[38] However, unlike HSG, it requires no use of X-ray images or iodine contrast.[38,39] Hy-Co-Sy can extend the use of ordinary ultrasound to include detailed evaluation of adnexal architecture, uterine cavity, myometrial assessment, and tubal patency.[38]

It is recommended that Hy-Co-Sy should be offered instead of HSG where appropriate expertise is available.[5] Some experts feel that Hy-Co-Sy should replace HSG as the first-line investigation of tubal patency.[39]

Sonohysterography (saline infusion sonography (SIS))

Sonohysterography (also known as saline infusion sonography (SIS) or intrauterine saline infusion) is an advanced form of ultrasound scan where saline fluid is injected into the uterus and the fallopian tubes, and concomitant ultrasound is carried out to visualize the uterine cavity and to observe if the fluid appears in the cul-de-sac.[3,38]

SIS is used to detect intrauterine pathology such as endometrial polyps,[3] submucous myomas,[3] synechiae,[3] fibroids,[41] endometrial scarring or adhesions,[41] malignancies,[41] and congenital defects.[41]

Although the test can be used to assess tubal patency, it does not differentiate between unilateral and bilateral patency.[3]

The advantage of SIS is that it allows assessment of intrauterine factors without the use of harmful contrast agents or ionizing radiation.[38]

Laparoscopy

Laparoscopy is the only way to directly visualize pelvic reproductive anatomy and, therefore, the only diagnostic method for confirming peritoneal factors that may contribute to subfertility (for example, endometriosis).[3] Usually, therapeutic correction of abnormal findings can be carried out at the same time.[38] However, it is a surgical procedure that requires general anaesthesia and has associated risks of adverse events, such as postoperative infection and/or adhesions, requires postoperative recovery, and is a costly procedure.[38]

Laparoscopy should only be offered to women who have signs and symptoms, such as pelvic pain, history of previous pelvic infection or surgery, abnormal HSG findings, and no other major indications for ART, for example, severe male factor infertility.[3,5] Asymptomatic younger women should only be offered laparoscopy if they have a history of more than 3 years of subfertility and no other recognized abnormalities because laparoscopy rarely yields abnormal findings in asymptomatic women.[3]

Laparoscopy with chromotubation or dye test (dilute solution of methylene blue or indigo carmine (preferred)) is an invasive tubal investigation. Laparoscopy provides more detailed information about the type of tubal pathology and, in some instances, allows the pathology to be corrected during the same procedure.[3]

Case study

Tests and investigations: Endometriosis

- Leona received 4 months of acupuncture treatment to help her conceive, initially without success.
- Leona had some signs of endometriosis, in particular, very painful periods. She was advised to go back to her doctor and discuss further investigations.
- Leona was referred for exploratory laparoscopy. During the procedure, endometrial lesions were found and treated. Leona returned for acupuncture treatment and conceived a month later.
- In this case, it was acceptable to try acupuncture and natural conception for three to four cycles because laparoscopy is very invasive and has procedural risks. However, once it became clear that natural conception was unlikely, further investigations were appropriate.

Fluoroscopic/hysteroscopic selective tubal cannulation

Fluoroscopic/hysteroscopic selective tubal cannulation can be carried out to confirm or exclude proximal tubal pathology previously suggested by HSG or laparoscopy with chromotubation.[3]

Hysteroscopy

Hysteroscopy is a direct and definitive method of assessing intrauterine pathology. A hysteroscope (long, thin, lighted telescope) is inserted through the cervix into the uterus. Gas or special fluids are then infused into the uterus. As a result, the uterine walls are stretched, allowing for good visual examination of the uterine cavity. As with many uterine assessment methods, hysteroscopy is usually done soon after menstruation so the uterine cavity can be more easily assessed. A directed biopsy can be done during the procedure, and therapeutic correction of certain pathologies can also be undertaken.[42] Antibiotics may be prescribed afterward to reduce the risk of infection.

When compared with transvaginal ultrasonography (a first-line noninvasive uterine cavity assessment), hysteroscopy has been shown to detect up to 19% more abnormal findings that were missed by an ultrasound.[43] Hysteroscopy can detect such abnormalities as cervical stenosis, endocervicitis, endocervical polyp, uterine cavity hypoplasia, uterine septum, intrauterine adhesions, intrauterine

foreign body, endometriosis, submucous myoma, endometrial polyp, polypoid endometrium, endometrial hyperplasia, and blocked ostia.[43]

Major guidelines on infertility investigations do not recommend hysteroscopy as a routine investigation because it is costly and invasive and should be reserved as a secondary investigation, for example, in patients with a history of IVF failures.[3,5] However, some experts call for hysteroscopy to be used as part of pre-IVF investigations.[43] Hysteroscopy during the cycle preceding the IVF treatment cycle has been shown to nearly double the chances of conception in patients with two or more than two failed IVF treatment cycles.[44]

MRI

Magnetic resonance imaging (MRI) can be used to assess uterine abnormalities. However, because of the high cost of MRI scans and their limited availability, it is not routinely offered.[42]

Endometrial biopsy

Endometrial biopsy should only be used to investigate strongly suspected specific endometrial pathology, such as neoplasia or chronic endometritis.[3] It is no longer indicated for evaluating luteal function or dating the endometrium.[3]

Chlamydia Antibody Test

The presence of antibodies to *Chlamydia trachomatis* has been associated with tubal disease.[3] CAT is a good noninvasive alternative to HSG. However, CAT is not as sensitive as laparoscopy.[3] If the CAT is normal, the likelihood of tubal obstruction is reduced to approximately 8%.[12] An abnormal result warrants laparoscopy.[12]

Genetic screening

Peripheral karyotyping should be done as part of infertility investigations or prior to ART treatment in women with amenorrhoea (primary and secondary, including premature ovarian failure), oligomenorrhoea with hypergonadotropism, and in apparently healthy women who have failed to conceive after 1 year.[45]

Maternal balanced translocation, maternal mosaic for numeric aberration, and maternal inversion are the most common anomalies identified by peripheral karyotyping in patients with recurrent miscarriages.[46] Balanced structural chromosomal abnormalities and Robertsonian translocations are identified in 2–5% of repeated miscarriages.[47] Peripheral karyotyping is therefore recommended in patients with repeated miscarriages.[45,47] Tests for repeated miscarriages are described in more detail in Chapter 12.

Chromosomal abnormalities are found in 1.3% of subfertile female patients.[48] This is higher than in the general population. Some experts recommend that all women should undergo genetic testing prior to IVF or Intracytoplasmic Sperm Insemination (ICSI) because the incidence of genetic abnormalities is higher in this patient group and, if transmitted, can lead to abnormalities in the offspring.[49] However, this recommendation is not supported by other studies.[50]

Preimplantation genetic diagnosis is one of the treatment options for detecting specific translocations, resulting in only unaffected embryos being transferred.[47] The use of donor gametes provides an alternative treatment option.[47]

It is also recommended that women with oligomenorrhoea caused by primary ovarian dysfunction (including premature ovarian failure) or apparently healthy women with poor response to ovarian stimulation during IVF should be tested for fragile X syndrome.[45] Other genetic tests may be indicated, depending on the medical history.[51]

Thrombophilia investigations

Overview

Thrombophilia is a group of different disorders that make blood clot abnormally.[52] Thrombophilia is linked to recurrent pregnancy loss and other pregnancy complications, such as foetal growth restriction, stillbirth, and severe preeclampsia.[52]

Routine testing for thrombophilias in subfertile and IVF populations is not currently recommended.[47,53] Screening is recommended in patients:

- With a history of venous thromboembolism (for example, developing postsurgery)[47]
- Who have a first-degree relative who is known or suspected to have high-risk thrombophilia[47]
- With a history of unexplained pregnancy loss ≥10 weeks' gestation[54]
- With a history of severe preeclampsia[54]
- With a history of severe intrauterine growth restriction (<5th percentile)[54]
- With a history of placental abruption[54]

Thrombophilia has been linked to other clinical conditions and, therefore, screening in these patient groups may be justified:

- Unexplained subfertility[55,56]
- Repeated Implantation Failure[55–58]
- Recurrent miscarriages[55,56,59,60]
- Autoimmune disease[59]

Types of thrombophilia

Thrombophilia may be acquired or secondary to other diseases, or it may be genetic or inherited (Table 4.5).

Table 4.5 Thrombophilia types

Acquired or secondary thrombophilia[52]	Inherited or genetic thrombophilia[52]
• Active cancer	• Antithrombin deficiency
• Chemotherapy	• Protein C deficiency
• Sickle cell disease	• Protein S deficiency[a]
• Oral contraceptives	• Activated protein C resistance[b]
• Oestrogen therapy	• Factor V Leiden (homozygous)[b]
• Pregnancy/ postpartum state	• Factor V Leiden (heterozygous)[a,b]
• Selective oestrogen receptor modulator therapy (tamoxifen and raloxifene)	• Prothrombin G20210A[b]
• Antiphospholipid antibodies[a,b]	• Homocystinuria
	• Increased plasma factors I (fibrinogen), II (prothrombin), VIII, IX, XI
• Inflammatory bowel disease	• Factor XIII polymorphisms
• Systemic lupus erythematosus	• Hyperhomocysteinaemia[b]
	• Dysfibrinogenemia
• Progesterone therapy	• Reduced tissue factor pathway inhibitor
• Infertility therapy	• Reduced protein Z and Z-dependent protease inhibitor
• Dehydration	• Tissue plasminogen activator deficiency
	• Increased plasminogen activator inhibin (PAI)-1
	• Increased thrombin-activatable fibrinolysis inhibitor
	• Hypoplasminogenemia and dysplasminogenemia
	• Hypofibrinolysis

[a] Strongly linked to late pregnancy loss.[61]
[b] Strongly linked to early pregnancy loss.[61]

Diagnostic tests for acquired or secondary thrombophilia

The main type of acquired thrombophilia is Antiphospholipid Syndrome (APS),[62] also known as Hughes syndrome and Lupus Anticoagulant Syndrome. It is associated with pregnancy loss in the first and the second trimesters. It is also associated with preeclampsia and intrauterine growth restriction.[62] Between 5% and 42% of women with recurrent pregnancy loss will test positive for antiphospholipid antibodies.[47] These antibodies affect the trophoblast and cause maternal inflammatory response.[47]

To confirm a diagnosis of APS, patients must have one or more of the clinical criteria and one or more of the laboratory criteria set out in Table 4.6. Other antibodies may be

---

Table 4.6 Criteria for diagnosing APS

Clinical criteria	Laboratory criteria*

• Vascular thrombosis: one or more clinical episodes of arterial, venous, or small vessel thrombosis in any tissue or organ. Thrombosis must be confirmed by objective validated criteria (i.e., unequivocal findings of appropriate imaging studies or histopathology). For histopathologic confirmation, thrombosis should be present without significant evidence of inflammation in the vessel wall.
  • Pregnancy morbidity:
    a. One or more unexplained deaths of a morphologically normal foetus at or beyond the 10th week of gestation, with normal foetal morphology documented by ultrasound or by direct examination of the foetus, or
    b. One or more premature births of a morphologically normal neonate before the 34th week of gestation because of:
      ▪ Eclampsia or severe preeclampsia defined according to standard definitions, or
      ▪ Recognized features of placental insufficiency, or
    c. Three or more unexplained consecutive spontaneous abortions before the 10th week of gestation, with maternal anatomic or hormonal abnormalities and paternal and maternal chromosomal causes excluded. In studies of populations of patients who have more than one type of pregnancy morbidity, investigators are strongly encouraged to stratify groups of subjects according to a, b, or c above.
	• Lupus anticoagulant (LA) present in plasma, on two or more occasions at least 12 weeks apart, detected according to the guidelines of the International Society on Thrombosis and Haemostasis (Scientific Subcommittee on LAs/phospholipid-dependent antibodies)
	• Anticardiolipin (aCL) antibody of IgG and/or IgM isotype in serum or plasma, present in medium or high titre (i.e., >40 GPL or MPL or more than the 99th percentile), on two or more occasions, at least 12 weeks apart, measured by a standardized ELISA
	• Anti-b2 glycoprotein-I antibody of IgG and/or IgM isotype in serum or plasma (in titre more than the 99th percentile), present on two or more occasions, at least 12 weeks apart, measured by a standardized ELISA, according to recommended procedures

Reprinted with permission from Ref.[63]

* Other antibodies may be linked to APS. However, they are not included in the diagnostic criteria because of nonstandardized testing.

---

linked to APS. However, they are not included in the diagnostic criteria because of nonstandardized testing.

CLINICAL TIPS

ANTIPHOSPHOLIPID SYNDROME (APS)

Patients with APS often have headaches or migraines, flashing lights in the eyes, memory problems (foggy brain), and balance problems.[64] About a fifth of patients have a mottled skin condition called *livedo reticularis*, described as 'a red or blue blotchy, lacy pattern usually on the knees, thighs, and upper arms', which can be more pronounced in cold weather.[65]

Therefore, if patients present with this type of pattern, it may be justifiable to screen for APS, even if they do not meet any other criteria for tests.

Diagnostic tests for genetic or inherited thrombophilia

There are numerous genetic clotting mutations, but not all have been linked to reproductive health issues. The following tests should be included in a basic inherited thrombophilia screening battery because the evidence of these genetic clotting mutations' involvement is strong:[54]

- Protein C levels (functional assay)
- Protein S levels (functional or free level)
- Antithrombin III (functional assay)
- Factor V Leiden (PCR)
- Prothrombin Gene Mutation (20210A) (PCR)
- Protein Z

Other genetic mutations have been linked to pregnancy complications, but the evidence for these is weaker:[54]

- Homocysteine
- Other FV mutations
- Thrombomodulin gene variants
- PAI-1 activity levels
- PAI-1 4G/4G polymorphism
- MTHFR C677T
- Factor evaluation (VII, VIII, IX, XI)

In addition, it is advisable to assess the platelet count as a screen for thrombocytosis and myeloproliferative disorders.[54]

Treatment

If diagnosed, treatment of thrombophilia usually consists of a combination of anticoagulation medication, such as low molecular weight heparin administered subcutaneously twice daily (for example, Clexane), and low dose aspirin, resulting in a 74.3% success rate in preventing pregnancy losses.[47] Routine administration of steroids (such as prednisone) is not recommended because of lack of evidence of steroid effectiveness and potential risk of complications such as gestation hypertension and gestational diabetes.[47]

TCM associations

- Blood-Stasis (with or without Heat)
- Cold
- Damp-Heat
- Phlegm
- Heat (not from Stasis)
- Liver Blood Deficiency with Stagnation
- Liver and/or Heart Qi Stagnation
- Kidney Yin Deficiency
- Kidney Yang Deficiency
- Kidney Jing (Essence) Deficiency

 Case study

Tests and Investigations: Thrombophilia

Zoe presented for acupuncture treatment to prepare for IVF. She was almost 39 years old.

Her reproductive history included one miscarriage at 10 weeks gestation and two miscarriages at about 4 weeks gestation, all within the last 1.5 years.

Orthodox Medical Diagnosis

Severe male factor infertility because of poor morphology and motility

Reduced ovarian reserve (FSH 15.2 IU/L, AMH 3.76 pmol/L)

Zoe conceived on her first round of IVF but miscarried at about 4 weeks gestation. Her IVF consultant very strongly recommended that she have donor eggs IVF as he felt Zoe was miscarrying due to her age-related poor ovarian reserve. I referred her for a second opinion to a reproductive consultant specializing in miscarriages.

Zoe underwent thrombophilia investigations and tested positive (heterozygote) for the MTHFR C677T mutation. Zoe's IVF consultant did not feel this mutation was causing Zoe's miscarriages but nevertheless agreed to try another round of IVF incorporating anticoagulation therapy (clexane). Following her second round of treatment, Zoe conceived, and this time the pregnancy progressed to full term. She had a healthy baby girl.

When her daughter was 7 months old, Zoe re-presented for acupuncture treatment to prepare for another round of IVF to try and conceive her second baby. We both were realistic about the chances of success being low because her ovarian reserve was likely to be even more depleted. To our surprise, Zoe conceived naturally after only 1 month of acupuncture treatment (while still breastfeeding her

Continued

 Case study—cont'd

daughter). She started to inject clexane as soon as she knew she was pregnant. This pregnancy also progressed to full term, and she had a healthy baby boy.

In Zoe's case, infertility was complicated by an inherited thrombophilia disease. Once Zoe was prescribed the correct anticoagulation therapy, she successfully carried her pregnancies to full term.

Infection screening

Infections in all parts of the female reproductive tract can lead to subfertility by causing pelvic inflammatory disease, adhesions, and tubal occlusion.[66] Many infections are asymptomatic. Therefore, it may be prudent to rule out infections before ART treatment.

Microbiological agents that affect female fertility are summarized in Table 4.7.

Some infections also lead to pregnancy complications. Bacterial vaginosis (BV) is linked with up to 40% of births before 32 weeks gestation,[67] and 75–95% of neonatal deaths occur as a result of premature delivery.[68] BV is also associated with early miscarriages after IVF.[69] Some experts recommend that one BV screening in early pregnancy is sufficient to identify women at risk of preterm birth.[70]

However, others argue that miscarriages associated with BV also happen around the time of implantation or shortly after implantation.[69] Therefore, it might be advisable to screen all women undergoing ART for BV before treatment starts and perhaps one more time shortly after embryo transfer in case infection is introduced during the medical procedures. Because the tests are cheap and simple to perform, whilst ART is very expensive, it makes logical sense to screen all women.

From the TCM point of view, infections are associated with:

- Liver Qi Stagnation transforming into Heat
- Spleen Qi Deficiency with Dampness
- Damp-Heat[20]

Immunological investigations

Researchers have proposed that several immunological conditions are involved in reproductive failure. Chapter 12 discusses reproductive immunology in detail.

TESTS AND INVESTIGATIONS: MALE

Twenty to thirty percent of infertility is caused by a male factor,[4,71,72] and 25–40% is caused by both male and female factors.[6,71,72] ASRM states that male factor

Table 4.7 Associations between some microbiological agents and anatomical location of female infertility[66]

Microorganism	Cervical/vaginal	Uterine	Tubal/pelvic
Bacteria			
C. trachomatis	Definite	Definite	Definite and very common
Neisseria gonorrhoeae	Definite, but less studied	Definite	Definite
Mycoplasma hominis	Probable	Possible	Still to be defined
Ureaplasma urealyticum	Probable	Possible	Still to be defined
Mycoplasma genitalium	Probable	Possible	Most probable
Bacteria associated with vaginosis	Possible	Possible	Probable; no associations with specific organisms
Escherichia coli	Doubtful	Possible	Possible
Yeastsx			
Candida spp.	Doubtful	Doubtful	Highly improbable
Protozoa			
Trichomonas vaginalis	Possible cofactor	Doubtful	Possible cofactor
Viruses			
Human papilloma virus	Defined through cervical intraepithelial neoplasia	Defined through cervical intraepithelial neoplasia	Improbable
Herpes simplex virus	Doubtful	Doubtful	Association needs further investigation

Adapted from Ref.,[66] with permission from Elsevier.

subfertility is defined 'by abnormal semen parameters but may be present even when the semen analysis is normal'.[4] The aim of male factor subfertility investigation is to identify the cause of abnormal semen and any underlying medical condition.[4] Chapter 8 discusses male factor infertility in greater detail.

CLINICAL TIPS

MALE FACTOR INVESTIGATIONS

If a male partner already has a child, it does not exclude the possibility of newly acquired secondary subfertility.[4] Therefore, male infertility investigations should still be undertaken.

Confirmed male factor does not exclude presence of a concomitant female factor; therefore, a female partner should still be evaluated.

Semen analysis

Semen analysis is the most fundamental part of the assessment of male factor subfertility. After 2–5 days of abstinence,

a semen sample can be collected usually by masturbation into a special container or by intercourse into a special condom.[4] The semen sample needs to be examined in the laboratory within an hour of collection.[4] WHO interpretation of semen analysis is provided in Table 4.8.

The finding of an abnormal semen analysis result should be followed up by another semen analysis, ideally 3 months later to allow sufficient time for new sperm to be formed.[5] However, if no sperm is found in the initial sample or there is an extremely low sperm concentration, a repeat semen analysis should be performed as soon as possible.[5]

Following two or more abnormal semen analyses or in cases with unexplained subfertility, additional assessment by a urologist and additional tests are indicated.[4] Additional tests may include:[4]

- Serial semen analyses
- Endocrine evaluation
- Postejaculatory urinalysis
- Ultrasound scan
- Specialized semen and sperm tests, such as sperm antibodies tests and sperm DNA fragmentation tests
- Genetic screening

Table 4.8 WHO interpretation of semen analysis (2010)[73]

Parameter	Reference range	Terminology relating to abnormal findings
Semen volume (mL)	≥1.5	Aspermia: no semen (or retrograde ejaculation)
Total sperm number (10^6 per ejaculate)	≥39	
Sperm concentration (10^6 per mL)	≥15	Azoospermia: absence of sperm in semen
		Oligospermia: total number of sperm below lower reference limit
		Severe oligospermia: sperm concentrations of <5 mil/mL
Total motility (progressive motility (PR) +NP, %)	≥40	Asthenozoospermia: sperm motility below reference limit
		Asthenoteratozoospermia: low percentage of progressive motile (PR) and normal sperm
Progressive motility (PR, %)	≥32	Oligoasthenozoospermia: low concentration and low percentage of progressively motile (PR) sperm
Vitality (live spermatozoa, %)	≥58	Necrozoospermia: low percentage of live and high percentage of immotile sperm
Sperm morphology (normal forms, %)	≥4	Teratozoospermia: percentage of normal sperm below reference limit
		Oligoteratozoospermia: low concentration and low normal forms
		Oligoasthenoteratozoospermia: low concentration, low percentage of progressively motile (PR) sperm and low normal forms
pH	≥7.2	
Peroxidase-positive leukocytes (10^6 per mL)	<1.0	Leukospermia (leukocytospermia, pyospermia): presence of leukocytes in the ejaculate above reference limit
MAR test (motile spermatozoa with bound particles, %)	<50	
Immunobead test (motile spermatozoa with bound beads, %)	<50	
Seminal zinc (μmol/ejaculate)	≥2.4	
Seminal fructose (μmol/ejaculate)	≥13	
Seminal neutral glucosidase (mU/ejaculate)	≥20	

Reproduced with the permission of the World Health Organization.
Men with semen parameters outside the reference range may still be fertile, and, equally, men with semen parameters within normal range may be subfertile.[4]

CLINICAL TIPS

TESTS AND INVESTIGATIONS: SEMEN ANALYSIS

Semen analysis results can be affected by many factors, including medication, period of abstinence, and fever in the 3 months preceding the test.

Endocrine investigations

An endocrine investigation is recommended for men with:

- Abnormal semen parameters (especially if concentration is ≤10 mil/mL)[4,74]
- Impaired sexual function[4]
- Other clinical findings suggesting hormonal involvement[4]

Table 4.9 interpretation of male factor hormone assessment[4]

Parameter	FSH	LH	Testosterone	Prolactin
Normal spermatogenesis	Normal	Normal	Normal	Normal
Hypogonadotropic hypogonadism	Low	Low	Low	Normal
Abnormal spermatogenesis[a]	High/normal	Normal	Normal	Normal
Complete testicular failure/hypergonadotropic hypogonadism	High	High	Normal/low	Normal
Prolactin-secreting pituitary tumour	Normal/low	Normal/low	Low	High

Reprinted from Ref.,[4] with permission from Elsevier.
[a] Elevated FSH always indicates abnormal spermatogenesis, but normal FSH levels may indicate abnormal spermatogenesis in some men.

ASRM recommends that FSH and total testosterone concentrations should be measured initially. Elevated FSH or FSH levels in the upper normal range suggest impaired spermatogenesis.[4] Inhibin B levels are better associated with semen parameters than FSH, but because of the cost of the inhibin B test, it is currently not recommended for screening purposes.[4]

If the total testosterone is ≤300 ng/mL, other hormones, such as a second measurement of total testosterone, free testosterone, LH, and prolactin, should be checked. Table 4.9 provides details on how to interpret hormonal levels in male partners.

TSH should be checked in men who require an even more thorough endocrine evaluation.[4]

Postejaculatory urinalysis

Normally, urine should contain no sperm. However, in cases of retrograde ejaculation (which is discussed in more detail in Chapter 8), sperm can be found in the urine.

Postejaculatory urinalysis is where a urine sample, after first being centrifuged, is checked for the presence of sperm. It is indicated for all men with a semen volume of <1.0 mL (except men diagnosed with hypogonadism or Congenital Bilateral Absence of the Vas Deferens (CBAVD)).[4] Inappropriate collection methods or short abstention intervals should be excluded before further tests.[4] Table 4.10 provides details on how to interpret postejaculatory urinalysis results.

Ultrasound scan

Ultrasound scanning is used in only a small number of cases. Transrectal ultrasound (TRUS) can be used for further evaluation of men with oligospermia (low sperm concentrations) and low semen volume, palpable vasa, and normal testosterone level and testicle size.[4]

Physical examination of the scrotum can identify most scrotal pathology. Scrotal ultrasound may be useful to help confirm the findings of a physical examination or to help

Table 4.10 ASRM interpretation of postejaculatory urinalysis[4]

Men with	Findings and interpretation
Azoospermia (no sperm) or aspermia (no semen)	• Any sperm: confirmed retrograde ejaculation • No sperm: consider ejaculatory duct obstruction, hypogonadism, or CBAVD (exclude incomplete semen collection)
Low ejaculate volume and oligospermia (low sperm concentration)	• Significant numbers of sperm: confirm retrograde ejaculation (significant is not defined) • No sperm or small numbers of sperm: consider ejaculatory duct obstruction, hypogonadism, or CBAVD (exclude incomplete semen collection)

evaluate men with anatomical anomalies where a physical examination is not possible.[4] Men with risk factors for testicular cancer (cryptorchidism or history of testicular neoplasm) also should undergo scrotal ultrasound examination.[4]

Table 4.11 summarizes possible findings of ultrasound scans and their implications.

Abnormal findings such as varicoceles, testicular masses, or spermatoceles may, in TCM terms, be associated with Blood-Stasis or Damp-Phlegm. Congenital anatomical abnormalities are likely to be caused by Kidney Jing (Essence) Deficiency.

Test of leukocytes in semen

Some semen analysis reports show a raised number of 'round cells' or 'white blood cells' but include within these

Table 4.11 ASRM interpretation of ultrasound examination of male factor subfertility[4]

Type of ultrasound	Findings	Interpretation and comments
Transrectal (TRUS)	• Dilated seminal vesicles or • Dilated ejaculatory ducts and/or • Midline cystic prostatic structures	• Indicates (but does not in itself establish): complete or partial ejaculatory duct obstruction • Complete obstruction typically presents as low semen volume, acidic ejaculate with no sperm or fructose • Partial obstruction may present as low semen volume, oligoasthenospermia (low sperm concentration and low motility), and poor progressive motility • Can also indicate CBAVD (caused by absent or atrophic seminal vesicles)
Scrotal ultrasound	• Varicoceles • Spermatoceles • Absent vasa • Epididymal induration • Testicular masses	Ultrasound results help to confirm findings of physical examination

numbers both white blood cells and immature germ cells. Truly raised white blood cells (>1 million leukocytes per mL), also referred to as pyospermia, may indicate genital tract infection or inflammation.[4] A number of tests are available to help differentiate between immature germ cells and white blood cells.

Antisperm antibodies tests

Antisperm antibodies (ASA) can form when the immune system is exposed to large quantities of sperm through a breach of the blood-testes barrier,[4] for example, following trauma, torsion, biopsy, and vasectomy (the latter being the most common cause seen in the authors' practices). Once formed, ASA can affect the motility of sperm and its interaction with the egg.[75]

As ASA rarely causes male subfertility, and ICSI successfully overcomes ASA problems, ASA tests are not recommended as part of routine screening.[4,5]

 Case study

Tests and Investigations: ASA

Jessica came to the clinic for acupuncture treatment to help her and her husband, Mat, conceive. Mat had one child from a previous relationship.

They had already tried to conceive for 9 months. After 3 months of acupuncture treatment and no conception, Jessica and Mat were advised to see their doctor and have some tests.

The tests revealed that Mat's semen contained ASA. Mat had had a vasectomy while he was in a previous relationship and had later undergone vasectomy reversal. However, ASA formed as a result of the procedure.

Jessica and Mat needed IVF treatment.

MSOME

In addition to standard semen analysis, an advanced sperm examination method called Motile Sperm Organelles Morphology Examination (MSOME) can be undertaken.[76] It is a newer method of sperm examination that is done under high magnification ($\geq 6,000\times$).[77] It can pick up morphological sperm abnormalities, which standard semen analysis may miss.

Among other factors examined, the individual spermatozoon's nucleus is checked to see if its shape is smooth, symmetric, and oval with an average length and width estimated to be around 4.75 ± 0.20 and $3.28 \pm 0.20\,\mu$m, respectively.[77] The chromatin mass, acrosome, and tail are also checked.[77] MSOME is commonly used with the Intracytoplasmic Morphologically Selected Sperm Injection fertilization method (see Chapter 6).

Sperm DNA fragmentation tests

Semen parameters (as measured by basic semen testing) do not directly correlate with fertility. One of the explanations is that sperm may have damaged DNA, which semen analysis does not detect.[78] DNA fragmentation is commonly detected in the sperm of subfertile men.[79] DNA damage has been linked to reduced rates of natural conception[80] and conception through Intrauterine Insemination,[80] IVF,[80–82] and, to a lesser extent, ICSI.[80,81] DNA fragmentation of the ejaculate is potentially a better marker of male fertility.[83] DNA damage can occur:[79]

• During spermatogenesis
• During sperm maturation
• By apoptosis or
• As a result of oxidative stress

There are different types of sperm DNA integrity tests, the most common being Sperm Chromatin Structural Assay

Table 4.12 Interpretation of sperm DNA tests

Type of test	Findings	Interpretation and comments
SCSA	≥27% DNA damage[85]	Unlikely to result in pregnancy
TUNEL	>36.5% DNA damage[82]	Significantly lower pregnancy rates
COMET	>50% DNA damage[86]	Significantly lower live-birth rates
	25–50% DNA damage[86]	Reduced live-birth rates

(SCSA), terminal deoxynucleotidyl transferase dUTP nick end labelling (TUNEL) assay, and the single-cell gel electrophoresis (Comet) assay.[4,84] Table 4.12 provides threshold values for DNA fragmentation tests.

ASRM does not recommend routine DNA fragmentation testing because treatment options are very limited and the prognostic value is questionable.[4,87] However, DNA testing may be useful in cases of unexplained infertility because it is estimated that as many as 40% of these cases may be related to sperm DNA damage.[88]

From the TCM point of view, syndromes linked to sperm DNA fragmentation may include:

- Kidney Jing (Essence) Deficiency
- Yin Deficiency
- Yang Deficiency
- Qi Deficiency
- Blood Deficiency
- Heat/Fire

INTERESTING FACTS

SPERM DNA DAMAGE

There is evidence that eggs may repair the DNA damage in sperm. However, in eggs that are compromised (for example, in women of advanced reproductive age), this function may be less efficient.[78]

Case study

Tests and Investigations: Sperm DNA Fragmentation

A young couple, Ryan and Emma, underwent a first round of IVF. Despite having a good quality blastocyst transferred, they still failed to conceive. Their other embryos failed to

---

Case study—cont'd

develop. They were advised to undergo further investigations before attempting any more IVF, including the SCSA sperm DNA fragmentation test.

The SCSA result showed 32% damage. Ryan was advised about how he could minimize further damage to his sperm DNA.

On their next IVF cycle, Ryan and Emma conceived twins.

Genetic screening

Genetic abnormalities can affect spermatogenesis or sperm transport. Men with nonobstructive azoospermia (absence of sperm in semen) and severe oligospermia (sperm concentration of <5 mil/mL) are particularly at risk of genetic abnormalities and, therefore, should undergo genetic screening.[4,45] Patients in whom genetic abnormalities are detected may need genetic counselling prior to IVF.

Cystic fibrosis gene mutation

The cystic fibrosis transmembrane conductance regulator (CFTR) gene is so strongly associated with CBAVD that ASRM recommends that all men with CBAVD should be assumed to have a CFTR gene mutation.[4] The CFTR mutation is also common in men with azoospermia (absence of sperm in semen) because of congenital bilateral obstruction of the epididymides and in men with unilateral congenital absence of the vas deferens.[4] Therefore, these men should be offered genetic testing.

Karyotyping

Chromosomal abnormalities in men can lead to a higher incidence of miscarriages and chromosomal abnormalities of children. The prevalence of chromosomal abnormalities is inversely proportionally related to sperm count; these abnormalities are more common in men with no sperm and very rare in men with normal sperm concentrations.[4] The most common chromosomal abnormalities are sex chromosomal aneuploidy (Klinefelter syndrome; 47,XXY) and structural autosomal abnormalities.[4,89]

ASRM recommends that all men with nonobstructive azoospermia (absence of sperm in semen) or severe oligospermia (sperm concentration of <5 mil/mL) should have high-resolution karyotyping evaluation before undergoing ART[45] or ICSI.[4]

Y-chromosome analysis

Y-chromosome microdeletions are more common in infertile men compared with fertile men and are even more common in men with azoospermia (absence of sperm in semen) or severe oligospermia (sperm concentration of

<5 mil/mL).[4] Karyotyping cannot detect this abnormality, but polymerase chain reaction techniques can be used instead. The degree and location of the deletion will affect the success of ART, even with ICSI. Sons of men with Y-chromosome microdeletions will inherit the abnormality.

ASRM recommends that Y-chromosome analysis should be offered to all men with nonobstructive azoospermia (absence of sperm in semen) or severe oligospermia (sperm concentration of <5 mil/mL) before undergoing ICSI.[4]

Infection screening

Infections can affect the male reproductive tract and potentially lead to blockage and infection affecting the semen.[66] Many infections are asymptomatic. Therefore, it may be prudent to rule out infections before ART treatment is started.

Microbiological agents, which affect male fertility, are summarized in Table 4.13.

Other tests

Other advanced tests have been developed, particularly in research settings, but they have limited clinical applications.

Some of these tests are listed here for information purposes only.

Sperm Penetration Assay/Hamster Egg Penetration Test

Sperm Penetration Assay, also known as the Hamster Egg Penetration Test, looks at the ability of sperm to penetrate a zona-free hamster egg. This test was originally developed in 1976. Despite its very good predictive value for fertilization, it is not widely used because it is expensive and technically demanding.[79] Tests results depend on the experience of the laboratory carrying out the test.[90] ASRM does not recommend the routine use of these tests because ICSI is widely adopted in male factor patients, and, therefore, the sperm's ability to penetrate the egg is less relevant.[4]

Hemizona Assay

Hemizona Assay (HZA) is a test developed in 1988 that examines sperm's ability to bind to the zona pellucida of a human egg. Many IVF cycles are believed to fail because

Table 4.13 Associations between some microbiological agents and male infertility[66]

Microorganism	Testes/ epididymus	Prostate/accessory glands	Semen alterations/sperm damage
Bacteria			
C. trachomatis	Definite	Doubtful	Possible
N. gonorrhoeae	Definite	Probable	Probable
M. hominis	Doubtful	Doubtful	Doubtful
U. urealyticum	Doubtful	Doubtful	Doubtful
M. genitalium	Doubtful	Doubtful	Attaches to human sperm
Bacteria associated with vaginosis	Doubtful	Doubtful	Doubtful
E. coli	Definite, common	Definite, common	Possible
Yeasts			
Candida spp.	Doubtful	Doubtful	Rare cases
Protozoa			
T. vaginalis	Doubtful	Doubtful	Probable under specific conditions
Viruses			
Human papilloma virus	Doubtful	Doubtful	Association needs further investigations
Herpes simplex virus	Doubtful	Doubtful	Probable

Adapted from Ref.,[66] with permission from Elsevier.

of faulty sperm–zona binding. HZA has a strong predictive value of clinical pregnancy.[79]

Acrosome Reaction assay

When the sperm reach the site of the egg, they undergo the acrosome reaction (AR), where the plasma membrane and the outer acrosomal membrane break down and merge; this change is required for the egg and sperm to fuse.[91] The AR test examines the AR status of sperm and can help to investigate fertilization failure in IVF cycles.[79]

Hyposmotic Swelling test

The Hyposmotic Swelling (HOS) test was first developed in 1984 and is used to examine sperm's plasma membrane integrity. In this test, sperm are exposed to hypo-osmolar fluid, and sperm with a healthy membrane are expected to swell, especially at the tail end. This correlates with their ability to penetrate denuded hamster eggs. The HOS is inexpensive and is used to noninvasively select viable sperm from nonmotile sperm for ICSI. However, it is not useful in assessing the fertilizing capacity of sperm.[79]

SUMMARY

- The role of fertility acupuncturists has evolved. One of our responsibilities as acupuncturists specializing in this discipline is to ensure that our patients are screened properly because this could ultimately make a difference to their treatment outcome. In some cases, appropriate tests are not done. In other cases, the tests are interpreted incorrectly. Fertility acupuncturists add another layer of quality control to infertility patients' conventional medical care.
- When no cause of infertility is found after basic tests are undertaken, more advanced infertility tests should be considered (for example, genetic tests, sperm DNA fragmentation, ASA tests).[75] However, in patients with no identified cause of subfertility, referral for advanced investigations is not always made by conventional medical care practitioners. In these cases, the referral may need to be initiated by fertility acupuncturists.
- Being able to interpret the test results can help to refine and enhance TCM diagnosis and treatment. For example, a woman with reduced ovarian reserve may benefit from Kidney Jing (Essence) support, even if there is no clinical evidence of Kidney Jing (Essence) Deficiency.

REFERENCES

1. Cochrane S, Smith CA, Possamai-Inesedy A. Development of a fertility acupuncture protocol: defining an acupuncture treatment protocol to support and treat women experiencing conception delays. J Altern Complement Med 2011;17:329–37.

2. Kamel RM. Management of the infertile couple: an evidence-based protocol. Reprod Biol Endocrinol 2010;8:21–8.

3. Practice Committee of American Society for Reproductive Medicine. Diagnostic evaluation of the infertile female: a committee opinion. Fertil Steril 2012;98:302–7.

4. Practice Committee of American Society for Reproductive Medicine. Diagnostic evaluation of the infertile male: a committee opinion. Fertil Steril 2012;98:294–301.

5. National Collaborating Centre for Women's and Children's Health, Commissioned by the National Institute for Health and Clinical Excellence 2013. Guideline summary. In: Fertility: assessment and treatment for people with fertility problems. NICE Clinical Guideline, 2nd ed. London: The Royal College of Obstetricians and Gynaecologist. p. 1–46 [chapter 1].

6. Wilkes S, Chinn DJ, Murdoch A, et al. Epidemiology and management of infertility: a population-based study in UK primary care. Fam Pract 2009;26:269–74.

7. Hull MG, Glazener CM, Kelly NJ, et al. Population study of causes, treatment, and outcome of infertility. Br Med J (Clin Res Ed) 1985;291:1693–7.

8. Wathen NC, Perry L, Lilford RJ, et al. Interpretation of single progesterone measurement in diagnosis of an ovulation and defective luteal phase: observations on analysis of the normal range. Br Med J (Clin Res Ed) 1984;288:7–9.

9. Jordan J, Craig K, Clifton DK, et al. Luteal phase defect: the sensitivity and specificity of diagnostic methods in common clinical use. Fertil Steril 1994;62:54–62.

10. Filicori M, Butler JP, Crowley WF. Neuroendocrine regulation of the corpus luteum in the human. Evidence for pulsatile progesterone secretion. J Clin Invest 1984;73:1638–47.

11. Beltran L, Fahie-Wilson MN, McKenna TJ, et al. Serum total prolactin and monomeric prolactin reference intervals determined by precipitation with polyethylene glycol: evaluation and validation on common immunoassay platforms. Clin Chem 2008;54:1673–81.

12. Collins JA. Evidence-based infertility: evaluation of the female partner. Int Congr Ser 2004;1266:57–62.

13. Prolactin: MedlinePlus medical encyclopedia. Available from: http://www.nlm.nih.gov/medlineplus/ency/article/003718.htm [accessed 19 April 2013].

14. ASRM Medication for inducing ovulation. A guide for patients. Report of the ASRM. ASRM, Birmingham, Alabama; 2012.

15. Montoya JM, Bernal A, Borrero C. Diagnostics in assisted human reproduction. Reprod Biomed Online 2002;5:198–210.

16. Practice Committee of the American Society for Reproductive Medicine. Testing and interpreting measures of ovarian reserve: a committee opinion. Fertil Steril 2012;98:1407–15.

17. Stricker R, Eberhart R, Chevailler MC, et al. Establishment of detailed reference values for luteinizing hormone, follicle stimulating hormone, estradiol, and progesterone during different phases of the menstrual cycle on the abbott ARCHITECT analyzer. Clin Chem Lab Med 2006;44:883–7.

18. Cahill DJ, Wardle PG. Management of infertility. BMJ 2002;325:28–32.

19. Song JJ, Yan ME, Wu XK, et al. Progress of integrative Chinese and Western medicine in treating polycystic ovarian syndrome caused infertility. Chin J Integr Med 2006;12:312–6.

20. Liang L. The pathology of infertility. In: Acupuncture & IVF. Boulder, CO: Blue Poppy Press; 2003. p. 9–16 [chapter 2].

21. Mutlu MF, Erdem M, Erdem A, et al. Antral follicle count determines poor ovarian response better than anti-Müllerian hormone but age is the only predictor for live birth in in vitro fertilization cycles. J Assist Reprod Genet 2013;30:657–65. Available from: http://dx.doi.org/10.1007/s10815-013-9975-3.

22. Fanchin R, Schonäuer LM, Righini C, et al. Serum anti-Müllerian hormone is more strongly related to ovarian follicular status than serum inhibin B, estradiol, FSH and LH on day 3. Hum Reprod 2003;18:323–7.

23. Maughan TA, Zhai X. The acupuncture treatment of female infertility – with particular reference to egg quality and endometrial receptiveness. J Chin Med 2012;98:13–21.

24. Elliott D. The treatment of elevated FSH levels with Chinese medicine. J Chin Med 2009;91:5–11.

25. Zhao LQ. TCM treatment of female infertility caused by high FSH. J Assoc Tradit Chin Med 2009;16:13–7.

26. Zhao L. Treating infertility by the integration of Traditional Chinese Medicine and assisted conception therapy. J Assoc Tradit Chin Med (UK) 2011;28:9–14.

27. National Collaborating Centre for Women's and Children's Health, Commissioned by the National Institute for Health and Clinical Excellence 2013. Investigation of fertility problems and management strategies. In: Fertility: assessment and treatment for people with fertility problems. NICE Clinical Guideline, 2nd ed. London: The Royal College of Obstetricians and Gynaecologists. p. 80–132 [chapter 6].

28. Kitajima M, Khan KN, Hiraki K, et al. Changes in serum anti-Müllerian hormone levels may predict damage to residual normal ovarian tissue after laparoscopic surgery for women with ovarian endometrioma. Fertil Steril 2011;95:2589–91.

29. Chang HJ, Han SH, Lee JR, et al. Impact of laparoscopic cystectomy on ovarian reserve: serial changes of serum anti-Müllerian hormone levels. Fertil Steril 2010;94:343–9.

30. Somigliana E, Berlanda N, Benaglia L, et al. Surgical excision of endometriomas and ovarian reserve: a systematic review on serum anti-Müllerian hormone level modifications. Fertil Steril 2012;98:1531–8.

31. Uncu G, Kasapoglu I, Ozerkan K, et al. Prospective assessment of the impact of endometriomas and their removal on ovarian reserve and determinants of the rate of decline in ovarian reserve. Hum Reprod 2013;28:2140–5.

32. Homburg R, Ray A, Bhide P, et al. The relationship of serum anti-Mullerian hormone with polycystic ovarian morphology and polycystic ovary syndrome: a prospective cohort study. Hum Reprod 2013;28:1077–83.

33. Seifer DB, Baker VL, Leader B. Age-specific serum anti-Müllerian hormone values for 17,120 women presenting to fertility centers within the United States. Fertil Steril 2011;95:747–50.

34. Lee JY, Jee BC, Lee JR, et al. Age-related distributions of anti-Müllerian hormone level and anti-Müllerian hormone models. Acta Obstet Gynecol Scand 2012;91:970–5.

35. Verhagen TE, Hendriks DJ, Bancsi LF, et al. The accuracy of multivariate models predicting ovarian reserve and pregnancy after in vitro fertilization: a meta-analysis. Hum Reprod Update 2008;14:95–100.

36. The Rotterdam ESHRE/ASRM-sponsored PCOS consensus workshop group. Revised 2003 consensus on diagnostic criteria and long-term health risks related to polycystic ovary syndrome (PCOS). Hum Reprod 2004;19:41–7.

37. National Collaborating Centre for Women's and Children's Health, Commissioned by the National Institute for Health and Clinical Excellence 2013. Introduction. In: Fertility: assessment and treatment for people with fertility problems. NICE Clinical Guideline, 2nd ed. London: The Royal College of Obstetricians and Gynaecologists. p. 47–49 [chapter 2].

38. Saunders RD, Shwayder JM, Nakajima ST. Current methods of tubal patency assessment. Fertil Steril 2011;95:2171–9.

39. Lim CP, Hasafa Z, Bhattacharya S, et al. Should a hysterosalpingogram be a first-line investigation to diagnose female tubal subfertility in the modern subfertility workup? Hum Reprod 2011;26:967–71.

40. Taşkın EA, Berker B, Ozmen B, et al. Comparison of hysterosalpingography and hysteroscopy in the evaluation of the uterine cavity in patients undergoing assisted reproductive techniques. Fertil Steril 2011;96:349–52.

41. Sonohysterography – ultrasound of the uterus (saline infusion sonography). Available from: http://www.radiologyinfo.org/en/info.cfm?pg=hysterosono [accessed 1 May 2013].

42. Pundir J, El Toukhy T. Uterine cavity assessment prior to IVF. Womens Health 2010;6:841–8.

43. El-Mazny A, Abou-Salem N, El-Sherbiny W, et al. Outpatient hysteroscopy: a routine investigation before assisted reproductive techniques? Fertil Steril 2011;95:272–6.

44. Bosteels J, Weyers S, Puttemans P, et al. The effectiveness of hysteroscopy in improving pregnancy rates in subfertile women without other gynaecological

symptoms: a systematic review. Hum Reprod Update 2010;16:1–11.

45. Foresta C, Ferlin A, Gianaroli L, et al. Guidelines for the appropriate use of genetic tests in infertile couples. Eur J Hum Genet 2002;10:303–12.

46. Carp H, Feldman B, Oelsner G, et al. Parental karyotype and subsequent live births in recurrent miscarriage. Fertil Steril 2004;81:1296–301.

47. The Practice Committee of the American Society for Reproductive Medicine. Evaluation and treatment of recurrent pregnancy loss: a committee opinion. Fertil Steril 2012;98:1103–11.

48. Riccaboni A, Lalatta F, Caliari I, et al. Genetic screening in 2,710 infertile candidate couples for assisted reproductive techniques: results of application of Italian guidelines for the appropriate use of genetic tests. Fertil Steril 2008;89:800–8.

49. Schreurs A, Legius E, Meuleman C, et al. Increased frequency of chromosomal abnormalities in female partners of couples undergoing in vitro fertilization or intracytoplasmic sperm injection. Fertil Steril 2000;74:94–6.

50. Papanikolaou EG, Vernaeve V, Kolibianakis E, et al. Is chromosome analysis mandatory in the initial investigation of normovulatory women seeking infertility treatment? Hum Reprod 2005;20:2899–903.

51. Crosignani PG, Rubin BL. Optimal use of infertility diagnostic tests and treatments. The ESHRE capri workshop group. Hum Reprod 2000;15:723–32.

52. Heit JA. Thrombophilia: common questions on laboratory assessment and management. Hematol Am Soc Hematol Educ Program 2007;2007 (1):127–35.

53. Baglin T, Gray E, Greaves M, et al. Clinical guidelines for testing for heritable thrombophilia. Br J Haematol 2010;149:209–20.

54. Paidas MJ, Ku D-HW, Langhoff-Roos J, et al. Inherited thrombophilias and adverse pregnancy outcome: screening and management. Semin Perinatol 2005;29:150–63.

55. Bellver J, Soares SR, Alvarez C, et al. The role of thrombophilia and thyroid autoimmunity in unexplained infertility, implantation failure and recurrent spontaneous abortion. Hum Reprod 2008;23:278–84.

56. Sauer R, Roussev R, Jeyendran RS, et al. Prevalence of antiphospholipid antibodies among women experiencing unexplained infertility and recurrent implantation failure. Fertil Steril 2010;93:2441–3.

57. Qublan HS, Eid SS, Ababneh HA, et al. Acquired and inherited thrombophilia: implication in recurrent IVF and embryo transfer failure. Hum Reprod 2006;21:2694–8.

58. Azem F, Many A, Yovel I, et al. Increased rates of thrombophilia in women with repeated IVF failures. Hum Reprod 2004;19:368–70.

59. Austin S, Cohen H. Antiphospholipid syndrome. Medicine 2006;34:472–5.

60. Beaman KD, Ntrivalas E, Mallers TM, et al. Immune etiology of recurrent pregnancy loss and its diagnosis. Am J Reprod Immunol 2012;67:319–25.

61. Robertson L, Wu O, Langhorne P, et al. Thrombophilia in pregnancy: a systematic review. Br J Haematol 2006;132:171–96.

62. McNamee K, Dawood F, Farquharson RG. Thrombophilia and early pregnancy loss. Best Pract Res Clin Obstet Gynaecol 2012;26:91–102.

63. Miyakis S, Lockshin MD, Atsumi T, et al. International consensus statement on an update of the classification criteria for definite antiphospholipid syndrome (APS). J Thromb Haemost 2006; 4(2):295–306.

64. About Hughes syndrome | APS | the brain. Available from: http://www.hughes-syndrome.org/about-hughes-syndrome/brain.php#.UYRdeZXS6fQ [accessed 4 May 2013].

65. About Hughes syndrome | APS | the skin. Available from: http://www.hughes-syndrome.org/about-hughes-syndrome/skin.php#.UYReZZXS6fQ [accessed 4 May 2013].

66. Pellati D, Mylonakis I, Bertoloni G, et al. Genital tract infections and infertility. Eur J Obstet Gynecol Reprod Biol 2008;140(1):3–11.

67. Goldenberg RL, Iams JD, Mercer BM, et al. The preterm prediction study: the value of new vs standard risk factors in predicting early and all spontaneous preterm births. NICHD MFMU network. Am J Public Health 1998;88:233–8.

68. Lee HJ, Park TC, Norwitz ER. Management of pregnancies with cervical shortening: a very short cervix is a very big problem. Rev Obstet Gynecol 2009;2:107–15.

69. Ralph SG, Rutherford AJ, Wilson JD. Influence of bacterial vaginosis on conception and miscarriage in the first trimester: cohort study. BMJ 1999;319:220–3.

70. Larsson PG, Fåhraeus L, Carlsson B, et al. Predisposing factors for bacterial vaginosis, treatment efficacy and pregnancy outcome among term deliveries; results from a preterm delivery study. BMC Womens Health 2007;7:20–6.

71. ESHRE ART fact sheet. Available from: http://www.eshre.eu/ESHRE/English/Guidelines-Legal/ART-fact-sheet/page.aspx/1061 [accessed 13 December 2012].

72. Thonneau P, Marchand S, Tallec A, et al. Incidence and main causes of infertility in a resident population (1 850 000) of three French regions (1988–1989)*. Hum Reprod 1991;6:811–6.

73. WHO. Reference values and semen nomenclature. In: WHO Laboratory Manual for the Examination and Processing of Human Semen. 5th ed. Geneva: World Health Organization; 2010. p. 223–6, Appendix 1.

74. Choy JT, Ellsworth P. Overview of current approaches to the evaluation and management of male infertility. Urol Nurs 2012;32:286–304.

75. Esteves SC, Miyaoka R, Agarwal A. An update on the clinical assessment of the infertile male. Clinics 2011;66:691–700.

76. Klement AH, Koren-Morag N, Itsykson P, et al. Intracytoplasmic morphologically selected sperm injection versus intracytoplasmic sperm injection: a step toward a clinical algorithm. Fertil Steril 2013;99:1290–3.

77. Oliveira JB, Petersen CG, Massaro FC, et al. Motile sperm organelle morphology examination (MSOME): intervariation study of

normal sperm and sperm with large nuclear vacuoles. Reprod Biol Endocrinol 2010;8:56.

78. Barratt CL, Aitken RJ, Björndahl L, et al. Sperm DNA: organization, protection and vulnerability: from basic science to clinical applications – a position report. Hum Reprod 2010;25:824–38.

79. Natali A, Turek PJ. An assessment of new sperm tests for male infertility. Urology 2011;77:1027–34.

80. Evenson D, Wixon R. Meta-analysis of sperm DNA fragmentation using the sperm chromatin structure assay. Reprod Biomed Online 2006;12:466–72.

81. Li Z, Wang L, Cai J, et al. Correlation of sperm DNA damage with IVF and ICSI outcomes: a systematic review and meta-analysis. J Assist Reprod Genet 2006;23:367–76.

82. Henkel R, Hajimohammad M, Stalf T, et al. Influence of deoxyribonucleic acid damage on fertilization and pregnancy. Fertil Steril 2004;81:965–72.

83. Barnhart KT. Epidemiology of male and female reproductive disorders and impact on fertility regulation and population growth. Fertil Steril 2011;95:2200–3.

84. Schulte RT, Ohl DA, Sigman M, et al. Sperm DNA damage in male infertility: etiologies, assays, and outcomes. J Assist Reprod Genet 2010;27:3–12.

85. Larson-Cook KL, Brannian JD, Hansen KA, et al. Relationship between the outcomes of assisted reproductive techniques and sperm DNA fragmentation as measured by the sperm chromatin structure assay. Fertil Steril 2003;80:895–902.

86. Simon L, Proutski I, Stevenson M, et al. Sperm DNA damage has a negative association with live-birth rates after IVF. Reprod Biomed Online 2013;26:68–78.

87. The Practice Committee of the American Society for Reproductive Medicine. The clinical utility of sperm DNA integrity testing: a guideline. Fertil Steril 2013;99:673–7.

88. Bungum M. Sperm DNA, integrity assessment: a new tool in diagnosis and treatment of fertility. Obstet Gynecol Int 2012;2012:531042.

89. Esteves SC, Hamada A, Kondray V, et al. What every gynecologist should know about male infertility: an update. Arch Gynecol Obstet 2012;286:217–29.

90. Practice Committee of the American Society for Reproductive Medicine. Report on optimal evaluation of the infertile male. Fertil Steril 2006;86:S202–9.

91. Speroff L, Fritz MA. Sperm and egg transport, fertilization, and implantation. In: Clinical gynecologic endocrinology and infertility. 7th ed. Philadelphia: Lippincott Williams & Wilkins; 2005. p. 233–59. [chapter 7].

Chapter | 5 |

Investigations from a TCM perspective

Clinical methods of diagnosis in Traditional Chinese Medicine (TCM) include looking and listening, pulse examination, inspection of the tongue, abdominal examination, and inquiry (medical history taking). These diagnostic methods help fertility acupuncturists to diagnose and correctly manage patients before, during, and after Assisted Reproductive Technology (ART) treatments such as *In Vitro* Fertilization (IVF).

MEDICAL AND FERTILITY HISTORY TAKING

In TCM, inquiry into the patient's medical history enables the acupuncturist to assess the state of health,[1,2] identify possible aetiology and causative factors, make a prognosis,[3] and then treat the disease. It may also help to prevent complications.[4]

In subfertility practice, medical history taking is very similar to that in general acupuncture practice, with an emphasis on fertility and ART history. This section presumes prior knowledge of how to take a TCM-related medical history. It therefore only covers specific questions relating to infertility and any previous ART treatments. Appendix I provides templates that can be used when taking medical and fertility history.

Personal information

Basic information should include:

- Patient's name
- Patient's date of birth and age
- Partner's date of birth and age

- Patient's contact details: address, telephone numbers, email address, etc.
- Family doctor's name and clinic
- ART clinic and consultant's name (if relevant)
- Confirmed associated co-morbid medical illnesses (such as diabetes, hypertension, thyroid disease, Polycystic Ovarian Syndrome (PCOS))
- Confirmed infertility diagnosis (if any)

For ethical and medico-legal purposes, it is useful to obtain your patient's and his or her partner's signed consent permitting you to liaise with medical professionals on their behalf.

Presenting complaint

This is a patient's chance to tell you his or her story of their subfertility journey thus far. Patients tend to begin with what they consider to be a priority, the aspects they see as key to their fertility. Some patients provide very detailed information; others may need prompting. Women may cry when they describe what they have been through and how they are feeling. Men may look and feel uncomfortable, especially if there is confirmed male factor subfertility. Therefore, some men may need reassurances and encouragement to 'open up' about their issues.

Specific information that can be established includes:

- How long a patient has been trying to conceive. The length of time is less relevant compared to the number of menstrual cycles and when sexual intercourse took place during the fertile window. For example, if a patient's partner travels a lot, they might only manage to have intercourse at the right time in the menstrual cycle three to four times a year. Or women with prolonged menstrual cycles may only have three to four chances of conception per year compared to women with regular 28-day cycles, who may have up to 13 opportunities in a year. So, in 3 years, one couple may make as many as 39 attempts, but another couple, only 9 attempts.

- Frequency and timing of intercourse (see Chapter 7).[5,6]
- Length of time since stopping contraception.[5]
- Any sexual intercourse issues, such as pain or bleeding during or after the intercourse,[5,6] any ejaculation or erectile issues,[5] low libido, relationship issues, or others. In some cases, IVF may not be necessary, and, instead, alternative methods of natural conception, such as self-insemination using a syringe (the 'turkey baster' method), could be tried (see Chapter 7 for more information).
- If the female patient produces fertile cervical mucus, how much, and for how many days. Many patients know about cervical mucus, but some may not. (The significance of this is discussed in the section on sexual intercourse in Chapter 7.)
- Lubrication usage.
- Frequency of sexual intercourse outside of the fertile window; this is relevant because men who ejaculate on a regular basis have healthier sperm.[7,8]

General health

This is where acupuncturists enquire into every aspect of a patient's health, including digestive, respiratory, cardiovascular, urinary, and musculoskeletal systems, energy levels, body temperature regulation, memory and concentration, headaches, and sleeping patterns.

Some specific findings, which may necessitate further Orthodox medical investigations relating to subfertility, include:

- Digestive symptoms such as pain and bloating may be related to inflammatory bowel disease (IBD), which is increasingly being linked to infertility,[9–11] possibly because of nutritional deficiencies caused by IBD absorption issues.
- Thirst and frequent urination could indicate diabetes.[12]
- Feeling cold with low energy levels could be due to hypothyroidism,[13,14] which can cause infertility and pregnancy loss.[13]
- Feeling unusually hot could be caused by hyperthyroidism[15] or early or premature menopause, especially if accompanied by short or irregular menstrual cycles.[16]
- Widespread joint pain may potentially indicate inflammation and autoimmune pathology.
- Migraines and/or problems with concentration could be caused by clotting issues such as Antiphospholipid Syndrome,[17] especially in patients who have a history of miscarriages or pregnancy loss.
- Vaginal discharges may be normal or pathologic. Abnormal discharge may be:[18]

- ■ White, curdy, and odourless
- ■ White/grey homogeneous coating of vaginal walls and vulva that has a fishy odour
- ■ Yellow-green frothy discharge with fishy odour.
- Breast discharges in men and women may be linked to high prolactin levels and, potentially, pituitary tumours; therefore, all affected patients (except breastfeeding women) should be referred for a magnetic resonance imaging scan.[19]
- Excessive body hair and/or acne in women could indicate PCOS.[20]

It is important to remember that these are only indicators of possible pathology and not proof of diseases. Therefore, care should be taken not to alarm your patients unnecessarily when discussing these symptoms with them.

Menstrual cycle

Questions relating to menstrual cycles should include the following (see the section on menstrual cycle regulation in Chapter 8 for details on how to use this information):

- Age at menarche.[6]
- Length and regularity of the menstrual cycle.[6]
- Any premenstrual symptoms, for example, breast tenderness, changes in bowels, bloating, lower back pain, mood swings, headaches, etc.
- Any menstrual pain and, if so, its severity, location, and type.[6] Does the patient have to take medication and if so, which one? (See Appendix VI for details on commonly used medications that can affect fertility.) All patients with period pain should be assessed for other signs of endometriosis, such as painful intercourse, cycle-related bowel or urinary changes, pelvic pain outside of period, ovulation pain, etc. (see the section on endometriosis in Chapter 8 for further information).
- Menses: their length, amount of blood flow (heavy or light), any spotting before or after menses, colour, clotting, consistency (see the section on menstrual cycle regulation in Chapter 8 for information about how to interpret these signs from the TCM point of view).
- Any recent changes to cycle length or bleeding patterns. These may indicate pathology, such as early stages of menopause, systemic disease, PCOS (see Chapter 8).
- If there is any bleeding outside of menses (for example, at ovulation time). This is considered a red flag, and women should be referred to their doctor for further investigations to exclude a sinister cause of midcycle bleeding.
- If a patient charts her Basal Body Temperature (BBT), it may be useful to review the charts (see section 'Introduction to BBT diagnosis' later in this chapter).

Past medical history

Past medical history may impact on fertility. Men should be asked about any history of:[5]

- Mumps
- Testicular trauma or torsion
- Surgery (for example, hernia or orchidopexy, vasectomy)
- Undescended testis
- Sexually transmitted diseases (STDs)

Women should be asked about any history of:[5]

- STDs
- Pelvic inflammatory disease or infections
- Pelvic surgery (for example, appendicitis or ovarian cysts)
- Cervical conization

Cancer treatments in either partner may cause subfertility.[5]

Medical tests and investigations

It is not unusual for patients to use phrases such as 'all the tests results were normal'. It is very important to request copies of all the test results and follow up on any abnormal or borderline results. In many cases, a referral for further investigations is necessary. Sometimes errors, such as incorrect timing of hormonal blood tests, can be identified. Such patients should be referred for a retest. In some cases, essential tests may not have been conducted. For example, patients with symptoms of thyroid disease do not always get tested to confirm or exclude the disease. Chapter 4 provides detailed information about Orthodox medical subfertility investigations and their interpretation.

Female patients need to confirm their rubella vaccination status and their cervical smear history.[5]

Chapter 4 provides detailed information about tests and investigations. Appendix I provides a test and investigation template form.

Family medical history

Female patients need to be asked about any history of maternal gynaecologic and obstetric problems. This is important to record because a woman tends to have the menopause at a similar age as her mother.[6,21] Therefore, if a patient's mother had early onset menopause, it may be prudent (if it has not already been done) to refer the patient for ovarian reserve investigations.

There is also some evidence that daughters of women with endometriosis are at higher risk of developing endometriosis.[22] Diabetes, PCOS,[23–26] and thyroid disease[27] can also have a familial link. Familial twin delivery may also be relevant.

A maternal history of recurrent miscarriages[6] may indicate family history of thrombophilia or autoimmune

disease. A family history of diabetes may put a female patient at higher risk of developing this disease. PCOS is also associated with diabetes.

Previous pregnancies and obstetric history

Both partners should be asked individually if they have achieved a pregnancy in the current or in previous relationships and the outcome of any pregnancies. It is important to remember that a past history of pregnancy does not exclude the possibility of current infertility.[28] For example, it is quite common for men who have previously fathered a child to have an abnormal semen analysis when trying for a baby with a new partner.

The emotional impact of any previous terminations can be evident decades later and should not be underestimated. It is important to ask if there were any post-termination complications, such as infections, that may have caused damage to the endometrial lining.

In women with a history of miscarriage(s) or pregnancy loss, it is important to find out the following:

- Do they know at which stage the baby stopped developing? This may be different from when they started bleeding or physically miscarried the pregnancy. If the foetus stopped developing during the second trimester, this outcome should have triggered investigations, even if the woman had only one miscarriage.[29] (Chapter 12 discusses miscarriages in greater detail.)
- If they had investigations undertaken to determine the cause of the miscarriage, what were the findings?
- How was the miscarriage managed: naturally, medically, or surgically? Surgical curettage may have affected the endometrium.[30]
- Were there any circumstances that could explain the miscarriage(s), such as an infection or a physical or emotional trauma? For example, if a miscarriage at 17 weeks was caused by physical trauma, it is likely to be a one-time event that will require no further investigations.
- Were there any lifestyle-related factors that were linked to the miscarriages (see Chapter 7)? For example, did the woman take any medication that is known to increase the risk of miscarriage? When asking questions, be very careful not make the patient feel guilty or as if she is being judged by the acupuncturist about something she may or may not have done or events that were out of her control or influence.

Sometimes a referral for miscarriage investigation may be indicated (see the section on miscarriages in Chapter 12 for further information).

In pregnancies that resulted in live birth, it is important to find out the following:

- Number of pregnancies
- Gestation at delivery
- Method of delivery (for example, caesarean sections may increase the risk of secondary infertility)[31]
- Complications during pregnancy (for example, preeclampsia)
- Complications postpartum (for example, infections that may cause endometrial scarring or post-natal depression)

With any history of pregnancies, it is useful to find out how long it took patients to conceive those pregnancies in order to ascertain their fertility potential.

It might also be useful to find out if the female patient ever suspected she was pregnant only to have a period arrive few days later. This may indicate an implantation issue (see the section on repeated implantation failure (RIF) in Chapter 12).

Modifiable lifestyle factors

Lifestyle factors in subfertility are important in both TCM[1] and Orthodox medicine. Factors that may impair fertility include:

- Excess or low weight
- Smoking
- Use of alcohol
- Use of caffeine
- Medications
- Use of recreational drugs
- Occupational and environmental factors
- Stress
- Nutritional deficiencies
- Lack of or too much exercise

Chapter 7 provides detailed information about which lifestyle factors affect fertility. Appendix I provides a lifestyle factors template form.

Assisted Reproductive Technology treatment (ART) history

By asking questions about a patient's past ART history, acupuncturists can assess what went well and what could have gone better, with both the TCM and Orthodox medical management. Preventative measures for future management can then be suggested to the patient. Appendix I provides an IVF audit tool template that can be used for auditing past ART cycles.

Previous ART treatment cycles: Basic information

How many and what type of ART cycles did the patient have and when? This reviews the severity of subfertility from both the Orthodox medical and TCM perspectives.

Preparation phase

Acupuncture treatment (if it was done)

Did the patient and/or his or her partner have acupuncture treatment in preparation for IVF? If so, was the treatment dose adequate (the number and timing of treatment sessions, etc.)? Was there an improvement in the identified syndromes? It is important to remember that a 'cure' is not always possible or necessary. In many cases, an improvement is all that is required to improve the outcome of ART treatment.

Orthodox medical treatment (if relevant)

Did the patient receive the correct medical treatment for any underlying medical conditions? Were there significant improvements in the condition(s) before ART treatment started? For example, if a patient has hypothyroidism, did the treatment succeed in bringing the Thyroid-Stimulating Hormone levels into the normal range?

If the medical treatment was not adequate or not provided at all, acupuncturists may need to make recommendations.

Lifestyle factors

Some lifestyle factors are known to influence IVF outcome. (Chapter 7 discusses lifestyle factors in detail.) It is important to ask if the patient took any specific steps to prepare for ART/IVF treatment, and, if so, which modifications were made. Did the patient make the changes long enough before the treatment began? Ideally, lifestyle modifications should be implemented at least 2–3 months beforehand.

If further lifestyle modifications are required, patients should be appropriately informed, and their progress should be monitored.

RIF prevention steps

Did the patient's ART clinic take steps to reduce the risk of implantation failure? This is especially relevant in patients who previously failed three or more times.

The following measures may reduce the risk of implantation failure (see Chapter 12 for more details):

- Hysteroscopy
- Endometrial scratch
- Interval (sequential) transfer
- Frozen Embryo Transfer
- Embryo glue
- Vaginal Viagra
- Subclinical infection treatment
- Immune treatments
- Thrombophilia treatment
- Intracytoplasmic morphologically selected sperm injection (IMSI) fertilization method
- Assisted hatching
- Day 2 versus 3 versus blastocyst
- Genetic screening of embryos

- Morphokinetic analysis (embryoscope, Early Embryo Viability Assessment or EEVA™)

Pretreatment stage (usually downregulation stage)

Acupuncture treatment (if it was done)

Was acupuncture treatment administered to one or both partners? If so, was it sufficient and appropriate?

Medication protocol

What ART/IVF medication was prescribed, what was the dose, and for how long was it taken?

Reaction to medication

Did the patient experience any reaction to the medication? For example:

- Mood swings or emotional imbalances such as worry or anxiety
- Physical side effects, commonly hot flushes, headaches, congestion, or dryness
- Medication-induced TCM pathology (for example, of the Liver, Kidney, Stomach, and Spleen) that could have negatively affected subsequent stages of the IVF process (see Chapter 9)

Ovarian stimulation phase

Baseline ultrasound scan (if carried out)

- The number of antral follicles on each ovary (gives an idea of the patient's follicular pool available for recruitment in that cycle)
- Thickness of the endometrium (if too thick in the beginning of the cycle, it may compromise the result)
- Oestrogen levels (if raised, the patient may need to downregulate for longer)
- Any cysts and their sizes

Acupuncture treatment (if it was done)

Was acupuncture treatment administered to one or both partners? If so, was it sufficient and appropriate?

Medication protocol

What ART/IVF medication was prescribed, what was the dose, and for how long was it taken?

Response to ovarian stimulation

Finding out the patient's level of response to ovarian stimulation will help to determine the extent to which acupuncture treatment and management may improve the patient's response. The ways to measure ovarian response include finding out:

- How many follicles were available for aspiration on each ovary and their sizes

- Peak oestrogen level (if raised, may indicate Ovarian Hyperstimulation Syndrome or OHSS (discussed in Chapter 11) or damaged endometrial receptivity (discussed in Chapter 12))
- Endometrial thickness and quality (see Chapter 10 for a discussion of what is considered a suboptimal endometrium)

Chapter 10 discusses in detail how to overcome obstacles during ART/IVF and Chapters 8 and 9 outline methods that may possibly improve a patient's response to ovarian stimulation. Chapter 6 discusses how acupuncture treatment may enhance each stage of ART/IVF treatment.

Complications

Did the patient experience any degree of OHSS (see Chapter 11)?

Ovulation induction

- What medication and what dose was used to 'trigger' final egg maturation?
- Was acupuncture administered between the 'trigger' and egg retrieval days (see Chapter 9)?

Egg retrieval

Day of egg retrieval

This helps to establish how many days of stimulation occurred before the patient underwent egg retrieval. In some cases, egg retrieval is carried out too early or too late (for reasons of logistical convenience of the ART units). Suboptimal timing of egg retrieval may result in a lower number of mature eggs or a lower number of eggs being retrieved (see Chapter 10).

Number and maturity of eggs at collection

- How many eggs were collected?
- Is it in accordance with the number of follicles? Most follicles ≥ 15 mm should contain a mature egg.
- How many eggs were mature and suitable for fertilization?
- How many eggs, if any, were matured with *In Vitro* Maturation?

Pain during egg retrieval

- What kind of anaesthesia was used?
- Did the patient experience any pain during or after the retrieval?

Semen parameters

If fresh semen was used, what were the semen parameters that day? (See Chapter 4 for semen analysis interpretation and Chapter 8 for information about male factor subfertility.)

Fertilization

- Which fertilization method was used: IVF, Intracytoplasmic Sperm Insemination (ICSI), IMSI, or some other method? (Chapter 6 discusses methods of fertilization.)
- How many eggs were suitable for fertilization, and how many of them were fertilized? Poor fertilization rate is discussed in Chapter 10.
- How many eggs fertilized abnormally?

Embryo development

- How many embryos were there, and what were their grades on days 2, 3, and 5 posttransfer?
- Did the clinic use an embryoscope or EEVA (see Chapter 12)?
- If embryos were genetically tested, what were the results (see Chapter 12)?

This information helps to ascertain whether TCM pathology may have influenced embryo development, for example, whether Pre- and/or Post-Natal Jing (Essence) Deficiency affected embryos. Chapter 6 discusses embryo grading, Chapter 3 discusses the Embryo's Qi and Chapter 10 discusses poor embryo development.

Embryo transfer

Acupuncture treatment (if it was done)

Was acupuncture treatment administered? If so, which protocol was used (if any), and when was it administered?

Complications during the transfer

- Was there any discomfort during the transfer?
- Were there any complications during the transfer, such as issues with ejecting the embryos from the catheter, pain, and so on? Chapter 10 discusses difficult embryo transfer.

Embryos

- How many embryos were transferred and on which day of their development?
- What were their grades?
- How many embryos were frozen (if any), and what were their grades?

If ART/IVF fails two or three times despite seemingly good quality embryos, RIF measures should be considered. (Chapter 12 discusses this both from the Orthodox and TCM points of view.)

Luteal phase

Acupuncture treatment (if it was done)

Was acupuncture treatment administered during this phase? If so, was it sufficient and appropriate?

Stress

During ART/IVF, patients are more vulnerable to fluctuating emotions, which may cause or exacerbate TCM disharmony. This is especially true during the luteal phase. For example, anger can Stagnate Liver Qi and negatively affect implantation.

It is important to ask open-ended questions such as 'How were you feeling?' and 'What were you doing?' and listen carefully to the patient's response and concerns whilst assessing the patient's behaviour.

Common negative emotions associated with key reproductive organs that may negatively affect implantation and the possibility of pregnancy can include:

- The Liver: instability of mood, crying, despair, hope
- The Heart, (Shen) Mind, and Spirit: reduced clarity of thought, anxiety
- The Kidney: fear of IVF failure
- The Spleen: worry, negativity, and/or constant thinking about the outcome

Physical symptoms

- Did the patient experience any unusual symptoms such as vaginal bleeding, abdominal cramping, breast tenderness, or tiredness?
- Did the patient experience any early pregnancy symptoms? These are not always reliable and may be caused by progesterone supplementation but, in the authors' experience, may include increased levels of tiredness, breast tenderness, and abdominal 'stitch-like' sensations.

Outcome(s)

What type of pregnancy test was used: a urine or blood test? If a blood test, what was the Human Chorionic Gonadotrophin (hCG) level? (The section on miscarriages in Chapter 12 discusses the significance of hCG levels.)

If there was a pregnancy, what was its outcome? For example, a live birth, a miscarriage, an ectopic pregnancy, or a stillbirth (see the section 'Previous pregnancies and obstetric medical history' earlier in this chapter).

CLINICAL OBSERVATIONS

In TCM, clinical observation and examination are broadly split into five categories:

- Jing-Shen examination
- The Five Phases examination
- Pulse diagnosis
- Tongue diagnosis
- Abdominal diagnosis

Jing-Shen examination in subfertility

The Jing-Shen examination is an assessment of a person's vitality.[32] It includes the evaluation of the patient's complexion, his or her eyes,[32] and Shen (Mind). A radiant complexion, shiny eyes, a clear Shen (Mind), and an assured presence is an external manifestation of a healthy Jing-Shen.

A good time to first assess Jing-Shen is during the initial consultation, when an acupuncturist often intuitively senses the patient's state of Jing-Shen. While taking the case history, the acupuncturist can observe the patient's eyes and complexion and assess whether the patient's personality, communications, and interactions are in accordance with each other. For example, if a patient discusses her history of miscarriages and tells the acupuncturist that she has accepted what happened to her, yet her eyes at that point look very dull and sad, this could potentially indicate a repressed emotion, which is a sign of pathology. The acupuncturist can then enquire further to ascertain the degree of grief still present and/or blocked. On further questioning, it is not unusual for a patient to open up and cry, which can have a therapeutic value. Other signs to look for include whether the patient is able to make eye contact and/or the movement patterns of the eyes.

The assessment of Jing-Shen can also be used prognostically. For example:

- In a woman in whom Jing-Shen becomes evident following the embryo transfer procedure, this may indicate that conception is taking place, particularly if Jing-Shen was not observable prior to that.
- Conversely, if, after a previous observation of Jing-Shen in a pregnant woman, there is a sudden change, such as a pale, dull, lustreless complexion with dullness of the eyes, this may coincide with the cessation of foetal development and an impending pregnancy loss.

The Five Phases examination in subfertility

The Five Phase doctrine divides Qi into Five Phases: Water, Wood, Fire, Earth, and Metal. Observation of the nature and the varied qualities of different types of people resulted in the generation of a system of correspondences[33] between the Spirit, emotions, tone of voice, odour, and colours of a patient and his or her state of health.

Figure 5.1 summarizes all Five Phase correspondences. Acupuncturists can use this as one of the tools to assess a subfertile patient and gain a different perspective of the patient's health.

For example, the Kidney is associated with the spirit Zhi (Will) and the emotion of fear. A patient with a healthy Kidney will have a strong Zhi (Will), which will enable that person to overcome fertility obstacles. Those patients who have a weak Zhi (Will) may give up after only one IVF failure because they fear another failure of the treatment. This fear may further injure an already weak Kidney. A weak Kidney may also result in poor-quality eggs, sperm, and/or embryos, or miscarriage because Kidney Qi, Jing (Essence), Yin, and Yang are important for egg and sperm production.

Another example is a very angry patient who shouts when speaking and has a green-blue (purplish) hue around the eyes and mouth and a fetid body odour, signs that the Wood phase or Liver is in distress. Such a patient may have issues with fertility because of disordered functioning of Liver Qi, which is required for growth, regeneration, and activity, thus affecting embryo development or implantation in the Uterus.

Recommended reading for those who are interested in learning more about the Five Phases is:

- Classical Five Element Acupuncture by John Worsley
- Five Element Constitutional Acupuncture by Angela Hicks, John Hicks, and Peter Mole

TCM pulse diagnosis in subfertility

Pulse examination of both wrists confirms the location of disorders[44] and pathology of the Zang organs.[45,46] The emotional disposition of the patient can also be identified. Pulse examination is usually combined with other methods of diagnosis; however, it can be used as the sole method of assessment.[47]

Pulse examination provides a baseline clinical reference of the state of health. Ongoing pulse examination helps to measure acupuncture treatment progress[48] and also identify new clinical issues that may need the administration of timely acupuncture treatment. This is especially important during all IVF stages because IVF medications, particularly downregulation and ovarian stimulation medications, may cause Qi, Yang, or Blood Deficiency, Stagnation, Dampness, and/or Fire. A new pathology initially may only be evident as a new pulse quality.

Pulse examination is both a diagnostic and prognostic tool, helping to formulate the treatment principles, needle techniques, dose, and frequency of acupuncture treatment. In complex cases, the predominance of an Empty or Full condition can be clarified. Table 5.1 lists pulse qualities and their associated syndromes commonly found in subfertile patients.

CLINICAL TIPS

PULSE DIAGNOSIS IN SUBFERTILITY IN TCM CLASSICAL LITERATURE

- A thin pulse reading in an overweight person may indicate the presence of Cold in the Uterus.[51]
- A deficient pulse reading on the right rear position indicates Mingmen (Fire of Life) is weak.[59]
- In TCM classical literature, it is said that a choppy, weak, and faint pulse indicates severe infertility.[51]
- According to Li Shi Zhen, a choppy pulse can indicate an inability of the mother's Blood to nourish the (embryo) or foetus,[49] potentially resulting in its demise. This is often observed in patients who have Blood Deficiency or patients who have diminishing ovarian reserve and/or implantation failure.
- A floating and tight pulse may indicate an impending miscarriage.[51]

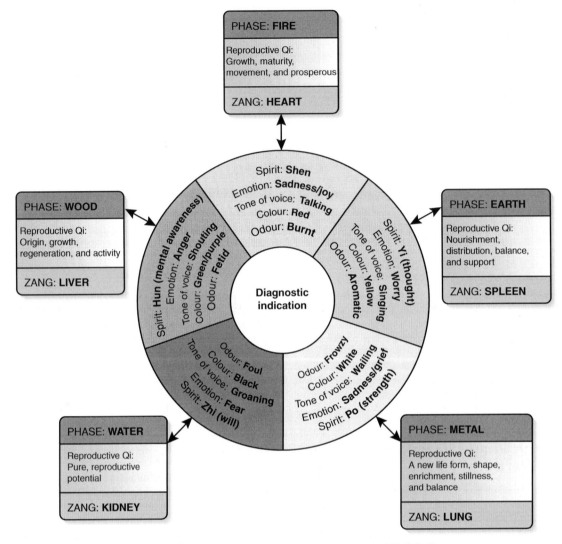

Figure 5.1 Diagnostic indications and correspondences within the Five Phase doctrine.[4,34–40,42,43]

TCM tongue diagnosis in subfertility

Examination of the tongue is an important clinical method of diagnosis, assessment, treatment, and management in TCM, particularly in identifying pathogenic factors. Tongue examination is generally conducted along with the examination of the pulse and collection of background data.[60,61] However, tongue diagnosis can show the presence of pathology (for example, Blood Stasis, Cold, Damp, or Phlegm) even in the absence of any other clinical manifestations. Tongue diagnosis also helps to determine the severity of a pathology and whether a pathology is chronic or of fairly recent onset. Figure 5.2 summarizes various tongue diagnosis correspondences.

Some of the common manifestations in subfertile patients include:

- Pale, dull tongue body can signify Blood Deficiency, which may indicate Blood Deficiency in the Uterus and endometrial lining problems.
- A red tongue usually indicates Heat and/or Fire (for example, in the Uterus), but it can also indicate a disordered Qi and Blood. For example, Blood Stasis may present as a dark red tongue body.
- A red tip may signify that excessive emotions are affecting the health of the patient,[60] causing Heat/Fire, which, in turn, may be disturbing the Uterus, Spirit and Mind and thus affecting implantation.

Table 5.1 Pulse qualities commonly found in subfertile patients and differential diagnosis

Pulse quality	Shen (Spirit) Deficiency	Jing (Essence) Deficiency	Qi Deficiency	Blood Deficiency	Cold	Damp	Phlegm	Heat/Fire	Damp-Heat	Stagnation or Blood Stasis	Yin Deficiency	Yang Deficiency
Choppy		√49,50	√48,51	√49–51	√Blood-Cold or Blood disorder52 or Cold-Damp48	√+Cold50				√48Blood Stagnation49	√Damage to Bodily Fluids49	
Deep			√49 Qi and Yang53		√49,53			√49,53		√Stasis of Qi and Blood53	√Yin Pulse54	√49 Qi and Yang53
Empty	√Shen (Spirit) Deficiency, causing fear or fright49	√49Damage to Jing (Essence) and Blood50	√49Qi and Blood,55 Yuan (Original) Qi Deficiency49	√Qi and Blood55				√50			√50	
Fine/thin	√The seven Emotions49	√49,50	√48,49	√49,50	√49	√48,49						√49
Knotted		√49	√49	√49	√+Stagnation49		√55			√55Blood and Qi55		
Moving	√Heart and Kidney Dysfunction49	√Jing (Essence) Deficiency in the male49			√49						√Yin Deficiency in the female49	
Overflowing		√49		√49				√Full or Empty Heat48			√+Empty Fire49	
Rapid	√Anger47							√Heat/Fire48,54			√Yin Fluid damaged, Empty-Heat49	
Slippery			√52			√53	√48,56 Rheum,52 (Floating and Rapid = Phlegm–Heat)48	√Internal Heat49,56	√49	√52,56		√Yang pulse50,54
Slow					√48,54	√49	√49					√49,57,58
Soft		√49	√49	√49	√Empty-Cold49,55	√49,55					√49	√49
Weak		√49,50	√49	√49,50+Floating48	√48,49		√49,56				√49,50	√49,50
Wiry					√48,49		√49,56	√+Rapid49		√49,56		
Leathery		√49		√49	√49							

105

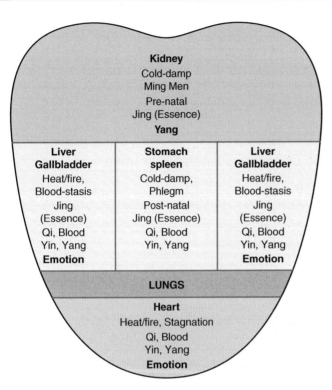

Figure 5.2 Tongue diagnosis and correspondences in subfertile patients.

- A purple tongue body indicates Blood Stasis,[61] as do swollen sublingual veins.[62] Stasis may be a result of Heat or Cold or Qi Stagnation.
- Even a slight blue tongue body signifies Cold. A bluish-purple colour can indicate that Cold has created Blood Stasis; therefore, treatment principles should include points rectifying Cold.
- Very few or subtle cracks in the tongue indicate Yin Deficiency. A thin tongue body may indicate Kidney Jing (Essence), Qi, or Yin Deficiency.[61] This often presents in patients with ovarian reserve issues.
- A thick white coating in the centre of the tongue indicates Cold–Damp[61] or Phlegm.[53] A thick white coating in the Kidney area may signify oppression of Mingmen (Fire of Life) as a result of these pathogenic factors.
- Heat spots (commonly observable in the Liver and Heart areas) indicate Blood Heat or Fire.[61] This can present with no other clinical manifestations or signs of extreme Heat. Large Heat spots may indicate Blood Stasis.[53]

CLINICAL TIPS

TONGUE DIAGNOSIS: ORTHODOX MEDICAL PERSPECTIVE

- ◆ A swollen tooth-marked tongue (macroglossia) may indicate hypothyroidism.[63]
- ◆ A pale tongue may indicate pernicious anaemia.[64]

CLINICAL TIPS—cont'd

- ◆ A red or pink tongue that is smooth and glossy in appearance (atrophic glossitis) may indicate nutritional deficiencies of such elements as iron, folic acid, or vitamin B12 and a riboflavin or niacin deficiency.[63]
- ◆ Thick, white patchy coating could indicate an oral fungal infection.[63]

Chapter 2 discussed the importance of healthy function of the Extraordinary Vessels in TCM reproductive medicine. Tongue diagnosis can help to determine the pathology of the Extraordinary Vessels. In the authors' experience, a purple tongue body can illustrate that the Chong (Penetrating) Vessel may be disordered because of Blood Stasis; a cracked tongue body indicating Yin Deficiency can mean that the Ren (Conception) Vessel may be impaired; a wet, swollen tongue body with a white coating can indicate that the Du (Governing) Vessel may be disordered.

Abdominal diagnosis in subfertility

Observation and palpation of the abdomen is also a useful diagnostic method. Abdominal palpation is integrated with other methods, helping to refine the diagnosis. Examples of commonly seen observations on abdominal palpation are shown in Figure 5.3 and outlined below:

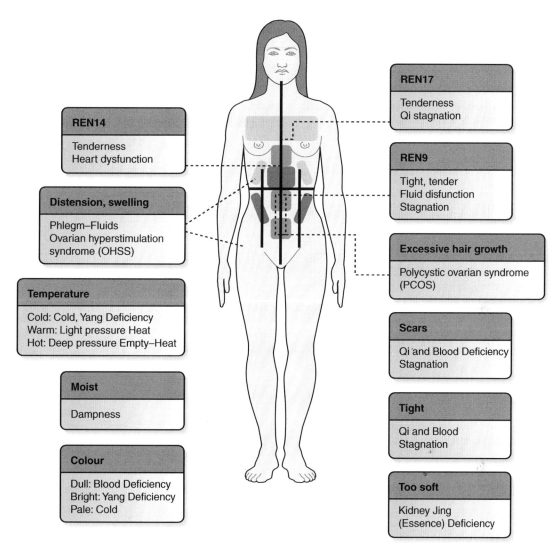

REN14

Tenderness
Heart dysfunction

Distension, swelling

Phlegm–Fluids
Ovarian hyperstimulation
syndrome (OHSS)

Temperature

Cold: Cold, Yang Deficiency
Warm: Light pressure Heat
Hot: Deep pressure Empty–Heat

Moist

Dampness

Colour

Dull: Blood Deficiency
Bright: Yang Deficiency
Pale: Cold

REN17

Tenderness
Qi stagnation

REN9

Tight, tender
Fluid disfunction
Stagnation

Excessive hair growth

Polycystic ovarian syndrome
(PCOS)

Scars

Qi and Blood Deficiency
Stagnation

Tight

Qi and Blood
Stagnation

Too soft

Kidney Jing
(Essence) Deficiency

Figure 5.3 A guide to abdominal diagnosis in subfertility.

- Abdominal pain, relieved on pressure: Empty condition,[65,66] for example, Empty Cold.
- Tenderness or pain felt with pressure: a Full condition,[65] for example, Qi Stagnation,[66] Blood Stasis, Cold, or Dampness.[67]
- Pain on pressure may also indicate Kidney Jing (Essence) Deficiency.[67]

From an integrated medical perspective, it is important to visually examine the abdomen. The presence of scars may suggest adhesions or other pelvic disease. Abdominal hair in a woman may suggest raised androgen levels, increasing the likelihood of PCOS. Tenderness on palpation can indicate endometriosis. A referral for further investigations may be appropriate in these cases (see Chapter 8).

INTERESTING FACTS

ABDOMINAL PALPATION AS A THERAPEUTIC TOOL

Abdominal palpation can be used therapeutically:
- If the Shen (Spirit) is deficient, palpate Luo connecting channels. Palpation transports Qi, and this reinforces the Shen (Spirit)[68] and facilitates Qi and Blood flow.
- Producing a reaction to palpation can help to reconnect Spirit (Shen) and Mind with the body.[66]
- Abdominal palpation (especially with warm hands) helps disperse Cold.[69]
- Palpation and massage tonifies Qi and facilitates the movement of Blood.[47]

TCM SYNDROMES DIAGNOSIS IN SUBFERTILE PATIENTS

The principles of syndromes in the management of ART patients

TCM syndromes are a prognostic indication of issues that may present during and after IVF. For example, the quality of Kidney Jing (Essence) or the presence of Liver and Heart Blood Deficiency may negatively impact the quality of eggs, sperm, and embryos and, therefore, negatively affect the likelihood of conception.

More often than not there are multiple syndromes with various degrees of pathology and associations. For example, Spleen and Stomach Qi Deficiency with minor Dampness, Liver and Heart Blood Deficiency, and Blood Stasis with Heat. Although the syndromes listed in this chapter are the ones most commonly seen in subfertile patients, it is important to note that other syndromes may be present. A thorough TCM diagnosis and an individualized prescription of treatment is essential.[70,71]

The nature of syndromes in subfertility and IVF practice:

- Syndromes are dynamic and change not only naturally but also as a result of acupuncture treatment and/or Orthodox medical treatment.
- IVF treatment stages may influence the planning of the treatment of syndromes.
- All syndromes have varying scales and degrees of severity. The same syndromes can have different effects on different people.
- Syndromes do not need to be totally resolved for conception to occur and result in a healthy pregnancy. Reducing the syndromes' severity (even a little) can often help the patient to conceive and have a healthy pregnancy. However, in some complex cases, it is only when syndromes are completely eradicated that the patient conceives.
- Some syndromes are very difficult to treat with acupuncture, and Orthodox medical intervention is essential in these cases. For example, patients with thyroid disease may need thyroxin replacement therapy in order to rapidly improve their pathology and, therefore, not unnecessarily delay their reproductive treatment. As this example demonstrates, the use of such an integrated approach enhances patient care and optimizes results.
- Sometimes Orthodox medical treatment and/or IVF/ART treatments fail to help patients. TCM treatment may be essential in helping such patients conceive. For example, in unexplained infertility, from the Orthodox medical point of view, everything functions as it should, yet patients still do not conceive. TCM syndromes may be identified in this patient group and addressed with acupuncture, potentially increasing chances of conception.

The following section reviews the signs and symptoms associated with the most common syndromes, the pathophysiology leading to these syndromes, and ART complications that in the authors' experience often occur with each syndrome.

Common syndromes in subfertility in contemporary TCM literature

In their 2011 study, Cochrane et al. attempted to establish a consensus amongst 12 TCM recognized experts in the field of female reproductive health on how best to manage women with fertility problems.[70] The experts agree that 'differential diagnosis should include the following patterns':

- Kidney Yang/Yin Deficiency
- Liver Blood Deficiency
- Heart Yin and/or Blood Deficiency
- Spleen Qi Deficiency
- Liver Qi Stagnation
- Blood Stasis
- Phlegm/Damp Accumulation
- Assessment of the Spirit

A study by Birkeflet et al. assessed common syndromes in fertile and infertile women.[72] They found that 'the most common syndromes in subfertile women were':[72]

- Liver Blood Stasis
- Spleen Yang Deficiency
- Kidney Yang Deficiency
- Qi and Blood Stagnation
- Cold

Interestingly, in the same study, some syndromes were less likely to be present in subfertile women compared with fertile women. These syndromes were:[72]

- Liver Yang Rising
- Kidney Yin Deficiency
- Heat
- Damp

There is a great deal of agreement amongst TCM practitioners regarding common pathology in female subfertility. These pathologies are:

- Kidney Jing (Essence) Deficiency[73,74]
- Kidney Yin and/or Yang Deficiency[73–79]
- (Liver) Qi Stagnation[73–79]
- Heart Qi Stagnation[73,74]
- Qi Deficiency[73,79]
- Blood Deficiency[73,75–79]
- Blood Stasis
- Cold Uterus[74,75,78]
- Damp[76,78]
- Phlegm–Damp[74,75,77–79]
- Blood Heat[78,79]

Although the preceding syndromes are commonly cited, it is important to note that other syndromes may be present. Also, more than one syndrome can be present in the same patient. Therefore, a fertility acupuncturist must make a thorough TCM diagnosis and individualize each treatment approach, rather than relying on a rote approach.

The following section provides a detailed TCM literature review of signs and symptoms associated with the most common syndromes.

Kidney syndromes

Kidney Jing (Essence) Deficiency

As discussed in Chapter 2, the Kidney has an important role in fertility as the basis for reproduction. The Kidney is related to Mingmen (the Gate of Life), connecting to the Chamber of Semen in the male and the Uterus in the female. Therefore, Kidney Jing (Essence) has a significant influence over the quality of sperm, eggs, and embryos.

Aetiology

The Kidney stores Jing (Essence) that fluctuates in yearly cycles. The age of patients and/or their supply of Pre-Natal Jing (Essence) may cause constitutional tendencies that influence the quality and supply of Kidney Jing (Essence) in their offspring.[80,81] Many couples begin trying for a baby at a later stage of life, when reserves of Kidney Jing (Essence) are in decline. In ART treatment, this can potentially result in failure because of egg and sperm issues.

It is not uncommon in today's society for people to work hard without a balance of rest and activity. Patients can consume their supply of Kidney Jing (Essence) through excessive demanding physical or mental strain and overwork.[81]

Constant and prolonged fear (for example, fear of not conceiving) can also consume Kidney Jing (Essence).

An inadequate diet and irregular eating contributes to an earlier decline of Kidney Jing (Essence) as Post-Natal Jing (Essence) supplements and supports Pre-Natal Jing (Essence).

Pathology

The Kidney's interrelationship with the Zangfu is often prevalent in subfertile patients undergoing ART. Such patients often have Kidney Jing (Essence) Deficiency associated with Liver and Uterus Blood Deficiency along with deficiencies of the Ren and Chong Mai (Conception and Penetrating Vessels). Liver Blood and Kidney Jing (Essence) are mutually engendering.[82] Subfertile women with histories of failed IVF caused by implantation failure after the transfer of seemingly good or poor-quality embryos have this dual pathology.

However, it is important to note that there are other syndromes that influence Kidney Jing (Essence) and reduce reproductive potential. For example, Kidney Jing (Essence) pathology can be secondary to Liver Qi Stagnation. Stagnation can block Kidney Jing (Essence), reduce sperm and egg quality and implantation potential, or lead to early pregnancy loss. Kidney Jing (Essence) Deficiency can also induce Liver Blood Deficiency.

Signs and symptoms

- Fear,[83,84] for example, of childlessness
- Dispirited Shen (Spirit)[85–88]
- Premature ageing,[81,85] for example, premature hair loss and/or greying[87,89]
- Weak constitution and physical strength,[85,86] low reserves of Qi[74]
- Forgetfulness[81,86,87,89]
- Sexual and reproductive decline[74,81,85,86,88,90]
- Thin vaginal discharge[87,91,92]
- Late onset of menarche[85]
- Amenorrhoea[81,93]
- Menstrual irregularities,[86,87,94–97] delayed[86,94,96,98] or early menses[98,99]
- Lower abdominal pain after menstruation[94]
- Spotting[86]
- Miscarriage(s)[87,100,101]
- Complexion: dull and dark[85,86]
- Lower back pain[74,83,89]
- Weak legs[85,86,102]
- Dizziness[81,87]
- Urination: frequent or dribbling of urine,[43,86] slight incontinence[74]
- Pulse: leathery,[49,103] weak,[49,74,80,81,87,96] deep,[80,81,96] fine[49,87]
- Tongue: white coating,[87,96] pale,[74,87] or red and peeled tongue body[80]

Potential consequences for reproduction and ART

- Poor ovarian reserve
- Poor response to ovarian stimulation (for example, low number of follicles, eggs, or poor-quality eggs)
- Abnormal sperm parameters or sperm DNA (may require ICSI fertilization method)
- Low fertilization rate (due to poor-quality sperm or eggs)
- Poor embryo grades or embryos that develop abnormally
- Genetic abnormalities in parents or embryos
- RIF
- Preclinical or first trimester pregnancy loss
- Potentially may result in a need for donor eggs and/or sperm

Acupuncture treatment

Table 5.2 lists acupuncture points that treat Kidney Jing (Essence) Deficiency and the rationale for using them.

Kidney Yin Deficiency

As discussed in Chapter 2, Yin plays a fundamental role in fertility because it is closely linked to the phases of the menstrual cycle. The Kidney is the source of Yin and Yang.[92] From an integrated viewpoint, Yin is responsible for the quality of follicles, eggs, and sperm. Kidney Yin is also the foundation for the quality and movement of Blood in the reproductive system.

Table 5.2 Kidney Jing (Essence) Deficiency acupuncture treatment	
Acupuncture points	**Rationale**
REN4	• Tonifies the Kidney, Yuan (Original) Qi[104,105] • Benefits Jing (Essence),[105] Qi and Blood, Yin and Yang[104,105] • Benefits the Uterus, assists with conception,[105] positively influences Dan Tian[104] in the male
KID12	• Tonifies the Kidney, astringes Jing (Essence)[106]
ST27	• Benefits the Kidney and firms Jing (Essence)[106]
KID3	• Benefits the Kidney[106] • Moxibustion at KID3 tonifies Qi, Blood, and Jing (Essence)[104] • Benefits the embryo and the foetus[104]
KID4	• Nourishes Jing, strengthens Shen (Spirit)[107]
SP8	• Stabilizes the Kidney[104] • Benefits fertility[104] • Benefits sperm Jing (Essence)[104]
LIV3	• Tonifies Jing (Essence) and sperm insufficiency in the male[108]
KID13	• Regulates the Ren and Chong Mai (Conception and Penetrating Vessels)[106] • Regulates the Uterus and Lower Jiao[106]
ST25	• Regulates menses, promotes fertility[104] • Regulates the Stomach and Spleen, Qi and Blood,[109] thus supporting Post-Natal Jing (Essence) and Kidney Jing (Essence)
BL23+BL52	• Tonifies the Kidney, benefits Jing (Essence) (with moxa)[104] • Benefits the Uterus[110] and Dan Tian[104]
DU4	• Tonifies Jing (Essence)[104] • Benefits fertility[104]
Moxa	• Warms the Kidney, tonifies Qi, and nourishes Blood[111]

Aetiology

Similar to Kidney Jing (Essence), Kidney Yin Deficiency can result from ongoing mental and physical overwork.[80] Couples of advanced reproductive age or who have a busy lifestyle, 'always on the go', tend to consume Kidney Yin, causing Deficiency.

Many people travel abroad for occupational and/or recreational reasons, and some patients may contract a febrile disease whilst abroad. Even though the illness may have happened many years ago, the Heat is often retained and, over time, consumes Bodily Fluids and damages Yin.[80] Therefore, these patients may present with marked Kidney Yin and/or Stomach Yin Deficiency with Empty Heat, which is usually reflected in the tongue presentation and the sensation of heat.

Kidney Yin is particularly affected by the person's emotional disposition. Many people find subfertility particularly anxiety provoking. In addition, it is not unusual for one or both partners to have had many years of psychological stress and emotional upset because of strained relationships with family members, friends, or work colleagues. These emotions may further exacerbate pre-existing Yin Deficiency, which often leads to Empty Heat or even Fire in severe cases.

Yin can also be depleted by previous ovarian stimulation (especially where there was pre-existing pathology) and failed IVF treatment.

Pathology

Deficiencies of other organs can negatively influence Kidney Yin and Yang.[112] Kidney Yin can be affected by pathology from the Heart and/or Liver because these organs are strongly linked to each other.[92,113]

For example, a subfertile patient diagnosed with Heart Yin Deficiency caused by long-standing anxiety may be at high risk of developing Kidney Yin Deficiency. This can result in a much higher risk of poor response to ovarian stimulation, fertilization issues, and IVF failure because Heart Yin compromises Kidney Yin. In turn, Kidney Yin Deficiency can compromise the Yin of the Liver and Heart and induce Fire.

Signs and symptoms

- Patient of 40 or more years old[83]
- Thin face[84] and body[74,87]
- Restlessness[74,84]
- Soreness in the lower back[87,88,90,114]
- Dryness,[88,115] for example, vagina, hair, or skin[74,90,97]
- Sleeping difficulties[74,87,90]
- Dizziness[81,87,88,90,114]
- Tinnitus[81,87,88,115]
- Premature ejaculation[81,87]
- Amenorrhoea[98,114]
- Dull lower abdominal pain during or after menstruation (if combined with Liver Yin Deficiency)[116]
- Irregular[87,96,100,117] or short menstrual cycles[94,98,114]
- Excessive[94] or scant[74,97,118] menstrual blood flow

Table 5.3 Kidney Yin Deficiency acupuncture treatment

Acupuncture points	Rationale
LU7 + KID6	• Opens Ren Mai (Conception Vessel)[120] • Nourishes Yin, promotes fertility[121] • Tonifies the ovaries[121] • Nourishes the embryo and foetus[121] • Benefits semen
REN4	• Nourishes Kidney Yin[105]
SP6	• Benefits Kidney Yin and Blood, Jing (Essence)[104,122] • Regulates the Uterus[107]
KID3	• Nourishes Kidney Yin[106]
KID1	• Tonifies Kidney Yin and Jing (Essence), enriches Yin[104] • Regulates Kidney function[106]
REN7	• Tonifies the Kidney[104] • Benefits the Ren and Chong Mai (Conception and Penetrating Vessels)[104]
KID6	• Nourishes the Kidney[106] • Supports Yin[107]

- Spotting[41,98,119]
- Pulse: fine and rapid[55,81,88] (with Empty Heat), weak[49,74]
- Tongue: red,[81,87,88,97] with cracks, no coating[81] or patchy coating,[74,87] small tongue body[74]

Potential consequences for reproduction and ART

- Poor follicular growth and poorer quality of eggs
- Poor sperm parameters
- Low fertilization rate
- Suboptimal embryo development
- Emotional symptoms during reproductive treatment
- RIF

Acupuncture treatment

Table 5.3 lists acupuncture points that treat Kidney Yin Deficiency and the rationale for using them.

Case study

Kidney Jing (Essence), Kidney Yin, Liver Blood Deficiencies, and Stagnation

Julie, age 38, had two miscarriages at 8 and 10 weeks' gestation and 2 years of subfertility following her last miscarriage.

Continued

Case study—cont'd

Signs and Symptoms

- Dispirited Shen (Spirit), a weak constitution, thin hair, lower back pain with weakness and neck problems (with a family history of this), tiredness, low libido.
- Menstrual cycles and menses: prolonged (7 days), with clots (first few days), premenstrual tender breasts.
- Pulse: fine, weak, and deep
- Tongue: short, pale, paler at sides

TCM Diagnosis

- Kidney Jing (Essence), Kidney Yin, and Liver Blood Deficiencies with Liver Qi Stagnation

Causes

Constitution, age, repeated miscarriages

First Acupuncture Point Prescription

REN4, KID3, HE7, KID13, and LIV3

Discussion

Julie chose not to have IVF. It took just over a year of acupuncture treatment before she conceived her daughter. She was treated up to 20 weeks' gestation because she suffered from spotting in pregnancy. Unfortunately, she suffered from post-natal depression. Patients with deficiencies of Jing (Essence), Qi, and Blood require continuous care and monitoring.

Kidney Yang Deficiency

Yang Deficiency in men or women may prevent new life forming. As discussed in Chapter 2, Yang is the motivating force for all physiological processes of transformation.[80] Kidney Yang has a wide range of catalytic functions and processes and is the foundation for all the Yang energies of the body. Kidney Yang warms the Uterus and is strongly related to the second phase of the menstrual cycle and embryonic development.

Aetiology

The interrelationship between Kidney Jing (Essence), Yin, and Yang means that constitutional tendencies are associated with Yang Deficiency, just as they are implicated in Jing (Essence) and Yin Deficiencies.[90] Other aetiologies include:

- Physical overwork may injure Kidney Yang.[80]
- Inappropriate sexual practices (for example, too much intercourse) may weaken the Kidney.[90] Chapter 7 discusses in detail sexual practices from a TCM perspective.
- Raw and cold foods (for example, salads and cold drinks) can injure Yang.[123]
- Invasion by External Pathogenic Factors (EPFs) such as Cold can damage Yang.[124]

- Miscarriage can result from Yang Deficiency[92] and may also cause or exacerbate Yang Deficiency.
- Generally, chronic illness can cause Kidney Yang Deficiency.[80]
- Fear and sadness, which are often seen in subfertile patients, may deplete Kidney Yang and injure the Shen (Spirit).

Pathology

Yang Deficiency can be a primary cause of subfertility. It can also induce or exacerbate secondary pathology. Kidney Yang Deficiency is associated with the decline of Mingmen (Fire of Life)[92] and with Du Mai (Governing Vessel) pathology.[125] Kidney Yang Deficiency can also result from its close associations with Yuan (Original) Qi, Jing (Essence), and Yin Deficiency. Yang Deficiency can also compromise Yin.[112]

Yang protects the body from EPFs. If Yang fails, EPFs can invade the body and combine with internal pathology. For example, External Wind Cold can combine with Internal Cold from Yang Deficiency, causing Blood Deficiency in women and Jing (Essence) Deficiency in men.[48]

Kidney Yang may also become deficient because of Spleen, Heart, or Lung Deficiency.[92] Conversely, Kidney Yang Deficiency may also induce deficiency in these organs.[92] For example, deficiency of Yang–Qi can affect the Heart and Shen (Spirit).[126] Subfertile patients often present with dispirited Shen (Spirit). This is particularly evident in women of advanced reproductive age (more than 40 years old) who are diagnosed with Kidney Yang Deficiency.

Women's physiology makes them prone to Dampness,[127] which can cause Kidney Yang Deficiency.[80]

Signs and symptoms

- Bright white complexion[81,88,90]
- Chilliness,[83,114] dislike of cold weather,[74,81,87,88,90] sensation of cold[81,87,88,90]
- Lethargy[74,84]
- Dispirited Shen (Spirit)[87,88,126]
- Low libido[74,81]
- Leucorrhoea[43,96,98,114]
- Overweight[74]
- Impotence[81,88,90]
- Lower backache[87,88,114]
- Urination: copious clear,[81,88,92] scant,[92,81,87,88] or nocturia[92,87,88]
- Pale menses,[97] tissue-type menstrual clots,[74] delayed menses,[97,128] spotting[87]
- Pulse: slow,[57,74,81,87] weak,[49,81] deep[81,87,121]
- Tongue: pale,[74,81,88] swollen,[74,88] wet,[121] thin white coating[81,87]

Potential consequences for reproduction and ART

- Poor sperm parameters, particularly motility
- Low fertilization rate or total fertilization failure

Table 5.4 Kidney Yang Deficiency acupuncture treatment	
Acupuncture points	**Rationale**
KID3	• Tonifies Kidney Yang[106]
KID2	• Regulates the Kidney and tonifies Kidney Yang[104,106]
DU20	• Regulates, raises,[129] and warms Yang • Tonifies Qi, calms the embryo and the foetus[104]
REN6	• Tonifies the Kidney, fortifies Yang[105] • Tonifies and regulates Qi[105]
DU4	• Tonifies the Kidney and Kidney Yang, warms Yang[104] • Benefits the embryo and foetus[104] • Regulates the Du Mai (Governing Vessel)[129]
BL23 + BL52	• Tonifies the Kidney, fortifies Yang, benefits Jing (Essence)[110] • Warms the Uterus[110] and Dan Tian
KID7	• Benefits the Kidney[106]
Moxa	• Warms the Kidney, strengthens Kidney Yang[111] • Warms Yang, especially moxa on REN8[105]

- Reproductive immunology issues
- RIF
- Early and/or recurrent miscarriages

Acupuncture treatment

Table 5.4 lists acupuncture points that treat Kidney Yang Deficiency and the rationale for using them.

Case study

Kidney Yang Deficiency and Jing (Essence) Deficiency

Joanne, age 35, and her partner John, age 40, had a 10-year history of infertility and one failed IVF cycle. All Orthodox medical tests' results were 'normal'. Their GP had advised them to keep on trying naturally. They decided to try acupuncture to help them achieve a pregnancy.

At the initial acupuncture consultation, John reported that he had had a vasectomy during his first marriage. I referred them to a local ART centre for further investigation, and it was later confirmed that he had developed sperm antibodies.

Case study—cont'd

Key Signs and Symptoms (Joanne)

♦ Joanne: white complexion. She was lethargic and dispirited, mainly because of the long duration of subfertility. She had a tendency to gain weight. She liked to wrap up to be warm and wore thick socks and several layers of clothing. She generally disliked the cold weather.

♦ Pulse: weak and deep in the right rear position

♦ Tongue: pale body, slightly swollen

TCM Diagnosis (Joanne)

Kidney Yang Deficiency

First Acupuncture Point Prescription (Joanne)

BL23+BL52, KID3, DU4, and BL15 (moxa)

Key Signs and Symptoms (John)

♦ John presented with complete loss of hair. He appeared very timid and fearful.

♦ Pulse: weak and deep, slightly fine quality

♦ Tongue: red

TCM Diagnosis (John)

Kidney Jing (Essence) Deficiency

First Acupuncture Point Prescription (John)

KID3, LIV3, GB40, REN4, and HE7.

Acupuncture treatment commenced 5 months prior to IVF/ICSI and continued throughout IVF. Joanne and John now have a son.

Discussion

John had sperm antibodies, and IVF/ICSI was their best treatment option. However, it is likely that John's TCM diagnosis of Jing (Essence) Deficiency and Joanne's TCM diagnosis of Kidney Yang Deficiency would compromise the outcome. They had already undergone one IVF cycle, during which they only had one embryo available for transfer, perhaps because of their TCM pathology. Therefore, acupuncture treatment was provided to both of them to increase the probability of conception.

Liver syndromes

Liver Blood Deficiency

As discussed in Chapter 2, the Liver is essential for conception. This is because the Liver has complex interrelationships with key reproductive organs (the Heart, Lung, Kidney, the Stomach and Spleen, and the Uterus) and the Extraordinary Vessels.

Aetiology

The same constitutional factors that cause Kidney Jing (Essence) and Yin Deficiency can also influence the supply and quality of Liver Blood.[130] This is because Kidney Jing (Essence) and Liver Blood share the same source[131] and Yin Deficiency can reduce Liver Blood.[131]

Heavy periods may cause or advance Liver Blood Deficiency. Miscarriages, physical trauma, and internal bleeding may also lead to Blood Deficiency.

Energy that is used by the Liver to 'get through the day' and nourish the body depends on an adequate breakfast, lunch, and dinner. A diet lacking in nourishment,[130] irregular meals, or dieting affects the Stomach and Spleen and can cause Liver Blood Deficiency. This is because the Stomach, Spleen, and Heart are involved with the production of Blood. Busy lifestyles, occupational influences such as night shifts, or working though lunchtimes and break periods can create unhealthy habits. These factors reduce Post-Natal Jing (Essence); induce pathology of the Kidney, Stomach, and Spleen; and subsequently reduce Blood stored by the Liver. Liver Blood Deficiency can result from Stomach Qi or Yin Deficiency.

Emotional dysfunction that injures the Heart and Shen Mind and Spirit may induce Liver Blood Deficiency. This is because the Heart governs Blood, and the Liver stores it. Emotion may Stagnate Qi and Blood; this then reduces Liver Blood and nourishment to the body, and these factors lead to Uterus Blood Deficiency.

Pathology

Liver Qi, Blood, and Yin Deficiency may compromise the function of the Heart.

Deficiency of Blood makes a woman more susceptible to invasion by EPFs, for example, Wind Cold.[132] When Cold enters the Uterus, fertility is reduced. Blood Deficiency creates Qi Stagnation and Blood Stasis.[132]

Blood (or Yin) Deficiency can cause Heat in the Blood,[133] thus potentially affecting implantation, causing excessive bleeding, and/or increasing the risk of miscarriages.

Signs and symptoms

- Dull complexion[81,90,115,134]
- Insomnia,[88] excessive dreaming[88,89,135,136]
- Blurred vision[81,88,89,137,138]
- Dull nails[89,136]
- Pale-red menstrual blood,[90,134,138,139] scant blood flow,[81,88,136] delayed[114,140] or suppressed menses,[141] amenorrhoea[81,96,138]
- Dizziness[81,88]
- Fear, agitation,[39,43,137,141] crying before period[83,142]
- Numbness,[81] for example, of limbs[130]

- Impotence[115,143]
- Pulse: choppy,[81,121] thin[49,81,121,136]
- Tongue: pale,[81,121,136] especially on the Liver area[130]

Potential consequences for reproduction and ART

- Poor ovarian response to stimulation
- Endometrial issues (for example, thin endometrium)
- RIF
- Reproductive immunological issues

Acupuncture treatment

Table 5.5 lists acupuncture points that treat Liver Blood Deficiency and the rationale for using them.

Table 5.5 Liver Blood Deficiency acupuncture treatment

Acupuncture points	Rationale
LIV8	• Invigorates Blood and benefits the Uterus[108] • Nourishes Blood and Yin[108] • Benefits the Dan Tian[108]
LIV3	• Nourishes Liver Blood and Yin[108] • Tonifies Qi, Jing (Essence)[108] • Invigorates sperm[108] • Regulates menses[108] • Spreads Liver Qi, facilitates Qi and Blood flow, calms the embryo and foetus[104]
LIV11	• Benefits the Uterus[108] • Regulates menses[108] • Promotes fertility (with moxa)[108] • Benefits the Dan Tian
ST36	• Regulates and tonifies Qi and Blood, facilitates Qi and Blood flow[104] • Calms the embryo and foetus[104] • Nourishes Blood Yin[109] • Tonifies Qi and Blood[104]
P6	• Invigorates Blood[104] • Calms the embryo and foetus[104]
BL18	• Regulates, spreads Liver Qi and Blood[104]
BL17	• Regulates and tonifies Blood[104]
Moxa	• Tonifies Qi and nourishes Blood[111]

Case study

Liver Blood Deficiency

Susan, aged 34, had a 3-year history of subfertility and two failed IVF cycles.

Orthodox Medical Tests and Diagnosis

Basic investigations: subfertility caused by low ovarian reserve (AMH = 6.4 pmol/L)
 Advanced clotting disorders tests: normal
 Reproductive immunology: not tested on advice of her consultant

Previous IVF History

Two IVF cycles; in each cycle, four eggs were retrieved, two eggs were fertilized by ICSI, and two embryos (medium and poor quality) were transferred each time.

Signs and Symptoms

- Mood: grumpy. It was difficult for her to open up and express her feelings; she pretended that she had no hope that IVF would work, yet, without fail, she attended weekly acupuncture treatments in preparation for the next IVF cycle.
- Floaters
- Breast tenderness
- Headaches toward the end of her period
- Pulse: left positions thin, small
- Tongue: pale, sides orangey

Lifestyle

- Four or more cups of coffee per day
- Tired because of a busy job, long work hours
- Nutrition: she did not like vegetables or chicken and ate at irregular times, often missing meals.

TCM Diagnosis

- Liver Blood Deficiency and Liver Qi Stagnation
- Kidney Jing (Essence) Deficiency

Causes

Poor diet, overwork, constitution, injury by emotion

First Acupuncture Point Prescription

LIV3, LIV8, P6, HE6, ZIGONG, ST29, and KID3
 Acupuncture treatment began 3 months prior to IVF. Susan responded better to ovarian stimulation. She had more follicles and achieved a higher fertilization rate. Four good-quality embryos reached blastocyst stage and two were transferred. Unfortunately, the cycle still failed.

Discussion

The ART team were pleased to note a significant improvement in the quality of embryos and achieved a blastocyst-stage transfer. But they could not explain why the

Case study—cont'd

treatment still failed. Susan and her husband may benefit from advanced investigations, such as reproductive immunology tests or a sperm DNA fragmentation test.

From a TCM point of view, the IVF cycle failed most likely because of the severity of Liver Blood and Kidney Jing (Essence) Deficiency. A busy lifestyle, shift work, and poor dietary habits were significant contributing factors.

Liver Qi Stagnation

As discussed in Chapter 2, the Liver regulates the menstrual cycle by moving Qi and Blood.[144] This promotes fertility. Healthy Liver Qi can optimize a woman's response to ovarian stimulation, regulate the embryo's development, and support the process of implantation and early pregnancy.

Aetiology

Liver Qi Stagnation can be a consequence of emotional and mental disharmony,[145] such as depression, anger, frustration, and resentment. Qi can also become stagnated as a result of excessive thought, anxiety, and fear.[146] Lack of emotional regulation causes complicated disorders in subfertility.[127]

Qi Stagnation (and Blood Stasis) may also result from a physical trauma,[145] for example, a surgical procedure. Invasion of EPFs such as Cold can also stagnate Qi.

Pathology

Liver Qi Stagnation can result from a complex underlying pathology of Spleen, Kidney, and Heart. For example, Spleen Qi Deficiency can lead to Dampness, and this can cause Liver Qi Stagnation.[131] Kidney Yang Deficiency can lead to Internal Cold, and this, in turn, can result in Liver Qi Stagnation.

Signs and symptoms

- Moodiness,[114,140] fluctuation in mental state,[93,102,137,140] irritability[81]
- Easily angered[83,90,93] or supressed anger[93]
- Depression,[81,90,147] jealously[93]
- Irregular menstrual cycles[88,96,138,140] or delayed menses,[96,140] sometimes scant[81] or sometimes heavy menses,[148] uneven flow of menstrual blood[140]
- Painful periods[88,96,149]
- Premenstrual breast tenderness[81,136] and emotional tension related to menstrual cycle[74]
- Abdominal distension[81,90]
- Pulse: wiry[49,81,90]
- Tongue: normal[81] or red[93,121]

Table 5.6 Liver Qi Stagnation acupuncture treatment

Acupuncture points	Rationale
LIV3	• Tonifies Liver Qi, Yang, Blood, and Yin,[104] thus regulating the Liver
LIV8	• Regulates and tonifies Liver Qi and Blood[104]
LIV14	• Spreads and regulates Liver Qi[108] • Invigorates Blood[108]
P6	• Regulates Liver Qi and invigorates Blood[104] • Regulates menses[104] • Calms the embryo and foetus[104]
ST30	• Regulates Qi in the Uterus and Lower Jiao[109] • Regulates the Chong Mai (Penetrating Vessel)[109]
ST29	• Regulates menstruation[104] • Promotes fertility[104] • Restores the Uterus's ability to function[104] • Treats impotence[104]

Potential consequences for reproduction and ART

- Poor or unpredictable ovarian response to stimulation
- Poor fertilization rate
- RIF
- Reproductive immunology issues
- Preclinical or early pregnancy loss

Acupuncture treatment

Table 5.6 lists acupuncture points that treat Liver Qi Stagnation and the rationale for using them.

Case study

Liver Qi Stagnation with Blood Heat

Lucy, aged 33, suffered 18 months of subfertility. She then conceived, but the 12-week scan showed that the baby had died. Lucy was shocked.

Orthodox Medical Diagnosis

- ◆ PCOS
- ◆ Mild endometriosis

Signs and Symptoms

- ◆ Complexion: dull
- ◆ Body: slender

Continued

Case study—cont'd

◆ Easily angered
◆ History of insomnia and excessive dreaming
◆ Fearful (different to direct Kidney pathology), but she had planned to be assertive and insist that the consultant conduct every test possible related to subfertility and miscarriage. She was frustrated and believed she was infertile.
◆ Menses: irregular menstrual cycle, PMT, and bloating
◆ Pulse: wiry
◆ Tongue: red with Heat spots in the Liver area

TCM Diagnosis

Liver Qi Stagnation with Blood Heat

First Acupuncture Point Prescription

LIV2, LIV3, LIV8, YINTANG, P6, P7, and LI11

Discussion

Lucy conceived after 2 months of acupuncture treatment and had a healthy baby boy. She conceived again when her baby was 5 months old and now has two children.

Liver Blood Stasis

Blood Stasis is a long-standing cause of subfertility.[132] In contemporary TCM fertility practice, Blood Stasis is often a secondary cause of subfertility.

Aetiology

Repressed emotions can lead to stagnation of Qi and Blood Stasis.[131]

Blood Stasis can also result from EPF Cold entering the Uterus.[131]

Physical trauma – for example, from pelvic surgery – can cause severe Blood Stasis in the Uterus,[131] which can be difficult to resolve with acupuncture alone.

Pathology

Blood Stasis is a pathogenic factor[150] that produces secondary complications in subfertile patients. For example, Blood Stasis can block the Chong and Ren Mai (Penetrating and Conception Vessels) and the 'Blood Vessels of the Uterus'.[131]

Warming and regulating Blood can promote fertility[132] when Blood Stasis is caused by Yang Deficiency or Cold. Other pathologies that can cause Blood Stasis include[131]:

- Qi Stagnation
- Qi Deficiency
- Blood Deficiency
- Blood Heat

Signs and symptoms

- Purple[89,93] (dark) circles under eyes, dark complexion[102,136,151]
- Insomnia and excessive dreaming[114]
- Poor blood circulation[152]
- Irregular or delayed menstruation[98]
- Menses: dark menstrual blood; large clots,[114] or clotted[151] thick consistency;[131] uneven menstrual flow; spotting;[74,93] prolonged,[153] heavy,[154] or scant flow[140,155]
- Lower abdominal pain, stabbing or dull,[97,154] fixed in location[151]
- Amenorrhoea[97,98]
- Pulse: choppy,[49,114,151] firm,[49,121] wiry[49,121]
- Tongue: dark red or purple[136,151] or purple areas,[74,151] bruised colour or appearance[136,151]

Possible consequences for reproduction and ART

- Associated with endometriosis,[74,114] uterine fibroids, polyps, blocked fallopian tubes,[74] ovarian cysts[114]
- Poor or unpredictable ovarian response to stimulation
- Poor egg quality and embryo development
- Poor fertilization rate
- RIF
- Reproductive immunology issues
- Thin or irregular endometrial lining
- Genetic issues
- Miscarriage(s)

Acupuncture treatment

Table 5.7 lists acupuncture points that treat Liver Blood Stasis and the rationale for using them.

Heart syndromes

Heart Blood Deficiency

As discussed in Chapter 2, the Heart is involved in the production and circulation of Blood around the body. If Heart Blood is deficient, the circulation of Qi and Blood to the reproductive systems is disordered and nourishment is reduced.

Aetiology

Emotions such as anxiety or worry can affect the Mind and consume Qi and Blood, leading to Heart Blood Deficiency.[157] The emotional consequences of IVF failures can affect the Shen (Mind) and Spirit and Jing (Essence) by weakening Qi and Blood.

Heavy blood loss (for example, from a threatened miscarriage) may lead to Heart Blood Deficiency, further complicated by the emotional stress.

A diet lacking Blood-nourishing properties can affect the Stomach and Spleen and be an indirect cause of Heart Blood Deficiency.[157]

Table 5.7 Liver Blood Stasis acupuncture treatment

Acupuncture points	Rationale
SP4 + P6	• Opens Chong Mai (Penetrating Vessel)[122] • Regulates Blood in the Uterus[156] • Nourishes Blood[156] • Benefits Jing (Essence)[156] • Regulates Qi[156] • Eliminates Blood Stasis[156] • Reduces pain[156]
LIV14	• Invigorates Blood, disperses masses[108]
ST29	• Regulates menses[109] • Warms the Uterus, invigorating Blood[109] • Restores the Uterus functions[109] • Influences physiology associated with the penis[109]
SP8	• Invigorates Blood[122] • Regulates menses[104]
KID14	• Regulates Qi and moves Blood Stasis[106] • Benefits the Uterus[106] • Alleviates pain[106] • Promotes fertility[106]
SP10	• Invigorates Blood and dispels Blood Stasis[122] • Cools Blood[122] • Benefits menses[122] and the embryo
BL17 + BL18	• Dispels Blood Stasis[110] • Cools Blood Heat[110] • Invigorates Blood[110] • Regulates and nourishes Liver Blood, spreads Qi[110]

Pathology

When Heart Blood is deficient, the entire body lacks nourishment.[101] The Heart has a close relationship with the Lung, Kidney, Spleen, and Stomach.[113] Combined syndromes, therefore, often occur in conjunction with Heart Blood Deficiency. The Heart can induce disorders in other organs.[126] Therefore, preventative measures in patients with Heart Blood Deficiency are essential to minimize the effects on other organs, especially during ovarian stimulation when the Zang organs are under strain.

The Heart and Uterus have a direct connection through the Bao Mai Vessel. This ensures that Qi and Blood are revitalized in the vessels and circulate effectively to the Uterus in women or the Chamber of Sperm or Bao in men. Therefore, Heart Blood deficiency can lead to Uterus Blood Deficiency.

Heart Yin and Yang, Qi, and Blood are mutually counterbalancing.[112,158] This means that the Yang function of the Heart is essential for the quality and circulation of Qi and Blood. Moxibustion can be used to nourish Blood and promote circulation in cases not complicated by Fire.

Signs and symptoms

- Disquieted Shen (Spirit),[88,159] sadness, sorrow[39]
- Complexion: dull, pale,[160] or pale white[88]
- Palpitations[83,90,158,160]
- Insomnia,[90,157] dream-disturbed sleep,[160] or frequent dreaming[88,90]
- Amenorrhoea[100,121] or delayed menses[134]
- Scant,[155] pale-red menses[161]
- Poor memory[90,160]
- Dizziness[88,162]
- Easily frightened,[160] anxious,[83,157] emotional disturbances[88,163]
- Pulse: weak,[49,159] fine,[49,88,157,160] or choppy[157]
- Tongue: pale[88,90,157,159,160]

Acupuncture treatment

Table 5.8 lists acupuncture points that treat Heart Blood Deficiency and the rationale for using them.

Possible consequences for reproduction and ART

- Low number of follicles
- Poor ovarian response to stimulation
- Poor egg quality
- Thin endometrial lining
- Poor fertilization rate
- Compromised embryo development
- RIF
- Reproductive immunology issues

 Case study

The Heart: Subfertility and Miscarriage

Kylie was diagnosed with PCOS. Her cycles were irregular and prolonged. Despite that (after years of trying), to her surprise, she conceived naturally. Unfortunately, she suffered a miscarriage. Following the miscarriage, Kylie suffered from continual bleeding. In her words, 'it was awful', as it reminded her of her loss. She was also keen to start trying to conceive again. She decided to have acupuncture to help stop the bleeding and help to prepare her for an Intra Uterine Insemination (IUI) treatment cycle.

Signs and Symptoms

- History of insomnia, dream-disturbed sleep, dizziness
- Pulse: fine, especially weak in left front position
- Tongue: pale and tooth marked

Continued

Case study—cont'd

Lifestyle Factors

She did not eat red meat but had a healthy balanced diet otherwise.

TCM Diagnosis

Heart Blood Deficiency and Spleen and Stomach Qi Deficiency

First Acupuncture Point Prescription

SP4+P6, SP1 with moxa, ST36, HE6, and DU20

The bleeding stopped the day after the first acupuncture treatment. Kylie felt much more positive. After eight acupuncture treatments, she conceived naturally and had a baby girl.

Discussion

Uncomplicated syndromes are often simple to resolve. In this case, disturbed Shen (Spirit) and emotions exacerbated bleeding.

Table 5.8 Heart Blood Deficiency acupuncture treatment

Acupuncture points	Rationale
HE6	• Regulates Heart Blood and calms the Shen (Spirit)[164]
P6	• Nourishes Heart Blood[104]
P5	• Benefits the Uterus[165]
P4	• Tonifies Shen (Spirit)[166]
HE7	• Regulates and tonifies Heart Blood[104] • Calms Shen (Spirit)[107]
SP4	• Fortifies the Spleen[122] • Benefits the Heart[122] • Invigorates Blood[104] • Regulates the Chong Mai (Penetrating Vessel)[104] • Calms the Shen (Spirit)[104]
REN14	• Regulates the Heart[164]
ST36	• Tonifies Qi, nourishes Blood[109]
BL15	• Regulates Qi, tonifies and nourishes the Heart[110] • Calms the Shen (Spirit)[110]
DU11	• Tonifies the Heart and Lung, calms the Shen (Spirit)[129]

Heart Yin Deficiency

Heart Yin has similar functions to that of Heart Blood. When the Yin of the Heart is Deficient, this can induce Heart Heat/Fire, which, in turn, can disturb the Shen (Spirit).[101]

Aetiology

Similar to the causes of Kidney Yin Deficiency,[157] a busy lifestyle, work, and family pressures with the added impact of mental stress damages the Mind and injures Yin.

Long-standing emotional upset such as anxiety or worry consumes Heart Yin.[157] Some women faced with subfertility issues and/or IVF failure find that the desire to become pregnant and have a family can become so overwhelming that it causes anxiety and intense emotional upset. The clarity of the mind and the Shen (Spirit) become injured, leading to Heart Yin Deficiency.

Women of advanced reproductive age are particularly prone to developing Heart Yin Deficiency as their Yin naturally declines.

Pathology

The syndromes Heart Qi and/or Blood Deficiency may eventually lead to Heart Yin Deficiency.[101]

In subfertile patients, Heart and Kidney Yin Deficiency often occur together.[101] When these patterns are combined, they have a significant negative impact on follicles, eggs, sperm, and embryos.

Signs and symptoms

• Complexion: facial flushing[101] or malar flush
• Disturbed Shen (Spirit): unease, restlessness, anxiety[88,159,160]
• Feeling of heat, night sweats[90,160]
• Dry mouth[90,160]
• Palpitations[90,157]
• Insomnia,[101] dream-disturbed sleep,[160] or frequent dreaming[90]
• Dizziness[88]
• Pulse: floating-empty,[49,157] rapid and thin,[88,157,160] or overflowing[157]
• Tongue: red body[88,90,157,160] with no coating on whole[160] or part of tongue. Red tip and/or deep midline crack reaching the tip of tongue body.[157,159]

Possible consequences for reproduction and ART

• Low number of antral follicles
• Follicular growth too quick
• Immature or poor-quality eggs
• Low fertilization rate
• Poor-grade embryos
• Poor endometrial lining
• RIF

Table 5.9 Heart Yin Deficiency acupuncture treatment	
Acupuncture points	**Rationale**
HE6	• Benefits Heart Yin and regulates Blood[164] • Clears Heat and Fire, calms the Shen (Spirit)[164]
P6	• Regulates, tonifies Heart Yin[104] • Clears Heat/Fire[104] • Calms the embryo and foetus[104]
P5	• Benefits the Uterus[165]
HE7	• Regulates and tonifies Heart Yin[104]
REN7	• Benefits Yin and the Uterus[166]
BL15	• Nourishes the Heart[110] • Calms the Shen (Spirit)[110] • Clears Heart Heat and Fire[110] • Cools Blood Heat[104]

Acupuncture treatment

Table 5.9 lists acupuncture points that treat Heart Yin Deficiency and the rationale for using them.

Heart Qi Stagnation

As discussed in Chapter 2, Shen (Spirit) is acquired when the body, Heart, and Mind are settled, calm, and 'properly aligned'.[167] A healthy Heart promotes and generates the Shen (Spirit) and revitalizes the Uterus. A good flow of Heart Qi positively influences the Shen, Mind, and Spirit, the menstrual cycle, the egg, sperm, fertilization, the embryo's Qi, and conception.

Aetiology

Worry and sadness can affect the Qi aspect of the Shen (Spirit). Heart Qi Stagnation can arise when the mind and emotional disposition of a patient restrict the normal flow of Qi.[146]

Pathology

Heart Qi Stagnation can compromise the flow and vitality of Jing (Essence), Qi, and Blood, influencing the well-being of the patient. Heart Qi invigorates and governs the circulation of Qi–Blood in the Uterus. Stagnation of Heart Qi can lead to Qi circulation issues in the Uterus, for example, in the case of amenorrhoea.[74]

Signs and symptoms

• Chronic anxiety, agitation[74]
• Sudden shock or emotional upset[74]
• Anovulation or amenorrhoea[74]

Table 5.10 Heart Qi Stagnation acupuncture treatment	
Acupuncture points	**Rationale**
HE5	• Regulates and tonifies Heart Qi[164] • Calms the Shen (Spirit)[164] • Benefits the Uterus[164]
P5+P7	• Regulates Heart Qi Stagnation[165] • Regulates the seven emotions[165] • Benefits the Uterus[165]
HE7	• Regulates the Heart, calms the Shen (Spirit)[164]
REN15	• Regulates the Heart, calms the Shen (Spirit)[164]

• Disturbed Heart and Shen (Spirit)[74]
• Palpitations[74]
• Insomnia[74]
• Pulse: choppy or tight, thready[74]
• Tongue: may have a red tip[74]

Possible consequences for reproduction and ART

• Imbalance of hormones (for example, FSH or Luteinizing Hormone (LH))[74]
• Low oestrogen levels[74]
• RIF

Acupuncture treatment

Table 5.10 lists acupuncture points that treat Heart Qi Stagnation and the rationale for using them.

Spleen and Stomach syndromes

Spleen Qi Deficiency

As discussed in Chapter 2, the Spleen plays an important role in fertility because it is the source of Qi and Blood. The Spleen influences the quality of sperm and eggs through Post-Natal Jing (Essence). Spleen Qi's main function after embryo transfer is the transformation and movement of fluids and nutrients to supply nutrition to the embryo.

Aetiology

Spleen Qi Deficiency is caused by overexertion, poor dietary habits, and/or emotional imbalances.[61]

Irregular eating,[155] consuming cold or raw foods and drinks, skipping meals, not eating enough, or overeating all weaken Spleen Qi.[168]

Overthinking, worrying, or feeling anxious can lead to mental strain and harm Spleen Qi.[155]

Dampness weakens the Spleen and creates Spleen Qi Deficiency.[168]

Pathology

Spleen Qi Deficiency may arise from Stomach Qi Deficiency[95] and Lung Qi Deficiency because these organs are closely linked. Conversely, Spleen Qi Deficiency may affect these organs. Therefore, it is important to assess the Lung and Stomach in patients who have been diagnosed with Spleen Qi Deficiency. Signs of Lung and/or Stomach Deficiencies may be evident only in the reading of the pulse. Spleen Qi Deficiency can also cause Stagnation.[158]

Signs and symptoms

- Complexion: yellow[83,90,169]
- Tiredness,[88,170] lassitude[84,169,170]
- Loose stools[84,88,90,169,170]
- Bearing down sensation in the lower abdomen[133]
- Poor digestion,[84,88] abdominal discomfort[169]
- Reduced appetite[84,90]
- Early menses, prolonged bleeding,[133] heavy menstrual flow,[121,133] midcycle spotting
- Prolapse of the Uterus[121]
- Pulse: empty,[55,121,169] soft,[55,88] fine,[55] slow[96,170]
- Tongue: pale[88,169] or normal colour,[168] may be slightly swollen,[90,121] tooth-marked edges[96]

Possible consequences for reproduction and ART

- RIF
- Early pregnancy loss

Acupuncture treatment

Table 5.11 lists acupuncture points that treat Spleen Qi Deficiency and the rationale for using them.

Spleen and Stomach Qi Deficiency

As discussed in Chapter 2, the Stomach and Spleen have a fundamental role in reproductive physiology. The Stomach is the source of Qi and Blood and closely linked to the Chong Mai (Penetrating Vessel). When the Spleen is Deficient, the Stomach becomes weak, too,[171] because the Spleen and Stomach are 'interlinked'.[112]

Aetiology

Emotions such as indignation, worry, and fear can harm the Stomach.[172]

Long-standing dietary irregularities cause Deficient Stomach Qi[155,171,173] and have long been associated with subfertility.[127] Energetically, Cold or Hot foods may injure the Spleen and Stomach.[171]

As discussed in Chapter 2, the functions of Qi are essential for reproduction. An irregular diet can damage Original (Yuan) Qi,[155,171] which reduces fertility and the possibility

Table 5.11 Spleen Qi Deficiency acupuncture management	
Acupuncture points	**Rationale**
REN12	• Regulates and tonifies Spleen Qi[104] • Regulates Stomach Qi and Yin[104] • Benefits the embryo and foetus[104]
SP3	• Regulates Stomach and Spleen Qi[104] • Strengthens the Spleen[104] • Regulates the Lower Jiao[104]
ST36	• Regulates Stomach and Spleen Qi[104] • Tonifies Spleen Qi and Blood (with moxa)[104] • Assists the flow of Qi and Blood[104] • Benefits the embryo and foetus[104]
SP1	• Regulates and tonifies the Spleen[107] • Stops uterine bleeding (with moxa)[122] • Facilitates the flow of Blood[104] • Regulates the Shen (Spirit) and emotion (resulting from Heart dysfunction)[122]
BL20+BL21	• Tonifies Spleen Qi[110] • Raises Spleen Qi[110] • Holds Blood[110] • Regulates the Stomach[110] • Supports Pre-Natal Jing (Essence)

of fertilization and can negatively influence the embryo's Qi and conception.

Pathophysiology

Spleen and Stomach Qi Deficiency can negatively affect the quality of Jing (Essence) and Blood.[95,171]

The Stomach is linked with the Liver and the Heart via Blood.[171] Deficient Stomach Qi can, therefore, cause Liver and Heart Blood Deficiency. Often, acupuncture points useful in treating Stomach and Spleen Qi Deficiency are also useful in treating the Shen (Spirit) and Heart Fire (see Table 5.12) because the Stomach can enrich Blood.[172]

Signs and symptoms

- Lassitude of Shen (Spirit)[171,174]
- Tiredness,[84,170,175] especially in the mornings[173]
- Reduced food intake[88]
- Discomfort after eating,[88] distension, feeling of fullness, or stomach pain[155]
- Poor appetite,[175] tastelessness of food[155]
- Thin body[171]
- Nausea[155]

Table 5.12 Stomach and Spleen Qi Deficiency acupuncture treatment	
Acupuncture points	Rationale
REN12	• Regulates, tonifies Spleen Qi[104] • Regulates Stomach Qi and Yin[104] • Benefits the embryo and foetus[104]
SP3	• Regulates Stomach and Spleen Qi[104] • Regulates the Lower Jiao[104] • Strengthens the Spleen[104]
ST36	• Regulates Stomach and Spleen Qi[104] • Tonifies Spleen Qi and Blood (with moxa)[104] • Assists Qi and Blood flow[104] • Benefits the embryo and foetus[104]
SP1	• Regulates the Spleen[107] • Nourishes the Stomach[107] • Nourishes the Shen (Spirit)[107] • Stops uterine bleeding (with moxa)[107,122] • Facilitates the flow of Blood[104]
ST25	• Regulates Stomach and Spleen Qi[104] • Generates Bodily Fluids[104] • Promotes fertility[104] • Regulates menses[104] • Regulates Blood, eliminates Stagnation[109]
BL20+BL21	• Tonifies Spleen Qi[110] • Raises Spleen Qi[110] • Holds Blood[110] • Regulates the Stomach[110] • Supports Post-Natal Jing (Essence)

• Any of the Spleen Qi Deficiency signs and symptoms (see above)
• Pulse: soft,[55,175] empty[49,173]
• Tongue: pale,[173,175] tooth marks, white coating[175]

Possible consequences for reproduction and ART
• Poor response to ovarian stimulation
• Poor-quality eggs and sperm
• Poor ovarian reserve
• Thin endometrial lining
• RIF

Acupuncture treatment
Table 5.12 lists acupuncture points that treat Stomach and Spleen Qi Deficiency and the rationale for using them.

Case study

Worry
Susan, aged 35, was about to undergo an IVF cycle to treat unexplained subfertility. She was friendly and chatty, with a singing tone to her voice. Susan confessed to being a worrier, constantly thinking and fussing about everything. She was tired and stressed because her work environment was 'getting her down'; she felt pressured and was easily irritated.

Other Significant Signs and Symptoms:
• Slight PMT, occasional premenstrual abdominal distension, uneven menstrual blood flow (it would stop and start).
• Pulse: both middle positions empty, soft (more so on the right).
• Tongue: pale, short, white coating, tooth-marked.

TCM Diagnosis
• Dampness and Spleen Qi Deficiency
• Blood Deficiency
• Liver Qi Stagnation

Cause
Worrying

First Acupuncture Prescription (Day 20 of Her Menstrual Cycle)
REN6, ST36, KID7, REN12, DU20, LIV8, and moxa
  Susan conceived naturally after 3 months of acupuncture treatment and had a little girl. At the time of this writing, she was pregnant with her second child.

Discussion
This case highlights the negative influence emotion and inappropriate Spirit (Yi) can have on fertility.

Pathogenic factors

Phlegm–Damp

Aetiology
As discussed in Chapter 1, Dampness can arise from environmental Damp conditions.[146]

Sun Si Miao stated that the nature of a woman's physiology means that women are prone to Dampness.[127] Women often weaken their Spleen through mental strain, worry, and anxiety. This results in failure of the Spleen's transforming functions,[146] which eventually generates Damp and Phlegm.

An excessive intake of sweet or fatty-rich foods damages and weakens the Stomach and Spleen, causing Damp–Phlegm.[161]

Pathology

Damp has a complex pathology. It may combine with Cold or retain Heat.[126] Dampness can reside in the Uterus, damaging its flesh.[146] With the passage of time, Damp gathers and forms Phlegm.[146]

Phlegm–Damp negatively affects the Stomach and Spleen[150] and thus Pre- and Post-Natal Jing (Essence). It impairs the proper movement and transformation function of the Spleen,[146] generating even more Dampness and Phlegm.

Damp–Phlegm causes stagnation and obstructs Blood, particularly in the Chong and Ren Mai (Penetrating and Conception Vessels),[161] the Uterus, the Bao Mai, and Bao Luo.

Signs and symptoms

- Copious white vaginal discharge[161]
- Menstrual irregularities,[161] for example, amenorrhoea[97]
- Scant menstrual flow,[100] thick or mucous menses[74]
- Overweight[97,161] and/or tendency for weight gain[74]
- Congestion[97]
- Reduced appetite[176]
- Dizziness[97,161]
- Fatigue,[176] sleepiness, desire to lay down[146]
- Palpitations[97]
- Diarrhoea[146]
- Pulse: soft,[49,177] slippery,[176] sinking–slippery,[49] slippery full,[74] wiry[49,53]
- Tongue: thick, greasy coating[74,177]

Table 5.13 Phlegm–Damp acupuncture treatment

Acupuncture points	Rationale
ST29	• Resolves Phlegm–Stagnation and restores the function of the Uterus[109]
ST40	• Transforms Phlegm and Damp[109]
SP6	• Resolves Phlegm and Damp[122]
REN3	• Drains Damp[105] • Benefits the Uterus[105]
ST36	• Resolves Damp[109]
GB26	• Drains Damp[179]
SP9	• Resolves Damp[122]
LIV5	• Clears Damp[108]
BL20	• Resolves Damp[110]
Moxa is indicated	

Possible consequences for reproduction and ART

- Ovarian cysts (with Blood Stasis)[178]
- Hydrosalpinx[74]
- Poor follicular recruitment
- RIF
- Early miscarriages
- Ectopic pregnancy
- Genetic issues
- Thyroid disease
- Severe depression in subfertile patients
- Complicated subfertility medical history with complex diagnoses

Acupuncture treatment

Table 5.13 lists acupuncture points that treat Phlegm–Damp and the rationale for using them.

 Case study

Phlegm–Damp–Cold and Blood Stasis

Rebecca, aged 33, had a history of one miscarriage and subsequently 2 years of subfertility. She had PCOS and was offered Intra-Uterine Insemination (IUI) as a first-line ART treatment, but she needed to lose weight before starting fertility treatment.

Menses

- ◆ Very irregular: only three periods in a year
- ◆ Dull backache and stabbing abdominal pain during a period
- ◆ Heavy blood flow, big clots

Other Signs and Symptoms

- ◆ Difficulty losing weight
- ◆ Talked in her sleep, had a lot on her mind, felt stressed and overwhelmed
- ◆ Soft stools
- ◆ Cold hands and feet
- ◆ Was lethargic and had mood swings
- ◆ Thick, white vaginal discharge
- ◆ Pulse: soft, wiry
- ◆ Tongue: phlegm lines, white bitty (like porridge) coating at the back of tongue body, pale and cracked

TCM Diagnosis

Phlegm–Damp, Blood Stasis, Kidney Yang Deficiency

First Acupuncture Prescription

ST40, LIV3+LI4, KID13, KID8, ST29, REN6, and HE5
    After 5 months of acupuncture treatment, she conceived naturally. She has a son.

Cold/Coolness

The pathophysiology of Cold is not easily overcome by IVF techniques. Patients diagnosed with Cold in the Uterus often have retained it for many years.

Cold can damage reproductive physiological processes by inducing irregular menstrual cycles and affecting the eggs and sperm. It can harden the egg and, thus, also affect fertilization. Although the ICSI fertilization technique may bypass this, Cold can still prevent embryonic development and implantation. If implantation does occur, Cold may lead to preclinical pregnancy loss as Internal Cold causes an 'inability to receive the foetus'.[132]

Aetiology

As discussed in Chapter 1, Cold can arise because of environmental Cold.[124] Wind-Cold may enter the Uterus directly. Cold drinks and/or raw foods may damage the Stomach and Spleen and cause Cold.

Pathology

Empty Cold can arise from Yang Deficiency,[124] particularly Kidney Yang. Conversely, Cold can damage Yang, causing Yang Deficiency.[180] Yang Deficiency may allow the invasion of External Cold, thus further complicating the Empty/Full Cold condition.

Cold often combines with Dampness. Cold–Damp causes Stagnation of Yang–Qi, which causes Cold in the flesh of the Uterus.[124] This occurs because the normal flow of Qi and Blood is prevented.

It is not uncommon to have mixed Hot/Cold conditions in subfertile patients. This commonly results from the emotional consequence of subfertility generating Heat from the Heart or Liver, whilst Cold remains in the Uterus (a type of 'Heat above and Cold below' syndrome).

Cold can transform into Heat disorders[48,181] and cause Stagnation or Blood Stasis.[124]

Signs and symptoms

- Complexion: dark white[124] or pale[121]
- Chilliness, aversion to Cold, cold limbs[124,150]
- Desire for warm drinks[124]
- Pale urine[124,150]
- Clear and thin vaginal discharge[150]
- Delayed cycle,[182] painful periods,[121,124] dull or gripping-type period pain, better with warmth[124]
- Dark clots[121,124] (if Full Cold), pale-red menstrual blood[133]
- Constricted,[124] scant menses[121]
- Pulse: tight and slow[121,124,176]
- Tongue: white tongue coating,[124,176] bluish-purple[121] or pale[121,176] tongue body

Possible consequences for reproduction and ART

- Hardening of egg's zona pellucida
- Poor semen parameters

Table 5.14 Internal Cold acupuncture treatment

Acupuncture points	Rationale
ST28	• Eliminates Stagnation of Cold in the Uterus[109] • Promotes fertility[109]
ST29	• Warms and benefits the Uterus[104] • Regulates menses, promotes fertility[109]
REN6	• Rectifies Cold Stagnation[105] • Warms Cold[104] • Regulates menses[104] • Benefits the embryo and foetus[104]
ST30	• Corrects Yang Deficiency with Cold[109] • Promotes fertility[109]
BL23	• Warms the Uterus[110]
DU4	• Warms Cold[104]
REN8 with moxa	• Warms Yang[105] • Disperses Cold[105] • Promotes fertility[105]
Moxa is indicated	

- Poor egg quality
- Low fertilization rates
- Poor embryo development
- RIF
- Reproductive immunology
- Compromises the environment of the Uterus and embryonic development

Acupuncture treatment

Table 5.14 lists acupuncture points that treat Internal Cold and the rationale for using them.

Case study

Cold–Coolness

Julia suffered 3 years of unexplained subfertility and was undergoing her first cycle of IVF. Her consultant decided to fertilize half of her eggs by ICSI and the other half by conventional IVF. With IVF, none of the eggs fertilized. ICSI resulted in the fertilization of three embryos. Two embryos were transferred on day 3 and resulted in conception and live birth.

TCM Diagnosis

Cold, Coolness mainly because the tongue body was light blue

Continued

Case study—cont'd

First Acupuncture Point Prescription

ST36, BL60, ZIGONG, REN4, and LI4 + moxa

Discussion

It is possible that chronic Cold hardened Julia's eggs' zona pellucida (outer shell), and fertilization was only possible by ICSI.

Heat/Fire

Heat is very common in subfertile patients and often manifests on the tongue body and in the pulse; it can also be confirmed by questioning the patient about menstruation. The intensity of Heat/Fire has various physiological and pathological influences. Gentle Fire reinforces Qi and is essential for life,[83] sperm potential, fertilization, and embryonic health and development whereas pathological Fire, which is too robust, weakens the body. Lower levels of Fire can at any time gain strength and injure the body.[83] Heat may also transform into Fire, remain low-grade Heat, or be supressed; all of these instances significantly compromise reproductive health.

Pathological Heat/Fire damages sperm, follicles, and eggs; affects fertilization; and injures the embryo. This is because Fire acts negatively on paternal and maternal Qi, Jing (Essence), and Blood and can consume Yin. Heat/Fire is associated with complex Orthodox medical conditions associated with RIF and reproductive immunology.

Aetiology

Heat can result from the invasion of EPFs.[41] In subfertility, Heat/Fire often arises from Liver or Heart pathology resulting from emotional disturbances.[41] Heat, in turn, also affects the Shen (Spirit).[101,158] Fire can occur when Heat increases in intensity.

Pathology

Heat reduces subfertility through various mechanisms. For example, it can consume Kidney Qi, Jing (Essence), and Yin; it may produce Phlegm by condensing fluids or create Blood Stasis.

Signs and symptoms

- Red complexion[101]
- Red eyes[101,150]
- Feeling hot, dislike of heat, preference for coolness[101]
- Agitation[101,150]
- Thirst[101,150]
- Desire for cold drinks[101]
- Constipation[101]
- Scant,[101,150] dark urine[150]
- Insomnia[41]

- Menses: early, heavy, bright red,[100,121] thick consistency[100]
- Pulse: overflowing, rapid,[101,121] full[150]
- Tongue: red body, yellow coating[101]

Possible consequences for reproduction and ART

- Infections
- Impact on the functioning, development, and maturity of eggs
- Affects the development of embryos
- Affects uterine receptivity
- Poor semen parameters
- RIF
- Reproductive immunology issues
- Early pregnancy loss

Acupuncture treatment

Table 5.15 lists acupuncture points that treat Heat/Fire and the rationale for using them.

Case study

Heat/Fire

Amelia experienced 3 years of subfertility and had a history of one miscarriage.

Signs and Symptoms

- Red, bloodshot eyes
- Waking at night feeling hot
- Menses: bright red, heavy, cycle length 26–35 days
- Pulse: fine, deep
- Tongue: heat spots on Liver and Heart, red body

TCM Diagnosis

Liver and Heart Fire

Cause

Emotions, due to ongoing relationship difficulties with her mother. These difficulties had started in Amelia's childhood.

First acupuncture prescription

SP10, SP6, ST36, SJ6, P7, LIV2, and LIV3

The IVF cycle resulted in the transfer of a blastocyst. The blastocyst split into two, and Amelia conceived identical twins. Interestingly, she had some vaginal bleeding in early pregnancy. She was treated weekly up to 20 weeks gestation, then every 2 weeks (on her request to help keep her calm). She delivered twin girls by an elective caesarean section at 38 weeks gestation.

Discussion

Acupuncture focused on draining Heat, but it took a while before the effect was noticeable.

Table 5.15 Heat or Fire acupuncture treatment

Acupuncture points	Rationale
LIV2	• Clears Liver Fire, modulates uterine bleeding[108] • Regulates emotions[108] • Regulates menses[108] • Calms the Shen (Spirit)[108] • Relaxes the Uterus • Cools Blood Heat and invigorates Blood[104]
P7	• Clears Fire/Heat and cools Blood[165] • Regulates the emotions and rebalances Shen (Spirit)[165]
SJ5	• Clears Heat from the Lower Jiao[183]
LIV4	• Clears Stagnant Heat[108] • Regulates the Lower Jiao[108]
REN3	• Cools Blood Heat and regulates the Uterus[104]
SP10	• Cools and invigorates Blood, resolves Blood Stasis[122] • Regulates menses[104] • Benefits the Uterus[104]
KID8	• Clears Blood Heat and cools Blood[104] • Benefits the Uterus[104] • Regulates the Ren and Chong Mai (Conception and Penetrating Vessels)[106]
ST44	• Clears retained Heat[109] in the Stomach[104] • Regulates Shen (Spirit)[109]
GB44	• Clears Heat from Liver and Gallbladder[179] • Calms the Shen (Spirit)[179] • Benefits the Heart[179] • Relaxes the Uterus
HE9	• Clears Heart Heat, calms the Shen (Spirit)[164]
P8	• Clears Heat, Cools Blood[165]
LI11	• Clears Heat, Cools Blood[184]

Empty Heat/Fire

Empty Heat/Fire can negatively affect reproductive health in a similar manner to Full Heat/Fire. Syndromes that can lead to Empty Heat (for example, Kidney Yin Deficiency, Liver Blood Deficiency, and Heart Blood or Heart Yin Deficiency)[41] are commonly diagnosed in subfertile patients.

Aetiology

The same causes that lead to Yin Deficiency may also lead to Empty Heat (see the section 'Kidney Yin Deficiency'). A busy lifestyle and the mental/emotional strain of subfertility can reduce Yin and eventually lead to Empty Heat/Fire. The emotional roller coaster that many patients suffer during IVF can initiate Empty Heat/Fire, especially in patients already deficient.

Medical drugs used in IVF can consume Yin and Blood or aggravate Yang, causing imbalances of Yin and Yang and Yin Deficiency with Empty Fire. Repeated IVF cycles can consume Yin and Kidney Jing (Essence) and lead to Empty Heat/Fire. These patients often produce a lower number of eggs with each subsequent IVF cycle.

Pathology and physiology

In a majority of cases, Empty Heat/Fire arises from Deficiency of Yin[171] or Blood.[91] Yin Deficiency in these instances can exhaust Jing (Essence).[80]

Empty Heat/Fire can affect the Chong and Ren Mai (Penetrating and Conception Vessels). This can lead to bleeding or the early arrival of menses.

Empty Heat can also Stagnate Blood[91] and negatively affect the Uterine environment.

Empty Heat deriving from the Kidney may flare upward and injure the Heart.[91]

Signs and symptoms

• Feeling of heat[121] in the chest area, on the palms, and/or on the soles of the feet[101]
• Red cheeks[150]
• Dry throat and/or mouth[185]
• Night sweats[121]
• Early, prolonged periods, menses: scarlet red colour[121]
• Pulse: rapid fine,[101] rapid floating empty,[150,157] or overflowing[157]
• Tongue: red body and peeled coating,[101,150] red tip[80,157]

Possible consequences for reproduction and ART

• Affects the functioning, development, and maturity of eggs
• Affects the development of embryos
• May affect uterine receptivity
• Poor semen parameters
• RIF
• Early pregnancy loss

Acupuncture treatment

Table 5.16 lists acupuncture points that treat Empty Heat/Fire and the rationale for using them.

125

Table 5.16 Empty Heat/Fire acupuncture treatment

Acupuncture points	Rationale
SP6	• Clears Heat or Fire[104] • Cools Blood[122] • Facilitates the flow of Blood, nourishes Blood[104] • Tonifies Kidney Yin, regulates Liver Yin[104]
KID6	• Clears Heat from Deficiency[106]
HE6	• Clears Fire, regulates and moderates Blood[164] • Calms the Shen (Spirit)[164] • Cools Blood Heat[104]
KID2 + KID3	• Clears Fire[106] • Regulates the Uterus[106] • Promotes fertility[106]
BL17	• Cools Blood Heat and nourishes Blood[110]

BBT CHARTING AS A DIAGNOSTIC AID

Introduction to BBT diagnosis

BBT is the temperature taken when the body is at rest (basal = rest), usually immediately on waking before any activity and after at least 3 consecutive hours of sleep. BBT is influenced by the reproductive hormones. In a healthy cycle, the rise in progesterone after ovulation causes a small increase in BBT,[186] and then the BBT drops to its pre-ovulatory level, usually a day before the start of the next period. Some couples use BBT charting as an ovulation detection method. BBT charts can also be used to monitor reproductive hormones at all stages in the menstrual cycle. This section will discuss how acupuncturists can use BBT charts as a diagnostic method and when optimizing reproductive health by means of the regulation of menstrual cycle pathologies.

Advantages and disadvantages of BBT charting as a diagnostic method

The use of BBT charting in a natural fertility acupuncture practice is potentially of great benefit, and these charts are used by many practitioners. However, the benefits of TCM BBT charting in preparation for and during ART treatment is debatable. Patients might not present early enough to chart BBTs for two or three menstrual cycles before commencement of their ART treatment.

Monitoring BBT during ART treatment can help obtain information that otherwise would be unavailable. For example, if a BBT Heart Fire pattern was observed on BBT charts during the ovarian stimulation phase, then, consequently, timely TCM treatment adjustment could be integrated. In addition, the BBT can be incorporated to help monitor the post-embryo transfer stage and early pregnancy. For example, a sudden drop in BBT may indicate Kidney Yang Deficiency and could be immediately addressed by acupuncture.[187]

A study by Lynch found that BBT charting was an agreeable technique for women to use, with only 1% saying they would be unwilling to chart their BBT.[188] However, BBT charting may not be suitable for all patients. One of the criticisms of BBT charting is that some women and their partners find it too stressful to take and record their temperature every morning. Some people may also attempt to self-diagnose, which will add to their anxiety levels. In some cases, BBT charting may be impractical, for example, in those women who already have young babies and have to get up frequently in the night to attend to the baby. Their temperature may not get to basal level because they may not sleep for a sufficient number of consecutive hours. Charting may also be impractical for women who work night shifts. Therefore, practitioners must take great care when deciding which patients would benefit from BBT charting and also review on a regular basis how their patients are coping with this technique.

If BBT charting is used during the preparation stage for ART, it can help monitor acupuncture treatment progress. Acupuncture treatment usually takes place over several months, and symptomatic changes are sometimes not evident until much later in the course of the treatment. With BBT charting, small positive changes in the charts can be observed earlier and, thus, can motivate the practitioner and the patient to continue the treatment.

Table 5.17 summarizes the main advantages and disadvantages of BBT charting as a diagnostic tool in ART acupuncture practice. As with all tools, it is up to an acupuncturist to decide if it is of benefit on a case-by-case basis.

Working with BBT charts

If the practitioner decides to use BBT charting with his or her patients, education in the correct BBT charting methods will be necessary (see Appendix II for a BBT template and patient instruction sheet).

Ideally, collect BBT charts for two or three menstrual cycles before analysing them. When analysing the temperature, exclude factors such as fever, alcohol, medication, poor sleep, or incorrect charting techniques when the temperature looks abnormal. Look for signs of stress in patients who are charting their BBT, and discontinue BBT charting if such signs are observed.

Figure 5.4 provides a step-by-step guide to using BBT charts in ART acupuncture practice.

Analysing BBT charts

BBT charting is one of many diagnostic tools that can help differentiate TCM syndromes.

Table 5.17 Advantages and disadvantages of BBT charting in ART acupuncture practice

Advantages	Disadvantages
• Simple and cheap to administer • Can help to confirm the diagnosis • May provide a TCM diagnosis that may not be available through other methods • May help to monitor treatment progress • Helps record and monitor other observations, such as cervical mucus secretions, timing and frequency of intercourse, etc. • Can be very accurate if used correctly and if factors that could affect the temperature are logged • May be useful for monitoring early pregnancy, especially in patients with a history of miscarriages • Provides different information than hormonal blood tests because BBT provides a day-by-day account of hormonal balance whereas blood tests provide a snapshot of hormones on a given day	• Can take a minimum of two or three menstrual cycles to identify patterns • Patients may find it too stressful to take and record their temperature daily because they forget to do it and also because they become anxious in response to every minor temperature fluctuation • Patients' partners may also dislike this technique because they may be awoken daily by a thermometer beeping • BBT may not be very accurate because it can be affected by many factors, such as poor sleep, alcohol intake, fever, medication, or poor charting techniques • It may be difficult for an inexperienced practitioner to identify patterns • It takes a lot of consultation time to review the latest BBT logs and give patients feedback • It can take a lot of the practitioner's time to train patients in correct BBT charting techniques • BBT charting is not highly regarded in conventional medical practice.

Figure 5.4 A step-by-step guide to using BBT charting in ART acupuncture practice.

STEP 1
• Decide if BBT charting will provide you with information that cannot be easily obtained elsewhere (for example, from BBT charts a patient may logged in the recent past).

STEP 2
• Estimate if there is sufficient time for a patient to chart before the beginning of ART treatment (minimum of 2–3 menstrual cycles).

STEP 3
• Assess patient's suitability and willingness to do BBT charting.
• Assess patient's partner's agreeableness to BBT charting.

STEP 4
• Train your patient in correct BBT charting techniques.
• Check that the patient has understood and remembered the techniques.
• Keep re-assessing if BBT charting is putting too much pressure on your patient.

STEP 5
• Review TCM diagnosis as soon as BBT pattern emerges and modify treatment principles if appropriate.
• Consider if a referral to another practitioner is necessary, for example, to an endocrinologist, if the temperature looks very abnormal.

The aim is to analyse BBT patterns and compare these with the Traditional Chinese Medicine diagnosis.

As already mentioned, BBT can be affected by bedroom temperature, alcohol and food ingestion, and emotional state.[189] Illness (especially febrile) can also affect the temperature. Therefore, these factors need to be excluded if the BBT looks abnormal. It is important to exercise extreme caution when using BBT charts to decide if a woman ovulates because there are some women who ovulate, but, for some reason, this is not reflected in their basal temperature.

BBT pathology during the follicular phase

There are six main types of BBT abnormalities during the follicular phase:

- Temperature is too low (see Table 5.18)
- Temperature is too high (see Table 5.19)
- Phase is too long (see Table 5.20)
- Phase is too short (see Table 5.21)
- Temperature is unstable (see Table 5.22)
- Temperature is initially too high (see Table 5.23)

BBT pathology during the ovulatory phase

Multiple markers of ovulation have more reliability than individual markers.[188] BBT charts as a method of predicting ovulation have proven to be an inadequate tool.[189,195] Urinary measures of ovulation such as LH detection kits show more reliability than BBT charts.[196] One study found that only 34% of gynaecologists were able to predict ovulation from BBT charts; however, 80% were able to retrospectively correctly interpret the presence or absence of ovulatory cycles.[197] Based on this, it is a reasonable presumption that couples and acupuncturists may also struggle to correctly predict ovulation from BBT charts. However, BBT charting is useful in retrospectively determining whether a woman has ovulated.[198] Therefore, BBT charts may help to determine whether an ovulatory cycle occurred but not as a prospective predictor of ovulation.

Usually, but not always, ovulatory BBT charts will have what is referred to as a *biphasic pattern*. This means that the temperature immediately after ovulation will rise by approximately 0.4–0.5°C (up to 1°F) and will remain at that level throughout most of the luteal phase, only dropping 1–2 days before menstruation.[190] The rise in BBT indicates a successful transformation from Yin to Yang.[190]

It is important to note that some women can still ovulate without a clear rise in luteal temperature; this is called a *monophasic pattern* (Table 5.24).[195,199] Whilst this is considered normal from an Orthodox medical point of view, for fertility acupuncturists, a monophasic pattern may be a pathological finding. For example, it could indicate Kidney Yang or Yin Deficiency.[187]

A low point on a BBT chart, referred to as *thermal nadir*, can occur 1 or 2 days before ovulation. Professionals and patients sometimes mistakenly believe that the presence of a thermal nadir confirms ovulation. However, its

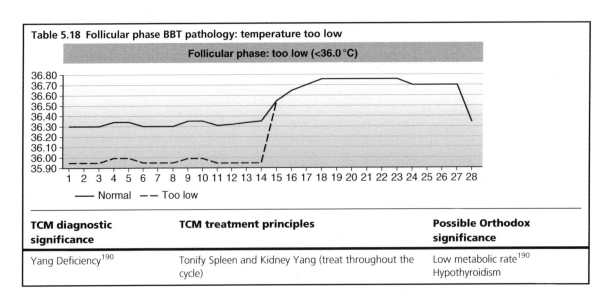

Table 5.18 Follicular phase BBT pathology: temperature too low

Follicular phase: too low (<36.0 °C)

— Normal   -- Too low

TCM diagnostic significance	TCM treatment principles	Possible Orthodox significance
Yang Deficiency[190]	Tonify Spleen and Kidney Yang (treat throughout the cycle)	Low metabolic rate[190] Hypothyroidism

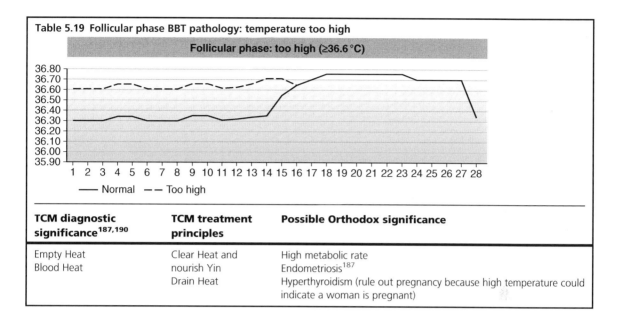

Table 5.19 Follicular phase BBT pathology: temperature too high

TCM diagnostic significance[187,190]	TCM treatment principles	Possible Orthodox significance
Empty Heat Blood Heat	Clear Heat and nourish Yin Drain Heat	High metabolic rate Endometriosis[187] Hyperthyroidism (rule out pregnancy because high temperature could indicate a woman is pregnant)

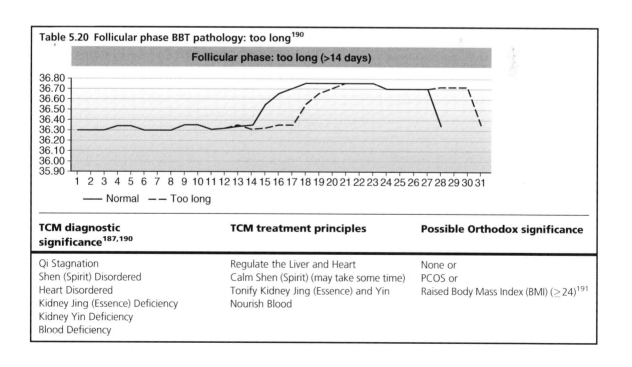

Table 5.20 Follicular phase BBT pathology: too long[190]

TCM diagnostic significance[187,190]	TCM treatment principles	Possible Orthodox significance
Qi Stagnation Shen (Spirit) Disordered Heart Disordered Kidney Jing (Essence) Deficiency Kidney Yin Deficiency Blood Deficiency	Regulate the Liver and Heart Calm Shen (Spirit) (may take some time) Tonify Kidney Jing (Essence) and Yin Nourish Blood	None or PCOS or Raised Body Mass Index (BMI) (≥ 24)[191]

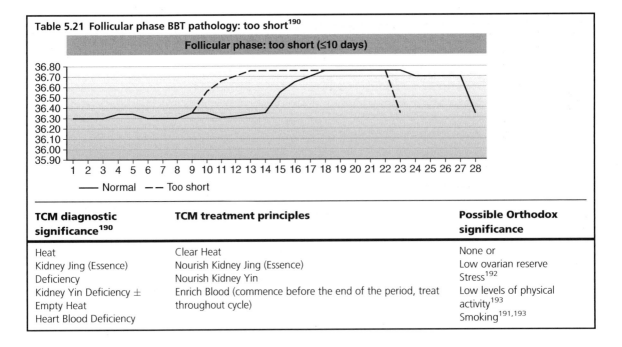

Table 5.21 Follicular phase BBT pathology: too short[190]

TCM diagnostic significance[190]	TCM treatment principles	Possible Orthodox significance
Heat	Clear Heat	None or
Kidney Jing (Essence) Deficiency	Nourish Kidney Jing (Essence) Nourish Kidney Yin	Low ovarian reserve Stress[192]
Kidney Yin Deficiency ± Empty Heat	Enrich Blood (commence before the end of the period, treat throughout cycle)	Low levels of physical activity[193]
Heart Blood Deficiency		Smoking[191,193]

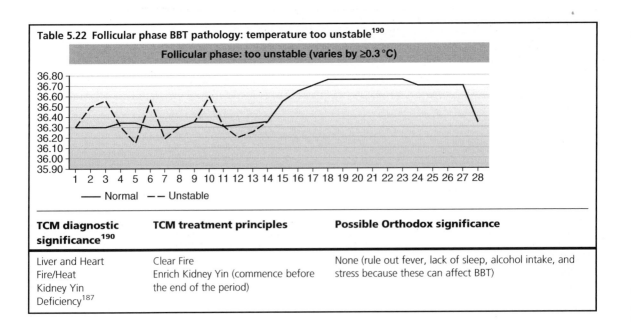

Table 5.22 Follicular phase BBT pathology: temperature too unstable[190]

TCM diagnostic significance[190]	TCM treatment principles	Possible Orthodox significance
Liver and Heart Fire/Heat	Clear Fire	None (rule out fever, lack of sleep, alcohol intake, and stress because these can affect BBT)
Kidney Yin Deficiency[187]	Enrich Kidney Yin (commence before the end of the period)	

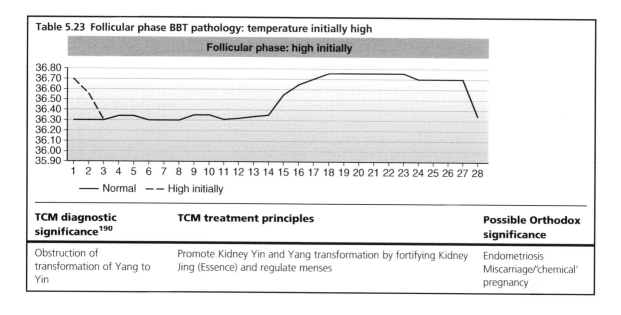

Table 5.23 Follicular phase BBT pathology: temperature initially high

TCM diagnostic significance[190]	TCM treatment principles	Possible Orthodox significance
Obstruction of transformation of Yang to Yin	Promote Kidney Yin and Yang transformation by fortifying Kidney Jing (Essence) and regulate menses	Endometriosis Miscarriage/'chemical' pregnancy

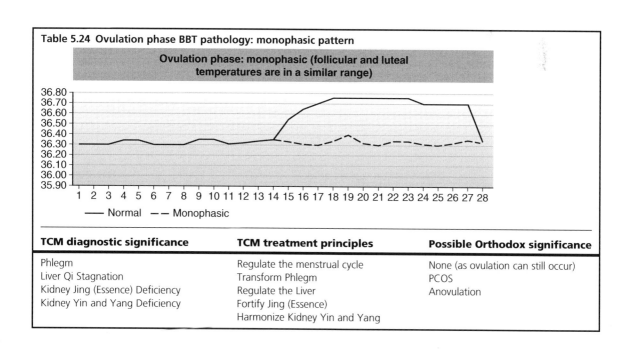

Table 5.24 Ovulation phase BBT pathology: monophasic pattern

TCM diagnostic significance	TCM treatment principles	Possible Orthodox significance
Phlegm Liver Qi Stagnation Kidney Jing (Essence) Deficiency Kidney Yin and Yang Deficiency	Regulate the menstrual cycle Transform Phlegm Regulate the Liver Fortify Jing (Essence) Harmonize Kidney Yin and Yang	None (as ovulation can still occur) PCOS Anovulation

presence or absence is not considered significant from either conventional medicine or by TCM; although one study found that the thermal nadir occurs in 72% of normal cycles and in 42% of abnormal cycles.[197]

BBT pathology during the luteal phase

The maintenance of pregnancy requires progesterone production by the corpus luteum after ovulation and during the first trimester. Cycles in which conception occurs have been shown to have a more rapid rise of progesterone and higher midluteal oestrogen and progesterone levels when compared to cycles in which there is no conception.[200]

Luteal phase deficiency (temperature too unstable or too low) has been associated with infertility, first trimester pregnancy loss, short cycle, premenstrual spotting, excessive exercise, stress, obesity, PCOS, endometriosis, thyroid dysfunction, and ovarian ageing.[200] Patients with evidence of luteal phase deficiency potentially need to be referred for conventional medical investigations to exclude more serious pathology.

The TCM view of the luteal phase is remarkably similar to that of conventional medicine. Once the BBT has risen by 0.4–0.5°C (up to 1°F), this level should preferably remain stable for between 11 and 14 days.[190] The luteal phase BBT should not fluctuate by more than 0.1°C (0.2°F). BBT should only drop the day before or on the day of the period.

Luteal phase pathology variants are ovulating early (i.e., having a shorter follicular phase) or possible inadequacy of the luteal phase.[190] Both may be pathological (i.e., Heat causing short follicular phase, or Kidney Yang Deficiency affecting the maternal environment or the viability of the embryo or both). The scale of Kidney Yang Deficiency is determined by the length of the luteal phase.[190]

There are six types of BBT abnormalities during the luteal phase:

- Phase is too short (see Table 5.25)
- Temperature is too low (see Table 5.26)
- Temperature is unstable
  - Sawtooth pattern (see Table 5.27)
  - Saddle pattern (see Table 5.28)
- Temperature rises too slowly (see Table 5.29)
- Temperature drops too early (see Table 5.30)

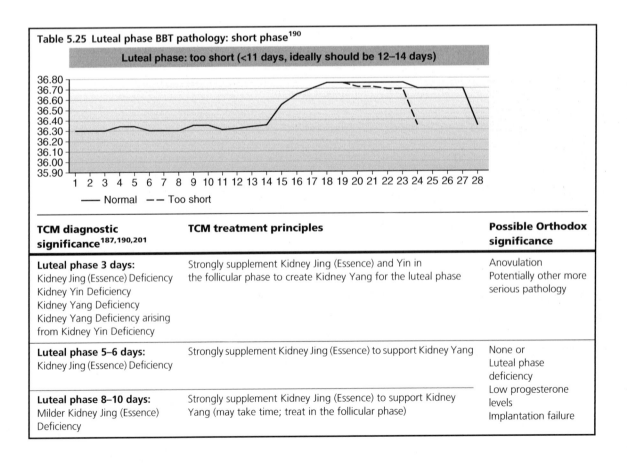

Table 5.25 Luteal phase BBT pathology: short phase[190]		
Luteal phase: too short (<11 days, ideally should be 12–14 days)		
— Normal − − Too short		
TCM diagnostic significance[187,190,201]	**TCM treatment principles**	**Possible Orthodox significance**
Luteal phase 3 days: Kidney Jing (Essence) Deficiency Kidney Yin Deficiency Kidney Yang Deficiency Kidney Yang Deficiency arising from Kidney Yin Deficiency	Strongly supplement Kidney Jing (Essence) and Yin in the follicular phase to create Kidney Yang for the luteal phase	Anovulation Potentially other more serious pathology
Luteal phase 5–6 days: Kidney Jing (Essence) Deficiency	Strongly supplement Kidney Jing (Essence) to support Kidney Yang	None or Luteal phase deficiency Low progesterone levels Implantation failure
Luteal phase 8–10 days: Milder Kidney Jing (Essence) Deficiency	Strongly supplement Kidney Jing (Essence) to support Kidney Yang (may take time; treat in the follicular phase)	

Table 5.26 Luteal phase BBT pathology: too low[190]

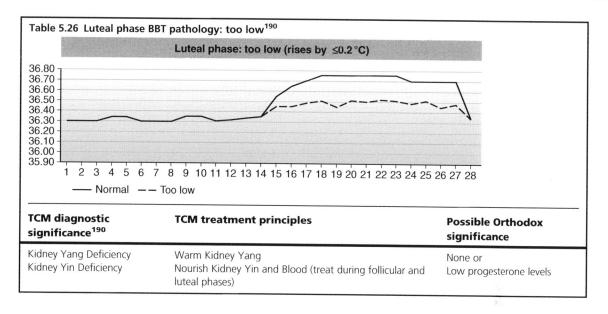

Luteal phase: too low (rises by ≤0.2 °C)

— Normal −− Too low

TCM diagnostic significance[190]	TCM treatment principles	Possible Orthodox significance
Kidney Yang Deficiency Kidney Yin Deficiency	Warm Kidney Yang Nourish Kidney Yin and Blood (treat during follicular and luteal phases)	None or Low progesterone levels

Table 5.27 Luteal phase BBT pathology: too unstable (sawtooth pattern)[190]

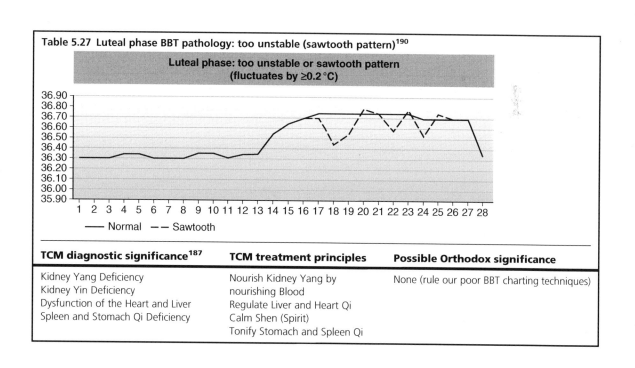

Luteal phase: too unstable or sawtooth pattern (fluctuates by ≥0.2 °C)

— Normal −− Sawtooth

TCM diagnostic significance[187]	TCM treatment principles	Possible Orthodox significance
Kidney Yang Deficiency Kidney Yin Deficiency Dysfunction of the Heart and Liver Spleen and Stomach Qi Deficiency	Nourish Kidney Yang by nourishing Blood Regulate Liver and Heart Qi Calm Shen (Spirit) Tonify Stomach and Spleen Qi	None (rule our poor BBT charting techniques)

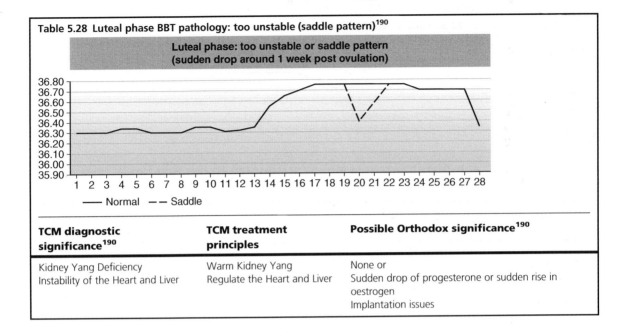

Table 5.28 Luteal phase BBT pathology: too unstable (saddle pattern)[190]

TCM diagnostic significance[190]	TCM treatment principles	Possible Orthodox significance[190]
Kidney Yang Deficiency Instability of the Heart and Liver	Warm Kidney Yang Regulate the Heart and Liver	None or Sudden drop of progesterone or sudden rise in oestrogen Implantation issues

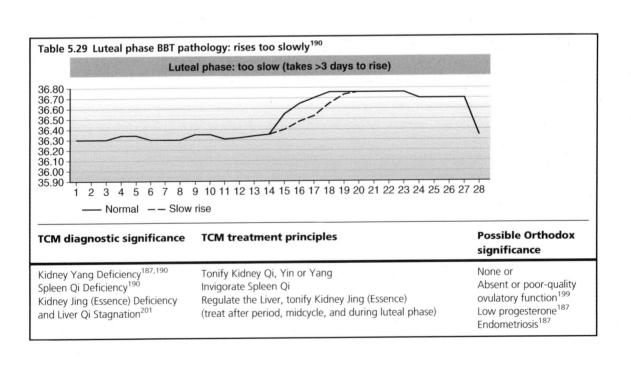

Table 5.29 Luteal phase BBT pathology: rises too slowly[190]

TCM diagnostic significance	TCM treatment principles	Possible Orthodox significance
Kidney Yang Deficiency[187,190] Spleen Qi Deficiency[190] Kidney Jing (Essence) Deficiency and Liver Qi Stagnation[201]	Tonify Kidney Qi, Yin or Yang Invigorate Spleen Qi Regulate the Liver, tonify Kidney Jing (Essence) (treat after period, midcycle, and during luteal phase)	None or Absent or poor-quality ovulatory function[199] Low progesterone[187] Endometriosis[187]

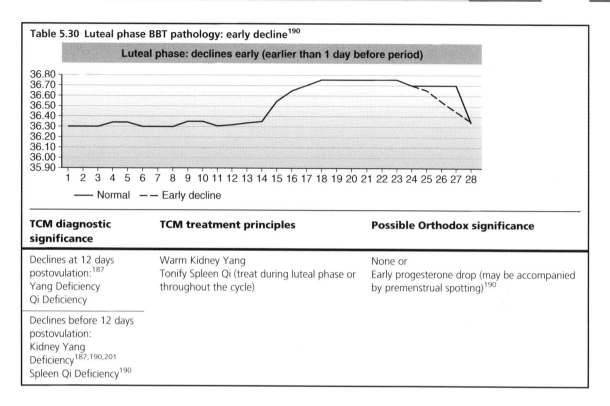

Table 5.30 Luteal phase BBT pathology: early decline[190]

Luteal phase: declines early (earlier than 1 day before period)

— Normal −− Early decline

TCM diagnostic significance	TCM treatment principles	Possible Orthodox significance
Declines at 12 days postovulation:[187] Yang Deficiency Qi Deficiency	Warm Kidney Yang Tonify Spleen Qi (treat during luteal phase or throughout the cycle)	None or Early progesterone drop (may be accompanied by premenstrual spotting)[190]
Declines before 12 days postovulation: Kidney Yang Deficiency[187,190,201] Spleen Qi Deficiency[190]		

SUMMARY

Conventional medicine and TCM investigations have similarities. For example, both medical systems use detailed medical histories and patient observation and examination.

The Orthodox medical model incorporates laboratory tests and imagery whereas TCM uses external sensory methods such as pulse examination and tongue diagnosis in order to determine what is happening inside the body.

Manifestations, which are significant for acupuncturists, may not be significant to an Orthodox medical practitioner. For example, subtle changes in tongue and pulse presentations are very important for acupuncturists but would make no difference to conventionally trained reproductive specialist. However, results of the laboratory tests and imaging can contribute to the acupuncturist's treatment and management strategy.

In some cases, TCM diagnosis can further refine an Orthodox medical diagnosis. For example, a patient who is not ovulating (as confirmed by progesterone test) can be further analysed from a TCM perspective and treated according to this refined TCM diagnosis.

In the authors' opinion, the integration of the interpretation of conventional medical tests and investigations and TCM diagnosis and syndrome identification is the key to effective treatment and management of subfertile patients.

REFERENCES

1. Lu HC. On loving natural life and total health. In: A complete translation of the Yellow Emperor's classics of internal medicine and the difficult classic (Nei-Jing and Nan-Jing). Vancouver: International College of Traditional Chinese Medicine; 2004. p. 151–4, Section two: Essential questions [Su Wen] [chapter 25].

2. Lu HC. Medical knowledge acquired from a master. In: A complete translation of the Yellow Emperor's classics of internal medicine and the difficult classic (Nei-Jing and Nan-Jing). Vancouver: International College of Traditional Chinese Medicine; 2004. p. 487–9,

Section three: Spiritual pivot [Ling Shu] [chapter 29].

3. Lu HC. On five kinds of careless faulty diagnosis. In: A complete translation of the Yellow Emperor's classics of internal medicine and the difficult classic (Nei-Jing and Nan-Jing). Vancouver: International College of Traditional Chinese Medicine; 2004. p. 359–61, Section two: Essential questions [Su Wen] [chapter 77].

4. Lu HC. Great treatise on regulation of spirits in harmony with the climates of the four seasons. In: A complete translation of the Yellow Emperor's classics of internal medicine and the difficult classic (Nei-Jing and Nan-Jing). Vancouver: International College of Traditional Chinese Medicine; 2004. p. 72–6, Section two: Essential questions [Su Wen] [chapter 2].

5. Infertility—NICE CKS. Available from: http://cks.nice.org.uk/infertility#! scenariorecommendation:2; 2013 [accessed 26 July 2013].

6. Practice Committee of American Society for Reproductive Medicine. Diagnostic evaluation of the infertile female: a committee opinion. Fertil Steril 2012;98:302–7.

7. Elzanaty S, Malm J, Giwercman A. Duration of sexual abstinence: epididymal and accessory sex gland secretions and their relationship to sperm motility. Hum Reprod 2005;20:221–5.

8. Levitas E, Lunenfeld E, Weiss N, et al. Relationship between the duration of sexual abstinence and semen quality: analysis of 9,489 semen samples. Fertil Steril 2005;83:1680–6.

9. Choi JM, Lebwohl B, Wang J, et al. Increased prevalence of celiac disease in patients with unexplained infertility in the United States. J Reprod Med 2011;56:199–203.

10. Zugna D, Richiardi L, Akre O, et al. A nationwide population-based study to determine whether coeliac disease is associated with infertility. Gut 2010;59:1471–5.

11. Machado AP, Silva LR, Zausner B, et al. Undiagnosed celiac disease in women with infertility. J Reprod Med 2013;58:61–6.

12. Diabetes—type 2—NICE CKS. Available from: http://cks.nice.org.uk/diabetes-type-2#!diagnosissub; 2013 [accessed 25 July 2013].

13. ASRM. Hypothyroidism. Available from: http://www.reproductivefacts.org/Hypothyroidism_factsheet/; 2013 [accessed 26 July 2013].

14. Hypothyroidism—NICE CKS. Available from: http://cks.nice.org.uk/hypothyroidism#!diagnosissub; 2013 [accessed 25 July 2013].

15. Hyperthyroidism—NICE CKS. Available from: http://cks.nice.org.uk/hyperthyroidism#!diagnosissub; 2013 [accessed 26 July 2013].

16. Menopause—NICE CKS. Available from: http://cks.nice.org.uk/menopause#!diagnosissub:1; 2013 [accessed 25 July 2013].

17. About hughes syndrome | APS | the brain. Available from: http://www.hughes-syndrome.org/about-hughes-syndrome/brain.php#.UYRdeZXS6fQ; 2013 [accessed 4 May 2013].

18. Vaginal discharge—NICE CKS. Available from: http://cks.nice.org.uk/vaginal-discharge#!diagnosissub:1; 2013 [accessed 25 July 2013].

19. Collins JA. Evidence-based infertility: evaluation of the female partner. Int Congr Ser 2004;1266:57–62.

20. Fauser BC, Tarlatzis BC, Rebar RW, et al. Consensus on women's health aspects of polycystic ovary syndrome (PCOS): the Amsterdam ESHRE/ASRM-sponsored 3rd PCOS consensus workshop group. Fertil Steril 2012;97:28–38.

21. Bentzen JG, Forman JL, Larsen EC, et al. Maternal menopause as a predictor of anti-Mullerian hormone level and antral follicle count in daughters during reproductive age. Hum Reprod 2013;28:247–55.

22. Dalsgaard T, Hjordt Hansen V, Hartwell D, et al. Reproductive prognosis in daughters of women with and without endometriosis. Hum Reprod 2013;28:2284–8.

23. Azziz R, Kashar-Miller MD. Family history as a risk factor for the polycystic ovary syndrome. J Pediatr Endocrinol Metab 2000;13(Suppl. 5): 1303–6.

24. Kahsar-Miller MD, Nixon C, Boots LR, et al. Prevalence of polycystic ovary syndrome (PCOS) in first-degree relatives of patients with PCOS* 1. Fertil Steril 2001;75:53–8.

25. Yildiz O. Glucose intolerance, insulin resistance, and hyperandrogenemia in first degree relatives of women with polycystic ovary syndrome. J Clin Endocrinol Metab 2003;88:2031–6.

26. Franks S, Webber LJ, Goh M, et al. Ovarian morphology is a marker of heritable biochemical traits in sisters with polycystic ovaries. J Clin Endocrinol Metab 2008;93:3396–402.

27. Ban Y, Tomer Y. Genetic susceptibility in thyroid autoimmunity. Pediatr Endocrinol Rev 2005;3:20–32.

28. Practice Committee of American Society for Reproductive Medicine. Diagnostic evaluation of the infertile male: a committee opinion. Fertil Steril 2012;98:294–301.

29. Royal College of Obstetricians and Gynaecologists 2011. GTG17 the investigation and treatment of couples with recurrent first-trimester and second-trimester miscarriage. Report of the Royal College of Obstetricians and Gynaecologists.

30. Shufaro Y, Simon A, Laufer N, et al. Thin unresponsive endometrium—a possible complication of surgical curettage compromising ART outcome. J Assist Reprod Genet 2008;25:421–5.

31. Gurol-Urganci I, Bou-Antoun S, Lim CP, et al. Impact of caesarean section on subsequent fertility: a systematic review and meta-analysis. Hum Reprod 2013;28:1943–52.

32. Wiseman N, Feng Y. E. A practical dictionary of Chinese medicine. 2nd ed. Brookline, MA: Paradigm Publications; 1998. p. 166–192.

33. Sivin N. Yin Yang and the five phases. In: Traditional medicine in contemporary China, science, medicine and technology in East Asia 2. USA: Center for Chinese Studies, University of Michigan; 1987. p. 203–12, Contents of translation [chapter 1].

34. Lu HC. Yin Yang and twenty-five categories of people. In: A complete translation of the Yellow Emperor's classics of internal medicine and the difficult classic (Nei-Jing and Nan-Jing). Vancouver: International College of Traditional Chinese Medicine; 2004. p. 541–6,

Section three: Spiritual pivot [Ling Shu] [chapter 64].

35. Worsley J. The five seasons: the Spirit of the elements. In: Wheeler J, editor. 3rd ed., Classical five-element acupuncture: the five elements and the officials. vol. 3. The Worsely Institute of Classical Five-Element Acupuncture; Jacksonville, Florida; 1998. p. 1–13 [chapter 1].

36. Lu HC. Acupuncture treatment in accord with the four seasons within a day. In: A complete translation of the Yellow Emperor's classics of internal medicine and the difficult classic (Nei-Jing and Nan-Jing). Vancouver: International College of Traditional Chinese Medicine; 2004. p. 508–10, Section three: Spiritual pivot [Ling Shu] [chapter 44].

37. Unschuld PU, translator and annotator. The depots and palaces. In: Janzen JM, Leslie C, editors. Nan-ching, the classic of difficult issues, medicine in China. London: University of California; 1986. p. 382–6 [chapter 3].

38. Larre C, Schatz J, Rochat de la Vallée E, et al. The differential energies. In: Survey of Traditional Chinese Medicine. 1 ed. Columbia Maryland: Institute Ricci; 1986. p. 111–39, Part 2 [chapter 3].

39. Lu HC. Spirit as the fundamental of needling. In: A complete translation of the Yellow Emperor's classics of internal medicine and the difficult classic (Nei-Jing and Nan-Jing). Vancouver: International College of Traditional Chinese Medicine; 2004. p. 402–4, Section three: Spiritual pivot [Ling Shu] [chapter 8].

40. Lu HC. On nine needles. In: A complete translation of the Yellow Emperor's classics of internal medicine and the difficult classic (Nei-Jing and Nan-Jing). Vancouver: International College of Traditional Chinese Medicine; 2004. p. 577–83, Section three: Spiritual pivot [Ling Shu] [chapter 78].

41. Wiseman N, Feng Y. F. A practical dictionary of Chinese medicine. 2nd ed. Brookline, MA: Paradigm Publications; 1998. p. 193–233.

42. Lu HC. Viscera and bowels (questions 30–47). In: A complete translation of the Yellow Emperor's classics of internal medicine and

the difficult classic (Nei-Jing and Nan-Jing). Vancouver: International College of Traditional Chinese Medicine; 2004. p. 606–12, Section four: Difficult classic [Nan Jing] [chapter 3].

43. Unschuld PU, Tessenow H, Jinsheng Z. Discourse on the true words in the golden chest. In: Huang Di Nei Jing Su Wen, vol. 1. Berkeley: University of California Press; 2011. p. 83–94 [chapter 4].

44. Unschuld PU. Huang Di Nei Jing Su Wen: nature, knowledge, imagery in an ancient Chinese medical text. J Altern Complement Med 2004;10:191–7.

45. Lu HC. From beginning to end. In: A complete translation of the Yellow Emperor's classics of internal medicine and the difficult classic (Nei-Jing and Nan-Jing). Vancouver: International College of Traditional Chinese Medicine; 2004. p. 405–10, Section three: Spiritual pivot [Ling Shu] [chapter 9].

46. Li Shi Zhen. Using the principal pulses to differentiate. In: Seifert GM, editor. Pulse diagnosis [Hoc Ku Huynh, Trans.]. Brookline: Paradigm Press; 1985. p. 10–1 [chapter 4].

47. Lu HC. Symptoms of disease of viscera and bowels by pathogens. In: A complete translation of the Yellow Emperor's classics of internal medicine and the difficult classic (Nei-Jing and Nan-Jing). Vancouver: International College of Traditional Chinese Medicine; 2004. p. 384–91, Section three: Spiritual pivot [Ling Shu] [chapter 4].

48. Li Shi-zhen. Four word rhymes. In: The lakeside master's study of the pulse [Flaws B, Trans.]. Boulder, CO: Blue Poppy Press; 1998. p. 1–60 [chapter 1].

49. Li Shi-zhen. The twenty-seven pulse states. In: Seifert GM, editor. Pulse diagnosis [Hoc Ku Huynh, Trans.]. Brookline: Paradigm Press; 1985. p. 61–101 [chapter 11].

50. Li Shi-zhen. Seven word rhymes. In: The lakeside master's study of the pulse [Flaws B, Trans.]. Boulder, CO: Blue Poppy Press; 1998. p. 65–123 [chapter 2].

51. Wang Shu-he. Book nine. In: The pulse classic [Yang S, Trans.]. A translation of the Mai Jing. Boulder,

CO: Blue Poppy Press; 1997. p. 319–49.

52. Wang Shu-he. Book ten. In: The pulse classic [Yang S, Trans.]. A translation of the Mai Jing. Boulder, CO: Blue Poppy Press; 1997. p. 351–79.

53. Maciocia G. Diagnosis. In: The foundations of Chinese medicine: a comprehensive text for acupuncturists and herbalists. Edinburgh, New York: Churchill Livingstone; 1989. p. 143–74 [chapter 16].

54. Lu HC. Pulse (questions 1–22). In: A complete translation of the Yellow Emperor's classics of internal medicine and the difficult classic (Nei-Jing and Nan-Jing). Vancouver: International College of Traditional Chinese Medicine; 2004. p. 592–601, Section four: Difficult classic [Nan Jing] [chapter 1].

55. Li Shi Zhen. Pulse description tables. In: Seifert GM, editor. Pulse diagnosis [Hoc Ku Huynh, Trans.]. Brookline: Paradigm Press; 1985. p. 102–15, Appendix A.

56. Li Shi Zhen. Pulses and associated diseases. In: Seifert GM, editor. Pulse diagnosis [Hoc Ku Huynh, Trans.]. Brookline: Paradigm Press; 1985. p. 20–5 [chapter 6].

57. Li Shi Zhen. Types of pulse. In: Seifert GM, editor. Pulse diagnosis [Hoc Ku Huynh, Trans.]. Brookline: Paradigm Press; 1985. p. 12–9 [chapter 5].

58. Li Shi Zhen. The pulse in complicated diseases. In: Seifert GM, editor. Pulse diagnosis [Hoc Ku Huynh, Trans.]. Brookline: Paradigm Press; 1985. p. 26–49 [chapter 7].

59. Wang Shu-he. Book one. In: The pulse classic [Yang S, Trans.]. A translation of the Mai Jing. Boulder, CO: Blue Poppy Press; 1997. p. 3–28.

60. Maciocia G. Clinical aspects of tongue diagnosis. J Chin Med 1995;48:17–20.

61. Wiseman N, Feng Y. T. A practical dictionary of Chinese medicine. 2nd ed. Brookline, MA: Paradigm Publications; 1998. p. 602–635.

62. Kirschbaum B. Observation of subligual veins. J Chin Med 2003;71:30–4.

63. Reamy BV, Derby R, Bunt CW. Common tongue conditions in primary care. Am Fam Physician 2010;81:627–34.

64. Glossitis: MedlinePlus medical encyclopedia. Available from: http://www.nlm.nih.gov/medlineplus/ency/article/001053.htm; 2013 [accessed 21 July 2013].

65. Liu G, Hyodo A, Cao Q. Four examination diagnostic methods in TCM. In: Fundamentals of acupuncture and moxibustion. Beijing: Huaxia Publishing House; 2006. p. 173–242 [chapter 5].

66. MacPherson H. Body palpation and diagnosis. J Chin Med 1994;44:5–11.

67. Maciocia G. Chest and abdomen. In: Diagnosis in Chinese medicine: a comprehensive guide. Edinburgh: Elsevier; 2004. p. 321–35 [chapter 38].

68. Lu HC. On regulating the meridians. In: A complete translation of the Yellow Emperor's classics of internal medicine and the difficult classic (Nei-Jing and Nan-Jing). Vancouver: International College of Traditional Chinese Medicine; 2004. p. 237–43, Section two: Essential questions [Su Wen] [chapter 62].

69. Lu HC. On pain of various kinds. In: A complete translation of the Yellow Emperor's classics of internal medicine and the difficult classic (Nei-Jing and Nan-Jing). Vancouver: International College of Traditional Chinese Medicine; 2004. p. 184–8, Section two: Essential questions [Su Wen] [chapter 39].

70. Cochrane S, Smith CA, Possamai-Inesedy A. Development of a fertility acupuncture protocol: defining an acupuncture treatment protocol to support and treat women experiencing conception delays. J Altern Complement Med 2011;17:329–37.

71. Huang ST, Chen AP. Traditional Chinese Medicine and infertility. Curr Opin Obstet Gynecol 2008;20:211–5.

72. Birkeflet O, Laake P, Vøllestad N. Traditional Chinese Medicine patterns and recommended acupuncture points in infertile and fertile women. Acupunct Med 2012;30:12–6.

73. Rosenthal L, Anderson B. Acupuncture and in vitro fertilisation: recent research and clinical guidelines. J Chin Med 2007;84:28–35.

74. Lyttleton J. Diagnosis and treatment of female infertility. In: Treatment of infertility with Chinese medicine. London: Churchill Livingstone; 2004. p. 83–164 [chapter 4].

75. Zhiqiang G, Baixiao C. Infertility. EJOM 1995;1:22–33.

76. Coyle M, Smith C. A survey comparing TCM diagnosis, health status and medical diagnosis in women undergoing assisted reproduction. Acupunct Med 2005;23:62–9.

77. Ke SX. Treating infertility in Traditional Chinese Medicine. EJOM 2008;6:10–1.

78. Maciocia G. Infertility. In: Obstetrics and gynecology in Chinese medicine. 2nd ed. Edinburgh: Elsevier Health Sciences; 2011. p. 685–734 [chapter 57].

79. Liang L. The pathology of infertility. In: Acupuncture & IVF. Boulder, CO: Blue Poppy Press; 2003. p. 9–16 [chapter 2].

80. Maciocia G. Kidney patterns. In: The foundations of Chinese medicine: a comprehensive text for acupuncturists and herbalists. Edinburgh, New York: Churchill Livingstone; 1989. p. 249–63 [chapter 25].

81. Ross J. Shen (Kidneys) and Pang Guang Bladder. In: Zang Fu, the organ systems of Traditional Chinese Medicine: functions, interrelationships and patterns of Disharmony in theory and practice. 2nd ed. Edinburgh: Churchill Livingstone; 1985. p. 65–82, Part 2 [chapter 7].

82. Wiseman N, Feng Y. L. A practical dictionary of Chinese medicine. 2nd ed. Brookline, MA: Paradigm Publications; 1998. p. 338–381.

83. Unschuld PU, Tessenow H, Jinsheng Z. Comprehensive discourse on phenomena corresponding to Yin Yang. In: Huang Di Nei Jing Su Wen, vol. 1. Berkeley: University of California Press; 2011. p. 95–126 [chapter 5].

84. Lu HC. Meridians. In: A complete translation of the Yellow Emperor's classics of internal medicine and the difficult classic (Nei-Jing and Nan-Jing). Vancouver: International College of Traditional Chinese Medicine; 2004. p. 411–37, Section three: Spiritual pivot [Ling Shu] [chapter 10].

85. Unschuld PU, Tessenow H, Jinsheng Z. Discourse on the true [Qi endowed by] Heaven in high antiquity. In: Huang Di Nei Jing Su Wen, vol. 1. Berkeley: University of California Press; 2011. p. 29–44 [chapter 1].

86. Liu F. Medical essays. In: The Essence of Liu Feng-Wu's gynecology. 1st ed. Boulder: Blue Poppy Press; 1998. p. 13–9, Section 2. A talk on the Kidneys [chapter 1].

87. Lu HC. Kidneys. In: Syndromes in Traditional Chinese Medicine. Marston: CreateSpace Independent Publishing Platform; 2013. p. 328–54 [chapter 30].

88. Wiseman N. Ellis. Organ pattern identification. In: Zhong Yi Xue Ji Chu, editor. Fundamentals of Chinese medicine. 2nd ed. MA: Paradigm Publications; 1996. p. 153–86 [chapter 9].

89. Unschuld PU, Tessenow H, Jinsheng Z. The generation and completion of the five depots. In: Huang Di Nei Jing Su Wen, vol. 1. Berkeley: University of California Press; 2011. p. 185–201 [chapter 10].

90. Liu G, Hyodo A, Cao Q. Diagnosis and treatment of TCM. In: Fundamentals of acupuncture and moxibustion. Beijing: Huaxia Publishing House; 2006. p. 243–342 [chapter 6].

91. Wiseman N, Feng Y. V. A practical dictionary of Chinese medicine. 2nd ed. Brookline, MA: Paradigm Publications; 1998. p. 645–657.

92. Wiseman N, Feng Y. K. A practical dictionary of Chinese medicine. 2nd ed. Brookline, MA: Paradigm Publications; 1998. p. 324–337.

93. Rochat de la Vallee E. Menstrual problems. In: Root C, editor. The essential women, female health and fertility in Chinese classical texts. Norfolk: Monkey Press; 2007. p. 92–127.

94. Fu Qing-zhu. Tiao Jing regulating the menses. In: Flaws B, editor. Fu Qing-Zhu's gynecology [Yang S, Liu D, Trans.]. 2nd ed. Chelsea: Blue Poppy Press; 1992. p. 29–54, Part 1 [chapter 3].

95. Liu F. Book one. Medical essays. The clinical significance of the Spleen and Stomach's upbearing and down bearing. In: The Essence of Liu Feng-Wu's gynecology. 1st ed. Boulder: Blue Poppy Press; 1998. p. 3–12.

96. Liu G, Hyodo A. Gynecological diseases. In: Clinical acupuncture

and moxibustion. Beijing: Huaxia Publishing House; 2006. p. 286–354, Part B [chapter 2].

97. Rochat de la Vallee E. Infertility. In: Root C, editor. The essential women, female hand fertility in Chinese classical texts. Norfolk: Monkey Press; 2007. p. 72–83.

98. Tan Y, Qi C, Zhang Q, et al. Etiology and pathogenesis of gynecological diseases. In: Gynecology of Traditional Chinese Medicine, Chinese-English bilingual textbooks for international students of Chinese TCM institutions. China: People's Medical Publishing House; 2007. p. 174–82 [chapter 3].

99. Maciocia G. Early periods. In: Obstetrics and gynecology in Chinese medicine. New York: Churchill Livingstone; 1998. p. 167–78 [chapter 8].

100. Wiseman N, Feng Y. M. A practical dictionary of Chinese medicine. 2nd ed. Brookline, MA: Paradigm Publications; 1998. p. 382–404.

101. Wiseman N, Feng Y. H. A practical dictionary of Chinese medicine. 2nd ed. Brookline, MA: Paradigm Publications; 1998, p. 251–294.

102. Unschuld PU, Tessenow H, Jinsheng Z. Discourse on the essentials of Vessels and the subtleties of the Essence. In: Huang Di Nei Jing Su Wen, vol. 1. Berkeley: University of California Press; 2011. p. 274–300 [chapter 17].

103. Maciocia G. Women's symptoms. In: Diagnosis in Chinese medicine: a comprehensive guide. Edinburgh: Elsevier; 2004. p. 395–409 [chapter 46].

104. Lade A. Point images and function. In: Acupuncture points: images and functions. Seattle, Wash: Eastland Press; 1989. p. 27–309 [chapter 3].

105. Deadman P, Al-Khafaji M, Baker K. The conception vessel. In: A manual of scupuncture. England: Journal of Chinese Medicine Publications; 1998. p. 493–526.

106. Deadman P, Al-Khafaji M, Baker K. The Kidney channel. In: A manual of acupuncture. England: Journal of Chinese Medicine Publications; 1998. p. 329–64.

107. Al-Khafaji M. Acupuncture prescriptions for tranquillising the

Heart and calming the Spirit. J Chin Med 1988;27:13–22.

108. Deadman P, Al-Khafaji M, Baker K. The Liver channel. In: A manual of acupuncture. England: Journal of Chinese Medicine Publications; 1998. p. 467–92.

109. Deadman P, Al-Khafaji M, Baker K. The Stomach channel. In: A manual of acupuncture. England: Journal of Chinese Medicine Publications; 1998. p. 123–74.

110. Deadman P, Al-Khafaji M, Baker K. The Bladder channel. In: A manual of acupuncture. England: Journal of Chinese Medicine Publications; 1998. p. 249–328.

111. Auteroche B, Gervais G, Auteroche M, et al. Moxibustion and other techniques. In: Zhong Yi Xue Ji Chu, editor. Acupuncture and moxibustion: a guide to clinical practice. Edinburgh: Churchill Livingstone; 1992. p. 75–92, Section 2 [chapter 1].

112. Wiseman N. Ellis. The bowels and viscera. In: Zhong Yi Xue Ji Chu, editor. Fundamentals of Chinese medicine. 2nd ed. MA: Paradigm Publications; 1996. p. 51–75 [chapter 4].

113. Maciocia G. Yin organ interrelationships. In: The foundations of Chinese medicine: a comprehensive text for acupuncturists and herbalists. Edinburgh, New York: Churchill Livingstone; 1989. p. 105–10 [chapter 12].

114. Maciocia G. Women's pathology. In: Obstetrics and gynecology in Chinese medicine. 2nd ed. Edinburgh: Elsevier Health Sciences; 2011. p. 49–74 [chapter 3].

115. Lu HC. Various types of energy. In: A complete translation of the Yellow Emperor's classics of internal medicine and the difficult classic (Nei-Jing and Nan-Jing). Vancouver: International College of Traditional Chinese Medicine; 2004. p. 489–90, Section three: Spiritual pivot [Ling Shu] [chapter 30].

116. Maciocia G. Painful periods. In: Obstetrics and gynecology in Chinese medicine. New York: Churchill Livingstone; 1998. p. 235–60 [chapter 14].

117. Maciocia G. Irregular periods. In: Obstetrics and gynecology in Chinese medicine. New York: Churchill Livingstone; 1998. p. 197–206 [chapter 10].

118. Maciocia G. Scanty periods. In: Obstetrics and gynecology in Chinese medicine. New York: Churchill Livingstone; 1998. p. 217–28 [chapter 12].

119. Maciocia G. Flooding and trickling. In: Obstetrics and gynecology in Chinese medicine. New York: Churchill Livingstone; 1998. p. 303–38 [chapter 17].

120. Deadman P, Al-Khafaji M, Baker K. The lung channel. In: A manual of acupuncture. England: Journal of Chinese Medicine Publications; 1998. p. 71–92.

121. Maciocia G. Women's pathology. In: Obstetrics and gynecology in Chinese medicine. New York: Churchill Livingstone; 1998. p. 31–49 [chapter 3].

122. Deadman P, Al-Khafaji M, Baker K. The Spleen channel. In: A manual of acupuncture. England: Journal of Chinese Medicine Publications; 1998. p. 175–206.

123. Lyttleton J. The menstrual cycle. In: Treatment of infertility with Chinese medicine. London: Churchill Livingstone; 2004. p. 7–46 [chapter 2].

124. Wiseman N, Feng Y. C. A practical dictionary of Chinese medicine. 2nd ed. Brookline, MA: Paradigm Publications; 1998. p. 53–107.

125. Li Shi Zhen. Diagnosing disorders of the eight curious channels. In: Seifert GM, editor. Pulse diagnosis [Hoc Ku Huynh, Trans.]. Brookline: Paradigm Press; 1985. p. 55–7 [chapter 9].

126. Unschuld PU, Tessenow H, Jinsheng Z. Discourse on how the generative Qi communicates with heaven. In: Huang Di Nei Jing Su Wen, vol. 1. Berkeley: University of California Press; 2011. p. 59–81 [chapter 3].

127. Sun Si-Miao. Translation. In: Bèi Jí Qian Jin Yào Fang. Essential prescriptions worth a thousand in gold for every emergency [Wilms S, Trans.], vol. 2. Portland: The Chinese Medicine Database; 2007. p. 52–216, 3 Volumes on Gynecology [chapter 2].

128. Maciocia G. Late periods. In: Obstetrics and gynecology in Chinese medicine. 2nd ed. Edinburgh: Elsevier Health Sciences; 2011. p. 211–25 [chapter 9].

129. Deadman P, Al-Khafaji M, Baker K. The governing vessel. In: A manual of acupuncture. England: Journal of Chinese medicine publications; 1998. p. 527–62.

130. Maciocia G. Liver patterns. In: The foundations of Chinese medicine: a comprehensive text for acupuncturists and herbalists. Edinburgh, New York: Churchill Livingstone; 1989. p. 215–29 [chapter 22].

131. Wiseman N, Feng Y. B. A practical dictionary of Chinese medicine. 2nd ed. Brookline, MA: Paradigm Publications; 1998. p. 14–52.

132. Sun Si-Miao. Prolegomena. In: Bèi Jí Qian Jin Yào Fang. Essential prescriptions worth a thousand in gold for every emergency [Wilms S, Trans.]. Portland: The Chinese Medicine Database; 2007. p. 4–50, [chapter 1]: 3 Volumes on Gynecology.

133. Tan Y, Qi C, Zhang Q, et al. Menstrual diseases. In: Gynecology of Traditional Chinese Medicine, Chinese-English bilingual textbooks for international students of Chinese TCM institutions. China: People's Medical Publishing House; 2007. p. 211–308 [chapter 7].

134. Maciocia G. Late periods. In: Obstetrics and gynecology in Chinese medicine. New York: Churchill Livingstone; 1998. p. 179–96 [chapter 9].

135. Unschuld PU, Tessenow H, Jinsheng Z. Discourse on the six terms [of a year] and on phenomena [associated with the condition] of the depots. In: Huang Di Nei Jing Su Wen, vol. 1. Berkeley: University of California Press; 2011. p. 163–84 [chapter 9].

136. Larre C, Rochat de la Vallee E. The Liver, syndromes of the Liver and Gallbladder. In: Root C, editor. The Liver. 1st ed. Norfolk: Monkey Press; 1994. p. 127–42.

137. Unschuld PU, Tessenow H, Jinsheng Z. Discourse on how the Qi in depots follow the pattern of the seasons. In: Huang Di Nei Jing Su Wen, vol. 1. Berkeley: University of California Press; 2011. p. 384–400 [chapter 22].

138. Larre C, Rochat de la Vallee E. Liver functions and related symptomatology. In: Root C, editor. The Liver. 1st ed. Norfolk: Monkey Press; 1994. p. 106–15.

139. Liu F. Medical essays. In: The essence of Liu Feng-Wu's gynecology. 1st ed. Boulder: Blue Poppy Press; 1998. p. 121–30, Section 10. A preliminary exploration of the treatment of menstrual irregulatory based on Chinese medical pattern discrimination [chapter 1].

140. Liu F. Medical essays. In: The essence of Liu Feng-Wu's gynecology. 1st ed. Boulder: Blue Poppy Press; 1998. p. 21–33, Section 3. Why is it said the Liver is the thief of the five viscera and six bowels [chapter 1].

141. Lu HC. Liver. In: Syndromes in Traditional Chinese Medicine. Marston: CreateSpace Independent Publishing Platform; 2013. p. 360–85 [chapter 32].

142. Maciocia G. Pre-menstrual syndrome. In: Obstetrics and gynecology in Chinese medicine. New York: Churchill Livingstone; 1998. p. 339–58 [chapter 18].

143. Soszka S. Liver and Gallbladder based erectile dysfunction: treatment by Chinese medicine (part one). J Chin Med 2002;68:5–14.

144. Rochat de la Vallee E. Zang and Fu. In: Root C, editor. The essential women, female health and fertility in Chinese classical texts. Norfolk: Monkey Press; 2007. p. 26–46.

145. Wiseman N, Feng Y. Q. A practical dictionary of Chinese medicine. 2nd ed. Brookline, MA: Paradigm Publications; 1998. p. 475–491.

146. Wiseman N, Feng Y. D. A practical dictionary of Chinese medicine. 2nd ed. Brookline, MA: Paradigm Publications; 1998. p. 108–165.

147. Unschuld PU, Tessenow H, Jinsheng Z. Wide promulgation of the five Qi. In: Huang Di Nei Jing Su Wen, vol. 1. Berkeley: University of California Press; 2011. p. 401–11 [chapter 23].

148. Fu Qing-zhu. Xue Beng/profuse uterine bleeding. In: Flaws B, editor. Fu Qing-zhu's gynecology [Yang S, Liu D, Trans.]. 2nd ed. Chelsea: Blue Poppy Press; 1992. p. 15–27, Part 1. [chapter 2].

149. Maciocia G. Painful periods. In: Obstetrics and gynecology in Chinese medicine. 2nd ed. Edinburgh: Elsevier Health Sciences; 2011. p. 255–85 [chapter 14].

150. Maciocia G. Identification according to pathogenic factors. In: The foundations of Chinese medicine: a comprehensive text for acupuncturists and herbalists. Edinburgh, New York: Churchill Livingstone; 1989. p. 293–302 [chapter 32].

151. Wiseman N. Ellis. Qi, blood, essence, and fluids. In: Zhong Yi Xue Ji Chu, editor. Fundamentals of Chinese medicine. 2nd ed. MA: Paradigm Publications; 1996. p. 17–28 [chapter 2].

152. Lu HC. Birth and growth of the five viscera. In: A complete translation of the Yellow Emperor's classics of internal medicine and the difficult classic (Nei-Jing and Nan-Jing). Vancouver: International College of Traditional Chinese Medicine; 2004. p. 108–11, Section two: Essential questions [Su Wen] [chapter 10].

153. Maciocia G. Long periods. In: Obstetrics and gynecology in Chinese medicine. New York: Churchill Livingstone; 1998. p. 229–34 [chapter 13].

154. Liu F. Medical essays. In: The Essence of Liu Feng-Wu's gynecology. 1st ed. Boulder: Blue Poppy Press; 1998. p. 45–60, Section 5. The treatment of Blood patterns in gynecology as learned through practice [chapter 1].

155. Wiseman N, Feng Y. S. A practical dictionary of Chinese medicine. 2nd ed. Brookline, MA: Paradigm Publications; 1998. p. 511–601.

156. Maciocia G. Women's physiology. In: Obstetrics and gynecology in Chinese medicine. New York: Churchill Livingstone; 1998. p. 7–29 [chapter 2].

157. Maciocia G. Heart patterns. In: The foundations of Chinese medicine: a comprehensive text for acupuncturists and herbalists. Edinburgh, New York: Churchill Livingstone; 1989. p. 201–13 [chapter 21].

158. Zhang Zhong-Jing. Greater Yang disease. In: Shang Han Lun. On Cold damage [Mitchell C, Feng Y, Wiseman N, Trans.]. Brookline, MA: Paradigm Publications; 1999. p. 33–295 [chapter 1].

159. Lu HC. Heart. In: Syndromes in Traditional Chinese Medicine. Marston: CreateSpace Independent Publishing Platform; 2013. p. 287–317 [chapter 27].

160. Ross J. Xin (Heart) and Xiao (Small Intestine). In: Zang Fu, the organ systems of Traditional Chinese Medicine: functions, interrelationships and patterns of disharmony in theory and practice 2nd ed. Edinburgh: Churchill Livingstone; 1985. p. 122–37, Part 2 [chapter 10].

161. Wiseman N, Feng Y. P. A practical dictionary of Chinese medicine. 2nd ed. Brookline, MA: Paradigm Publications; 1998. p. 423–474.

162. Lu HC. Cold and hot diseases. In: A complete translation of the Yellow Emperor's classics of internal medicine and the difficult classic (Nei-Jing and Nan-Jing). Vancouver: International College of Traditional Chinese Medicine; 2004. p. 464–6, Section three: Spiritual pivot [Ling Shu] [chapter 21].

163. Unschuld PU, Tessenow H, Jinsheng Z. Discourse on the hidden canons in the numinous orchid [chambers]. In: Huang Di Nei Jing Su Wen, vol. 1. Berkeley: University of California Press; 2011. p. 155–62 [chapter 8].

164. Deadman P, Al-Khafaji M, Baker K. The Heart channel. In: A manual of acupuncture. England: Journal of Chinese Medicine Publications; 1998. p. 207–24.

165. Deadman P, Al-Khafaji M, Baker K. The Pericardium channel. In: A manual of acupuncture. England: Journal of Chinese Medicine Publications; 1998. p. 365–84.

166. Deadman P, Al-Khafaji M. Some acupuncture points which treat disorders of blood. J Chin Med 1994;21–9.

167. Kirkland R. Varieties of Taoism in ancient China: a preliminary comparison of themes in the Nei Yeh and other Taoist classics. Available from: http://www.optim.ee/mati/Taoism/VARIETIES.pdf.

168. Maciocia G. Spleen patterns. In: The foundations of Chinese medicine: a comprehensive text for acupuncturists and herbalists. Edinburgh, New York: Churchill Livingstone; 1989. p. 241–8 [chapter 24].

169. Ross J. Pi (Spleen) and Wei (Stomach) Bladder. In: Zang Fu, the organ systems of Traditional Chinese Medicine: functions, interrelationships and patterns of disharmony in theory and practice. 2nd ed. Edinburgh: Churchill Livingstone; 1985. p. 83–100, Part 2 [chapter 8].

170. Li Dong-Yuan. Treaties on food damage to the Spleen. In: Li Dong-Yuan's treatise on the Spleen and Stomach: a translation of the Pi Wei Lun [Yang S, Li J, Trans.]. Boulder, CO: Blue Poppy Press; 1993. p. 153–4, [chapter 3]. Section 13.

171. Li Dong-Yuan. Treaties on the transmutation of vacuity and repletion of the Stomach and Spleen. In: Li Dong-Yuan's treatise on the Spleen and Stomach: a translation of the Pi Wei Lun [Yang S, Li J, Trans.]. Boulder, CO: Blue Poppy Press; 1993. p. 3–9, Section 1 [chapter 1].

172. Li Dong-Yuan. Book two. In: Li Dong-Yuan's treatise on the Spleen & Stomach: a translation of the Pi Wei Lun [Yang S, Li J, Trans.]. Boulder, CO: Blue Poppy Press; 1993. p. 55–105 [chapter 2].

173. Maciocia G. Stomach patterns. In: The foundations of Chinese medicine: a comprehensive text for acupuncturists and herbalists. Edinburgh, New York: Churchill Livingstone; 1989. p. 265–72 [chapter 26].

174. Lu HC. Verbal questions. In: A complete translation of the Yellow Emperor's classics of internal medicine and the difficult classic (Nei-Jing and Nan-Jing). Vancouver: International College of Traditional Chinese Medicine; 2004. p. 481–7, Section three: Spiritual pivot [Ling Shu] [chapter 28].

175. Lu HC. Spleen and Stomach. In: Syndromes in traditional Chinese medicine. Marston: CreateSpace Independent Publishing Platform; 2013. p. 415–25 [chapter 43].

176. Wiseman N. Ellis. Disease-evil pattern identification. In: Zhong Yi Xue Ji Chu, editor. Fundamentals of Chinese medicine. 2nd ed. MA: Paradigm Publications; 1996. p. 187–223 [chapter 10].

177. Lu HC. Dampness. In: Syndromes in Traditional Chinese Medicine. Marston: CreateSpace Independent Publishing Platform; 2013. p. 46–66 [chapter 4].

178. Wing TA. The treatment of ovarian cysts with Traditional Chinese Medicine. J Assoc Tradit Chin Med Acupunct UK 2012;19:21–4.

179. Deadman P, Al-Khafaji M, Baker K. The Gall Bladder channel. In: A manual of acupuncture. England: Journal of Chinese Medicine Publications; 1998. p. 415–66.

180. Lu H. Causes of diseases. In: Terminology of Traditional Chinese Medicine. Milton Keynes: Lightening Source UK Ltd; 2013. p. 99–112 [chapter 4].

181. Zhang Zhong-Jing. Introduction. In: Shang Han Lun. On Cold damage [Mitchell C, Feng Y, Wiseman N, Trans.]. Brookline, MA: Paradigm Publications; 1999. p. 1–25.

182. Tan Y, Qi C, Zhang Q, et al. Outline of treatment. In: Gynecology of Traditional Chinese Medicine, Chinese-English bilingual textbooks for International students of Chinese TCM institutions. China: People's Medical Publishing House; 2007. p. 189–202 [chapter 5].

183. Deadman P, Al-Khafaji M, Baker K. The San Jiao channel. In: A manual of acupuncture. England: Journal of Chinese Medicine Publications; 1998. p. 385–414.

184. Deadman P, Al-Khafaji M, Baker K. The Large Intestine channel. In: A manual of acupuncture. England: Journal of Chinese Medicine Publications; 1998. p. 93–122.

185. Wiseman N. Ellis. Eight principle pattern identification. In: Zhong Yi Xue Ji Chu, editor. Fundamentals of Chinese medicine. 2nd ed. MA: Paradigm Publications; 1996. p. 127–43 [chapter 7].

186. Grimes DA, Gallo MF, Grigorieva V, et al. Fertility awareness-based methods for contraception.

Cochrane Database Syst Rev 2004;
(4):CD004860.

187. Wood V. Infertility and the use of basal body temperature in diagnosis and treatment. J Chin Med 1999;61:33–41.

188. Lynch CD, Jackson LW, Buck Louis GM. Estimation of the day-specific probabilities of conception: current state of the knowledge and the relevance for epidemiological research. Paediatr Perinat Epidemiol 2006;20:3–12.

189. Lang Dunlop A, Schultz R, Frank E. Interpretation of the BBT chart: using the "gap" technique compared to the coverline technique. Contraception 2005;71:188–92.

190. Lyttleton J. Charting the menstrual cycle. In: Treatment of infertility with Chinese medicine. London: Churchill Livingstone; 2004. p. 47–82 [chapter 3].

191. Rowland AS, Baird DD, Long S, et al. Influence of medical conditions and lifestyle factors on the menstrual cycle. Epidemiology 2002;13:668–74.

192. Fenster L, Waller K, Chen J, et al. Psychological stress in the workplace and menstrual function. Am J Epidemiol 1999;149:127–34.

193. Liu Y, Gold EB, Lasley BL, et al. Factors affecting menstrual cycle characteristics. Am J Epidemiol 2004;160:131–40.

194. Jukic AM, Weinberg CR, Baird DD, et al. Lifestyle and reproductive factors associated with follicular phase length. J Womens Health (Larchmt) 2007;16:1340–7.

195. Barron ML, Fehring RJ. Basal body temperature assessment: is it useful to couples seeking pregnancy? MCN Am J Matern Child Nurs 2005;30:290–6, quiz 297–8.

196. Dunson DB, Baird DD, Wilcox AJ, et al. Day-specific probabilities of clinical pregnancy based on two studies with imperfect measures of ovulation. Hum Reprod 1999;14:1835–1839.

197. Lenton EA, Weston GA, Cooke ID. Problems in using basal body temperature recordings in an infertility clinic. Br Med J 1977;1:803–5.

198. ASRM. Infertility: an overview. A guide for patients. Alabama, US: Report of the ASRM; 2012

199. Practice Committee of the American Society for Reproductive Medicine. Optimal evaluation of the infertile female. Fertil Steril 2006;86:S264–S267.

200. The Practice Committee of the American Society for Reproductive Medicine. The clinical relevance of luteal phase deficiency. Fertil Steril 2012;98:1112–7.

201. Lian F. TCM treatment of luteal phase defect—an analysis of 60 cases. J Tradit Chin Med 1991;11:115–20.

Chapter 6

The fundamentals of ART

INTRODUCTION

Depending on the underlying cause(s) of subfertility, patients may be offered one of the following treatment options to help them conceive:

- Surgery (for example, where endometriosis is suspected)
- Hormonal treatment (for example, if semen quality and/or quantity are affected by hormonal imbalance)
- Ovulation induction with Clomiphene Citrate (CC) (for example, in anovulatory patients)
- Assisted Reproductive Technology (ART) treatment

ART is defined as 'any treatment that deals with means of conception other than vaginal coitus; frequently involving the handling of gametes or embryos'.[1] *In Vitro* Fertilization (IVF) is probably the most well-known type of ART treatment. However, several other types of ART treatment are available (Figure 6.1):

- Intrauterine Insemination (IUI)
- IVF
- Frozen Embryo Transfer (FET)
- *In Vitro* Maturation (IVM)
- Gamete Intrafallopian Transfer (GIFT)
- Zygote Intrafallopian Transfer (ZIFT)
- Third-party ART (for example, IVF using sperm or egg donor or a surrogate)

The next sections review the most common types of ART treatments and discuss patients' suitability for them. Chapter 9 provides more detailed information about various treatment protocols and how to treat patients undergoing these procedures with acupuncture.

The most important outcome measure of any ART treatment is the birth of a healthy baby to a healthy mother. Such outcomes are referred to as live birth or delivery rates. Some research studies only report embryo implantation and/or clinical pregnancy rates and not live birth rates. Some clinics only treat women who are likely to have a good prognosis, thus manipulating their success rates. Therefore, it is important to critically analyse the success rates quoted by research studies and by fertility clinics. It is also advisable for acupuncturists to become familiar with the success rates of ART clinics within their vicinity or those fertility clinics where patients are most frequently treated.

ART statistics also vary by physician, classification of subfertility, patients' age, and other factors. The section 'Repeated Implantation Failure' in Chapter 12 provides further information on what could affect ART treatment outcome rates.

TYPES OF ART TREATMENT

Ovulation induction

Approximately 20–32% of infertility is due to anovulation (failure to release a mature egg).[2,3] Anovulation is the most common cause of infertility. Treatment of ovulatory disorders depends on the underlying cause and may include administration of medications such as:[4]

- Luteinizing hormone-releasing hormone/ Gonadotrophin-Releasing Hormone (GnRH) delivered via pulsed pump
- Gonadotrophins with Luteinizing Hormone (LH) activity

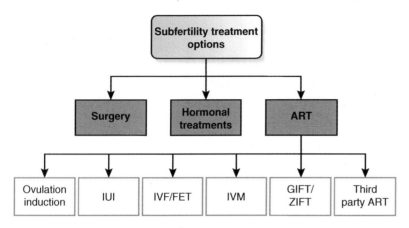

Figure 6.1 Overview of subfertility treatment options.

- CC
- Follicle-Stimulating Hormone (FSH) gonadotrophins
- Dopamine agonist medication

Surgical options, such as ovarian drilling, can also be used. Third-party ART treatment, such as donated eggs, is indicated in cases where anovulation is caused by Premature Ovarian Failure (POF).[4]

Success rates with ovulation induction depend on the treatment used and causes of subfertility.

IUI

Overview

IUI (sometimes referred to as artificial insemination) is a procedure that places the partner's or donor's prepared sperm into a woman's uterus via a soft catheter around the time of ovulation (Figure 6.2). IUI was developed in the 1940s and was one of the first successful ART techniques.

IUI helps to increase the chances of conception by increasing the number of sperm able to reach the egg.[5] It is different from IVF, where fertilization takes place in the laboratory. In IUI, the fertilization takes place in the female reproductive tract.[6]

Semen is produced by masturbation or ejaculated into a special condom following coitus. Semen samples are collected a few hours before the scheduled time of insemination.[7] Alternatively, previously frozen sperm can be used. The sperm is washed, and the seminal fluid is removed.[8]

IUI can be done in a spontaneous (natural) cycle or as part of a stimulated (medicated) cycle. In a stimulated cycle, the ovaries are stimulated with gonadotrophins, CC, or other antioestrogens. This increases the number of eggs ovulated in that cycle from just one to either two or three.[9]

Indications for IUI in a natural cycle are:

- Unexplained subfertility[7,9]
- Male factor subfertility
  - Low sperm count[10] but must have a minimum of one million motile spermatozoa[9]

- Retrograde ejaculation[9]
- Anejaculation[9]
- Erectile dysfunction[9]
- Sperm antibodies (because of previous infection or a vasectomy, making sperm clump together)[9]
- Cervical factors (for example, mucus or cervical hostility).[9,10]
- Minimal, but not severe,[11] endometriosis; IUI shortly after laparoscopic excision can be effective[12]
- Third-party reproduction (for example, donor sperm insemination in severe male factor infertility, for a single woman or a homosexual couple, or when IVF is not an option due to religion or personal preference)

Indications for a stimulated IUI are the same as for a natural IUI, and this is recommended for patients who fail to conceive with six rounds of natural IUI (although different clinics may apply their own criteria).[9]

IUI is contraindicated in:[13]

- Women with cervical atresia
- Women with cervicitis
- Women with endometritis or bilateral tubal obstruction
- Most cases of amenorrhoea
- Men with severe oligospermia

The pregnancy rate with natural IUI is about 8% per cycle,[9] with CC about 7% per cycle, and with gonadotrophin stimulation about 12% per cycle.[13]

IVF

IVF is an ART procedure that involves fertilization of an egg by sperm in a laboratory dish (Figure 6.2).[14]

As discussed in Chapter 2, in a natural reproductive cycle, several ovarian follicles are recruited each month. The body produces FSH, which is sufficient for only one follicle to grow and develop. Hence, only the strongest follicle

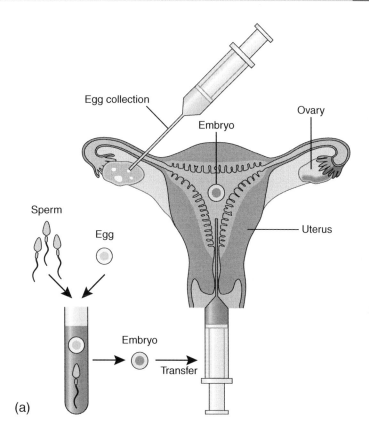

(a)

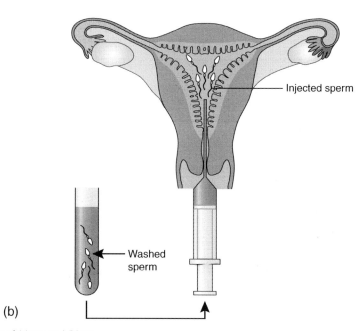

(b)

Figure 6.2 Comparisons of (a) IVF and (b) IUI.

survives and releases a mature egg in the process called *ovulation* (Table 6.1).

Originally, the main indication for IVF was blockage of the fallopian tubes. Now IVF is used to treat many other causes of subfertility (also see Table 6.2):

- Tubal pathology[15,16]
- Unexplained subfertility[15,16]
- Endometriosis[15,16]
- Cervical factors[15]
- Uterine factors[16]
- Immunological infertility (for example, autosperm antibodies in man's sperm, presence of sperm antibodies in the female partner's mucus)[15,16]
- Hormonal disorders (including ovulation dysfunction)[15,16]
- Male factor (by Intracytoplasmic Sperm Injection (ICSI))[15,16]
- Age-related subfertility (for example, Diminished Ovarian Reserve)[15,16]
- Donor treatment[15,16]
- Other reasons (chromosomal abnormalities, cancer chemotherapy, serious illnesses)[16]
- When other ART techniques fail[15]

The European Society of Human Reproduction and Embryology data from 32 European countries, 998 clinics, 117,318 IVF cycles, and 232,844 ICSI cycles performed in 2006 found an IVF clinical pregnancy rate of 32.4% per embryo transfer. If the ICSI fertilization technique was used, the pregnancy rate was a little higher at 33%.[17] Live birth rates per egg retrieval were 21.5% in IVF cycles and 18.4 in IVF–ICSI cycles.[17] Worldwide, a similar live birth rate of 20.2% per egg retrieval was reported in 2004 by 52 countries and 2,184 clinics.[18] Data also show that success rates continue to rise every year.[17]

Many factors can affect the success rate of IVF (see the section 'Repeated Implantation Failure' in Chapter 12). Patients often have an expectation that they will conceive after just one IVF cycle. However, research shows that some women (especially those over the age of 35) require more than one treatment cycle before they conceive, sometimes up to 10 cycles of treatment.[19]

Frozen Embryo Transfer

In an FET, previously frozen embryos are thawed and transferred into the uterus. Embryos can be frozen (cryopreserved) at the pronuclear (one cell), cleavage (2–10 cells), or blastocyst stage. The first successful pregnancy after FET was reported in 1983.[20] Worldwide data from 52 countries showed that, in 2004, FET represented 31% of all initiated IVF cycles.[18]

Reasons for cryopreservation of embryos include:

- Surplus of embryos from fresh IVF cycle[15]
- Unexpected complications or findings in a fresh IVF cycle that need to be resolved before embryos can be transferred (for example, Ovarian Hyperstimulation

Table 6.1 Comparison of natural and artificial ovulation and fertilization

Stage	Natural cycle (*in vivo*)	ART cycle (*in vitro*)
Follicular phase	Only enough FSH is secreted for one out of about 20 follicles to develop	A high dose of FSH is injected daily, allowing for more than one follicle to develop
Ovulation and fertilization	Ovulation is triggered by a raised LH level. An egg is picked up by the fallopian tube, and it travels into the ampulla part of the tube where it is fertilized by sperm deposited earlier	Ovulation is triggered by injecting the human Chorionic Gonadotrophin (hCG) hormone (which is similar in action to LH). Eggs are retrieved surgically 36 h later
		In the meantime, sperm is provided by a male partner who masturbates and ejaculates into a container. Alternatively, previously frozen or donor sperm can be used
		The retrieved eggs are fertilized by one of the following two methods: • IVF: Eggs are placed in a Petri dish with 50,000–100,000 sperm • Intracytoplasmic Sperm Injection (ICSI): One spermatozoon is injected directly into the egg
Postfertilization stage	The fertilized egg travels down the fallopian tube while undergoing division; it enters the uterus approximately 3.5 days later and attempts to implant after day 5	Fertilized eggs are left in the laboratory to divide. Embryo(s) can be transferred into the uterus on days 2, 3, or 5 postfertilization where they may then implant

Table 6.2 Indications for IVF and how IVF helps to overcome them

Indication for IVF	Explanation	How IVF helps with conception
Tubal factor	Blocked or damaged tubes make it difficult for the sperm to travel to fertilize the egg and for the embryo to travel into the uterus	IVF bypasses these issues by surgically extracting the eggs, fertilizing them in the lab, and replacing embryo(s) in the uterus
Endometriosis	Endometrial tissue outside of the uterus may affect fertilization of the egg and implantation of the embryo	
Cervical factors	Cervical issues may make it difficult for the sperm to reach the egg	
Immunological infertility	The immune system destroys sperm	
Unexplained infertility	No cause of infertility has been identified	IVF may help to overcome unknown or unidentified causes of infertility
Uterine factor	A disorder, either functional or structural, that reduces fertility	Medication and/or use of a surrogate helps with infertility caused by uterine factors
Hormonal disorders	Ovaries struggle to produce eggs normally; diminished ovarian reserve reduces the ability of the ovary to produce eggs	Ovarian development and ovulation is controlled entirely by IVF medication, thus eliminating the need for natural hormones
Male factors	Sperm are unable to fertilize the egg under normal conditions because of a low sperm count or issues with sperm function	Fertilization can be achieved using the ICSI technique, even in severe male factor infertility

Syndrome (OHSS), poor endometrial development, uterine polyps)

* Fertility preservation (for example, in oncology patients)

FET cycles can be done with or without hormonal preparation of the endometrium. Uncontrolled (natural) FET is only suitable for patients with regular ovulatory cycles. Pregnancy rates are similar in different protocols.[21] European data from 32 countries on ART treatments carried out in 2006 showed FET pregnancy rates as 19.1% and live birth rates as 12.7% per thawing.[17] Worldwide data for 52 countries showed that, in 2004, FET live birth rates were 16.6% per egg retrieval.[18]

It is important to note that cryopreservation techniques have improved over the last few years. The section 'Repeated Implantation Failure' in Chapter 12 discusses how FET may potentially be preferable in certain patient groups compared to fresh IVF cycles.

IVM

In IVF, eggs develop and mature under the influence of gonadotrophin stimulation *in vivo* (inside the female body) and are retrieved already matured. During IVM, immature eggs are retrieved from nonstimulated or minimally stimulated ovaries and are then matured and fertilized *in vitro* (in the laboratory). The fertilized embryos are then transferred into the uterus and/or cryopreserved.

The first attempts at IVM were reported by Edwards *et al.* in the 1960s. However, it was not until the 1980s when the first baby was born following stimulated IVM and as late as the 1990s following a nonstimulated IVM.[22]

Indications for IVM include:

* Poor responses to ovarian stimulation. For example, in women diagnosed with ovarian resistance to FSH (also known as ovary resistant syndrome) who may present with amenorrhoea and a menopausal range of FSH but have normal antral follicle count (AFC) and Anti-Müllerian Hormone (AMH) levels. These women are often misdiagnosed with POF.[23]
* Fertility preservation (for example, in patients undergoing cancer treatment or women wishing to reduce the risk of subfertility due to endometriosis).[23]
* Women at risk of OHSS (for example, patients with Polycystic Ovary Syndrome (PCOS) or Polycystic Ovaries (PCO)).[24]
* Women diagnosed with hormonally sensitive tumours or other contraindications for prolonged elevations of oestrogen levels.[24]

Implantation rates following IVM range from 5.5% to 21.6% and are lower compared to IVF.[24] IVM is still classed as an experimental treatment and is only recommended in research settings.[24]

GIFT

GIFT is a technique where gametes (an egg and sperm) are transferred into a woman's fallopian tubes via a laparoscopic procedure. This technique was first introduced in the 1980s and seemed to show promise for unexplained infertility.

GIFT accounts for <1% of ART procedures in the United States.[25] It requires at least one healthy fallopian tube and is not suitable in severe male factor infertility.[26] Some couples choose GIFT for religious or moral reasons because the egg is not fertilized outside the body. However, this is a drawback of GIFT because fertilization cannot be confirmed. Sometimes, surplus eggs are fertilized in the lab for subsequent freezing.[26] If there is a good rate of fertilization in the lab eggs, then fertilization is also assumed to have taken place in the fallopian tubes. However, a successful pregnancy is the only definitive proof.

Indications for GIFT include:[26]

- Pelvic adhesions unrelated to pelvic inflammatory disease
- Endometriosis
- Cervical factor infertility
- Oligoanovulatory infertility
- Unexplained infertility
- Religious or social reasons

Contraindications for GIFT include:[26]

- Pelvic inflammatory disease
- Tubal infertility
- Severe male factor infertility
- Contraindications for laparoscopy

Success rates of GIFT vary, depending on the underlying causes of subfertility and the patient's age, with average pregnancy rates per embryo transfer about 30%.[27]

ZIFT

ZIFT is a procedure similar to GIFT, but the egg is fertilized in the laboratory. Then the fertilized egg (zygote) is transferred into the fallopian tubes by a laparoscopic procedure. In the United States, ZIFT is performed in <1.5% of ART cases.[25] As in GIFT, ZIFT can only be performed in women who have at least one patent fallopian tube. In ZIFT, two laparoscopic procedures need to be performed: one for oocyte collection and one for embryo transfer.[26]

Indications for ZIFT are the same as for GIFT. The only difference is that patients with severe male factor infertility can have ZIFT as the eggs can be fertilized with an ICSI technique (see the section 'Intracytoplasmic Sperm Injection' later in this chapter).[26]

Average pregnancy rates per embryo transfer are 42% in ZIFT–ICSI cycles and are 37% in ZIFT–non-ICSI cycles.[27]

Third-party ART

There are two main types of third-party ART treatment: One type is where a couple uses donor eggs and/or sperm or embryos; the second involves the use of a surrogate to carry the foetus.

Donor ART

Donor ART is indicated in couples that have problems with their eggs and/or sperm. Donor ART is very tightly regulated. Donors must undergo extensive medical and genetic screening. Donated sperm is frozen and quarantined for 6 months and retested for the AIDS virus. Eggs, however, do not freeze as well, and the same AIDS virus screening is not possible in donated eggs. Donors can be financially compensated for their donation with varied national legislation relating to this. There is generally a shortage of egg donors. In the United Kingdom, a 'share' scheme exists where egg recipients pay for their donor's IVF treatment in return for half of the donor's eggs. Some couples choose their own donor. Often, the donor is a friend or a relative.

Egg donors have to undergo ovarian stimulation and egg retrieval as in standard IVF. The donated eggs are then fertilized with the recipient's partner's or donor's sperm. Concurrently, the recipient's uterus is prepared to receive the fertilized embryos.

Egg donation IVF accounts for nearly 10% of all ART cycles in the United States. Its overall success rate is very high at about 50%.[25]

Because the child will not be genetically related to one or both members of the couple, it can thus be a very difficult decision for a couple to make. There are also complex legislative issues relating to anonymity of donors. Donor ART is usually reserved as a procedure of last resort. However, for some couples, it is the only way to have a baby. All involved parties must undergo psychological counselling before starting the treatment. As acupuncturists, we are likely to treat a small proportion of the recipients and donors.

Surrogacy/gestational carrier

If a woman is unable to carry a baby, it can be carried for her by another woman. A 'traditional surrogate' is where a foetus is carried by the egg donor, whereas a 'gestational carrier' is where a foetus is carried by a woman who is not genetically related to the baby. A traditional surrogate carrier can conceive via insemination alone or via IVF. A gestational carrier will require IVF in order to get pregnant. In this case, the eggs are retrieved from the biological mother, fertilized in the lab with her partner's sperm and then transferred into the carrier's uterus. As with all third-party ART, legislation tightly controls this type of treatment, and all parties are required to undergo psychological counselling before any treatment takes place.

PHARMACOLOGICAL DRUGS USED IN ART

As described in Chapter 2, the Hypothalamic–Pituitary–Ovarian Axis (HPOA) is responsible for the development of follicles and eggs. In ART treatments, pharmacological drugs are given to alter HPOA function in order to enhance fertility. The next sections describe the main ART drugs and how they work. A summary table is provided in Appendix V.

Ovulation induction medication

CC therapy

CC is one of the most frequently prescribed ovulation drugs. It is used in women who do not ovulate or ovulate infrequently, for example, in PCOS patients. It can also be used in IUI.[28] In poor countries, CC has been used to induce ovulation in IVF patients. CC works by making the pituitary gland secrete more FSH. This encourages more follicles to develop. The usual dose of CC is 50–100 mg, but doses up to 200 mg can be prescribed in women who fail to respond to standard doses.[28] Women who do not ovulate because of hypothalamic disorders or have very low oestrogen levels should not be prescribed CC.[28]

INTERESTING FACTS

CC AND TCM ENERGETICS

It has been suggested that, in the long term, CC injures Yin and may exacerbate Heat symptoms in patients who have pre-existing Heat Syndrome, especially Liver Heat.[29]

Aromatase inhibitors

Aromatase inhibitors such as letrozole and anastrozole are drugs that reduce oestrogen levels and are commonly used in oestrogen-sensitive cancers. Their function and effectiveness is similar to CC.[28]

Insulin-sensitizing drugs (commonly used in patients with PCOS)

Insulin-sensitizing drugs (such as metformin and, less commonly, rosiglitazone and pioglitazone) are prescribed for women with PCOS either on their own or to enhance the function of CC.

Gonadotrophins

Gonadotrophins are medicines that are used as FSH or LH monotherapy or in combination, usually in injectable form. Gonadotrophins are prescribed for women who fail to respond to CC or who do not produce adequate amounts of FSH and LH. Gonadotrophins are also prescribed in IUI and IVF to induce multiple follicle (and egg) development. They are usually administered from day 2 to 3 of the menstrual cycle. The dose varies from 75–100 units a day in non-IVF cycles[28] and up to 450 units a day in IVF cycles.[30] The dose prescribed will depend on factors such as past response, the potential risk of developing OHSS (see Chapter 11), and a patient's ovarian reserve. The dose can be altered, depending on the patient's ovarian response, which is monitored by ultrasound and by checking blood oestrogen levels.

hCG

Human Chorionic Gonadotrophin (hCG) mimics LH and is used to induce or 'trigger' final egg maturation and ovulation. Following hCG injection, ovulation or egg retrieval occurs about 36 h later. hCG remains in the system for several days. Sometimes, it is responsible for a woman having a false-positive pregnancy test for up to 10 days after the injection.[28]

Dopamine agonists

High levels of prolactin supress FSH and LH production. This can stop women from ovulating. Dopamine agonists, commonly Bromocriptine and Cabergoline, may be prescribed. Dopamine agonists return prolactin levels to normal in 90% of women. In women who do not respond, CC may be prescribed along with dopamine agonists.[28]

GnRH

The hypothalamus normally releases GnRH in a pulsatile manner, approximately every 90 min. GnRH stimulates the pituitary to secrete LH and FSH. In women who do not ovulate or ovulate irregularly, small amounts of GnRH can be injected subcutaneously using a pump delivery system (see Chapter 8 for more details).

GnRH analogues (agonists and antagonists)

GnRH analogues are synthetic drugs similar to natural GnRH. There are two main types: agonists and antagonists. They are used in IVF in order to gain control of the reproductive cycle and to prevent undesired natural secretion of LH and, therefore, ovulation. GnRH analogues are ineffective if taken orally.

Agonists' mode of action is to stimulate the pituitary gland to secrete FSH and LH. Unlike natural GnRH, which is secreted in a pulsatile manner, synthetic agonists have a constant pharmacokinetic action.[28] After a period of about 10 days, the pituitary gland is desensitized, resulting in reduced FSH and LH production, which in turn stops undesired ovulation. Agonists are usually administered as a nasal spray or via injection.

Antagonists also supress FSH and LH production, but unlike agonists, they do so without the initial stimulation.[28] Antagonists are usually injected.

The benefits of using agonists or antagonists are the subject of much research and debate. GnRH analogues are discussed further in Chapters 9 and 12.

Luteal/endometrial support medication

Progestogens are commonly used to support the luteal phase of IVF cycles and in early pregnancy. They are available as a gel, pessaries, or injections,[31] and they can be used alone or in combination with oestrogen.[32] Progestogens are the most commonly used and the most effective form of luteal supplementation.[33]

Oestrogen can also be prescribed to promote the growth of the endometrial lining, for example, during the follicular phase of FET.

Other luteal support medications include hCG and GnRH agonists. However, hCG is linked to an increased risk of OHSS, and, therefore, most fertility clinics avoid using it.[33]

Other medications

In some patients, blood-thinning medication (antiplatelets and anticoagulation drugs such as aspirin, Clexane, and Lovenox) are prescribed as part of IVF treatment. Such medication is commonly prescribed in women who have been diagnosed with thrombophilia disorders[34] or empirically in patients with Repeated Implantation Failure[35] or repeated miscarriages.

Contraceptive pills can be used to help PCOS patients regulate their cycle prior to IVF.[36] They can also be used to alter the timing of a woman's menstrual cycle in such a way that it suits the clinic's logistical needs with respect to scheduling the patient's treatments.[37]

EMBRYO GRADING

Importance of embryo grading

The quality of the embryo is the best predictor of pregnancy in IVF.[38] One study analysed 1000 IVF embryo transfers and found that women with a low AFC (1–5 follicles) were able to achieve pregnancy at high rates with good embryos, suggesting that the quality of embryos may be a better predictor of pregnancy than ovarian reserve.[39] Another study analysed data from 44,437 day 3 embryo transfers and found that poor-quality embryos resulted in fewer conceptions, irrespective of maternal age.[40]

Embryo-grading principles

Different clinics use different grading methods. The basic principles of grading are the same; these principles are:

- Embryos should have the correct number of blastomeres (cells) that correspond to the day of their development, and
- Embryos should have as little fragmentation as possible.

Developing cleavage-stage embryos should normally divide every 18–20 h. Slower or faster division may signify metabolic and/or chromosomal defects.[41]

Fragmentation is defined as 'splintering, and consists of particles of a blastomere that is falling apart'.[15] It is considered to be an essential parameter when scoring embryos.[41] The fragmentation of embryos is associated with their necrosis and apoptosis.[42]

The degree of fragmentation is classified into mild, moderate, and severe:[41]

- Mild: <10%
- Moderate: 10–25%
- Severe: >25%

In their review, Prados et al. concluded that severe fragmentation is associated with implantation failure, reduced blastocyst formation, and reduced pregnancy rates. A minor amount of fragmentation may have no negative influence.[41]

Cleavage-stage embryo scoring systems

Several scoring systems exist, and different clinics adopt different systems. At a 2010 workshop in Istanbul, members reached a consensus on embryo grading. It is expected that this grading system will be adopted by most IVF laboratories worldwide.

The Istanbul consensus workshop established the following schedule for optimal cleavage rates:[43]

- Day 2 (44 ± 1 h): four cells
- Day 3 (68 ± 1 h): eight cells

Prados et al. concluded that transfers of embryos on day 2 with four cells and day 3 embryos with eight cells result in better implantation rates and fewer miscarriages. If the first division happens before 26 ± 1 h in ICSI and by 28 ± 1 h in IVF, better numbers and quality of blastocysts and higher pregnancy rates result.[41] Another parameter related to cell division is that regularly shaped blastomeres (cells) also result in increased pregnancy outcome.[41]

Table 6.3 Istanbul consensus on a scoring system for cleavage-stage embryos (in addition to cell numbers)[43]

Grade	Rating	Description
1	Good	• <20% fragmentation • Stage-specific cell size • No multinucleation
2	Fair	• 10–25% fragmentation • Stage-specific cell size for majority of cells • No evidence of multinucleation
3	Poor	• Severe fragmentation (>25%) • Cell size not stage specific • Evidence of multinucleation

Alpha Scientists in Reproductive Medicine and ESHRE Special Interest Group of Embryology. The Istanbul consensus workshop on embryo assessment: proceedings of an expert meeting. Human Reproduction 2011;26(6):1270–83, by permission of Oxford University Press and ESHRE.

In addition to cell division, embryos are assessed for fragmentation and other factors; this is shown in Table 6.3.

Figures 6.3 and 6.4 show good-quality and poor-quality embryos on days 2 and 3, respectively.

Blastocyst scoring systems

Grading of embryos at the blastocyst stage is based on the morphology of the inner cell mass, trophectoderm, degree of expansion of the blastocyst cavity, and hatching status.[43]

A similar consensus was reached by the 2010 workshop in Istanbul for cleavage-stage embryo scoring. It was agreed that embryos should be assessed on day 4 at the morula stage (Table 6.4) and on day 5 (Table 6.5).

Implications for acupuncturists

Most fertility patients like to know about the grade of their embryo(s). Acupuncturists benefit from this information, too. Knowing the grading can help in auditing the results of acupuncture treatment. For example, if, in previous ART cycles without acupuncture, a patient produced fewer and lower-grade embryos, yet in the cycle with acupuncture better-quality embryos developed, this should be considered a successful acupuncture treatment outcome even if a subsequent pregnancy test is negative.

Assessments have their limits, and lower-grade embryos can implant and result in pregnancies. Acupuncturists interested in embryology can liaise with the embryologist at the patient's ART unit. Once appropriate consent issues are resolved, the embryologist should be able to advise about specific details of a particular patient's embryos. The development of embryos can change quickly, and embryos that initially may be slow to develop may eventually become top-quality embryos.

ADVANCED ART TECHNIQUES

Over the last 35 years, many new adjunctive techniques have been developed to further increase the chances of successful conception.

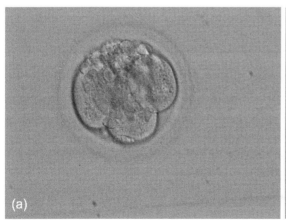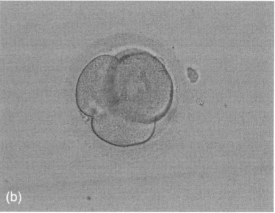

Figure 6.3 Day 2 embryos: (a) poor quality and (b) good quality.
Courtesy of Care Fertility, Nottingham, UK

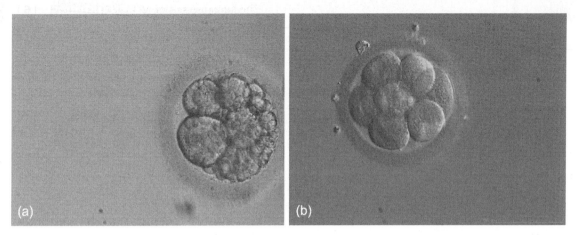

Figure 6.4 Day 3 embryos: (a) poor quality and (b) good quality.
Courtesy of Care Fertility, Nottingham, UK

Table 6.4 Istanbul consensus on scoring system for day 4 embryos[43]		
Grade	**Rating**	**Description**
1	Good	• Entered into a fourth round of cleavage • Evidence of compaction that involves virtually all the embryo volume
2	Fair	• Entered into a fourth round of cleavage • Compaction involves the majority of the volume of the embryo
3	Poor	• Disproportionate compaction involving less than half of the embryo, with two or three cells remaining as discrete blastomeres

Alpha Scientists in Reproductive Medicine and ESHRE Special Interest Group of Embryology. The Istanbul consensus workshop on embryo assessment: proceedings of an expert meeting. Human Reproduction 2011;26(6):1270-83, by permission of Oxford University Press and ESHRE.

Table 6.5 Istanbul consensus on scoring system for blastocysts[43]			
	Grade	**Rating**	**Description**
Stage of development	1		Early
	2		Blastocyst
	3		Expanded
	4		Hatched/hatching
ICM (inner cell mass)	1	Good	Prominent, easily discernible, with many cells that are compacted and tightly adhered together
	2	Fair	Easily discernible, with many cells that are loosely grouped together
	3	Poor	Difficult to discern, with few cells
TE (trophectoderm)	1	Good	Many cells forming a cohesive epithelium
	2	Fair	Few cells forming a loose epithelium
	3	Poor	Very few cells

Alpha Scientists in Reproductive Medicine and ESHRE Special Interest Group of Embryology. The Istanbul Consensus Workshop on Embryo Assessment: Proceedings of an Expert Meeting. Human Reproduction 2011;26(6):1270-83, by permission of Oxford University Press and ESHRE.

Assisted hatching

On day 6 or 7 postfertilization[44] or 72 h after the embryo enters the uterus,[45] it continually expands and contracts and eventually breaks through the zona pellucida (its shell). This process is called *embryo hatching* and is sometimes referred to as the 'first birth'. The embryo is then ready to implant. One of the possible causes of failed IVF treatment is the embryo's failure to hatch. In Assisted Hatching (AH), on day 3, the zona is partially dissected; it is drilled using acidified Tyrode's solution or piezo technology or thinned using laser technology.[46]

Evidence about the effectiveness of AH is mixed. The UK's National Institute for Health and Clinical Excellence 2013 guidelines do not recommend AH.[47] A 2012 Cochrane review of 31 studies (1992 clinical pregnancies out of 5728) concluded that AH offers a significantly increased chance of clinical pregnancy; however, in the studies that reported live birth rates, results were not significant.[48]

The American Society for Reproductive Medicine does not recommend routine AH.[49] However, it acknowledges that AH may be suitable in cases of:[49]

- Two or more failed IVF cycles
- Poor embryo quality
- Older women ($\geq$38 years of age)

Risk factors associated with AH include possible damage to the embryo, contamination with foreign material during AH, and chemical exposure.[49]

Specialist sperm retrieval methods

When a man produces no sperm on ejaculation, it might be possible to obtain spermatozoa from the epididymis using Percutaneous Epididymal Sperm Aspiration (PESA) or from the testes using Testicular Sperm Extraction (TESE) methods.

In PESA, a needle is inserted into the epididymis and the contents are aspirated. TESE involves cutting the testicular skin and extracting samples of the testes. Any extracted material is checked for spermatozoa. If found, spermatozoa are then frozen to be used in IVF, usually using the ICSI fertilization technique (see the section 'Intracytoplasmic Sperm Injection').[50] Variations on PESA/TESE have been developed, but it is not clear which technique is more effective.[51] Figure 6.5 shows indications for each technique.

ICSI

In conventional IVF, fertilization is achieved by placing eggs in a Petri dish with 50,000–100,000 sperm. Intracytoplasmic Sperm Injection (ICSI) is a fertilization technique in which an egg is fertilized by injecting a single seemingly intact sperm into the egg (Figure 6.6).[14,52]

With ICSI, fertilization can be achieved regardless of sperm concentration, motility, or morphology.[53] ICSI was first introduced in 1992,[54] and it is now the most commonly used method of egg fertilization *in vitro*. It is performed in 66% of ART cycles in the United States and Europe.[16,17]

ICSI is indicated in most types of male factor infertility.[52,54] Increasingly, ICSI is being used to treat infertility caused by other problems, but the evidence is mixed (see Table 6.6).

IMSI

Intracytoplasmic Morphologically Selected Injection (IMSI) is a fertilization method in which spermatozoa are selected using Motile Sperm Organelles Morphology Examination

Figure 6.5 PESA/TESE indications.[50]

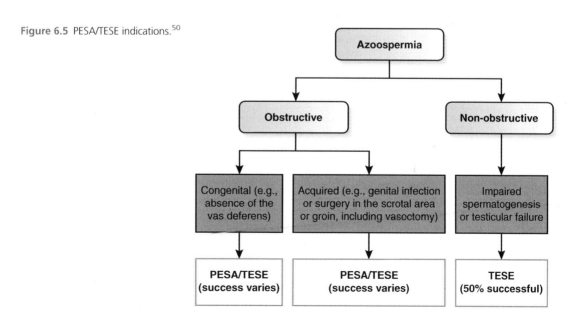

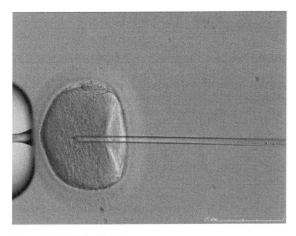

Figure 6.6 ICSI fertilization.
Courtesy of Care Fertility, Nottingham, UK

(MSOME) (see Chapter 4 for further information on MSOME).[57] In one study, 64.8% of spermatozoa, which were classed as normal for ICSI purposes, were classed as abnormal when examined for IMSI.[58]

IMSI appears to make no difference to implantation, pregnancy, or live birth rates in patients who undergo a first round of treatment,[59] but it has been shown to increase pregnancy and live birth rates almost threefold in patients who previously failed to conceive with ICSI.[57] As yet, there are no specific indications for IMSI.[60]

THE ROLE OF ACUPUNCTURE IN ART

Physiological effects of acupuncture in reproductive medicine and fertility

The following effects of acupuncture have been proposed:

- Modulating endocrine[61] and neuroendocrine factors[61–63]
- Increasing blood flow to the uterus and ovaries[62,63]
- Modulating cytokines[62]
- Modulating endogenous regulatory systems, including the sympathetic nervous system[61]
- Reducing stress, anxiety, and depression[62,63]

A 2007 Cochrane review paper summarized the physiological function of acupuncture as follows: 'Acupuncture has

Table 6.6 Indications for ICSI and the evidence for each indication

Indications[54]	Comments	Evidence
Male factor subfertility	Only a single sperm is required in order to fertilize the egg. Therefore, even severe male factor cases can be treated[54]	High
Unexplained subfertility	Unknown fertilization barriers may be overcome by ICSI[54]	Low
Poor-quality eggs	Poor-quality eggs may be more difficult for sperm to penetrate. ICSI bypasses this by injecting sperm directly into an egg	Not known
Low number of retrieved eggs	Poor fertilization rate or total fertilization failure is more likely to happen if the number of available eggs is low. Some experts believe that ICSI may help to increase the fertilization rate and therefore the number of embryos[54]	Low
Advanced maternal age	Eggs from older women are theorized to have structural defects, which ICSI is thought to overcome[54]	Not known
History of fertilization failure with conventional IVF	Patients who have a history of total fertilization failure are at a higher risk of future failure.[55] Using ICSI instead of conventional IVF may help to reduce the risk of total fertilization failure[54]	High
Routine use	Some believe that all infertility patients, irrespective of aetiology, would benefit from ICSI. However, evidence of routine use of ICSI is currently weak[56]	Low
In Pre-implantation Genetic Testing (PGT)	ICSI may be justifiable to avoid contamination from extraneous sperm attached to the zona pellucida[54]	High
In IVM	Eggs matured *in vitro* (known as IVM) are believed to potentially have features that may make them difficult for sperm to fertilize (for example, a faulty zona pellucida). ICSI is thought to overcome this problem[54]	Low
In frozen eggs	Eggs that have been previously cryopreserved will have had the cells that surround them (cumulus cells) stripped. This can compromise the eggs' potential for fertilization using conventional methods[54]	Not known

been shown to alter plasma beta-endorphin levels which in turn can affect the hypothalamic–pituitary–adrenal (HPA) axis by altering the release of hypothalamic GnRH and pituitary gonadotrophin secretion'.[64]

Role of acupuncture at key stages of ART

In the authors' experience, acupuncture treatment helps at every stage of the ART treatment process.

Preparation phase (3–6 months before the ART/IVF treatment cycle begins)

As described in Chapter 2, ovarian follicles take around 360 days to develop from their dormant stage to the ovulatory stage. During the preparation phase, acupuncture may improve the follicular development by increasing the blood flow to the ovaries, especially if regular acupuncture is administered in the 190 days prior to ovulation/egg retrieval.

The preparatory phase is also a very important time for any lifestyle modifications to be adopted by patients. Acupuncturists are often the only easily accessible source of reliable evidence-based information on what patients can do to increase their chances of conception (see Chapter 7 for further details).

During this 3- to 6-month preparation stage, acupuncture treatment can help to reduce the severity of pre-existing conditions known to negatively impact ART treatment, for example, PCOS,[63] endometriosis,[63] or male factor infertility[65] (see Chapter 8 for further details).

Pretreatment phase (up to 3 weeks before the ART/IVF treatment cycle)

During the pretreatment phase (often referred to as down-regulation), acupuncture can help to reduce a woman's stress levels and relieve some of the side effects of medication. In our opinion, it may also help to recruit more follicles for the treatment cycle.

The ART/IVF treatment cycle: Ovarian stimulation phase

This is the time when women inject a high dose of FSH in order to produce more than one egg. We believe acupuncture may help to enhance the ovarian response to medication.

Acupuncture can also help with endometrial lining development during this phase.[66–68]

The ART/IVF treatment cycle: Ovulation trigger and final egg maturation

When women inject the 'trigger' medication, this forces the follicles to grow further and the eggs within them to mature. In the authors' experience, administering acupuncture treatment between the trigger injection and the egg retrieval procedure helps with the final egg maturation, and, therefore, more mature eggs can potentially be retrieved. This has been noted by other authors.[63]

The ART/IVF treatment cycle: Egg retrieval

Research suggests that acupuncture can be used as an effective pain-relieving method during the egg retrieval procedure.[69–71] However, in our experience, this may be difficult to achieve as many ART clinics prefer to use other 'conventional' methods of pain relief.

The ART/IVF treatment cycle: Embryo transfer

There are numerous studies that show that acupuncture treatment around the time of embryo transfer helps to increase success rates of IVF although there are also studies that do not demonstrate this effect. In the authors' opinion, administering acupuncture only at the time of embryo transfer (as is done in majority of studies) fails to maximize the effect of acupuncture at other phases of IVF treatment. The section on embryo transfer in Chapter 9 explores this topic further.

The ART/IVF treatment cycle: Luteal phase and early pregnancy

Stress levels are probably at their highest in patients during the luteal phase (the dreaded '2-week wait'). Therefore, acupuncture and emotional support are extremely important during this stage. In addition, in our experience, using pregnancy-supporting acupuncture points helps to prevent miscarriage.

The role of fertility acupuncturists

The main role of fertility acupuncturists is to treat patients in preparation for, during, and after ART treatment. However, in contemporary subfertility acupuncture practise, patients expect more from their acupuncturists.

Advisory role

Helping patients understand their condition or test results or walking them through every aspect of the arduous ART treatment journey has become an integral part of the contemporary fertility acupuncturists' role.[63]

Patients expect their acupuncturists to provide up-to-date advice on factors that could influence the treatment outcome, such as nutrition or exercise.[63]

Emotional support

As discussed in Chapter 7, fertility patients are under immense pressure and experience high stress levels during ART treatment. Acupuncturists can help to reduce patients' stress levels by offering emotional support, not just through treatment but also through appropriate reassurances and explanations.[63]

Helping patients come to terms with failed treatments is one of the less enjoyable, but extremely important, roles acupuncturists have.

Referral

Fertility acupuncturists are expected to identify dangerous red flag signs and symptoms and refer patients to other practitioners when appropriate. They may also need to refer patients for further opinions or for additional investigations.

Prevention

Fertility acupuncturists should anticipate which possible barriers each individual patient may experience in trying to have a baby and take prophylactic action to reduce the impact of these barriers (see Chapter 10).

FUTURE ADVANCES IN ART: A POTENTIAL ROLE FOR ACUPUNCTURE?

Reproductive ageing and fertility preservation

There is a lot of interest in how to preserve or extend reproductive lifespan in women. Some believe that the reproductive lifespan depends on the innate number of follicles while others think that it is the rate of follicular atresia that is ultimately responsible for the duration of reproductive age.[72] Currently, researchers are focusing on slowing down the rate of atresia. Does regular acupuncture treatment have any potential to help to slow down the rate of follicular atresia and thus extend the reproductive lifespan? If so, by what underlying mechanisms?

Another major development in ART is the improvement in ovarian tissue and egg freezing techniques. Freezing eggs is no longer classed as an experimental treatment.[73] A meta-analysis showed that vitrified eggs result in the same fertilization and ongoing pregnancy rates as fresh eggs.[74] There is no evidence that babies born from previously frozen eggs are at higher risk of abnormalities although more research is necessary.[73] However, the ability of these preserved eggs to be fertilized and produce a viable embryo depends on their quality at the time of freezing and on the age of the woman when the eggs are retrieved, with greater chances of success in women <36 years old.[75]

The ethics of freezing eggs for social purposes (for example to delay parenthood) are extensively debated. In our experience, women who decide to freeze their eggs for fertility preservation may benefit from acupuncture to help them produce more and/or better quality eggs.

Case study

Egg Freezing for Fertility Preservation Reasons

Melanie was 38 years old when her relationship with her long-term partner ended. She decided to undergo an egg freezing procedure as a 'backup', in case her fertility had significantly declined by the time she was in a new relationship.

Melanie presented for acupuncture treatment to improve her response to ovarian simulation and help her cope emotionally with the procedure.

Her hormone profile was very good for someone of her age:

♦ FSH = 9 IU/L

♦ LH = 6 IU/L

♦ Oestrogen = 171 pmol/L

♦ AMH = 14.7 pmol/L

TCM Diagnosis

♦ *Kidney Yang Deficiency*: disliked cold, copious frequent urination, can be lethargic, lower back pain, weak pulse, especially on the third right position.

♦ *Liver Blood Stasis*: poor circulation (cold hands and feet), menstrual cramping requiring medication, clotted menstruation.

♦ *Some signs of Heat*: redness to the neck, red tongue, especially the tip, short menstrual cycles (26 days), tendency to anxiety.

Basic Acupuncture Points Prescription

SP4 + P6, KID7, KID3, LIV2, ST29, SP8, SP10

Melanie received 12 acupuncture treatments during the preparation phase, when she was also advised about lifestyle factors that would help to improve the treatment outcome. She also had acupuncture treatment during the ovarian stimulation phase. Melanie had 21 follicles from which 17 eggs were retrieved; 13 were suitable for freezing. This was a much better response than her clinic had expected.

Mitochondria replacement techniques

Mitochondria replacement techniques are very controversial, and ethics and safety are major concerns. The DNA replacement technique available includes 'spindle transfer' and pronuclear transfer (the nucleus from the diseased egg is transferred into a denucleated healthy egg). Another technique, known as 'nuclear genome transfer', has been recently reported.[76] These procedures are relatively new, and some are not even approved for day-to-day clinical use. It remains to be seen if acupuncture can enhance the effectiveness of these treatments.

SUMMARY

The role of fertility acupuncturists has evolved. In addition to providing acupuncture treatment, patients expect their acupuncturist to understand and advise about:

- Various ART treatments, their indications, and success rates
- Specialist techniques and why they are used
- Pharmaceutical drugs, their actions, and side effects
- Significance and interpretation of embryo grading

REFERENCES

1. National Collaborating Centre for Women's and Children's Health, Commissioned by the National Institute for Health and Clinical Excellence. Introduction. In: Fertility: assessment and treatment for people with fertility problems. NICE clinical guideline. 2nd ed. London: The Royal College of Obstetricians and Gynaecologists; 2013. p. 47–9 [chapter 2].

2. Wilkes S, Chinn DJ, Murdoch A, et al. Epidemiology and management of infertility: a population-based study in UK primary care. Fam Pract 2009;26:269–74.

3. Hull MG, Glazener CM, Kelly NJ, et al. Population study of causes, treatment, and outcome of infertility. Br Med J (Clin Res Ed) 1985;291:1693–7.

4. Broekmans F. The initial fertility assessment: a medical check-up of the couple experiencing difficulties conceiving. In: de Haan N, Spelt M, Gobel R, editors. Reproductive medicine: a textbook for paramedics. Amsterdam: Elsevier Gezondheidszorg; 2010. p. 21–39 [chapter 1].

5. Park SJ, Alvarez JR, Weiss G, et al. Ovulatory status and follicular response predict success of clomiphene citrate-intrauterine insemination. Fertil Steril 2007;87:1102–7.

6. Lucchini C, Volpe E, Tocci A. Comparison of intrafollicular sperm injection and intrauterine insemination in the treatment of subfertility. J Assist Reprod Genet 2012;29:1103–9.

7. Tonguc E, Var T, Onalan G, et al. Comparison of the effectiveness of single versus double intrauterine insemination with three different timing regimens. Fertil Steril 2010;94:1267–70.

8. ASRM patient fact sheet: Intrauterine insemination (IUI). Available from: http://www.reproductivefacts.org/intrauterine_insemination_IUI/; 2013 [accessed 27 June 2013].

9. Kosterman M. Intrauterine insemination. In: de Haan N, Spelt M, Gobel R, editors. Reproductive medicine: a textbook for paramedics. Amsterdam: Elsevier Gezondheidszorg; 2010. p. 101–4 [chapter 7].

10. Zadehmodarres S, Oladi B, Saeedi S, et al. Intrauterine insemination with husband semen: an evaluation of pregnancy rate and factors affecting outcome. J Assist Reprod Genet 2009;26:7–11.

11. Dmowki WP, Pry M, Ding J, et al. Cycle-specific and cumulative fecundity in patients with endometriosis who are undergoing controlled ovarian hyperstimulation-intrauterine insemination or in vitro fertilization-embryo transfer. Fertil Steril 2002;78:750–6.

12. Werbrouck E, Spiessens C, Meuleman C, et al. No difference in cycle pregnancy rate and in cumulative live-birth rate between women with surgically treated minimal to mild endometriosis and women with unexplained infertility after controlled ovarian hyperstimulation and intrauterine insemination. Fertil Steril 2006;86:566–71.

13. ESHRE Capri Workshop Group. Intrauterine insemination. Hum Reprod Update 2009;15:265–77.

14. Assisted Reproductive Technology (ART) – glossary. Available from: http://www.eshre.eu/ESHRE/English/Guidelines-Legal/ART-glossary/page.aspx/1062; 2013 [accessed 26 January 2013].

15. Blok L, Kremer J. In vitro fertilisation and intracytoplasmic sperm injection. In: de Haan N, Spelt M, Gobel R, editors. Reproductive medicine: a textbook for paramedics. Amsterdam: Elsevier Gezondheidszorg; 2010. p. 105–26 [chapter 8].

16. Centres for disease control and prevention, American society for reproductive medicine, society for assisted reproductive technology 2012 assisted reproductive technology national summary report. Report of the centres for disease control and prevention, American society for reproductive medicine, society for assisted reproductive technology. Atlanta: US department of health and human services; 2010.

17. de Mouzon J, Goossens V, Bhattacharya S, et al. Assisted reproductive technology in Europe, 2006: results generated from European registers by ESHRE. Hum Reprod 2010;25:1851–62.

18. Sullivan EA, Zegers-Hochschild F, Mansour R, et al. International committee for monitoring assisted reproductive technologies (ICMART) world report: assisted reproductive technology 2004. Hum Reprod 2013;28:1375–90.

19. Verit FF, Verit A. How effective is in vitro fertilization, and how can it be improved? Fertil Steril 2011;95:1677–83.

20. Trounson A, Mohr L. Human pregnancy following cryopreservation, thawing and transfer of an eight-cell embryo. Nature 1983;305:707–9.

21. Ghobara T, Vandekerckhove P. Cycle regimens for frozen-thawed embryo transfer. Cochrane Database Syst Rev 2008;23:CD003414.

22. Le Du A, Kadoch IJ, Bourcigaux N, et al. In vitro oocyte maturation for the treatment of infertility associated

with polycystic ovarian syndrome: the French experience. Hum Reprod 2005;20:420–4.

23. Grynberg M, El Hachem H, de Bantel A, et al. In vitro maturation of oocytes: uncommon indications. Fertil Steril 2013;99:1182–8.

24. The Practice Committees of the American Society for Reproductive Medicine and the Society for Assisted Reproductive Technology. In vitro maturation: a committee opinion. Fertil Steril 2013;99:663–6.

25. ASRM. Assisted reproductive technologies. A guide for patients. Report of the ASRM. Birmingham, Alabama: ASRM; 2008.

26. Friel KS, Penzias AS. Intratubal gamete transfer. In: Collins RL, Seifer DB, editors. Office-based infertility practice. London: Springer; 2012. p. 184–94 [chapter 18].

27. American Society for Reproductive Medicine. Assisted reproductive technology in the United States: 2001 results generated from the American society for reproductive medicine/ society for assisted reproductive technology registry. Fertil Steril 2007;87:1253–66.

28. ASRM. Medication for inducing ovulation. A guide for patients. Report of the ASRM. Birmingham, Alabama: ASRM; 2012.

29. Shefer A, Sela K. The Chinese energetics on clomiphene citrate – an introduction to "pharmakoenergetics". Available from: http://medigogy.com/ archives/chinese-energetics-clomiphene-citrate-introduction-pharmakoenergetics; 2011 [accessed 13 July 2011].

30. MD024: Female Infertility Pharmacotherapy-Stimulation Protocols. ASRM elearning course notes; Birmingham, Alabama: ASRM; 2010.

31. Practice Committee of American Society for Reproductive Medicine in collaboration with Society for Reproductive Endocrinology and Infertility. Progesterone supplementation during the luteal phase and in early pregnancy in the treatment of infertility: an educational bulletin. Fertil Steril 2008;90:S150–3.

32. Gelbaya TA, Kyrgiou M, Tsoumpou I, et al. The use of estradiol for luteal phase support in in vitro fertilization/intracytoplasmic sperm injection cycles: a systematic review and meta-analysis. Fertil Steril 2008;90:2116–25.

33. van der Linden M, Buckingham K, Farquhar C, et al. Luteal phase support in assisted reproduction cycles. Hum Reprod Update 2012;18:473.

34. McNamee K, Dawood F, Farquharson R. Recurrent miscarriage and thrombophilia: an update. Curr Opin Obstet Gynecol 2012;24:229–34.

35. Urman B, Ata B, Yakin K, et al. Luteal phase empirical low molecular weight heparin administration in patients with failed ICSI embryo transfer cycles: a randomized open-labeled pilot trial. Hum Reprod 2009;24:1640–7.

36. Essah PA, Arrowood JA, Cheang KI, et al. Effect of combined metformin and oral contraceptive therapy on metabolic factors and endothelial function in overweight and obese women with polycystic ovary syndrome. Fertil Steril 2011;96:501. e2–504.e2.

37. Griesinger G, Venetis CA, Marx T, et al. Oral contraceptive pill pretreatment in ovarian stimulation with GnRH antagonists for IVF: a systematic review and meta-analysis. Fertil Steril 2008;90:1055–63.

38. Terriou P, Sapin C, Giorgetti C, et al. Embryo score is a better predictor of pregnancy than the number of transferred embryos or female age. Fertil Steril 2001;75:525–31.

39. Hsu A, Arny M, Knee AB, et al. Antral follicle count in clinical practice: analyzing clinical relevance. Fertil Steril 2011;95:474–9.

40. Vernon M, Stern JE, Ball GD, et al. Utility of the national embryo morphology data collection by the society for assisted reproductive technologies (SART): correlation between day-3 morphology grade and live-birth outcome. Fertil Steril 2011;95:2761–3.

41. Prados FJ, Debrock S, Lemmen JG, et al. The cleavage stage embryo. Hum Reprod 2012;27(Suppl. 1):i50–71.

42. Chi HJ, Koo JJ, Choi SY, et al. Fragmentation of embryos is associated with both necrosis and apoptosis. Fertil Steril 2011;96:187–92.

43. Alpha Scientists in Reproductive Medicine and ESHRE Special Interest Group of Embryology. The Istanbul consensus workshop on embryo assessment: proceedings of an expert meeting. Hum Reprod 2011;26:1270–83.

44. Weima S. Embryology. In: de Haan N, Spelt M, Gobel R, editors. Reproductive medicine: a textbook for paramedics. Amsterdam: Elsevier Gezondheidszorg; 2010. p. 79–92 [chapter 5].

45. Norwitz ER, Schust DJ, Fisher SJ. Implantation and the survival of early pregnancy. N Engl J Med 2001;345:1400–8.

46. Hammadeh ME, Fischer-Hammadeh C, Ali KR. Assisted hatching in assisted reproduction: a state of the art. J Assist Reprod Genet 2011;28:119–28.

47. National Collaborating Centre for Women's and Children's Health, Commissioned by the National Institute for Health and Clinical Excellence. Procedures used during in vitro fertilisation treatment. Fertility: assessment and treatment for people with fertility problems. NICE clinical guideline. 2nd ed. London: The Royal College of Obstetricians and Gynaecologists; 2013. p. 267–382 [chapter 15].

48. Carney S-K, Das S, Blake D, et al. Assisted hatching on assisted conception (in vitro fertilisation (IVF) and intracytoplasmic sperm injection (ICSI)). Cochrane Database Syst Rev 2012;12. Available from: http://dx.doi.org/10.1002/ 14651858.CD001894.pub5.

49. Practice Committee of American Society for Reproductive Medicine. The role of assisted hatching in in vitro fertilization: a review of the literature. A committee opinion. Fertil Steril 2008;90:S196–S198.

50. Kastrop P. Laboratory aspects of male infertility. In: de Haan N, Spelt M, Gobel R, editors. Reproductive medicine: a textbook for paramedics. Amsterdam: Elsevier Gezondheidszorg; 2010. p. 57–72 [chapter 3].

51. Esteves SC, Miyaoka R, Agarwal A. Sperm retrieval techniques for

assisted reproduction. Int Braz J Urol 2011;37:570–83.

52. Oehninger S. Clinical management of male infertility in assisted reproduction: ICSI and beyond. Int J Androl 2011;34:1–11.

53. Mahutte NG, Arici A. Failed fertilization: is it predictable? Curr Opin Obstet Gynecol 2003;15:211–8.

54. The Practice Committees of the American Society for Reproductive Medicine and Society for Assisted Reproductive Technology. Intracytoplasmic sperm injection (ICSI) for non-male factor infertility: a committee opinion. Fertil Steril 2012;98:1395–9.

55. Barlow PP, Englert YY, Puissant FF, et al. Fertilization failure in IVF: why and what next? Hum Reprod 1990;5:451–6.

56. Bhattacharya S, Hamilton MP, Shaaban M, et al. Conventional in-vitro fertilisation versus intracytoplasmic sperm injection for the treatment of non-male-factor infertility: a randomised controlled trial. Lancet 2001;357:2075–9.

57. Klement AH, Koren-Morag N, Itsykson P, et al. Intracytoplasmic morphologically selected sperm injection versus intracytoplasmic sperm injection: a step toward a clinical algorithm. Fertil Steril 2013;99:1290–3.

58. Wilding M, Coppola G, di Matteo L, et al. Intracytoplasmic injection of morphologically selected spermatozoa (IMSI) improves outcome after assisted reproduction by deselecting physiologically poor quality spermatozoa. J Assist Reprod Genet 2011;28:253–62.

59. Leandri RD, Gachet A, Pfeffer J, et al. Is intracytoplasmic morphologically selected sperm injection (IMSI) beneficial in the first ART cycle? A multicentric randomized controlled trial. Andrology 2013;1:1–6.

60. Setti AS, de Braga DPAF, Iaconelli A, et al. Twelve years of MSOME and IMSI: a review. Reprod Biomed Online 2013;27:338–52.

61. Stener-Victorin E, Wu X. Effects and mechanisms of acupuncture in the reproductive system. Auton Neurosci 2010;157:46–51.

62. Anderson BJ, Haimovici F, Ginsburg ES, et al. In vitro fertilization and acupuncture: clinical efficacy and mechanistic basis. Altern Ther Health Med 2007;13:38–48.

63. Anderson B, Rosenthal L. Acupuncture and in vitro fertilization: critique of the evidence and application to clinical practice. Complement Ther Clin Pract 2013;19:1–5.

64. Cheong YC, Hung Yu Ng E, Ledger WL. Acupuncture and assisted conception. Cochrane Database Syst Rev 2008;8:CD006920.

65. Huang DM, Huang GY, Lu FE, et al. Acupuncture for infertility: is it an effective therapy? Chin J Integr Med 2011;17:386–95.

66. Ho M, Huang LC, Chang YY, et al. Electroacupuncture reduces uterine artery blood flow impedance in infertile women. Taiwan J Obstet Gynecol 2009;48:148–51.

67. Stener-Victorin E, Waldenström U, Andersson SA, et al. Reduction of blood flow impedance in the uterine arteries of infertile women with electro-acupuncture. Hum Reprod 1996;11:1314–7.

68. Isoyama Manca di Villahermosa D, Dos Santos LG, Nogueira MB, et al. Influence of acupuncture on the outcomes of in vitro fertilisation when embryo implantation has failed: a prospective randomised controlled clinical trial. Acupunct Med 2013;31:157–61.

69. Humaidan P, Stener-Victorin E. Pain relief during oocyte retrieval with a new short duration electro-acupuncture technique – an alternative to conventional analgesic methods. Hum Reprod 2004;19:1367–72.

70. Sator-Katzenschlager SM, Wölfler MM, Kozek-Langenecker SA, et al. Auricular electro-acupuncture as an additional perioperative analgesic method during oocyte aspiration in IVF treatment. Hum Reprod 2006;21:2114–20.

71. Humaidan P, Brock K, Bungum L, et al. Pain relief during oocyte retrieval – exploring the role of different frequencies of electro-acupuncture. Reprod Biomed Online 2006;13:120–5.

72. Barnhart KT. Epidemiology of male and female reproductive disorders and impact on fertility regulation and population growth. Fertil Steril 2011;95:2200–3.

73. Society for Assisted Reproductive Technology. Mature oocyte cryopreservation: a guideline. Fertil Steril 2013;99:37–43.

74. Cobo A, Diaz C. Clinical application of oocyte vitrification: a systematic review and meta-analysis of randomized controlled trials. Fertil Steril 2011;96:277–85.

75. Cil AP, Bang H, Oktay K. Age-specific probability of live birth with oocyte cryopreservation: an individual patient data meta-analysis. Fertil Steril 2013;100, 492.e3–499.e3.

76. Paull D, Emmanuele V, Weiss KA, et al. Nuclear genome transfer in human oocytes eliminates mitochondrial DNA variants. Nature 2013;493:632–7.

Chapter | 7 |

Preconception care in preparation for ART

Patients with subfertility are possibly one of the most motivated groups of patients that acupuncturists are ever likely to treat. They are keen to do all they can to maximize their chances of conception. Patients with subfertility seek out information on anything that they consider will help them conceive and then diligently follow through on what they consider to be helpful.

However, the vast quantity of information (both good and bad) available to people trying to conceive can often become a burden to them. It is not unusual to have patients who initially present who take a handful of supplements several times a day, have a very restrictive diet, and generally put their lives on hold while undergoing Assisted Reproductive Technology (ART) treatment.

This chapter will provide fertility acupuncturists with a detailed evidence-based review of the most important lifestyle modifications, from both an Orthodox medical perspective as well as from a Traditional Chinese Medicine (TCM) perspective, that are beneficial to patients trying to conceive. Appendix IV provides factsheets on lifestyle factors that affect fertility.

WEIGHT

Maternal weight

Maternal weight and infertility

The American Society for Reproductive Medicine (ASRM) states that 12% 'of all infertility cases are a result of the woman either weighing too little or two much'.[1] The World Health Organization (WHO) classifies weight according to Body Mass Index (BMI). BMI is calculated by dividing weight by the square of the height in metres (kg/m^2) and is categorized as follows (BMI table provided in Appendix III):[2]

- BMI <18.50 = underweight
- BMI 18.50–24.99 = normal weight
- BMI 25.00–29.99 = overweight
- BMI ≥ 30.00 = obese

With obesity levels increasing, it has been estimated that up to 50% of women of reproductive age will be in the obese category in the near future.[3] The importance of excess weight as a factor in fertility was illustrated in a prospective survey of 2112 consecutive pregnant women, which found that a BMI of >25 kg/m^2 significantly increased the time to conception.[4]

Maternal weight and comorbidities

Obesity is associated with a number of comorbidities such as Polycystic Ovary Syndrome (PCOS), endometriosis, and fibroids, all of which are linked with subfertility.[3] Obesity is thought to disrupt the menstrual cycle, affect ovulation, and raise insulin levels, which in combination leads to increased ovarian androgen production and elevated circulating oestrogen levels.[5] High BMI has been associated with long menstrual cycles, with effects seen even in women with BMIs of 24–25 kg/m^2 and rising with each increase in BMI.[6]

Maternal weight and ART

Overweight women undergoing reproductive treatments require more gonadotrophin stimulation, have a poorer response rate, and produce fewer eggs.[5] Several recent reviews have found evidence that maternal obesity negatively affects the quality of eggs.[7–9] This is thought to be from a disruption of the maternal endocrine system, and also through a direct effect on the developing egg.[7]

A meta-analysis of 33 studies and 47,976 *In Vitro* Fertilization (IVF)/Intracytoplasmic Sperm Injection (ICSI) cycles found that a BMI ≥ 25 kg/m^2 resulted in significantly lower clinical pregnancy and live birth rates and significantly higher miscarriage rates.[10] Another analysis of 45,163 embryo transfers found that higher BMI was significantly associated with a reduced chance of clinical pregnancy and live birth in women using their own eggs but not in donor egg recipients.[11] An analysis of a smaller sample size of 4609 cycles of IVF or ICSI found that women with BMI ≥ 30 kg/m^2 had a significantly lower chance of implantation and clinical pregnancy and a 60% lower chance of a live birth.[12] The odds of an IVF cycle cancellation are also higher in women with a BMI ≥ 25 kg/m$^{2.13}$

Being underweight is also detrimental for fertility. A study of 2362 IVF embryo transfers found that a maternal BMI of <19 kg/m^2 resulted in significantly lower implantation rates compared to a BMI of 19–28 kg/m^2 (26% vs. 40%).[14] A smaller study of 465 IVF patients had similar findings, where maternal BMI ≤ 19.9 kg/m^2 was associated with significantly reduced pregnancy rates compared to BMIs of 20–27.9 kg/m^2 (34.8% vs. 52.3%).[15]

Maternal weight and miscarriages

For women, being over- or underweight is also linked to miscarriages. A study of 23,821 women found that BMI <18.5 and ≥ 25 kg/m^2 significantly increased the risk of miscarriage.[16] A meta-analysis of 16 studies concluded that maternal BMI ≥ 25 kg/m^2 significantly increased the risk of miscarriage, even in egg donation recipients.[17] Early pregnancy Human Chorionic Gonadotrophin (hCG) levels are also lower in obese women.[18] Obesity has also been linked with an increased risk of developing pregnancy complications, such as gestational diabetes, hypertension, and spontaneous abortions. Babies of obese mothers may be large for their gestational age, may have an open neural tube defect, or may have congenital heart disease.[19]

Paternal weight

Paternal weight and infertility

Male weight is also important for fertility. A 2012 systematic review and meta-analysis of 21 studies (involving a sample of 13,077 men) concluded that being overweight or obese significantly increased the risk of azoospermia (no sperm) or oligozoospermia (low sperm concentration).[20] An earlier meta-analysis of 31 studies did not find such associations, but this study's findings were limited as data from most studies could not be aggregated.[21]

Paternal weight and ART

A study of 12,566 couples and 25,191 IVF or ICSI cycles found that couples with both partners having a BMI ≥ 25 kg/m^2 or couples who had a combined average BMI ≥ 25 kg/m^2 had a significantly lower rate of live birth following IVF but not following ICSI.[22] A smaller study of 345 couples undergoing ART found a significant linear reduction in clinical pregnancy and live birth rates with increasing paternal BMI.[23]

Paternal weight and miscarriages

Increased paternal BMI is linked to pregnancy loss based on a study of 345 couples undergoing ART.[23]

Recommendation

Because excess weight is detrimental to fertility and the outcome of reproductive treatment, it is vital that both male and female patients maintain their weight within normal BMI (19–24 kg/m^2).[24]

Regular exercise (at least 30 min of moderately intense exercise a minimum of 3 days a week) and a low calorie diet (1000–1200 kcal/day) is recommended by authoritative bodies as a first-line treatment of obesity.[5,25] However, one study showed that men who attempted to lose weight while undergoing IVF–ICSI had reduced success rates.[26] So overweight patients should attempt weight loss before starting ART treatments.

Some patients may need to be referred to dieticians or weight management programmes to help them lose or gain weight prior to undergoing ART.

SMOKING

The effects of smoking on reproductive health

Research shows that smoking is consistently associated with subfertility.[27] A major review of the effect of smoking on the reproductive system found that smoking impairs every stage of the reproductive process.[28] A prospective survey of 2112 consecutive pregnant women showed that when either partner smoked more than 15 cigarettes a day, it significantly increased the time to conception.[4] Women who smoke have decreased follicular phase length.[6,29]

ASRM reviewed the effects of smoking on reproductive health and found that:[27]

- Smoking reduces female reproductive lifespan by 1–4 years
- Smoking increases the risk of ectopic pregnancies and miscarriages

- Smokers require almost twice as many IVF cycles as nonsmokers
- Smokers have poorer semen parameters

A meta-analysis of 21 studies concluded that smoking by women undergoing ART significantly lowered the odds of clinical pregnancy and live birth and increased the odds of ectopic pregnancy and spontaneous miscarriage.[30]

Smoking by male partners also significantly reduces fertilization rates[26] and success rates of IVF and ICSI.[26,31]

Exposure to second-hand smoke is detrimental to female fertility.[27]

There are significant risks of birth defects as a result of maternal smoking. Most of the baby's developing bodily systems can be malformed as a result of exposure to smoke.[32]

The TCM view of smoking

Smoking injures the Qi of the Lungs and Heart, both of which play an important role in conception. Smoking can weaken Jing (Essence) and may also cause Heat, which, in turn, may consume Yin (see Chapter 2).

Recommendation

From both the Orthodox medical and TCM perspectives, smoking causes damage to reproductive health. Therefore, both male and female patients should be encouraged to give up smoking while attempting to conceive. According to ASRM, the negative effects of smoking are reversed after smoking cessation.[27] The latest National Institute of Clinical Excellence (NICE) guidelines recommend that both men and women should stop smoking while attempting to conceive.[33]

Understanding the ART patient's lifetime history of exposure to cigarette smoke should help the fertility acupuncturist appreciate what impact there may have been upon the patient's Jing (Essence), Lungs, and Heart and the extent to which acupuncture treatment principles may need to be modified accordingly.

ALCOHOL

The effects of alcohol on reproductive health

A prospective study of 7393 women reported that drinking 2 units of alcohol per day significantly increased the risk of infertility.[34]

Another study of 7760 healthy women found that infertility was not associated with alcohol intake in younger women. However, in women older than 30, the risk of infertility was higher in women who consumed seven or more drinks per week compared to those who consumed fewer than one.[35]

Another study that followed 18,555 women without a known history of infertility for 8 years found that alcohol intake was not associated with infertility when it was caused by ovulatory disorders.[36]

A study involving 39,612 pregnant women also found there was no link between low, moderate, or high alcohol intake and how long it took to conceive. Interestingly, women who reported no alcohol intake took slightly longer to conceive compared to women who consumed 0.5–2 units of alcohol per week.[37]

Drinking alcohol has been shown to affect sperm morphology and sperm production. The effect is more pronounced with increased intake.[38] In a prospective survey of 2112 consecutive pregnant women, researchers found that if the male partner drank more than 20 units of alcohol a week, it significantly increased the couple's time to conception.[4]

Effects of alcohol on IVF outcome

Low levels of alcohol intake may reduce live birth rates following IVF. A prospective cohort study of 2545 couples and 4729 IVF cycles found that women who drank ≥4 units of alcohol per week while undergoing IVF reduced their odds of live birth by 16%.[39] The same study found that when each of the partners drank ≥4 units of alcohol per week, the likelihood of live birth was 21% lower compared to couples in which each partner drank <4 units of alcohol per week.[39]

The effect of alcohol on the risk of miscarriages

The alcohol intake of both male and female partners in the preconception period is linked to miscarriage. For example, in a study of 430 couples and 186 pregnancies, researchers found that both male and female alcohol intake of 10 or more drinks per week during the week of conception significantly increased the risk of early pregnancy loss.[40]

In a study of 330 women with spontaneous miscarriages and 1168 pregnant women, researchers found that consumption of ≥5 units of alcohol per week resulted in increased risk of miscarriages.[41] A larger study of 24,679 pregnant women also reported increased first trimester miscarriage in those women who consumed five or more alcoholic drinks per week.

Drinking even low amounts of alcohol during pregnancy increases the risk of spontaneous miscarriage before 16 weeks gestation, according to the findings of a very large study of 92,719 Danish women.[42]

The TCM view of alcohol

Alcohol is pungent, sweet, and hot in nature, may induce Heat or Fire, and can weaken Kidney Jing (Essence),[43] the Stomach, and Liver. Drinking alcohol may damage the embryo or foetus.[44] When planning a pregnancy, the couple is advised not to drink alcohol as it reduces fertility.[43,44]

However, in some cases, the occasional glass of wine may be advantageous because it invigorates Blood vessels, dispels External Pathogenic Factors (EPFs), reduces tension, and can eliminate Blood Stasis. Couples trying to conceive who choose to continue to have an occasional drink should:[43]

- Limit the intake
- Drink a small glass of wine with food
- Drink alcohol slowly
- Avoid sexual intercourse when drunk as this damages Jing (Essence)[45]

Recommendations

On the basis of the research available, the following recommendations can be made:

- There is very little evidence to suggest that a low intake of alcohol reduces chances of conception. However, moderate and high alcohol intake has been shown to affect both male and female reproductive health.
- NICE guidelines recommend that women attempting to conceive should drink no more than 1–2 units of alcohol one to two times per week, and men should limit their intake to 3–4 units per day.[46]
- NICE guidelines also recommend that people undergoing reproductive treatment (e.g., IVF) should not drink more than 1 unit of alcohol per day because it reduces the effectiveness of the treatment.[47]
- The ASRM recommends that couples trying to conceive do not exceed two drinks per day.[48]
- Alcohol intake during pregnancy should be avoided altogether because it affects foetal health and is also linked to miscarriages.

CAFFEINE

Effect on female fertility

Women who consume more than six cups of coffee and/or tea a day have been shown to have increased time to conception.[4] A review by Homan et al. found that there is some evidence linking caffeine consumption to miscarriages and stillbirths.[49] NICE guidelines state that maternal caffeine consumption reduces success rates of reproductive treatment (e.g., IVF) and, therefore, caffeine consumption should be discouraged.[33] However, the ASRM advises that 1–2 cups of caffeinated beverages a day before or during pregnancy is not detrimental to fertility or pregnancy.[48]

Effect on male fertility

A large meta-analysis concluded that there is no strong evidence that moderate caffeine intake by men significantly affects their fertility.[50]

RECREATIONAL DRUGS

Orthodox medicine

The use of recreational drugs is also strongly associated with subfertility in both men and women[19] and can increase the risk of infertility by 70%.[48]

TCM

Recreational drug use compromises fertility and reproductive potential by depleting Jing (Essence).

Recommendation

It is important to ask a patient if he or she is currently using or has previously used recreational drugs. Those who are still using recreational drugs should be encouraged to stop and referred to appropriate supporting services. Specialist referral may be necessary to help patients overcome their dependence. When planning fertility treatment for patients who used recreational drugs in the past, Jing (Essence) should be supported in order to improve their reproductive health.

MEDICATION

Female fertility

Certain prescription medications are known to affect follicular rupture and ovulation and cause impairment of tubal function, implantation, and sexual and luteal functions (see Appendix VI for common types of medication known to affect fertility).[19]

Women should also take care over what medications they take during pregnancy. For example, the use of nonaspirin nonsteroidal anti-inflammatory drugs or NSAIDs (diclofenac, naproxen, celecoxib, ibuprofen, and rofecoxib), even in small doses, during pregnancy is associated with an increased risk of miscarriage.[51]

Male fertility

Certain prescription and nonprescription medications may affect male reproductive functions (such as sperm production, ejaculation, and/or erectile difficulties) and produce changes in male hormone levels and libido.[19] See Appendix VI for common types of medications that are known to affect fertility.

The negative effects of medication may be reversed when the medication is discontinued or changed to a medication that does not affect semen parameters.[19,52]

Recommendation

All patients should be asked what prescription or nonprescription medication they take. Acupuncture practitioners may not always be aware of what medications could harm reproductive functions. Therefore, practitioners may need to seek specialist advice; for example, patients could ask their pharmacists or doctors to review their medications.

If a patient takes medication that is known to affect reproductive function, he or she should be asked to see the doctor who prescribed that medication in order to discuss possible substitution or discontinuation.

Red flag
Medication that affects reproduction
Acupuncturists must never tell patients to stop medications because we are not qualified to do so. Refer them back to their medical doctors for a review of their medications.

ENVIRONMENTAL AND OCCUPATIONAL FACTORS

Environmental factors

Pollution can affect fertility and reproductive processes at different stages and in different ways. Exposure to environmental contaminants can happen *in utero*, during childhood and adolescent developmental years (when the reproductive organs grow and mature), and also in adulthood. Certain environmental hazards are linked to sperm issues, menstrual cycle irregularities, hormonal changes, miscarriages, foetal loss, early menopause, malformations of the reproductive tract, endometriosis, fibroids, altered puberty, and other reproductive changes.[53]

Contaminants that have been linked to reproductive system changes include:[53]

- Air pollution (carbon monoxide, lead, ground-level ozone, particulate matter, nitrogen dioxide, and sulphur dioxide)
- Bisphenol A (used to line metal food and drink cans, plastic baby bottles, baby pacifiers, baby toys, certain microwavable and reusable food and drink containers, and other products)
- Disinfection by-products
- Ethylene oxide (sterilant used in dental and medical practices)

- Glycol ethers (used in paints, varnishes, thinners, printing inks, cosmetics, perfumes)
- Pesticides (includes insecticides, fungicides, herbicides, rodenticides, fumigants; exposure can arise from consuming affected food or water)
- Phthalates (can be found in cosmetics, perfumes, toys, pharmaceuticals, medical devices, lubricants, and wood finishers)
- Solvents (exposure occurs primarily through breathing contaminated air from many different sources, including detergents, drugs, glues, paints, fingernail polish, insulation, fibreglass, food containers, carpet backing, cleaning products, and others)
- Perfluorinated compounds (PFOS, PFOA) (accumulated in the environment and food chain; used in making fabrics and carpets stain resistant and water repellent and used in cooking pan coating, floor polish, and food wrap coating)
- Polybrominated diphenyl ethers (used to make detergents, pesticides, paints; exposure mainly through consuming water contaminated by sewage and wet-weather runoff)
- Chlorinated hydrocarbons such as dioxins/furans, polychlorinated biphenyls, organochlorine pesticides, pentachlorophenol (some are banned in the United States but remain in the environment, sometimes for decades)
- Metals such as lead, mercury, manganese, cadmium (found in various household products, paints, and in the food chain (in particular, mercury is found in seafood))

(Adapted from Ref. 53, with permission from Elsevier).

Men are possibly affected by exposure to environmental oestrogens, both at puberty and continually through their lives. Environmental oestrogen may have an effect on the Hypothalamic–Pituitary Axis and spermatogenesis.[3] However, the current evidence is primarily based on animal models, and further investigations are warranted.[54,55]

Situations that increase scrotal temperature (for example, sauna use,[56] sitting down for prolonged periods, hot baths, using a laptop computer placed on the lap) can alter sperm production and should be avoided.[33,57] There is no strong evidence that tight-fitting underwear reduces male fertility.[33,57]

Occupational factors

Some occupations have been linked to reduced fertility. Therefore, it is important to enquire into both partners' occupations.

Male occupations most strongly associated with subfertility include:[46]

- Welders, bakers, drivers, or any other occupations involving increase in scrotal temperature

- Radiotherapists (due to X-ray radiation)
- Engine drivers, diggers (due to vibrations)
- Agricultural workers (due to chemical exposure)
- Chemists, laboratory workers, and painters (due to solvent exposure)

Female occupations most strongly associated with subfertility include:[46]

- Hospital workers or any other occupations involving shift work, intense physical workload, and long working hours
- Nurses, pharmacists (due to exposure to mercury and cadmium)
- Anaesthetists, theatre nurses, and dental nurses (due to exposure to nitrous oxide)
- Woodworkers (due to exposure to formaldehyde)

Recommendation

Patients should be asked about their occupational, home, and community exposure to environmental hazards.[19] Some of these hazards are unavoidable, but the effects of others can be minimized or avoided. Advise patients about steps they can take to reduce the amount of their exposure. For example:

- House decoration and renovations should be delayed until after completion of reproductive treatment.
- The use of plastic containers and food wrapping and canned food should be minimized.
- Ideally, organically grown food should be eaten, and fruits and vegetables should be thoroughly washed to reduce exposure to pesticides.
- Whenever possible, natural cosmetics and cleaning products should be used.
- When preparing fish, trimming the fat, removing or puncturing the skin, and not frying it may help to reduce exposure to chemicals and metals.[58]
- Patients with occupational exposure should consider changing their job or take steps to reduce their exposure.

NUTRITION AND SUPPLEMENTATION

Nutritional imbalances and excessive or insufficient intake of certain nutrients can contribute to difficulties conceiving and/or miscarriages. Some nutrients are most essential in female and male fertility. However, acupuncturists should be careful about advising patients regarding their diet and supplements because this is considered to be an area outside of acupuncture professional competence.

Micronutrients and female fertility

Folic acid and vitamin B

Women attempting to conceive should take 0.4 mg/day of folic acid before conception and for up to 12 weeks postconception. A higher dose of 5 mg/day is recommended for women who have previously had a baby with a neural tube defect, women who take anti-epileptic medication, and women who are diabetic.[33] Women with Hyperhomocysteinaemia (elevated Homocysteine), commonly found in patients with the methyl tetrahydrofolate reductase gene mutation,[59] should also take a higher dose of folic acid together with vitamins B6 and B12.[60]

Both folic acid[61] and vitamin B12[61] supplementation may help to reduce the risk of ovulatory subfertility. Good sources of folic acid include dark green leafy vegetables, fruits, nuts, beans, peas, dairy, poultry, eggs, seafood, and grains.[62] The best sources of vitamin B12 are beef liver and clams, fish, meat, poultry, and dairy.[63]

Vitamin D

Vitamin D is a fat-soluble vitamin that is synthesized in the body. It comes mainly from exposure to sunlight and certain foods, such as fish-liver oils, oily fish, egg yolks, and mushrooms.[64–66] Exposing the skin of the face and forearms to the midday sun for 20-30 min produces about 2000 IU of vitamin D.[65]

Vitamin D reduces inflammation, plays a role in cell differentiation and immune function, and is important for proper foetal development.[67] Research suggests that low levels of vitamin D are prevalent in women of childbearing age in the United States,[68] and it is estimated that 87% of the UK's population have suboptimal levels of vitamin D in winter and spring.[69]

Low vitamin D levels are linked to endometriosis,[70] antiphospholipid syndrome,[71] lower clinical pregnancy rates following IVF,[72,73] and PCOS.[74,75]

Reference ranges for vitamin D levels are provided in Table 7.1.

The American Endocrine Society's clinical guidelines recommend that all adults and pregnant and lactating women require a minimum of 600 IU (15 µg) per day of vitamin D but may require an even higher dose of 1500–2000 IU (37.5–50 µg) per day in order to maintain a blood level of 25-OHD above 75 nmol (30 ng/mL).[66] A dose of 10,000 IU (250 µg) per day may be required to correct

Table 7.1 Vitamin D reference ranges[65,66]	
Serum 25-OHD concentrations	**Status**
<25 nmol/L (<10 ng/mL)	Severely deficient
25–50 nmol/L (10–20 ng/mL)	Deficient
50–75 nmol/L (20–30 ng/mL)	Adequate[65] or insufficient[66]
>75 nmol/L (>30 ng/mL)	Optimal

vitamin D deficiency.[65,66] The guidelines state that levels of 4000 IU (100 μg) per day can be taken without medical supervision.[66]

Iodine

Maternal iodine intake helps with foetal neurological development.[19,76] It is also important for thyroid function because iodine is a significant component of the thyroid hormones (T4 and T3).[76]

According to WHO, 54 countries are still affected by iodine deficiency, even in places where food is supplemented with iodized salt.[76] Maternal iodine deficiency can lead to health problems, including hypothyroidism.[76] Iodine deficiency can also affect the foetus, leading to miscarriages, stillbirths, congenital anomalies, increased perinatal mortality, and endemic cretinism.[76]

Therefore, it is recommended that all women who are attempting to conceive or who are pregnant should take 250 μg of iodine supplement.[19,77,78] They should also eat foods rich in iodine, such as cow's milk, yoghurt, eggs, cheese, white fish, oily fish, shellfish, meat, and poultry.[78]

!	Red flag

Iodine supplementation

Women who have thyroid disease or take thyroid medication should consult their doctor before taking iodine supplements.

Iodine supplements should not be taken at the same time of the day as iron.

Vitamin A

Excessive amounts of vitamin A are harmful during pregnancy.[19] It is recommended that women who are trying to conceive should avoid taking vitamin A supplements and not eat foods rich in vitamin A (e.g., crustaceans and liver) during the luteal phase of the menstrual cycle and during pregnancy.[19]

Vitamin E

Vitamin E is a powerful antioxidant. It has been shown to improve the thickness of the endometrial lining, if taken at a high dose (400–500 IU/day) from day 3 of ovarian stimulation to hCG trigger.[79] Foods naturally rich in vitamin E include nuts, seeds, and vegetable oils.[80]

Omega 3

Omega 3 is a type of essential fatty acid that can only come from the diet. Omega 3 helps to reduce inflammation and blood coagulation[81] and reduces the risk of preterm birth.[81,82] It may improve egg quality and slow ovarian ageing,[83] improve embryo morphology,[84] and help to reduce the risk of miscarriages.[85]

In the Western world and increasingly in the developing world, people tend to have diets high in omega 6 and low in omega 3. Docosahexaenoic acid (DHA) and Eicosapentaenoic acid (EPA) are the most beneficial types of omega 3. During pregnancy, women should consume between 200 and 300 mg of DHA plus EPA per day.[81] Oily fish (salmon, sardines, herring, catfish, halibut, canned tuna) is particularly high in omega 3.[81,82] Fish high in mercury (tilefish, shark, swordfish, king mackerel, fresh or frozen tuna steaks (not canned), orange roughy, marlin, Spanish mackerel) should be avoided.[81] Non-fish eaters can take fish oil supplements with sufficiently high EPA and DHA levels; these supplements must be purified to filter out toxins.[81] Cod liver oil should be avoided because it is high in vitamin A.[81] Fish that feed on algae are a rich source of omega 3; thus, algal oil supplements are an alternative source of omega 3 for vegan patients.[81]

!	Red flag

Omega 3 and blood-thinning medication

Patients who take blood-thinning medication (for example, aspirin or clexane) should not increase their omega 3 intake without first checking with their doctor or nutritionist because omega 3 can also thin the blood.[86]

Selenium

Low selenium levels have been linked to recurrent pregnancy loss.[77,87] Selenium substitution and treatment with selenomethionine has been suggested to lower thyroid antibody (TPO-Ab) levels in euthyroid women, which are strongly linked to pregnancy loss.[77,88] Brazil nuts and fish (yellowfin tuna, halibut, sardines) are rich sources of selenium.[89]

Iron

Women of childbearing age are at risk of iron deficiency anaemia because of menstrual blood loss, poor diet, and pregnancies.[90] Iron deficiency has been linked to ovulatory problems.[91] Therefore, it is recommended that women trying to conceive should supplement their iron intake.[91] There are two types of iron: heme and nonheme. Heme iron is easier to absorb and is found in most meat-based products (chicken liver, canned oysters, beef liver, beef, turkey). Nonheme iron sources are fortified cereals, lentils, and kidney beans.[92]

Micronutrients and male fertility

Antioxidants that help with DNA sperm damage (vitamin C, vitamin E, vitamin A, omega 3)

DNA damage is common in subfertile men.[93] It is linked with reduced rates of natural conception[94] and conception through Intra Uterine Insemination (IUI),[94] IVF,[94–96] and, to a lesser extent, ICSI.[94,95] Oxidative stress is thought to damage sperm DNA.[93] Antioxidant therapy may help to reduce DNA damage, but, as yet, it is not clear exactly what type and dose of antioxidants is most optimal.[97]

However, some good quality evidence is beginning to emerge. Taking 1 g vitamin C and 1 g vitamin E daily for 2 months significantly reduces sperm DNA damage.[97] A daily combination of 30 mg of beta-carotene (a type of vitamin A), 180 mg of alpha-tocopherol (a type of vitamin E), 1 g of DHA, 0.25 g of gammalinolenic acid, and 0.10 g of arachidonic acid has been shown to significantly reduce oxidative damage.[98]

Foods naturally rich in vitamin E include nuts, seeds, and vegetable oils.[80] Vitamin C-rich foods are citrus fruits, red and green peppers, kiwifruit, broccoli, strawberries, canta-loupe, baked potatoes, and tomatoes.[99]

Omega 3

Omega 3 may also improve sperm's ability to fertilize an egg.[100] For more details on omega 3, see the Section 'Micronutrients and female fertility'.

Zinc

Zinc is important for sperm production and motility.[101] Zinc deficiency is associated with low testosterone levels and low sperm counts.[101]

Supplementing with 200 mg of zinc sulphate taken twice daily has been shown to improve sperm motility and sperm DNA fragmentation.[102] In another study, 24 mg/day of elemental zinc from zinc sulphate taken for 45–50 days significantly improved sperm count in infertile men.[103] In yet another study, 220 mg/day of oral zinc sulphate taken for 4 months significantly improved sperm count, motility, and morphology.[104]

Food sources of zinc are oysters (the richest source of zinc), red meat, poultry, and seafood (crab, lobster).[105]

Vitamin D

Vitamin D deficiency is associated with lower sperm parameters.[106] Vitamin D is a fat-soluble vitamin, which comes mainly from exposure to sunlight and certain foods, such as fish-liver oils, oily fish, egg yolks, and mushrooms.[64–66] Exposing the skin of the face and forearms to the midday sun for 20-30 min produces about 2000 IU of vitamin D.[65]

Vitamin B12

In his review of nutrients and male subfertility, Sinclair concluded that doses of vitamin B12 between 1000 µg/day and 6000 µg/day taken for 2–3 months help to improve sperm count.[101] The best sources of vitamin B12 are beef liver, clams, fish, meat, poultry, and dairy.[63]

Other

Other micronutrients that are also important for male fertility are carnitine, arginine, glutathione, selenium, and coenzyme Q10.[100,101] However, more better-quality and larger studies are needed to establish exact dosages and duration of supplementation.

Diet

Female fertility

A study of 18,555 women found that a diet with a high intake of low-fat dairy increased the risk of anovulatory infertility whereas a high dietary intake of high-fat dairy reduced the risk.[107] This finding was unrelated to the intake of lactose, calcium, phosphorus, and vitamin D.[107]

In the same cohort of women, researchers found that high-carbohydrate intake and higher dietary glycaemic load were linked to anovulatory infertility, even after adjusting for age, BMI, smoking, parity, physical activity, recency of contraception, total energy intake, protein intake, and other dietary variables.[108]

Dietary adherence to a Mediterranean-type diet (a high intake of vegetable oil, vegetables, fish, and legumes) has been shown to reduce the risk of infertility[109] and improve the odds of conception following IVF/ICSI.[110]

We would therefore suggest that to improve their fertility, women should:

- Eat a Mediterranean-type diet (plenty of vegetables, vegetable oil, fish, and legumes)
- Consume full-fat dairy
- Eat a low refined carbohydrates and low glycaemic load diet

Male fertility

A dietary pattern high in full-fat dairy has a negative effect on sperm morphology,[111] progressive motility,[111] and concentration.[112] Low-fat dairy does not have a negative effect on sperm.[112,113]

A diet rich in processed meat and sweets reduces sperm motility, but a diet high in fruit, vegetables, poultry, and seafood lowers the risks of motility problems.[113] In another study, researchers found that men who consumed high amounts of fruits and grains had better sperm motility and concentrations.[26] Sperm concentration is reduced in men who consume a high carbohydrate and high glycaemic load diet.[114]

Eating 75 mg of whole-shelled walnuts per day (potentially because of the high omega 3 content) improves vitality, motility, and morphology of sperm in healthy men, according to a recent study.[115]

Therefore, to ensure healthy sperm, men should:

- Eat a diet rich in vegetables, fruits, grains, poultry, and seafood
- Reduce their intake of foods that have high amounts of carbohydrates (particularly with a high glycaemic index) and high sugar content, and also reduce their intake of processed meats
- Replace full-fat dairy with low-fat dairy

TCM

General dietary advice

Good nutrition supports the Zang organs[43] and protects the body. Yin Yang balance, Kidney Jing (Essence),[116] Blood, and Qi can be promoted by good dietary practice, for example, by nourishing Stomach Qi and supporting Wei (Defensive) Qi.[44]

A balanced, moderate, and consistent approach to nutrition is advisable.[44,45] Patients should not get too hungry or too full. Excessive eating consumes Jing (Essence).[117] Eating regularly supports the Stomach and Spleen[44] and, therefore, the quality of Qi, Blood, and Jing (Essence). Eating late at night damages the Stomach. Eating slowly and enjoying meals nourishes Qi and Zang organs.[44]

It is advisable to eat according to the individual's syndromes and Hot/Cold nature. Hot foods may cause pathological Heat, which may injure Yin-Fluids and/or exacerbate Heat (in a hot person). Cold foods, especially if consumed by a person with Cold pathology, may injure his or her Yang Qi further[43,44] and exacerbate Cold. Well-cooked food (for example, stews and soups) is more warming in nature. To improve digestion, meat should be eaten with vegetables.[44] Dairy products and greasy fried foods may exacerbate Damp-Phlegm conditions and, therefore, should be avoided by patients with fertility issues and corresponding pathology.

Drinking plenty of water is very important for men and women. For women, this is especially true during menstruation as reduced fluid intake may induce Blood-Heat and/or injure Yin.

When menstruating, women should avoid icy cold drinks and foods as these may stagnate Blood.[43] Woman should also avoid hot and spicy foods, as these may create Blood-Heat.

An inadequate diet following ovulation and in early pregnancy may stagnate the embryo's Qi.[44] It is advisable to avoid greasy, hot, and spicy foods[44] to prevent Dampness and pathological Heat.

Foods beneficial in Qi Deficiency syndromes

- Eggs, milk[118]
- Grain, rice, millet[118]

- Chicken,[118] pork,[116] mutton[116]
- Carrots,[119] sweet potatoes,[118] potatoes,[44] chestnuts, chives[116]
- Mackerel[118]
- Apricots[116]
- Large-shaped beans[116]

Foods beneficial in Blood Deficiency syndromes

- Pork, chicken, duck eggs,[119] beef,[116] liver (pork, chicken, sheep,[120] ox)[43]
- Spinach, carrots,[119] beetroot,[118] edible black fungus,[44] mushrooms (shitake)
- Cuttlefish[119]
- Mulberry fruit, blackberries, raspberries,[120] red grapes,[119] dates[116]
- Sesame seeds[120]
- Milk[119]
- Rice[116]

Foods beneficial in Yin Deficiency syndromes

- Mulberry fruit, wolfberry fruit, peaches, apples,[118] dates, figs, pears, pomegranate,[121] mango[122]
- Walnuts, sesame[118]
- Wheat, barley, rice,[121] millet[116]
- Mung beans, sweet potato, asparagus, spinach[118]
- Crab, fish, oyster, cuttlefish[122]
- Milk,[121] especially goat's milk[123]
- Duck eggs, duck, beef,[121,122] chicken[116]
- Royal jelly,[121] honey[118]

Foods beneficial in Yang Deficiency syndromes

- Walnuts,[122] chestnuts[124]
- Shrimp, lobster,[124] trout[118]
- Pork,[124] chicken,[116] mutton, kidney[118]
- Cherries, apricots, raspberries[124]
- Dill seeds,[118] fennel, cinnamon,[124] cloves,[122] dried ginger, basil, cumin, caraway,[123] garlic[44]

Foods beneficial in Jing (Essence) Deficiency syndromes

- Almonds, walnuts,[118] pistachio nuts[122]
- Artichoke leaf[118]
- Bone marrow, chicken, kidney, liver[118]
- Eggs,[118] milk[125]
- Oysters, mussels,[118] clams, mackerel,[126] scallops[122]
- Nettle,[118] rose hip leaves, micro-algae, cereal grass, millet, sweet rice[125]
- Royal jelly[118]
- Sesame seeds,[118] soybeans with seaweed, blackbeans,[125] cassia fruits[122]

- Raspberries, blackberries, mulberries, strawberries, grapes, cherries, dates[126]

Foods beneficial in Qi Stagnation syndromes

- Vinegar[120]
- Hawthorne,[44] rose[44]
- Orange peel[118]
- Radish leaves, turnips, mushrooms, onions[120]
- Basil, cumin, turmeric, bay leaf, fennel, dill seeds, garlic, caraway seeds[118]

Foods beneficial in Blood Stasis syndromes

- Orange peel, hawthorne,[43] vinegar[44]
- Onions,[120] soybeans, eggplant, basil, saffron,[119] chestnuts,[118] turmeric[119]
- Mango, kiwi,[120] peach,[118] hawthorn berry[118]
- Brown sugar[119,120]

Foods beneficial in Heat/Fire syndromes

- Watermelon, pears, bananas, apples,[123] strawberries[127]
- Peppermint[124]
- Spinach, asparagus, bamboo shoots[127]
- Cucumbers, tomatoes, lettuce, radishes, celery, asparagus, broccoli, cauliflower[123]
- Mung beans, millet, barley, wheat[123]
- Extreme Heat: peas, bean curd, lentils, red beans[43]
- Blood-Heat: lotus root, eggplant[43]

Foods beneficial in Phlegm-Dampness syndromes

- Kelp, onions, (purple) turnips,[118] celery, radish roots[128]
- Almonds[44]
- Broad beans,[128] kidney beans[118]
- Mustard seeds, black pepper[118]
- Bamboo shoots[128]
- Pears, orange and lemon peel[118]

Foods beneficial in Cold syndromes

- Ginger, dill seeds, mustard seeds, pepper,[118] star anise, cinnamon, cloves[128]

EXERCISE AND REST

Orthodox medical perspective

Exercise and female fertility

Fertility can be improved by the judicious use of exercise. Regular exercise may help with weight management and, therefore, indirectly reduce the risk of subfertility. Exercise can reduce the risk of ovulatory infertility by increasing insulin sensitivity, which, in turn, improves ovarian function.[19,49]

For example, a study of 3628 women found that intensive exercise increases fertility in women with BMI ≥ 25 kg/m^2 but decreases fertility in women with BMI below that level.[129] Women with BMI < 25 kg/m^2 have slight improvement in fertility with moderate exercise levels.[129]

In their paper, Homan et al., after reviewing which lifestyle factors affect reproductive health, concluded that moderate exercise is beneficial for general health and reproductive health.[49]

However, overexercising may cause some people's BMI to decrease too much, which may contribute to subfertility.

Exercise and male fertility

In one study, researchers found that men who exercised for ≥ 15 h a week had 73% higher sperm concentrations compared to men who exercised <5 h a week.[130] The study also found that men who spent more than >20 h a week watching TV had 44% lower sperm counts compared to men who did not watch any TV.[130]

However, another study of 2261 men and 4565 semen samples found no association between exercise and semen parameters, except that bicycling ≥ 5 h per week was associated with low sperm concentrations.[131]

As discussed in the section on weight earlier in this chapter, both male and female obesity is linked to subfertility. Therefore, regular exercise may help overweight and obese men manage their excess weight.

Activity levels after the embryo transfer

A recent review found that there was no evidence to support routine use of bed rest following embryo transfer.[132] However, there is also some evidence that overexertion at the time of ovulation (and presumably, therefore, embryo transfer) may cause miscarriages.[133]

Sleep and fertility

Regular and adequate sleep is very important for female fertility. Female shift workers suffer from more menstrual cycle irregularities[134–136] and, therefore, are potentially at an increased risk of subfertility.[136,137] A large European multicentre study interviewed 6630 women and found that shift work by female partners (but not male partners) was significantly associated with subfertility.[138] Therefore, as much as they can, women trying to conceive should maintain regular sleeping routines.

Exposure to light during the night can modify reproductive hormones (through light's effect on the hormone melatonin).[139] Therefore, it is recommended that couples minimize exposure to light at night time (for example, ensuring they sleep in darkened rooms and use alarm clocks with a red light because humans are sensitive to green and blue lights).[140]

TCM perspective

Exercise

TCM posits that exercise helps with the flow of Qi, Blood, and Jing (Essence), preventing Stagnation.[43] It is good for the Heart, Shen (Spirit), and promotes health and well-being. Exercise in the morning rather than evening can help to preserve Kidney Jing (Essence) and Yin.[117] Exercise in the morning is especially beneficial for Yang-deficient patients. Patients should avoid exercising on an empty Stomach or immediately after they have eaten.[43] Table 7.2 provides details of common types of exercises and the TCM syndromes they benefit.

Rest

Overwork and overexercising can compromise Qi and weaken the Kidney and Spleen.[117]

Conversely, too much rest can also injure the body as Jing (Essence) fails to circulate and Qi Stagnates.[43] Qi Stagnation may lead to Blood Stagnation.[116]

Table 7.2 Exercise recommendations according to TCM syndrome differentiation[44]

TCM syndromes	Recommendations
Phlegm–Damp	Outdoor activities in warm weather help Phlegm–Damp. Jogging, walking, dancing, aerobic exercise, or swimming is beneficial as these help to disperse congestion. The best time to exercise is between 2 and 4 pm
Stagnation	Outdoor activities (for example, running) regulate and disperse Qi and Blood
Blood Stasis	Any sport promotes circulation of Qi and Blood
Yin Deficiency	Avoid strenuous exercise and overwork. Gentle exercise is recommended, for example, qigong, walking, gentle cycling, or gentle swimming
Blood Deficiency	Gentle exercise such as walking is recommended in order to reduce the loss of Blood through excessive sweating
Yang Deficiency	Avoid strenuous exercise to conserve Yang Qi and avoid profuse sweating. Exercise in warm weather or indoors. Avoid swimming in cold water as the cold water temperature may injure Yang further. Instead, walk or skip as these forms of exercise activate Yang Qi

Therefore, in early pregnancy, both overwork and too much rest may have a detrimental influence on the embryo. Too much rest may Stagnate Qi, but overwork consumes Qi.

Sleep

Adequate sleep helps to strengthen the individual's constitution, tonifies Qi,[43] and nourishes Yin.[44] The following sleeping routines are recommended by one TCM text:[44]

- Try to sleep for 8 h per night
- The best time to go to sleep is 10:00 pm to 10:30 pm
- The best time to wake is at 6:30 am
- A 1.5 h nap is recommend if the previous night's sleep was disturbed

Recommendation

A balanced approach to exercise and rest is important.[45] From an Orthodox medical point of view, intensive exercise is beneficial for patients who need to lose weight.

From the TCM point of view, different types of exercise may be suggested, depending on the individual's constitution, syndromes, and ability. For example, in cases of severe Kidney Deficiency and high-risk pregnancies, it may be advisable to preserve Jing (Essence), and, therefore, rest is indicated. In cases of Stagnation from Blood Deficiency, gentle exercise during the early stages of the stimulation phase of IVF treatment can help to promote the flow of Qi and Blood and free Jing (Essence).

STRESS

Stress as a cause of infertility

The longer it takes for a couple to conceive, the more stress they may experience.[141] However, the evidence that stress causes infertility is mixed.

Stress has been shown to significantly reduce the probability of conception each day during the fertile window.[142] In their review paper, Nakamura et al. state that the growing body of evidence suggests that stress might be involved in reproductive failure.[143] In his review paper, Campagne argues that there is sufficient evidence to state that stress may be a primary or secondary cause of infertility.[141]

However, this is not a universally held view.[144] Campagne argues that the failure to find links between stress and infertility in part might be caused by incorrect inclusion of other terms and diagnostic categories by researchers.[141] For example, 'depression' and 'anxiety' should not be included with the term 'stress'. He argues that these anxiety and depressive disorders should be investigated separately.

Effects of stress on the reproductive system

Stress affects the Hypothalamic–Pituitary–Gonadal Axis. It decreases the Gonadotrophin Releasing Hormone (GnRH) pulse amplitude. It also decreases the Luteinizing Hormone (LH) pulse amplitude through decreasing the pituitary's responsiveness to GnRH, caused by the stress hormone cortisol.[145] Stress increases testosterone levels in both men and women.[146] Stress has also been shown to reduce menstrual cycle length, but it does not affect other cycle parameters.[147]

Although the mechanisms are not fully understood, there is a link between psychosocial stress (including anxiety) and testicular function and sperm quality.[148–152] A meta-analysis of 57 studies with 29,914 participants found that psychological stress lowers sperm concentration and progressive motility and increases the amount of abnormal forms of sperm.[153]

Stress has been shown to significantly reduce the probability of natural conception.[142] A meta-analysis of 31 studies found a small but significant association between stress and reduced pregnancy rates following ART.[154] Stress may also increase the risk of miscarriages.[155,156]

Prevalence of stress in ART patients

Reproductive treatment causes distress, with psychological stress cited as a common reason why couples discontinue fertility treatments.[157] The more anxious and depressed that a woman feels before commencing IVF treatment, the more likely it is that she will terminate subfertility treatment after one failed cycle.[158] Those undergoing infertility treatment can have further exacerbations of stress levels because of financial, physical, and emotional reasons.[141,159] At the same time, patients are aware that such psychological factors may not be helpful to their chances of conception.[160]

Women undergoing IUI or IVF have been shown to experience emotional distress,[160–162] which may persist into pregnancy.[163] One in three women who undergoes fertility treatment admits being worried about becoming pregnant; anxiety about having treatment injections and concern about deterioration in the relationship with her partner is usually the main source of her stress.[164]

Women who have undergone ART to conceive and then miscarry in the first trimester experience more stress and emotional trauma for at least 3 months afterward than women who have conceived naturally and who then miscarry.[165]

Practical tips to reduce stress

Various approaches are used in Orthodox medicine to manage patients with psychological distress.[158,166,167]

It is likely that patients who have less emotional support may have more intense psychological symptoms.

Campagne believes that stress management should be used as part of fertility treatment.[141] Couples may need support during the infertility treatment process to help cope with their emotions and decision making.[161] Pessimism appears to be associated with IVF treatment failure.[168] Therefore, where appropriate, reducing negative preconceptions about IVF outcome by encouraging and emphasizing a pragmatically positive perception of fertility outcome may be useful.

Couples need to learn effective relaxation and stress management techniques. An RCT involving 100 women undergoing IVF found that a significantly higher proportion of women (52% vs. 20%) became pregnant using such techniques.[169]

A meta-analysis of 21 studies comparing psychological interventions in infertile patients found no significant effect on mental health scores, but pregnancy rates were improved in patients not undergoing ART.[170] Interventions included were counselling, individual or group support programmes, and behavioural therapy.

Other techniques couples could try include positive autogenic visualization, self-hypnosis, and relaxation exercises. Alice Domar's book, *Conquering Infertility* (ISBN 0142002011), is probably the most comprehensive resource to help those patients who need a deeper empathic understanding of the effects that stress, anxiety, and depression have on fertility.

CLINICAL TIPS

SIMPLE STEPS TO HELP REDUCE STRESS AND ANXIETY IN PATIENTS

- Explain test results so patients may better understand their situation and/or treatment.
- Reinforce that most patients are not infertile but subfertile, which means, unless they have been diagnosed with complete sterility, they can still have a child.
- Quote statistics to your patients that eventually most couples conceive and have babies. Between 82% and 92% of couples will conceive within 12 menstrual cycles of trying, and between 90% and 98% of couples will conceive within 24 menstrual cycles of trying.[171]
- Explain that it can take up to 3 years for some couples to conceive, especially older couples, who may need to keep trying for longer.[171]

The TCM view of stress, mind, and emotion

Chapter 1 described how emotions may be a cause of subfertility, and Chapter 2 discussed how emotions affect the reproductive system from a TCM point of view.

The stress response can encompass a range of emotions, including sadness, anger, frustration, and feeling out of control. Stress can weaken the Heart and Shen (Spirit).[43] Stress affects Qi and Blood movement, creating Stagnation[172] (especially during menses), so the arrival of menstruation can be upsetting for subfertile patients. Emotional disturbance impairs Kidney Jing (Essence) and Yin Yang.[43] Negative emotions may exacerbate existing syndromes[43] and, therefore, subfertility.

Regulating emotions helps to prevent physiological and pathological changes. The avoidance of emotional disturbances enhances Heart function and preserves Kidney Jing (Essence).

Calming a patient's Shen (Spirit) will help with the smooth flow of Qi[173] and Blood and will support the patient's Jing (Essence). Acupuncturists should aim to regulate the Mind to nourish the Shen (Spirit)[43] and Jing (Essence).[45]

Taking time out for hobbies and leisure activities strengthens the person's constitution and Mind,[43] thus helping to reduce stress levels. Therefore, couples should be advised to pursue their interests and hobbies as one of the ways to reduce stress levels, provided that their hobbies are not in themselves physical stressors or psychologically stress inducing.

Research on acupuncture and stress and/or anxiety in fertility patients

The ASRM recommends that patients experiencing infertility-related stress should try, among other things, acupuncture.[159]

An RCT of 43 IVF female patients found that acupuncture treatment significantly reduced anxiety symptoms in the active treatment group. Treatment consisted of 4 weekly acupuncture sessions using acupuncture points HE7, P6, REN17, DU20, and YINTANG.[174] In another observational study of 15 women receiving fertility acupuncture treatment, acupuncture improved self-efficacy and psychological coping parameters.[175] A pilot study of 57 IVF/ICSI patients showed that acupuncture was associated with significantly lower stress levels before and after embryo transfer, and preliminary data also suggested improved pregnancy rates.[176] It has been suggested that the acupuncture mode of action in improving IVF outcomes works by reducing prolactin and cortisol levels.[177]

RELATIONSHIP AND SEXUAL ISSUES

Sexual intercourse

The next few sections apply to patients who are still trying to conceive naturally during the preparation phase. It is easy to assume that patients presenting for ART treatment will have had sufficiently frequent intercourse at the right time in the menstrual cycle. However, research shows that couples struggle to identify their fertile time.[178] Therefore, each couple should be screened to determine if ART is an appropriate next step to take. If, after taking the reproductive history, it is clear that the couple did not have enough intercourse or did not time the intercourse correctly, they should be given information about the fertile window and different methods of detecting ovulation and be advised to keep trying during the preparatory stage of the ART treatment cycle.

For sterile couples, this is inappropriate advice. For example, if there are serious issues with sperm, then no amount of additional sexual intercourse will result in a pregnancy. Great care should be taken to advise couples where the woman is of advanced reproductive age, ensuring that months of valuable time are not wasted trying to conceive naturally when it is clear that because of the woman's age, the couple may require ART.

Fertile window and timing of intercourse

Conception is possible if intercourse takes place during the fertile window, beginning around 6 days before and ending on the day of ovulation.[179] During this 6-day period, a woman produces sperm-friendly mucus. This sperm-friendly mucus helps to nourish and support sperm inside the fallopian tubes until the egg is released.[180] The length of the fertile window is not determined or affected by a woman's age.[181] Men are also more sexually attracted to women who are about to ovulate, possibly in response to chemical messages released by women.[182,183] Women's behaviour also changes when they are most fertile, for example, they may dress more provocatively,[184] consume fewer calories,[185] and have increased sexual desire.[186] Couples will naturally increase the frequency of their intercourse during the fertile window.[187]

Several studies have shown that the chance of conception is great if intercourse takes place within 5 days of ovulation, and the chance of conception is even greater if intercourse takes place within 4 days of ovulation (Figure 7.1).[181]

While it is clear that frequent and well-timed intercourse helps to increase probability of conception, both clinicians and couples need to be aware that timed intercourse has been linked to stress, erectile dysfunction (in 42.8% of men), and even extramarital affairs (10.7% of men).[188] Sexual stress, such as loss of sexual self-esteem, the pressure of scheduling intercourse, and loss of enjoyment of sexual relations, affects both men and women in similar ways.[189] Therefore, advice on frequency and timing of sexual intercourse should be modified to take into account the individual circumstances of each couple.

Frequency of intercourse

Frequency of intercourse during the fertile window is important. It is generally accepted that the optimal intercourse frequency for conception is once every 1–2 days.[48,179] One study analysed data from 708 menstrual cycles provided by 221 couples and found that the probability of conception was highest with daily intercourse (37%), still good with intercourse that occurred every other day (33%), but was significantly lower with intercourse that took place only once a week (15%) (Figure 7.2).[190]

A common misconception is that frequent intercourse is damaging to sperm. In fact, when the sperm count is high, the hormone inhibin is released, and sperm production slows.[191] Sperm also degrades when retained in the body for long periods. A large study, which assessed 9489 semen samples obtained from 6008 patients, found that

men with male factor infertility (defined as oligozoospermia) should not abstain for more than 1 day if they want to achieve the best possible sperm motility and morphology. Even after only 2 days abstinence, sperm in these men started to degrade. Men with normal semen parameters do not appear to suffer from deterioration of sperm so soon into abstinence, but should not abstain for more than 7–10 days.[192]

Coital practices

Many couples engage in coital rituals in the belief that doing so will increase their chances of conception.

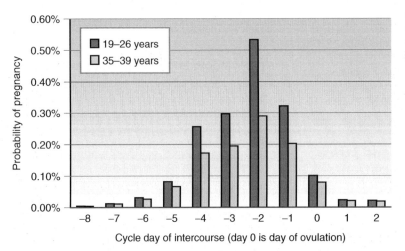

Figure 7.1 Probability of pregnancy from a single act of intercourse relative to ovulation.[181]

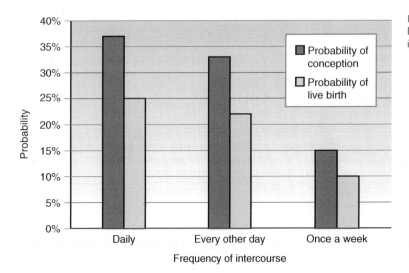

Figure 7.2 Probability of conception and live birth relative to frequency of intercourse.[190]

Common examples are women lying with their legs raised in the air for 20 min following intercourse, adopting certain sex positions, having intercourse at specific times in the day, and many other ways. However, none of these practices has sufficient evidence of efficacy.

Men's sexual arousal appears to make a difference to the quality of their ejaculate. Men's arousal is heightened by visual stimulation. This can be achieved, for example, by leaving the lights on when having sex, watching an erotic movie, seeing their female partner highly aroused or dressed in erotic underwear.[179] Longer periods of arousal are also associated with better quality ejaculation.[193]

The level of arousal in women is also important. Higher levels of arousal result in better mucus production, which is essential for survival of the sperm and also will make the act of intercourse more comfortable by allowing easier sliding of the penis.[179] This is important because most lubricants, such as KY Jelly, olive oil, and even saliva, are damaging to sperm integrity. Mineral oils (such as canola oil) and Hydroxyethylcellulose-based lubricants (such as Pre-Seed®) do not appear to have a damaging effect on sperm.[48]

Many subfertile couples use euphemistic terms such as 'baby dancing' or 'baby sex' when discussing intercourse during the fertile window. However, they should be encouraged to engage in 'fun sex' and to avoid thinking of it as sex for the purpose of conception. In some cases, when there are psychological issues, a referral to a sex therapist may be justified.

For couples for whom traditional sexual intercourse is not possible, a 'turkey baster' method can be used. In this method, sperm is ejaculated into a dish or a condom, usually after masturbation, and then inserted inside the vagina with a pipette or a turkey baster. This method is commonly used by couples when a woman's fertile period starts during menstruation and for religious or other reasons couples are unable to have intercourse during this time. Also, lesbian couples use this method with donated sperm. Strictly speaking, this method falls into the 'assisted insemination' category.

Case study

Unexplained Subfertility and Natural Conception Before IVF

Julie, aged 34, and Todd, aged 37, had been trying for 1.5 years to conceive. They were treated with acupuncture for just over 4 months.

Summary of Medical Test Findings

Semen sample: slightly low motility

Continued

Case study—cont'd

Julie's hormone blood tests results:
   progesterone = 32 nmol/L, FSH = 10 IU/L (slightly raised), AMH = 3 pmol/L (low).

Medical Diagnosis

Unexplained subfertility and reduced ovarian reserve. Julie and her husband were placed on a waiting list for IVF.

TCM Diagnosis

- EPF Wind-Cold: feeling chilly
- Phlegm: mucus on chest
- Yang Deficiency and Empty-Cold: white tongue coating, felt cold, liked warm drinks, wrapped up warm, weak pulse.
- Liver Qi Stagnation and Lung and Spleen Qi Deficiency: wheezing, loose stools or constipated, spotting before menses, irritable, tearful, PMT, irrational, cold hands and feet, abdominal bloating, 'worried and stressed out' about fertility
- Kidney Yin Deficiency and Liver Blood Deficiency: slight night sweating, scant period lasting only 1 day, early periods (23–27 days).
- Pulse: floating, wiry, thin, weak on third right position
- Tongue: pale, short

Weekly Acupuncture Point Prescription

LI4, LU7, ST36, LIV3, KID3

Modifications

- Phlegm: ST40, KID7, REN9, SP9, SP1
- Liver Qi Stagnation and Liver Blood Deficiency: SP4 + P6, SP10, P6, LIV8, ST25, ST37, HE5, GB26, P5, YINTANG
- Kidney Yin and Yang Deficiency: LU7 + KID6, REN6, REN12, KID4, KID13, REN7, ST25, SP3, REN6, ZIGONG

Two weeks before IVF was due to commence, Julie announced she had conceived naturally. Julia gave birth to a baby boy. The combination of acupuncture treatment and evidence-based lifestyle advice (particularly with respect to intercourse timing) assisted Julie and Todd's conception.

Ovulation detection methods

Previous sections have illustrated that timing sexual intercourse relative to ovulation and the fertile window is likely to increase the chance of conception. However, research shows that while most women appear to be aware of the importance of having intercourse during the fertile window, few identify it correctly.[178] Many couples resort to technological aids to help them to identify the fertile window or ovulation and to time their intercourse accordingly. This section reviews some of the most common ovulation detection methods used by couples.

Cervical mucus

Cervical mucus is secreted in larger quantities when plasma oestrogen levels rise. This is around 5–6 days before ovulation and peaks around 2–3 days before ovulation.[194] At this time, before ovulation, cervical mucus looks clear and stretchy, like egg whites, and it is sperm friendly. After ovulation, when progesterone levels rise, the mucus appears sticky and scanty; this a nonfertile type of mucus and is not sperm friendly.

While pregnancy is possible without it, fertile mucus helps to facilitate sperm transportation and survival in the female reproductive tract. A prospective analysis of 193 women and 161 conception cycles and 2594 nonconception cycles showed that the probability of conception is highest on fertile mucus days (30%) and lowest on dry days (0.3%) (Figure 7.3).[195]

Research shows that women are able to monitor their cervical mucus very accurately.[196] So this may be the simplest, most accurate, and least expensive method of ovulation monitoring.

Both Orthodox medicine and TCM associate cervical mucus with fertility. In TCM, egg-white slippery mucus around the time of ovulation illustrates good function of Bodily Fluids and Yin. If a female has a sparse amount of fertile mucus (and is using correct methods to check for it), Kidney Yin Deficiency should be suspected.

Ovulation predictor kits

There are two common types of ovulation detection test kits:

- LH ovulation detection test kit (more frequently used and less expensive)
- Estrone-3-glucuronide (E3G) and LH ovulation detection test kit

LH ovulation detection kits work by monitoring urinary LH levels. Urinary levels of LH rise approximately 12–36 h before ovulation.[197] This gives a couple a potential 1–2 day window for having intercourse for the purpose of conception.

However, research shows that the fertile window spans a period of up to 5 days before ovulation.[181] Therefore, relying completely on the LH ovulation detection kits may result in couples missing some of the fertile window.

E3G-based fertility monitors solve this problem. E3G mimics the rise of oestradiol during the follicular phase,[198] which occurs a few days before surge of LH. This helps couples identify the whole of the fertile window. Therefore, they can potentially maximize their chances of conception by having more intercourse during the whole time of the fertile window.

Basal body temperature (BBT) charting

BBT charting is an old, long-established technique used to monitor ovulation. It is based on the principle that higher

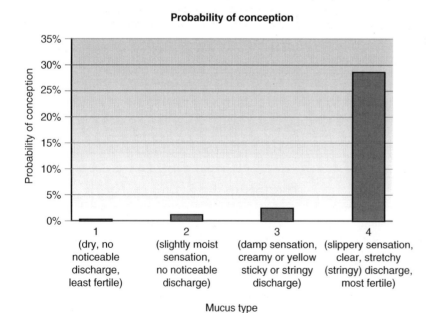

Probability of conception

Figure 7.3 Probability of conception based on mucus type on the day of intercourse.[195]

progesterone levels following ovulation make the body temperature rise by 0.5°F.[197] While it is an effective method of confirming when ovulation has taken place, it does not predict when the fertile window begins.

BBT is affected by factors such as fever, lack of sleep, and alcohol. So couples need to learn as much as they can about BBT charting in order to gather accurate information.

For acupuncturists, BBT charts may provide additional information to help them formulate the diagnosis. Chapter 5 discusses BBT charting in greater detail.

Other methods

Other ovulation detection methods used by couples include the salivary ferning test. In this test, saliva is evaluated under the microscope for signs of ferning, which is associated with ovulation. However, this method is difficult to interpret.[199]

Timing intercourse according to the days of the menstrual cycle is reliable in women whose menstrual cycles are fairly regular.[197] Ovulation usually takes place 14 days before the onset of the next menstruation. So women with regular 28 days menstrual cycles are likely to ovulate on day 14 and their fertile phase will begin around day 9.

The TCM view of sexual intercourse

Reproduction relies on a good relationship between a male and a female partner, and coitus for the purpose of reproduction ought to occur at a time when Blood and Qi are strong.[200] Yet, when a couple try to conceive, they need to have very frequent intercourse, even if they do not feel like it or if they are tired or ill.

Sexual intercourse is important for good physical and mental well-being. Yin, Yang, Qi, Blood, and Jing (Essence) may congeal in the absence of sexual intercourse.[43] Coitus regulates Qi and Blood.[43] Healthy sexual practice reduces tension and supports a relationship between the couple.[43] Sexual intercourse should occur when emotional well-being is not disturbed.[43]

Weak sexual desire and inability to enjoy sex or reach an orgasm is related to Kidney Deficiency, in particular Kidney Yang Deficiency.[201] Therefore, if patients are having difficulties with their sexual relationship, the affected partner may benefit from strengthening his or her Kidney energy. Excessive sexual desire is a result of Kidney Yin Deficiency and Empty-Fire Rising; nourishing Kidney Yin may be beneficial in these patients.[201] Excessive desire consumes Qi.[45]

Male and female 'sexual Essences' are manifestations of Kidney Jing (Essence). Sexual 'energy' of the male pertains to Kidney Jing (Essence) and the female more to Blood. Therefore, ejaculation is more of a direct loss of Kidney Jing (Essence).[201] Ejaculation, age, and the health of the man are therefore important sexual practice considerations.[202]

Gratification of 'sexual desires' and/or excessive sexual desire (even if no ejaculation takes place) can also consume Kidney Jing (Essence) and Shen (Spirit) in the male. Subfertile couples who engage in frequent intercourse in hopes of conceiving, therefore, benefit from lifestyle (preserving Mind, Spirit, and emotion) and dietary advice (supplementation of Jing (Essence), Qi, and Blood). Acupuncture treatments that support Kidney Jing (Essence), Yin Yang, Qi, and Blood are also useful, especially if these are already deficient. Supporting these vital substances avoids the need to advise patients to significantly reduce their frequency of sexual intercourse, which would reduce their potential chances of conception.

INTERESTING FACTS

TESTOSTERONE IN MEN AND YANG ENERGY

Interestingly, testosterone levels in men are highest in the morning.[204] From a TCM perspective, male fertility is said to fluctuate, with Yang energies rising in the morning.[205]

Recommendation

Daily intercourse is most likely to result in conception. Timing intercourse relative to the fertile window is necessary. The most reliable methods of ovulation detection are fertile mucus days or E3G-based ovulation detection kits.

Intercourse should be fun with an emphasis on foreplay, visual stimulation, and high and prolonged arousal. It is necessary for men to ejaculate on a regular basis even outside of the fertile window in order to reduce damage to sperm.

SUMMARY

Treating patients in preparation for ART provides acupuncturists with a unique opportunity to inform and educate patients about lifestyle modifications, which might significantly improve their chances of conception.

Being under- or overweight, smoking, drinking large amounts of alcohol, drinking large amounts of caffeine, using recreational drugs, taking certain prescriptions or over-the-counter medication, being exposed to environmental toxins, working in certain occupations, eating a poor diet or having a deficiency in certain micronutrients, exercising too much or not enough, and having high levels of stress have all been shown to affect reproductive health.

REFERENCES

1. ASRM. Quick facts about infertility. Available from: http://www.asrm.org/detail.aspx?id=2322 (accessed 16 January 2012).

2. WHO. Global database on body mass index. Available from: http://apps.who.int/bmi/index.jsp?introPage=intro_3.html (accessed 15 April 2013).

3. Barnhart KT. Epidemiology of male and female reproductive disorders and impact on fertility regulation and population growth. Fertil Steril 2011;95:2200–3.

4. Hassan MA, Killick SR. Negative lifestyle is associated with a significant reduction in fecundity. Fertil Steril 2004;81:384–92.

5. Practice Committee of American Society for Reproductive Medicine. Obesity and reproduction: an educational bulletin. Fertil Steril 2008;90:S21–9.

6. Rowland AS, Baird DD, Long S, et al. Influence of medical conditions and lifestyle factors on the menstrual cycle. Epidemiology 2002;13:668–74.

7. Purcell SH, Moley KH. The impact of obesity on egg quality. J Assist Reprod Genet 2011;28:517–24.

8. Robker RL. Evidence that obesity alters the quality of oocytes and embryos. Pathophysiology 2008;15:115–21.

9. Cardozo E, Pavone ME, Hirshfeld-Cytron JE. Metabolic syndrome and oocyte quality. Trends Endocrinol Metab 2011;22:103–9.

10. Rittenberg V, Seshadri S, Sunkara SK, et al. Effect of body mass index on IVF treatment outcome: an updated systematic review and meta-analysis. Reprod Biomed Online 2011;23:421–39.

11. Luke B, Brown MB, Stern JE, et al. Female obesity adversely affects assisted reproductive technology (ART) pregnancy and live birth rates. Hum Reprod 2011;26:245–52.

12. Moragianni VA, Jones SM, Ryley DA. The effect of body mass index on the outcomes of first assisted reproductive technology cycles. Fertil Steril 2012;98:102–8.

13. Luke B, Brown MB, Missmer SA, et al. The effect of increasing obesity on the response to and outcome of assisted reproductive technology: a national study. Fertil Steril 2011;96:820–5.

14. Sherbahn R. Effect of low and high body mass index (BMI) on embryo development, implantation and live birth rates. Fertil Steril 2011;96:S190.

15. Nichols JE, Miller PB, Boone WR, et al. Effects of extremes of body mass index (BMI) on in vitro fertilization (IVF) pregnancy rates. Fertil Steril 2001;76:S74.

16. Helgstrand S, Andersen AM. Maternal underweight and the risk of spontaneous abortion. Acta Obstet Gynecol Scand 2005;84:1197–201.

17. Metwally M, Ong KJ, Ledger WL, et al. Does high body mass index increase the risk of miscarriage after spontaneous and assisted conception? A meta-analysis of the evidence. Fertil Steril 2008;90:714–26.

18. Eskild A, Fedorcsak P, Mørkrid L, et al. Maternal body mass index and serum concentrations of human chorionic gonadotropin in very early pregnancy. Fertil Steril 2012;98:905–10.

19. Anderson K, Nisenblat V, Norman R. Lifestyle factors in people seeking infertility treatment – a review. Aust N Z J Obstet Gynaecol 2010;50:8–20.

20. Sermondade N, Faure C, Fezeu L, et al. BMI in relation to sperm count: an updated systematic review and collaborative meta-analysis. Hum Reprod Update 2013;19:221–31.

21. MacDonald AA, Herbison GP, Showell M, et al. The impact of body mass index on semen parameters and reproductive hormones in human males: a systematic review with meta-analysis. Hum Reprod Update 2010;16:293–311.

22. Petersen GL, Schmidt L, Pinborg A, et al. The influence of female and male body mass index on live births after assisted reproductive technology treatment: a nationwide register-based cohort study. Fertil Steril 2013;99:1654–62.

23. Bakos HW, Henshaw RC, Mitchell M, et al. Paternal body mass index is associated with decreased blastocyst development and reduced live birth rates following assisted reproductive technology. Fertil Steril 2011;95:1700–4.

24. ASRM patient fact sheet. Weight and fertility. Available from: http://www.asrm.org/Weight_and_Fertility_factsheet/ (accessed 15 April 2013).

25. National Institutes of Health 1998 Clinical guidelines on the identification, evaluation, and treatment of overweight and obesity in adults: the evidence report. US: National Heart, Lung and Blood Institute; 1998.

26. Braga DP, Halpern G, Figueira Rde C, et al. Food intake and social habits in male patients and its relationship to intracytoplasmic sperm injection outcomes. Fertil Steril 2011;97:53–9.

27. The Practice Committee of the American Society for Reproductive Medicine. Smoking and infertility: a committee opinion. Fertil Steril 2012;98:1400–6.

28. Dechanet C, Anahory T, Mathieu Daude JC, et al. Effects of cigarette smoking on reproduction. Hum Reprod Update 2011;17:76–95.

29. Liu Y, Gold EB, Lasley BL, et al. Factors affecting menstrual cycle characteristics. Am J Epidemiol 2004;160:131–40.

30. Waylen AL, Metwally M, Jones GL, et al. Effects of cigarette smoking upon clinical outcomes of assisted reproduction: a meta-analysis. Hum Reprod Update 2009;15:31–44.

31. Zitzmann M, Rolf C, Nordhoff V, et al. Male smokers have a decreased success rate for in vitro fertilization and intracytoplasmic sperm injection. Fertil Steril 2003;79:32.

32. Hackshaw A, Rodeck C, Boniface S. Maternal smoking in pregnancy and birth defects: a systematic review based on 173 687 malformed cases and 11.7 million controls. Hum Reprod Update 2011;17:589–604.

33. National Collaborating Centre for Women's and Children's Health, Commissioned by the National Institute for Health and Clinical Excellence. Guideline summary. In: Fertility: assessment and treatment for people with fertility problems. NICE clinical guideline. 2nd ed. London: The Royal College of Obstetricians and Gynaecologists; 2013. p. 1–46 [Chapter 1].

34. Eggert J, Theobald H, Engfeldt P. Effects of alcohol consumption on female fertility during an 18-year period. Fertil Steril 2004;81:379–83.

35. Tolstrup JS, Kjaer SK, Holst C, et al. Alcohol use as predictor for infertility in a representative population of Danish women. Acta Obstet Gynecol Scand 2003;82:744–9.

36. Chavarro JE, Rich-Edwards JW, Rosner BA, et al. Caffeinated and alcoholic beverage intake in relation to ovulatory disorder infertility. Epidemiology 2009;20:374–81.

37. Juhl M, Nyboe Andersen AM, Grønbaek M, et al. Moderate alcohol consumption and waiting time to pregnancy. Hum Reprod 2001;16:2705–9.

38. Gaur DS, Talekar MS, Pathak VP. Alcohol intake and cigarette smoking: impact of two major lifestyle factors on male fertility. Indian J Pathol Microbiol 2010;53:35–40.

39. Rossi BV, Berry KF, Hornstein MD, et al. Effect of alcohol consumption on in vitro fertilization. Obstet Gynecol 2011;117:136–42.

40. Henriksen TB, Hjollund NH, Jensen TK, et al. Alcohol consumption at the time of conception and spontaneous abortion. Am J Epidemiol 2004;160:661–7.

41. Rasch V. Cigarette, alcohol, and caffeine consumption: risk factors for spontaneous abortion. Acta Obstet Gynecol Scand 2003;82:182–8.

42. Andersen AM, Andersen PK, Olsen J, et al. Moderate alcohol intake during pregnancy and risk of fetal death. Int J Epidemiol 2012;41:405–13.

43. Liu Z, Ma L. Common methods used in health preservation of TCM. In: Health preservation of Traditional Chinese Medicine. Beijing: People's Medical Publishing House; 2007. p. 294–442 [Chapter 2].

44. Liu Z, Ma L. Guidance for practice in health preservation of TCM. In: Health preservation of Traditional Chinese Medicine. Beijing: People's Medical Publishing House; 2007. p. 443–568 [Chapter 3].

45. Lu HC. On the heavenly truth. In: A complete translation of the Yellow Emperor's classics of internal medicine and the difficult classic (Nei-Jing and Nan-Jing). Vancouver: International College of Traditional Chinese Medicine; 2004. p. 65–72, Section two: Essential questions [Su Wen] [Chapter 1].

46. National Collaborating Centre for Women's and Children's Health, Commissioned by the National Institute for Health and Clinical Excellence. Initial advice to people concerned about delays in conception. In: Fertility: assessment and treatment for people with fertility problems. NICE Clinical Guideline. 2nd ed. London: The Royal College of Obstetricians and Gynaecologists; 2013. p. 64–79 [Chapter 5].

47. National Collaborating Centre for Women's and Children's Health, Commissioned by the National Institute for Health and Clinical Excellence. Prediction of IVF success. In: Fertility: assessment and treatment for people with fertility problems. NICE Clinical Guideline. 2nd ed. London: The Royal College of Obstetricians and Gynaecologists; 2013. p. 217–29 [Chapter 13].

48. Practice Committee of American Society for Reproductive Medicine in collaboration with Society for Reproductive Endocrinology and Infertility. Optimizing natural fertility. Fertil Steril 2008;90:S1–6.

49. Homan GF, Davies M, Norman R. The impact of lifestyle factors on reproductive performance in the general population and those undergoing infertility treatment: a review. Hum Reprod Update 2007;13:209–23.

50. Peck JD, Leviton A, Cowan LD. A review of the epidemiologic evidence concerning the reproductive health effects of caffeine consumption: a 2000–2009 update. Food Chem Toxicol 2010;48:2549–76.

51. Nakhai-Pour HR, Broy P, Sheehy O, et al. Use of nonaspirin nonsteroidal anti-inflammatory drugs during pregnancy and the risk of spontaneous abortion. CMAJ 2011;183:1713–20.

52. Hayashi T, Miyata A, Yamada T. The impact of commonly prescribed drugs on male fertility. Hum Fertil (Camb) 2008;11:191–6.

53. Woodruff TJ, Carlson A, Schwartz JM, et al. Proceedings of the summit on environmental challenges to reproductive health and fertility: executive summary. Fertil Steril 2008;89:281–300.

54. Fisher JS. Environmental anti-androgens and male reproductive health: focus on phthalates and testicular dysgenesis syndrome. Reproduction 2004;127:305–15.

55. Akingbemi BT, Hardy MP. Oestrogenic and antiandrogenic chemicals in the environment: effects on male reproductive health. Ann Med 2001;33:391–403.

56. Garolla A, Torino M, Sartini B, et al. Seminal and molecular evidence that sauna exposure affects human spermatogenesis. Hum Reprod 2013;28:877–85.

57. Jung A, Schuppe HC. Influence of genital heat stress on semen quality in humans. Andrologia 2007;39:203–15.

58. Louis GM, Cooney MA, Lynch CD, et al. Periconception window: advising the pregnancy-planning couple. Fertil Steril 2008;89:e119–21.

59. Jauniaux E, Farquharson RG, Christiansen OB, et al. Evidence-based guidelines for the investigation and medical treatment of recurrent miscarriage. Hum Reprod 2006;21:2216–22.

60. Li TC, Makris M, Tomsu M, et al. Recurrent miscarriage:

aetiology, management and prognosis. Hum Reprod Update 2002;8:463–81.

61. Chavarro JE, Rich-Edwards JW, Rosner BA, et al. Use of multivitamins, intake of B vitamins, and risk of ovulatory infertility. Fertil Steril 2008;89:668–76.

62. Dietary supplement fact sheet. Folate – health professional fact sheet. Available from: http://ods.od.nih.gov/factsheets/Folate-HealthProfessional/ (accessed 19 June 2013).

63. Vitamin B12 – quickfacts. Available from: http://ods.od.nih.gov/factsheets/VitaminB12-QuickFacts/ (accessed 19 June 2013).

64. De-Regil LM, Palacios C, Ansary A, et al. Vitamin D supplementation for women during pregnancy. Cochrane Database Syst Rev 2012;2, CD008873.

65. Pearce H, Cheetham D. Diagnosis and management of vitamin D deficiency. BMJ 2010;340:142–7.

66. Holick MF, Binkley NC, Bischoff-Ferrari HA, et al. Evaluation, treatment, and prevention of vitamin D deficiency: an Endocrine Society clinical practice guideline. J Clin Endocrinol Metab 2011;96:1911–30.

67. Hovdenak N, Haram K. Influence of mineral and vitamin supplements on pregnancy outcome. Eur J Obstet Gynecol Reprod Biol 2012;164:127–32.

68. Ginde AA, Sullivan AF, Mansbach JM, et al. Vitamin D insufficiency in pregnant and nonpregnant women of childbearing age in the United States. Am J Obstet Gynecol 2010;202:436.e1–8.

69. Hyppönen E, Power C. Hypovitaminosis D in British adults at age 45 y: nationwide cohort study of dietary and lifestyle predictors. Am J Clin Nutr 2007;85:860–8.

70. Harris HR, Chavarro JE, Malspeis S, et al. Dairy-food, calcium, magnesium, and vitamin D intake and endometriosis: a prospective cohort study. Am J Epidemiol 2013;177:420–30.

71. Andreoli L, Piantoni S, Dall'Ara F, et al. Vitamin D and antiphospholipid syndrome. Lupus 2012;21:736–40.

72. Ozkan S, Jindal S, Greenseid K, et al. Replete vitamin D stores predict reproductive success following in vitro fertilization. Fertil Steril 2010;94:1314–9.

73. Rudick B, Ingles S, Chung K, et al. Characterizing the influence of vitamin D levels on IVF outcomes. Hum Reprod 2012;27:3321–7.

74. Li HW, Brereton RE, Anderson RA, et al. Vitamin D deficiency is common and associated with metabolic risk factors in patients with polycystic ovary syndrome. Metabolism 2011;60:1475–81.

75. Wehr E, Pilz S, Schweighofer N, et al. Association of hypovitaminosis D with metabolic disturbances in polycystic ovary syndrome. Eur J Endocrinol 2009;161:575–82.

76. WHO. Iodine deficiency, health consequences, assessment and control. In: Andersson M, de Benoist B, Darnton-Hill I, Delange F, editors. Iodine deficiency in Europe: a continuing public health problem. Geneva: WHO Press; 2007. p. 8–19.

77. De Groot L, Abalovich M, Alexander EK, et al. Management of thyroid dysfunction during pregnancy and postpartum: an Endocrine Society clinical practice guideline. J Clin Endocrinol Metab 2012;97:2543–65.

78. The British Dietetic Association. Food fact sheet. Iodine. Available from: http://www.bda.uk.com/foodfacts/Iodine.pdf (accessed 10 June 2013).

79. Cicek N, Eryilmaz OG, Sarikaya E, et al. Vitamin E effect on controlled ovarian stimulation of unexplained infertile women. J Assist Reprod Genet 2012;29:325–8.

80. Vitamin E – health professional fact sheet. Available from: http://ods.od.nih.gov/factsheets/VitaminE-HealthProfessional/ (accessed 19 June 2013).

81. Jordan RG. Prenatal omega-3 fatty acids: review and recommendations. J Midwifery Womens Health 2010;55:520–8.

82. Coletta JM, Bell SJ, Roman AS. Omega-3 fatty acids and pregnancy. Rev Obstet Gynecol 2010;3:163–71.

83. Nehra D, Le HD, Fallon EM, et al. Prolonging the female reproductive lifespan and improving egg quality with dietary omega-3 fatty acids. Aging Cell 2012;11:1046–54.

84. Hammiche F, Vujkovic M, Wijburg W, et al. Increased preconception omega-3 polyunsaturated fatty acid intake improves embryo morphology. Fertil Steril 2011;95:1820–3.

85. Rossi E, Costa M. Fish oil derivatives as a prophylaxis of recurrent miscarriage associated with antiphospholipid antibodies (APL): a pilot study. Lupus 1993;2:319–23.

86. Fish oil. MedlinePlus supplements. Available from: http://www.nlm.nih.gov/medlineplus/druginfo/natural/993.html#DrugInteractions (accessed 28 July 2013).

87. Al-Kunani AS, Knight R, Haswell SJ, et al. The selenium status of women with a history of recurrent miscarriage. BJOG 2001;108:1094–7.

88. Gärtner R, Gasnier BC, Dietrich JW, et al. Selenium supplementation in patients with autoimmune thyroiditis decreases thyroid peroxidase antibodies concentrations. J Clin Endocrinol Metab 2002;87:1687–91.

89. Dietary supplement fact sheet. Selenium – health professional fact sheet. Available from: http://ods.od.nih.gov/factsheets/Selenium-HealthProfessional/ (accessed 19 June 2013).

90. Gardiner PM, Nelson L, Shellhaas CS, et al. The clinical content of preconception care: nutrition and dietary supplements. Am J Obstet Gynecol 2008;199:S345–56.

91. Chavarro JE, Rich-Edwards JW, Rosner BA, et al. Iron intake and risk of ovulatory infertility. Obstet Gynecol 2006;108:1145–52.

92. Dietary supplement fact sheet. Iron – health professional fact sheet. Available from: http://ods.od.nih.gov/factsheets/Iron-HealthProfessional/ (accessed 19 June 2013).

93. Natali A, Turek PJ. An assessment of new sperm tests for male infertility. Urology 2011;77:1027–34.

94. Evenson D, Wixon R. Meta-analysis of sperm DNA fragmentation using

the sperm chromatin structure assay. Reprod Biomed Online 2006;12:466–72.

95. Li Z, Wang L, Cai J, et al. Correlation of sperm DNA damage with IVF and ICSI outcomes: a systematic review and meta-analysis. J Assist Reprod Genet 2006;23:367–76.

96. Henkel R, Hajimohammad M, Stalf T, et al. Influence of deoxyribonucleic acid damage on fertilization and pregnancy. Fertil Steril 2004;81:965–72.

97. Greco E, Iacobelli M, Rienzi L, et al. Reduction of the incidence of sperm DNA fragmentation by oral antioxidant treatment. J Androl 2005;26:349–53.

98. Comhaire FH, Christophe AB, Zalata AA, et al. The effects of combined conventional treatment, oral antioxidants and essential fatty acids on sperm biology in subfertile men. Prostaglandins Leukot Essent Fatty Acids 2000;63:159–65.

99. Vitamin C – quickfacts. Available from: http://ods.od.nih.gov/factsheets/VitaminC-QuickFacts/ (accessed 19 June 2013).

100. Comhaire FH, Mahmoud A. The role of food supplements in the treatment of the infertile man. Reprod Biomed Online 2003;7:385–91.

101. Sinclair S. Male infertility: nutritional and environmental considerations. Altern Med Rev 2000;5:28–38.

102. Omu AE, Al-Azemi MK, Kehinde EO, et al. Indications of the mechanisms involved in improved sperm parameters by zinc therapy. Med Princ Pract 2008;17:108–16.

103. Netter A, Hartoma R, Nahoul K. Effect of zinc administration on plasma testosterone, dihydrotestosterone, and sperm count. Arch Androl 1981;7:69–73.

104. Tikkiwal M, Ajmera RL, Mathur NK. Effect of zinc administration on seminal zinc and fertility of oligospermic males. Indian J Physiol Pharmacol 1987;31:30–4.

105. Zinc – quickfacts. Available from: http://ods.od.nih.gov/factsheets/Zinc-QuickFacts/ (accessed 19 June 2013).

106. Jensen MB, Bjerrum PJ, Jessen TE, et al. Vitamin D is positively associated with sperm motility and increases intracellular calcium in human spermatozoa. Hum Reprod 2011;26:1307–17.

107. Chavarro JE, Rich-Edwards JW, Rosner B, et al. A prospective study of dairy foods intake and anovulatory infertility. Hum Reprod 2007;22:1340–7.

108. Chavarro JE, Rich-Edwards JW, Rosner BA, et al. A prospective study of dietary carbohydrate quantity and quality in relation to risk of ovulatory infertility. Eur J Clin Nutr 2009;63:78–86.

109. Toledo E, Lopez-del Burgo C, Ruiz-Zambrana A, et al. Dietary patterns and difficulty conceiving: a nested case – control study. Fertil Steril 2011;96:1149–53.

110. Vujkovic M, de Vries JH, Lindemans J, et al. The preconception Mediterranean dietary pattern in couples undergoing in vitro fertilization/intracytoplasmic sperm injection treatment increases the chance of pregnancy. Fertil Steril 2010;94:2096–101.

111. Afeiche M, Williams PL, Mendiola J, et al. Dairy food intake in relation to semen quality and reproductive hormone levels among physically active young men. Hum Reprod 2013;28:2265–75.

112. Afeiche M, Mendiola J, Jørgensen N, et al. Dairy food intake in relation to semen quality among active young men. Fertil Steril 2012;98:S41.

113. Eslamian G, Amirjannati N, Rashidkhani B, et al. Intake of food groups and idiopathic asthenozoospermia: a case-control study. Hum Reprod 2012;27:3328–36.

114. Chavarro JE, Afeiche M, Mendiola J, et al. Carbohydrate intake and semen quality among young men. Fertil Steril 2012;98:S47.

115. Robbins WA, Xun L, FitzGerald LZ, et al. Walnuts improve semen quality in men consuming a Western-style diet: randomized control dietary intervention trial. Biol Reprod 2012;87:1–8.

116. Unschuld PU, Tessenow H, Jinsheng Z. Discourse on how the Qi in depots follow the pattern of the seasons. In: Huang Di Nei Jing Su Wen, vol 1. Berkeley: University of California Press; 2011. p. 384–400 [Chapter 22].

117. Unschuld PU, Tessenow H, Jinsheng Z. Further discourse on the conduit vessels. In: Huang Di Nei Jing Su Wen, vol 1. Berkeley: University of California Press; 2011. p. 369–81 [Chapter 21].

118. Leggett D. Patterns of disharmony: deficiency and excess. In: Helping ourselves: a guide to traditional chinese food energetics. 2nd ed. Totnes: Meridian; 1995. p. 21–35 [Chapter 2].

119. Lu HC. Blood. In: Syndromes in Traditional Chinese Medicine. Marston: CreateSpace Independent Publishing Platform; 2013. p. 163–84 [Chapter 20].

120. Lu HC. Liver. In: Syndromes in Traditional Chinese Medicine. Marston: CreateSpace Independent Publishing Platform; 2013. p. 360–85 [Chapter 32].

121. Lu HC. Yin. In: Syndromes in Traditional Chinese Medicine. Marston: CreateSpace Independent Publishing Platform; 2013. p. 96–100 [Chapter 12].

122. Lu HC. Kidneys. In: Syndromes in Traditional Chinese Medicine. Marston: CreateSpace Independent Publishing Platform; 2013. p. 328–54 [Chapter 30].

123. Pitchford P. The roots of diagnosis and treatment. In: Healing with whole foods: Asian traditions and modern nutrition. 3rd ed. Berkeley, California: North Atlantic Books; 2002. p. 47–102 [Chapter 1].

124. Lu HC. Yang. In: Syndromes in Traditional Chinese Medicine. Marston: CreateSpace Independent Publishing Platform; 2013. p. 101–16 [Chapter 13].

125. Pitchford P. The five element and organ system. In: Healing with whole foods: Asian traditions and modern nutrition. 3rd ed. Berkeley, Calif: North Atlantic Books; 2002. p. 303–68 [Chapter 3].

126. Lu HC. Deficiency. In: Syndromes in Traditional Chinese Medicine. Marston: CreateSpace Independent Publishing Platform; 2013. p. 135–47 [Chapter 17].

127. Lu HC. Fire. In: Syndromes in Traditional Chinese Medicine. Marston: CreateSpace Independent

Publishing Platform; 2013. p. 75–82 [Chapter 6].

128. Lu HC. Cold. In: Syndromes in Traditional Chinese Medicine. Marston: CreateSpace Independent Publishing Platform; 2013. p. 31–40 [Chapter 2].

129. Wise LA, Rothman KJ, Mikkelsen EM, et al. A prospective cohort study of physical activity and time to pregnancy. Fertil Steril 2012;97:1136–42e4.

130. Gaskins AJ, Mendiola J, Afeiche M, et al. Br J Sports Med Published Online First: February 2013. http://dx.doi.org/10.1136/bjsports-2012-091644.

131. Wise LA, Cramer DW, Hornstein MD, et al. Physical activity and semen quality among men attending an infertility clinic. Fertil Steril 2011;95:1025–30.

132. Li B, Zhou H, Li W. Bed rest after embryo transfer. Eur J Obstet Gynecol Reprod Biol 2011;155:125–8.

133. Hjollund NHI, Jensen TK, Bonde JPE, et al. Spontaneous abortion and physical strain around implantation: a follow-up study of first-pregnancy planners. Epidemiology 2000;11:18–23.

134. Attarchi M, Darkhi H, Khodarahmian M, et al. Characteristics of menstrual cycle in shift workers. Glob J Health Sci 2013;5:163–72.

135. Labyak S, Lava S, Turek F, et al. Effects of shiftwork on sleep and menstrual function in nurses. Health Care Women Int 2002;23:703–14.

136. Lawson CC, Whelan EA, Lividoti Hibert EN, et al. Rotating shift work and menstrual cycle characteristics. Epidemiology 2011;22:305–12.

137. Nurminen T. Shift work and reproductive health. Scand J Work Environ Health 1998;24(Suppl. 3): 28–34.

138. Bisanti L, Olsen J, Basso O, et al. Shift work and subfecundity: a European multicenter study. European study group on infertility and subfecundity. J Occup Environ Med 1996;38:352–8.

139. Barron ML. Light exposure, melatonin secretion, and menstrual cycle parameters: an integrative review. Biol Res Nurs 2007;9:49–69.

140. Barron ML. Fertility literacy for women in primary care settings. J Nurse Pract 2013;9:161–5.

141. Campagne DM. Should fertilization treatment start with reducing stress? Hum Reprod 2006;21:1651–8.

142. Louis GM, Lum KJ, Sundaram R, et al. Stress reduces conception probabilities across the fertile window: evidence in support of relaxation. Fertil Steril 2011;95:2184–9.

143. Nakamura K, Sheps S, Clara Arck P. Stress and reproductive failure: past notions, present insights and future directions. J Assist Reprod Genet 2008;25:47–62.

144. Catherino WH. Stress relief to augment fertility: the pressure mounts. Fertil Steril 2011;95:2462–3.

145. Wagenmaker ER, Breen KM, Oakley AE, et al. Psychosocial stress inhibits amplitude of gonadotropin-releasing hormone pulses independent of cortisol action on the type II glucocorticoid receptor. Endocrinology 2009;150:762–9.

146. King JA, Rosal MC, Ma Y, et al. Association of stress, hostility and plasma testosterone levels. Neuro Endocrinol Lett 2005;26:355–60.

147. Fenster L, Waller K, Chen J, et al. Psychological stress in the workplace and menstrual function. Am J Epidemiol 1999;149:127–34.

148. Hall E, Burt VK. Male fertility: psychiatric considerations. Fertil Steril 2012;97:434–9.

149. Jóźków P, Mędraś M. Psychological stress and the function of male gonads. Endokrynol Pol 2012;63:44–9.

150. Gollenberg AL, Liu F, Brazil C, et al. Semen quality in fertile men in relation to psychosocial stress. Fertil Steril 2010;93:1104–11.

151. Fenster L, Katz DF, Wyrobek AJ, et al. Effects of psychological stress on human semen quality. J Androl 1997;18:194–202.

152. Vellani E, Colasante A, Mamazza L, et al. Association of state and trait anxiety to semen quality of in vitro fertilization patients: a controlled study. Fertil Steril 2013;99: 1565–72.

153. Li Y, Lin H, Li Y, et al. Association between socio-psycho-behavioral factors and male semen quality: systematic review and meta-analyses. Fertil Steril 2011;95:116–23.

154. Matthiesen SM, Frederiksen Y, Ingerslev HJ, et al. Stress, distress and outcome of assisted reproductive technology (ART): a meta-analysis. Hum Reprod 2011;26:2763–76.

155. Li W, Newell-Price J, Jones GL, et al. Relationship between psychological stress and recurrent miscarriage. Reprod Biomed Online 2012;25:180–9.

156. Nepomnaschy PA, Welch KB, McConnell DS, et al. Cortisol levels and very early pregnancy loss in humans. Proc Natl Acad Sci USA 2006;103:3938–42.

157. Olivius C, Friden B, Borg G, et al. Why do couples discontinue in vitro fertilization treatment? A cohort study. Fertil Steril 2004;81:258–61.

158. Domar AD. Impact of psychological factors on dropout rates in insured infertility patients. Fertil Steril 2004;81:271–3.

159. ASRM. Patient fact sheet. Stress and infertility. Available from: http://www.asrm.org/Stress_and_Infertility_factsheet; 2008 (accessed 20 June 2013).

160. Cwikel J, Gidron Y, Sheiner E. Psychological interactions with infertility among women. Eur J Obstet Gynecol Reprod Biol 2004;117:126–31.

161. Salmela-Aro K, Suikkari AM. Letting go of your dreams—adjustment of child-related goal appraisals and depressive symptoms during infertility treatment. J Res Pers 2008;42:988–1003.

162. Beaurepaire J, Jones M, Thiering P, et al. Psychosocial adjustment to infertility and its treatment: male and female responses at different stages of IVF/ET treatment. J Psychosom Res 1994;38:229–40.

163. Vahratian A, Smith YR, Dorman M, et al. Longitudinal depressive symptoms and state anxiety among women using assisted reproductive technology. Fertil Steril 2011;95:1192–4.

164. Domar AD, Conboy L, Denardo-Roney J, et al. Lifestyle behaviors in women undergoing in vitro fertilization: a prospective study. Fertil Steril 2012;97: 697–700, e1.

165. Cheung C, Chan C, Ng E. Stress and anxiety-depression levels following first-trimester miscarriage: a comparison between women who conceived naturally and women who conceived with assisted reproduction. BJOG 2013;120:1090–7. Available from: http://dx.doi.org/10.1111/1471-0528.12251.

166. Cousineau TM, Domar AD. Psychological impact of infertility. Best Pract Res Clin Obstet Gynaecol 2007;21:293–308.

167. Schmidt L. Psychosocial burden of infertility and assisted reproduction. Lancet 2006;367:379–80.

168. Bleil ME, Pasch LA, Gregorich SE, et al. Fertility treatment response: is it better to be more optimistic or less pessimistic? Psychosom Med 2012;74:193–9.

169. Domar AD, Rooney KL, Wiegand B, et al. Impact of a group mind/body intervention on pregnancy rates in IVF patients. Fertil Steril 2011;95:2269–73.

170. Hämmerli K, Znoj H, Barth J. The efficacy of psychological interventions for infertile patients: a meta-analysis examining mental health and pregnancy rate. Hum Reprod Update 2009;15:279–95.

171. Dunson DB, Baird DD, Colombo B. Increased infertility with age in men and women. Obstet Gynecol 2004;103:51–6.

172. Maciocia G. Early periods. In: Obstetrics and Gynecology in Chinese medicine. 2nd ed. Edinburgh: Elsevier Health Sciences; 2011. p. 201–11 [Chapter 8].

173. Unschuld PU, Tessenow H, Jinsheng Z. Discourse on the true [Qi endowed by] Heaven in high antiquity. In: Huang Di Nei Jing Su Wen, vol. 1. Berkeley: University of California Press; 2011. p. 29–44 [Chapter 1].

174. Isoyama D, Cordts F.B, de Souza van Niewegen AM. Effect of acupuncture on symptoms of anxiety in women undergoing in vitro fertilisation: a prospective randomised controlled study. Acupuncture Med 2012;30:85–8.

175. Kovárová P, Smith CA, Turnbull DA. An exploratory study of the effect of acupuncture on self-efficacy for women seeking fertility support. Explore (NY) 2010;6:330–4.

176. Balk J, Catov J, Horn B, et al. The relationship between perceived stress, acupuncture, and pregnancy rates among IVF patients: a pilot study. Complement Ther Clin Pract 2010;16:154–7.

177. Magarelli PC, Cohen M, Cridennda DK. Proposed mechanism of action of acupuncture on IVF outcomes. Fertil Steril 2006;86:S174–S175.

178. Hampton KD, Mazza D, Newton JM. Fertility-awareness knowledge, attitudes, and practices of women seeking fertility assistance. J Adv Nurs 2013;69:1076–84. Available from: http://dx.doi.org/10.1111/j.1365-2648.2012.06095.x.

179. Gianotten W, Schade A. Sexuality and fertility issues. In: de Haan N, Spelt M, Gobel R, editors. Reproductive medicine: a textbook for paramedics. Amsterdam: Elsevier Gezondheidszorg; 2010. p. 167–78 [Chapter 13].

180. Bigelow JL, Dunson DB, Stanford JB, et al. Mucus observations in the fertile window: a better predictor of conception than timing of intercourse. Hum Reprod 2004;19:889–92.

181. Dunson DB, Colombo B, Baird DD. Changes with age in the level and duration of fertility in the menstrual cycle. Hum Reprod 2002;17: 1399–403.

182. Gildersleeve KA, Haselton MG, Larson CM, et al. Body odor attractiveness as a cue of impending ovulation in women: evidence from a study using hormone-confirmed ovulation. Horm Behav 2012;61:157–66.

183. Singh D, Bronstad PM. Female body odour is a potential cue to ovulation. Proc Biol Sci 2001;268:797–801.

184. Durante KM, Li NP, Haselton MG. Changes in women's choice of dress across the ovulatory cycle: naturalistic and laboratory task-based evidence. Pers Soc Psychol Bull 2008;34:1451–60.

185. Fessler DM. No time to eat: an adaptationist account of periovulatory behavioral changes. Q Rev Biol 2003;78:3–21.

186. Tarín JJ, Gómez-Piquer V. Do women have a hidden heat period? Hum Reprod 2002;17:2243–8.

187. Wilcox AJ, Baird DD, Dunson DB, et al. On the frequency of intercourse around ovulation: evidence for biological influences. Hum Reprod 2004;19:1539–43.

188. Bak CW, Lyu SW, Seok HH, et al. Erectile dysfunction and extramarital sex induced by timed intercourse: a prospective study of 439 men. J Androl 2012;33:1245–53.

189. Peterson BD, Newton CR, Feingold T. Anxiety and sexual stress in men and women undergoing infertility treatment. Fertil Steril 2007;88:911–4.

190. Wilcox AJ, Weinberg CR, Baird DD. Timing of sexual intercourse in relation to ovulation. Effects on the probability of conception, survival of the pregnancy, and sex of the baby. N Engl J Med 1995;333:1517–21.

191. Starr C, McMillan B. Reproductive systems. In: Human biology. Belmont, CA: Brooks/Cole Cengager Learning; 2012. p. 307–30, Chapter 15.

192. Levitas E, Lunenfeld E, Weiss N, et al. Relationship between the duration of sexual abstinence and semen quality: analysis of 9,489 semen samples. Fertil Steril 2005;83:1680–6.

193. Pound N, Javed MH, Ruberto C, et al. Duration of sexual arousal predicts semen parameters for masturbatory ejaculates. Physiol Behav 2002;76:685–9.

194. Stanford JB, White GL, Hatasaka H. Timing intercourse to achieve pregnancy: current

evidence. Obstet Gynecol 2002;100:1333–41.

195. Scarpa B, Dunson DB, Colombo B. Cervical mucus secretions on the day of intercourse: an accurate marker of highly fertile days. Eur J Obstet Gynecol Reprod Biol 2006;125:72–8.

196. Cortesi S, Rigoni G, Zen F, et al. Correlation of plasma gonadotrophins and ovarian steroids pattern with symptomatic changes in cervical mucus during the menstrual cycle in normal cycling women. Contraception 1981;23:629–41.

197. Ovulation detection. ASRM. Fact sheets and info booklets. Available from: http://www.intute.ac.uk/healthandlifesciences/cgi-bin/fullrecord.pl?handle=2024927.

198. Tanabe K, Susumu N, Hand K, et al. Prediction of the potentially fertile period by urinary hormone measurements using a new home-use monitor: comparison with laboratory hormone analyses. Hum Reprod 2001;16:1619–24.

199. Guida M, Tommaselli GA, Palomba S, et al. Efficacy of methods for determining ovulation in a natural family planning program. Fertil Steril 1999;72:900–4.

200. A translation of Zhu Dan-xi's Ge Zhi Yu Lun. Admonitions on sexual desire. In: Extra treatises based on investigation and inquiry: Translated by Yang Shou-zhong, Duan Wu-jin. Edited by: Flaws B. Boulder, CO: Blue Poppy Press; 1994. p. 3–4.

201. Maciocia G. The causes of disease. In: The foundations of Chinese medicine: a comprehensive text for acupuncturists and herbalists. Edinburgh, New York: Churchill Livingstone; 1989. p. 127–42 [Chapter 15].

202. Wilms S. Nurturing life in classical Chinese medicine: sun Simiao on healing without drugs, transforming bodies and cultivating life. J Chin Med 2010;5–13.

203. Lu HC. Spirit as the fundamental of needling. In: A complete translation of the Yellow Emperor's classics of internal medicine and the difficult classic (Nei-Jing and Nan-Jing). Vancouver: International College of Traditional Chinese Medicine; 2004. p. 402–4, Section three: Spiritual pivot [Ling Shu] [Chapter 8].

204. Dray F, Reinberg A, Sebaoun J. Biological rhythm of plasma free testosterone in healthy adult males: existence of a circadian variation. C R Acad Sci Hebd Seances Acad Sci D 1965;261:573–6.

205. Furth C. The development of Fuke in the Song Dynasties. In: A Flourishing Yin: Gender in China's Medical History, 960–1665. California and Los Angeles: University of California Press; 1999. p. 59–93 [Chapter 2].

Chapter | 8 |

Identification and management of conditions detrimental to IVF outcome

Conditions such as ovulatory dysfunction, tubal pathology, endometriosis, thyroid disease, and male factor subfertility reduce the chances of natural conception and may adversely affect Assisted Reproductive Technology (ART) treatment outcomes and/or pregnancy. Acupuncture treatment in preparation for ART treatment may help to reduce the severity of these conditions and, therefore, increase the chances of live birth.

TUBAL PATHOLOGY

Overview

As described in Chapters 2 and 3, successful conception occurs when sperm travel through the fallopian tube to the egg and fertilize it, and then the resulting embryo travels down the fallopian tube and implants in the uterus. If the fallopian tube is blocked or if it hypofunctions, tubal factor subfertility will be the result. One or both tubes can be affected.

Prevalence

Tubal disorders contribute to 14–26% of infertility.[1–3]

Aetiology

Pelvic inflammatory disease secondary to infection (for example, gonorrhoea or chlamydia), severe endometriosis, and postsurgical adhesions or nonpelvic infections (for example, from appendicitis or diverticulitis) can cause tubal factor infertility.[4] Hydrosalpinx (or hydrosalpinges if both sides are affected) damages fertility through distal

tubal obstruction; the accumulating fluid can leak into the uterus and is believed to be toxic to the embryo.[4]

Diagnosis

Tubal disease can be diagnosed by ultrasound, Hysterosalpingography (HSG), Hysterosalpingo-contrast-ultrasonography, Sonohysterography, Laparoscopy with dye, and Fluoroscopic/hysteroscopic selective tubal cannulation. The Chlamydia Antibody Test (CAT) checks for the presence of antibodies to *Chlamydia trachomatis*, which is associated with tubal disease. If the CAT is normal, the likelihood of tubal obstruction is reduced to approximately 8%.[5] The merits of each diagnostic technique are discussed in Chapter 4.

> **INTERESTING FACTS**
>
> **TUBAL BLOCKAGE**
>
> Interestingly, about 60% of patients diagnosed by HSG with proximal tubal blockage are subsequently shown to have patent tubes on the next HSG[6] or laparoscopy.[7]
>
> HSG may have a therapeutic role, with higher pregnancy rates reported in the months following HSG.[8]

Orthodox medical treatment

Treatment options for tubal blockage are corrective surgery or IVF. There are no Randomized Controlled Trials (RCTs) comparing the benefits of corrective surgery with no treatment or IVF.[9,10]

According to the Practice Committee of the American Society for Reproductive Medicine (ASRM), corrective surgery may be beneficial, depending on factors such as:[10]

- Woman's age and ovarian reserve
- Quality and quantity of sperm
- Site and extent of tubal disease
- Other infertility factors
- Risk of ectopic pregnancy
- Patient's preference
- Success rates and cost of IVF

In the United Kingdom, the National Institute for Health and Clinical Excellence recommends that women with mild tubal disease may benefit from surgery.[9]

Impact on ART treatment

Blocked fallopian tubes

Fallopian tube blockage does not affect the success rates of IVF because the egg(s) are surgically removed and are then fertilized with sperm in the laboratory. The embryo(s) are subsequently transferred directly into the uterus.

Hydrosalpinges

Hydrosalpinx is defined as a 'collection of watery fluid in the uterine tube, occurring as the end-stage of pyosalpinx'.[11] It is strongly associated with reduced implantation rates.[11] The fluid within the tube is believed to be toxic to the embryo. The mechanical washout of the embryo by the fluid is another possible explanation for reduced implantation rates.[11] Laparoscopic salpingectomy (removal of the affected fallopian tube(s)) prior to IVF improves IVF and pregnancy outcomes.[11,12]

The role of the acupuncturist

Acupuncture treatment

As already stated, about 60% of patients diagnosed by HSG with proximal tubal blockage are subsequently shown to have patent tubes on the next HSG[6] or laparoscopy.[7] Therefore, fallopian tube obstruction is not always permanent. If a patient wishes, a course of 3–4 months of corrective acupuncture treatment may be attempted before IVF to improve patency of the fallopian tubes and, therefore, increase the chances of natural conception. Treatment with acupuncture should only be attempted if:

- There are no other indications for IVF (for example, male factor subfertility).
- Fallopian tubes have not been previously surgically removed (for example, following ectopic surgery).
- Fallopian tubes are not absent (for example, because of an anatomical birth defect).
- The damage to the fallopian tubes is not permanent (such as extensive adhesions or scarring).

In Traditional Chinese Medicine (TCM), healthy functioning of the fallopian tubes depends on the free movement of Liver Qi and the moving function of Kidney Yang. Liver Qi Stagnation leads to Blood Stasis.[13,14] Deficiency of Kidney Yang leads to Damp-Phlegm accumulation in the fallopian tubes.[13] Damp-Heat may be implicated in patients whose tubal blockage is caused by infection(s).[13,15] Table 8.1 lists acupuncture points that can be used in the treatment of mild tubal factor infertility. Chapter 5 describes TCM syndromes in greater detail.

Referral for hydrosalpinges surgery

In our experience, not all patients with evidence of hydrosalpinges are adequately managed by the Orthodox medical team. Some patients undergo and fail several cycles of IVF without realizing that the failed IVF may

Table 8.1 Acupuncture points prescriptions for mild tubal factor infertility

Syndromes	Points	Rationale
Liver Qi Stagnation + Blood Stasis	LIV3, LIV4, LIV5	Regulate Qi in the lateral abdomen and the fallopian tubes[15,16] Moxibustion may be applicable if Stagnation is caused by Cold
	P7, P5	Calm Shen (Spirit) if emotions lead to Liver Qi Stagnation[16]
Kidney Yang Deficiency + Damp-Phlegm	ST28, SP9, SP6, REN9, BL32	Resolve Damp and drain Dampness from the genital system[14]
Damp-Heat	GB41R + SJ5L + GB26	Regulate Dai Mai (Girdle Vessel) and resolve Damp-Heat in the genital system[14]
	LIV5 + LIV8	Clear Damp-Heat and eliminate Blood Stasis in the Lower Jiao[16]
Other prescriptions relevant for all syndromes		• Electroacupuncture: BL32 (negative pole) + REN4 (positive pole)[14] • Acupuncture: ZIGONG + REN3, REN14 SP12 + SP13[16] • Moxibustion: REN8, REN4, REN3 and on the area corresponding to fallopian tubes[17]

be caused by the presence of hydrosalpinges. Therefore, all utero-tubal investigation reports should be carefully reviewed to see if hydrosalpinges were observed, and any identified patients should be referred for possible corrective surgery.

Referral for IVF

Patients with tubal obstruction who do not conceive naturally after a course of 3–4 months of acupuncture should be referred for IVF. Figure 8.1 summarizes the tubal factor infertility patient management pathway.

Figure 8.1 Algorithm of tubal factor infertility patient management with acupuncture.

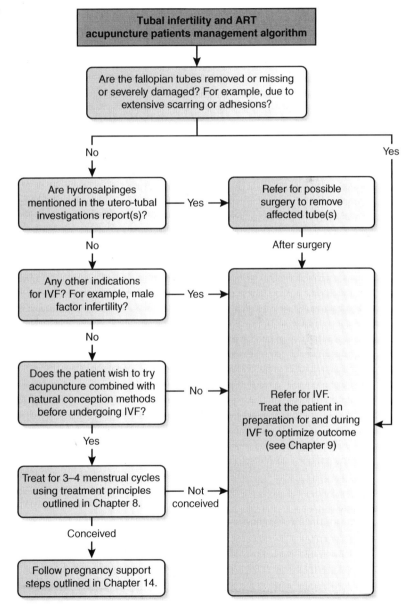

INTERESTING FACTS

EFFECTIVENESS OF ACUPUNCTURE DURING IVF IN PATIENTS WITH TUBAL INFERTILITY

Acupuncture has been shown to increase IVF implantation rates in patients with tubal factor infertility compared to a control group (48% and 12%, respectively).[18] In another study, acupuncture in patients with idiopathic and tubal-uterine factors increased implantation rates fivefold compared to the control group.[19]

 Case study

Tubal Factor Infertility

Julie was 35 years old and had a 2-year history of subfertility caused by blockage of her right fallopian tube. She had one pregnancy at the age of 21, which resulted in a termination.

Julie and her husband were considering IVF. However, their GP had suggested they continue trying to conceive naturally because there was still a chance of natural conception as her left tube was functional. Julie decided to try acupuncture.

Manifestations

- Menses: small clots, red menstrual blood, brown at the end of menstruation
- Ovulation pain
- Loose stools
- Frequent and a large amount of urine
- Felt the cold; liked a hot bath
- Disturbed sleep, a lot of dreams
- Anxious and worried because everyone around her was having babies
- Observations: Shen Mind and Spirit appeared depressed
- Pulse: fine, right rear position deep and weak
- Tongue: red, swollen, some Heat spots around the tip

TCM Diagnosis

- Spleen Qi Deficiency with Dampness
- Stagnation
- Kidney Yang Deficiency with some Cold
- Heart Heat

First Acupuncture Treatment Prescription

SP4 + P6, ST29, ST36, ZIGONG (moxa), and LI4 + LIV3
Julie became pregnant after 3 months of acupuncture treatment and has a healthy daughter.

OVULATORY DISORDERS

Overview

Ovulatory dysfunction is one of the most common causes of female infertility and is identified in approximately 20–32% of infertile women.[1,2] A menstrual history of regular 25- to 35-day cycles is usually sufficient to assume normal ovulation. Cycles of between 35 and 180 days are referred to as oligomenorrhoea, and such cycle patterns are likely to be associated with an ovulation disorder. Cycles over 180 days are classified as amenorrhoea and are very strongly associated with an absence of ovulation.[20] Anovulation can be confirmed by checking progesterone levels at the midluteal phase (see Chapter 4).

The World Health Organization (WHO) classifies anovulatory disorders into three categories. Table 8.2 compares these three categories.

WHO grade I ovulation disorders

The most beneficial treatment for this group of patients is the use of a Luteinizing Hormone Releasing Hormone (LHRH)/ Gonadotrophin Releasing Hormone (GnRH) pulse pump system. LHRH is injected intravenously via a mini pump at 90 min intervals. This induces an increased production of Follicle Stimulating Hormone (FSH) and LH, resulting in improved pituitary–ovarian feedback. Alternatively, FSH treatment (gonadotrophins) may be used if LHRH fails.[20] Chapter 9 provides an acupuncture treatment protocol for ovulation induction with the LHRH pulse pump system.

Patients who have high prolactin levels may be administered a dopamine agonist to lower these levels; this re-establishes LHRH release. Ovulation returns in 80% of patients, and 65% of them will eventually conceive.[20]

WHO grade II ovulation disorders and clomiphene citrate treatment

Eighty-five percent of ovulatory disorders meet this classification criteria;[20] 85% of these patients have Polycystic Ovary Syndrome (PCOS).[20] Many grade II ovulation disorder patients are overweight, and this often affects their hormonal balance. Therefore, weight loss should be a first-line treatment for these patients.[20] If lifestyle modifications are not successful in reducing weight, then other treatment options may need to be considered. For example, the ASRM considers ovulation induction with Clomiphene Citrate (CC) (sometimes referred to by its brand name Clomid) to be 'the best initial treatment for the large majority of anovulatory infertile women'.[21] CC works by increasing GnRH pulse frequency (in ovulatory women)[21,22] or pulse amplitude (in anovulatory women, such as PCOS patients).[21,23] CC causes both LH and FSH to rise during the course of treatment.

Table 8.2 WHO classification of ovulatory disorders

	Grade I Hypogonadotrophic hypogonadal anovulation	Grade II Normogonadotrophic normooestrogenic anovulation	Grade III Hypergonadotrophic hypooestrogenic anovulation
Incidence	Affects 10% of women with ovulatory disorders. Associated with low weight, excessive exercise, or stress-induced amenorrhea.[20]	Affects 85% of women with ovulatory disorders and is mostly associated with Polycystic Ovary Syndrome (PCOS), stress, or obesity.[20]	Affects 5% of ovulatory disorders. Associated primarily with ovarian failure.[20]
Menstrual cycle	History of amenorrhoea	History of oligomenorrhoea or possible history of amenorrhoea	Possible history of amenorrhoea
Oestrogen	Low[20]	Normal[20]	Low[20]
FSH	Normal or low	Normal[20]	High[20]
LH	Normal or low	Normal or high[20]	High[20]
Prolactin	Normal or high (in hyperprolactinaemia)[20]	Normal	Normal
Other	Low Gonadotrophin Releasing Hormone (GnRH) or unresponsive pituitary, leading to low Follicle Stimulating Hormone (FSH) and Luteinizing Hormone (LH) Negative response to progestogen challenge test (no withdrawal bleed)	Positive response to progestogen challenge test (withdrawal bleed)	

Indications for CC are:

- Anovulation (WHO grade II)[20]
- Luteal phase deficiency[21]
- Unexplained infertility[21]

The ASRM guidelines state that CC therapy is of no value to women with high FSH levels, those with hypothalamic/pituitary dysfunction, and those with uterine or tubal factors. Therefore, the presence of these conditions needs to be excluded before a patient starts CC therapy. Severe male factor infertility also needs to be excluded.[21] Chapter 9 provides the acupuncture treatment protocol for ovulation induction with CC.

In 'clomiphene-resistant' patients (patients who fail to regain ovulatory cycles after 150 mg of CC), in 'clomiphene-failure' patients (patients who have regained ovulatory cycles, but no pregnancy has been achieved after 6–8 ovulatory cycles), and in patients who experience severe adverse effects caused by CC (such as headaches, abdominal pain, and visual disturbances), CC plus Metformin, Laparoscopic Electrocoagulation of the Ovaries (LEO), and FSH gonadotrophins are indicated:

- In addition to usual CC therapy, Metformin can be taken daily (500–2000 mg, split into two to three doses) until a positive pregnancy test is achieved. It is effective in PCOS patients because it increases insulin

sensitivity. The expectation is that pregnancy should be achieved within 6–8 ovulatory cycles.[20]

- LEO, or 'ovarian drilling', is indicated for patients with enlarged ovaries with an excessive number of follicles. The ovary is injected with an electrocoagulation needle in 3–6 places with the intention of destroying some ovarian tissues and therefore reducing the number of follicles. This, in turn, is believed to normalize androgen, LH, and insulin levels. LEO is effective in achieving ovulation in 50% of cases.[20]

- Ovulation induction with FSH is recommended in patients who fail to conceive following CC therapy. This treatment protocol is 90% successful in achieving ovulation and has a 50% pregnancy rate. It can be repeated for a total of 6–8 cycles.[20,24] Chapter 9 provides the acupuncture treatment protocol for treating patients undergoing FSH ovulation induction therapy.

WHO grade III ovulation disorder

WHO grade III disorder is referred to as *depleted ovarian reserve*. The only treatment available for this disorder is third-party ART, such as IVF using donated oocytes.

Figure 8.2 summarizes the treatment pathway in ovulatory disorder patients.

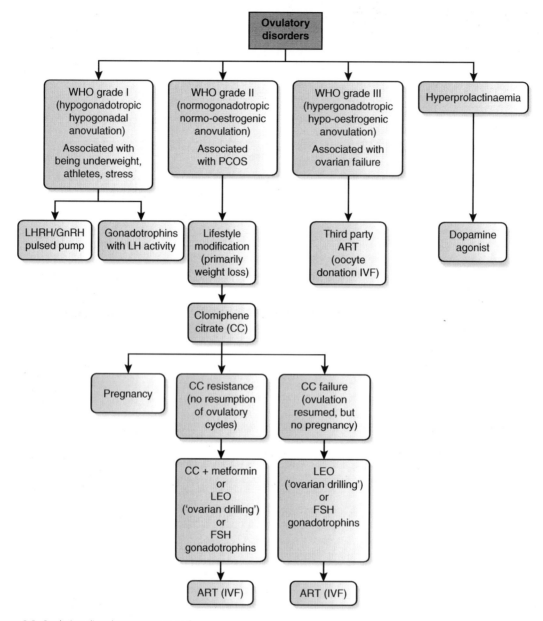

Figure 8.2 Ovulation disorders treatment pathway.

POLYCYSTIC OVARY SYNDROME

Overview and diagnosis

PCOS is a disorder characterized by a broad spectrum of signs and symptoms, including anovulation, menstrual irregularities, signs of androgen excess (hyperandrogenism), insulin resistance, and hyperinsulinaemia.

At the 2003 European Society of Human Reproduction and Embryology (ESHRE)/ASRM-sponsored PCOS consensus workshop group held in Rotterdam, it was agreed that patients should be diagnosed with PCOS if they have two of three of the following:[25]

- Oligo- and/or anovulation
- Clinical and/or biochemical signs of hyperandrogenism (hirsutism is the most reliable

sign). Biochemical assessment of hyperandrogenism should include 'free testosterone (T) or the free T (free androgen) index'.

- Polycystic ovaries (PCO): the presence of 12 or more follicles in each ovary that measure 2–9 mm in diameter and/or increased ovarian volume (>10 mL). 'Only one ovary fitting this definition is sufficient to define PCO'.

Other diseases with similar presentation (for example, congenital adrenal hyperplasias, androgen-secreting tumours, Cushing syndrome) should be excluded.[25]

Oligomenorrhoea and amenorrhoea are strong predictors of PCOS, and up to 90% of women with these menstrual abnormalities are diagnosed with PCOS.[26] Women with oligomenorrhoea and amenorrhoea may still experience spontaneous ovulation.[26] The greater the severity of menstrual irregularities, the greater the severity of PCOS.[26] As women with PCOS become older, their cycles become more regular.[26]

Hirsutism is present in about 70% of women with PCOS and is a reliable marker of hyperandrogenemia although blood tests should always be carried out in all women suspected of having PCOS.[26] Acne and alopecia are not reliable markers of hyperandrogenemia.[26]

CLINICAL TIPS

HIRSUTISM AND PCOS

Hirsutism is the most reliable sign of androgen excess. However, many women with hirsutism will have had it treated with laser treatment or may use creams or epilators to remove excess hair. Therefore, it is important to ask patients if they have ever suffered from excess facial or abdominal hair.

There are several different phenotypes of PCOS, presenting with various degrees of metabolic disorder, insulin resistance, menstrual cycle abnormalities, weight issues, hirsutism, and subfertility.[26]

Women with PCOS are at increased risk of developing diabetes. Therefore, an oral glucose tolerance test should be done in obese women with PCOS and/or women with increased visceral adiposity, as measured by waist circumference.[26]

Prevalence

PCOS is the most common endocrine disorder in women, affecting up to 15% of women.[20] WHO grade II ovulation disorders represent 85% of ovulatory disorders, and PCOS patients account for 85% of grade II ovulation disorders.[20]

Pathology

Extensive evidence shows that reproductive dysfunction in PCOS patients is caused directly by hyperinsulinaemia.[26] PCOS is also associated with metabolic syndrome.[26] Many PCOS patients are overweight, and this often affects their hormonal balance.[20]

Effect on reproduction

Ovarian reserve

The reproductive lifespan of women with PCOS can extend on average 2 years beyond that of women with normal ovulatory cycles.[27]

Miscarriages

There is conflicting data on PCOS and miscarriages[26,28] and no strong evidence that PCOS *per se* increases rates of miscarriage.[26,28] However, women with PCOS are often overweight or obese; this increases their risk of miscarriage and pregnancy loss.[29]

Pregnancy

Pregnant women who are diagnosed with PCOS are at risk of developing gestational diabetes,[26,30,31] preeclampsia,[26,31] and cardiovascular disease,[31] which are all associated with poorer pregnancy outcomes. The rate of preterm delivery is also higher in women with PCOS.[30]

There may be epigenetic implications for an embryo or foetus that develops in a high-androgen maternal environment. The high circulatory levels of androgens may have an effect on the subsequent genetic expression of the neonate's reproductive and metabolic physiology when it reaches reproductive maturity.[26]

Mental–emotional health

Women with PCOS are at an increased risk of psychological and behavioural disorders and experience a poorer quality of life.[26] Therefore, the medical management of PCOS should include psychological and behavioural therapeutic approaches.[26,32]

Orthodox medical management of PCOS

The optimal treatment of women with PCOS has still not been defined. Proposed treatments include lifestyle and dietary modifications, pharmaceutical treatment (for example, CC therapy as discussed earlier), surgical procedures (for example, ovarian drilling), and ART.[33]

Lifestyle and dietary modifications

Many PCOS patients are overweight, which often affects their hormonal balance[20,26] and their menstrual regularity and is associated with hyperandrogenemia and hirsutism.[26] Greater abdominal or visceral adiposity is linked to greater insulin resistance, which exacerbates PCOS.[26] Therefore, weight reduction through diet and exercise should be a first-line approach for these patients.[20,33]

A 2007 ESHRE/ASRM-Sponsored PCOS Consensus Workshop Group in Thessaloniki recommended that obese women with PCOS should follow a hypocaloric diet (with a 500 kcal/day deficit) with reduced glycaemic load. If such a regimen cannot be adopted, then any calorie-restricted diet that achieves a 5% weight loss should be used.[33]

A 2013 systematic review of various dietary approaches in the management of PCOS found that no dietary plan is preferable for women with PCOS. All of the investigated dietary plans led to improvements in pregnancy rate, menstrual regularity, ovulation, hyperandrogenism, insulin resistance, lipids, and quality of life.[34] However, the review did find that a low glycaemic index (GI) diet resulted in increased menstrual regularity compared with a 'healthy weight loss diet', and both low a GI diet and a low carbohydrate diet resulted in a decrease in insulin resistance.[34]

Women with PCOS tend to have lower baseline activity levels, which further exacerbates their symptomatology. Therefore, increased physical activity is recommended.[33]

In our experience, some women with PCOS can have very low BMI. These women tend to very carefully monitor their weight. Some of these women may be underweight and, therefore, may need to gain weight (see Chapter 7 for recommended BMI cut off points).

Ovulation induction

CC is the first choice treatment to induce ovulation in anovulatory women with PCOS.[33] If the treatment with CC fails, ovulation induction with gonadotrophins and GnRH analogues should be tried.[33] These treatments were discussed in detail earlier in this chapter.

Metformin

Some research suggests that patients with PCOS may benefit from metformin therapy. However, a 2012 consensus report reviewed the evidence for the use of metformin in women with anovulatory PCOS and found that metformin did not enhance live birth rates or reduce pregnancy complications. Therefore, its routine use is not recommended.[26]

Metformin may, however, have a role in prevention of Ovarian Hyperstimulation Syndrome (OHSS). A parallel, randomized, double-blind, placebo-controlled clinical trial concluded that metformin reduces the risk of OHSS by modulating the ovarian response to stimulation with FSH.[35]

Metformin should also be prescribed for PCOS women with frank diabetes.[26]

Surgery

Surgical procedures used in the management of PCOS include wedge resection, laparoscopic ovarian diathermy or laser, and multiple ovarian puncture or ovarian drilling.[33] Surgery is indicated in patients:[33]

- Resistant to CC
- With persistently high LH levels
- Who need laparoscopic assessment for other reasons

IVF

IVF is only recommended in women with PCOS if all other treatment methods fail or if they have other indications for IVF (for example, fallopian tube blockage, male factor infertility, severe endometriosis).[33]

The IVF cycle cancellation rate is higher in PCOS patients, and the duration of stimulation is longer.[36] This may be because PCOS is associated with excess weight. As discussed in Chapter 7, overweight women undergoing reproductive treatments require more gonadotrophin stimulation, have a poorer response rate, and produce fewer eggs.[37] Hyperandrogenism and hyperinsulinaemia may promote premature granulosa cell luteinization, alter the follicular environment, and, therefore, affect egg maturation.[26]

Not all women with a diagnosis of PCOS will be affected. Many women with PCOS still produce high-quality eggs and have comparable fertilization and implantation rates to those of women without PCOS.[26]

The rates of severe OHSS are higher in women with PCOS (15.4%) compared to women with normal ovaries (2.7%).[38] Women with PCO without PCOS are also at an increased risk of developing OHSS.[39] A systematic review found a significant and consistent relationship between PCO and OHSS. The reviewers concluded that interventions to moderate ART treatment are justified.[40]

Live birth rates per IVF cycle are similar in women with PCOS (37%) and in women with normal ovaries (40%).[38]

In Vitro Maturation

Recently, *In Vitro* Maturation (IVM) has been shown to be potentially a viable ART technique for PCOS patients. A prospective cohort clinical trial involving women with PCOS found improved implantation, clinical pregnancy, and live birth rates with a single embryo transfer by the use of an optimized IVM protocol.[41]

Vitamin D supplementation

Approximately 67–85% of women with PCOS are deficient in vitamin D.[42] In women with PCOS, low vitamin D levels are associated with obesity and metabolic and endocrine disturbances.[43] Therefore, it may be prudent to screen all women with PCO/PCOS for vitamin D deficiency. Vitamin D supplementation should be offered to those patients found to be deficient on the assumption that it may improve menstrual frequency and metabolic disturbances.[43]

Acupuncture treatment of PCOS

Research on acupuncture and PCOS

Conventional medical treatment of PCOS has inconsistent results, is expensive, and is associated with an increased risk of multiple gestation pregnancy; there are also other associated adverse effects.[44] Acupuncture is a safe, viable alternative.[44] In their review paper, Lim and Wong state that acupuncture may help to increase blood flow to the ovaries, reduce ovarian volume and the number of ovarian cysts, and control hyperglycaemia by increasing insulin sensitivity and decreasing blood glucose and insulin levels. Acupuncture's mode of action is by modulation of endogenous regulatory systems, including the sympathetic nervous system and the endocrine and the neuroendocrine systems.[45]

One small study of 66 women diagnosed with PCOS who were undergoing IVF showed that, in the group ($n = 32$ cases) undergoing electroacupuncture (EA), there was a significantly higher fertilization rate, cleavage rate, and high-quality embryo rate compared to an observation group ($n = 34$). The clinical pregnancy rate was also higher in the EA group, but this did not reach statistical significance. EA was administered once daily on acupuncture points REN4, REN3, SP6, ZIGONG, and KID3 during one menstrual cycle before and during the IVF ovarian stimulation phase.[46]

In another trial, 62 women diagnosed with PCOS who were undergoing an IVF/Intracytoplasmic Sperm Injection (ICSI) cycle of treatment were randomized into the EA group ($n = 31$) and a control group ($n = 31$). The EA group received five sessions of EA (at the start of downregulation, start of stimulation, 2 days before egg retrieval, and immediately before and after embryo transfer). In the first three sessions, the following acupuncture points were used: LI4, SP6, LIV3, REN4, DU20, ST36, and the Ovary and Uterus auricular points, bilaterally. In the pre- and post-embryo transfer sessions the following acupuncture points were used: LIV3, SP10, P6, ST29, and the Shenmen auricular point, bilaterally. The EA group had a significantly higher number of good-quality embryos, but all other outcome measures were comparable.[47]

In a nonrandomized, longitudinal, prospective study, 24 women with PCOS each received 10–14 sessions of EA. EA was administered twice a week for 2 weeks and once a week thereafter. Acupuncture points were selected in the 'somatic segments common to the innervation of the Ovary and Uterus (Th12–L2, S2–S4)'. One-third of women re-established regular ovulatory cycles following EA treatment. EA was more effective in women with lower BMIs, waist-to-hip circumference ratios, and serum testosterone concentrations.[48]

Acupuncture treatment

The greater the severity of menstrual irregularities, the greater the severity of PCOS.[26] Therefore, one of the aims of acupuncture treatment is to improve menstrual cycle regularity.

One way to do this is to help overweight patients lose weight, which, in turn, will improve their hormonal balance and menstrual cycle regularity. The TCM pathology associated with obesity includes Kidney Yang Deficiency and Damp-Phlegm. Acupuncture points particularly useful for obesity associated with PCOS include ST40, ST36, SP9, LIV3, ST25, GB26, ST29, KID14, and KID3 (moxa and EA can be useful adjuncts).

The Section 'The importance of menstrual cycle regulation' provides detailed treatment algorithms for various menstrual cycle irregularities.

PCOS can have a significant effect on patients' mental–emotional health. Acupuncture can be used to address this because pathology associated with PCOS (Damp-Phlegm, Stagnation, Yang, Yin imbalances and Blood Deficiency) is also associated with emotional and psychological ill health.

Common syndromes associated with PCOS include Kidney Yang Deficiency, Damp-Phlegm, Blood Stasis, Kidney Yin Deficiency, and Blood Deficiency. Treating these syndromes may help to reduce the severity of the patient's PCOS symptoms and, therefore, potentially increase the patient's chances of spontaneous conception.

In the authors' opinion, acupuncture treatment should be attempted for 4–8 menstrual cycles, depending on the patient's age and the length of menstrual cycles. If regular ovulatory cycles are not re-established or if no conception occurs, these patients should be referred for Orthodox ovulation induction therapy such as CC.

Table 8.3 lists TCM syndromes common in patients with PCOS and their treatment with acupuncture; Figure 8.3 provides a PCOS patient management algorithm.

Table 8.3 Common TCM syndromes in patients with PCOS and their treatment with acupuncture

	Kidney Yang Deficiency with Damp-Phlegm	Phlegm-Damp with Blood Stasis	Kidney Yin Deficiency, Liver Blood Deficiency, Stagnation/Blood Stasis
Manifestations	No or scant periods[49] Anovulation[50] Infrequent menstruation[50] Obesity[49–51] Excessive vaginal discharge[49] Feeling of heaviness in the abdomen[49] or generally[51] Cold limbs, aversion to cold[51] Dispirited, depressed	The same as Kidney Yang Deficiency with Damp-Phlegm plus Abdominal pain[49]	Irregular or infrequent ovulation[50] Infrequent menstruation[50] Thin body shape[50] Restlessness[50] Stress, depression, tearfulness[51]
Pulse	Weak, slippery[49]	Weak, slippery,[49] wiry	Wiry, fine,[51] may be rapid
Tongue	Pale,[51] swollen, sticky white coating[49]	Pale-purple or pale-blue, swollen, sticky white coating[49]	Red[51]
Treatment principles	Resolve Damp-Phlegm Warm and tonify Kidney Yang and Qi (with moxa)	Resolve Phlegm and Damp Tonify and warm Kidney Yang Eliminate Stasis Regulate Qi and Blood (with moxa)	Nourish Kidney Yin Regulate and tonify Qi and Blood
Acupuncture points and rationale	SP6: Invigorates Blood, harmonizes the Lower Jiao, regulates the menstrual cycle, calms Shen (Spirit), promotes fertility, and resolves Damp[52] KID3: Benefits the Kidneys, regulates the Chong (Penetrating) and Ren (Conception) Mai and the menstrual cycle, and promotes fertility[53] LIV3: Spreads Liver Qi, regulates menstruation and the Lower Jiao[52] LU7 + KID6: Opens and regulates the Ren Mai (Conception Vessel),[54] reinforces the Kidney, and tonifies the ovaries[55] SP4 + P6: Opens the Chong Mai (Penetrating Vessel),[52] regulates Blood in the Uterus, nourishes Blood, benefits Jing (Essence), regulates Qi, and eliminates Blood Stasis[56] ZIGONG 'Palace of the Child (Uterus)': tonifies deficiency[57] ST36: Tonifies and promotes Qi, resolves Dampness, and supports the Spleen and Kidney[58]		
	ST40: Transforms Phlegm-Damp, supports the Shen (Spirit), benefits the Spleen,[58] and may help with weight loss ST29: Regulates the menstrual cycle, warms the Lower Jiao (with moxa), and promotes fertility[58] ST28: Benefits the Uterus, regulates the Lower Jiao, dispels Stagnation (caused by Phlegm-Damp/Cold in the Uterus), and promotes fertility[58] SP9: Regulates the Spleen, resolves Dampness, and benefits the Lower Jiao[52] GB26: Regulates the Dai (Girdle), the Chong (Penetrating), and Ren (Conception) Mai (Vessels); drains Dampness; regulates the menstrual cycle; and promotes fertility[59] TITUO: Raises Qi and supports Qi in the Lower Jiao (heaviness due to Damp-Phlegm)[57] P5: Transforms Phlegm, regulates the menstrual cycle, and benefits the Heart and Uterus axis[60]		REN4: Nourishes Kidney Yin[61] REN7: Benefits the Ren and Chong Mai (Conception and Penetrating Vessels)[61] LIV8: Invigorates and nourishes Blood and Yin, benefits the Uterus[62]
		KID14: Regulates Qi, eliminates Blood Stasis, regulates the menstrual cycle, and promotes fertility[53] ST30: Regulates the Chong Mai (Penetrating Vessel), regulates the Lower Jiao and the menstrual cycle, and promotes fertility[58]	

Electroacupuncture (EA) is a useful auxiliary treatment method for PCOS.[46,48,63–65]

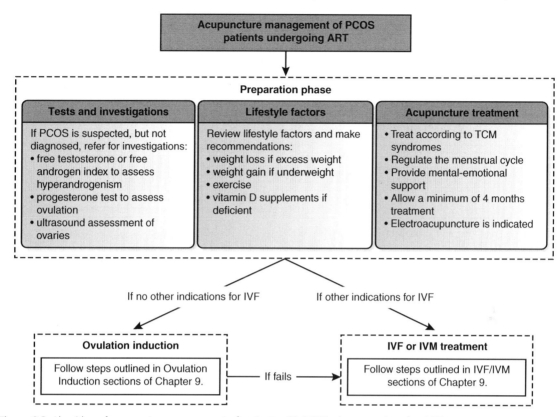

Figure 8.3 Algorithm of acupuncture management of patients with PCOS who are undergoing ART.

INTERESTING FACTS

HIRSUTISM AND PCOS

CLASSICAL TCM AND CONTEMPORARY ORTHODOX MEDICAL PHYSIOLOGY

- The Chong and Ren Mai (Penetrating and Conception Vessels) influence the abdomen, chest, face, and the area around the mouth.[66] In women with PCOS, these areas commonly show excessive hair growth; this is referred to as male pattern hair growth or hirsutism. This suggests that, in TCM, PCOS is linked to Chong and Ren Mai pathology.

- In TCM, men have facial and body hair because they do not have regular menstrual cycles. Thus, males have an abundance of Blood in the Chong and Ren Mai, which nourishes the abdomen, chest, and face, resulting in body hair growth.[66]

- In women diagnosed with PCOS, pathogenic factors such as Phlegm-Damp, Qi Stagnation, and/or Blood Stasis may obstruct the Chong and Ren Mai, resulting in no or infrequent periods. This obstruction creates an overabundance of Blood similar to that in men[66] and leads to male pattern hair growth or hirsutism.

Case study

PCOS

Victoria (age 31) and her husband had been trying to conceive for three and a half years. Victoria had previously been diagnosed with PCOS. She had a history of three miscarriages (all occurred at around 5–6 weeks' gestation), and her consultant believed the miscarriages were associated with the PCOS.

Nine cycles of ovulation induction with CC failed to help Victoria and her husband conceive. They were referred for IVF. Victoria sought acupuncture to help reduce her stress levels while undergoing IVF and to potentially improve her chances of conception.

Manifestations

◆ Menstrual cycle: irregular, bleeds for 3 days, light to medium flow, breast tenderness a week before menses, occasional menstrual spotting
◆ Appetite: can be low
◆ Bowels: loose (due to metformin medication)
◆ Energy levels: 'sluggish' in the afternoon
◆ Emotional disposition: nervous, anxious, tendency to become stressed easily
◆ Eyes: floater in left eye
◆ BMI: normal
◆ Pulse: right rear position weak, deep, and thin; right middle position weak; left rear and middle positions weak and thin
◆ Tongue: pale, especially in the Liver-Gallbladder area, slightly swollen, few small Heat spots at the tip

TCM Diagnosis

◆ Some Dampness and Spleen Qi Deficiency
◆ Liver Blood Deficiency with Qi Stagnation
◆ Kidney Yang and Yin Deficiency
◆ Heart Heat

First Acupuncture Prescription

SP6, P6, KID3, KID6, HE7, LIV3, and ST36

Acupuncture treatment principle included regulation of the menstrual cycle.

IVF1

Two good-quality embryos were transferred. However, Victoria suffered from early vaginal bleeding (around the time of implantation).

I recommended that, because of her history of miscarriages and early bleeding during the luteal phase of IVF, Victoria discuss undergoing advanced immune testing with her consultant. Her consultant authorized the tests, and the results were positive. Therefore, her consultant added immune and anticoagulation therapy to her second IVF treatment protocol.

IVF2

Two good-quality embryos were transferred 3 days after egg retrieval, and four embryos developed to blastocyst stage and were frozen. Victoria's pregnancy test was positive.

In view of Victoria's history of miscarriages, I continued treating her until 36 weeks gestation (once weekly up to 12 weeks gestation, then every 2 weeks up to 20 weeks, then every other month). She had a healthy baby girl delivered by caesarean section.

Conclusion

This case highlights that patients can present with multifactorial infertility. Immune and anticoagulant support together with acupuncture ensured a successful outcome.

THYROID DISEASE

Overview

Thyroid disease is characterized by either the under- or overproduction of thyroid hormone. The thyroid gland, which is located in the neck, produces two thyroid hormones: triiodothyronine (T3) and thyroxin (T4). Their production is regulated by Thyroid Stimulating Hormone (TSH), which is produced by the pituitary gland. Thyroid hormones regulate the body's metabolism and, hence, its ability to convert food into energy.[67]

Hypothyroidism is the underproduction of thyroid hormones by the thyroid gland.[67] Hyperthyroidism is the result of an overactive thyroid gland that produces excessive thyroid hormones.[68]

Thyroid autoimmunity (where immune antibodies destroy cells in the thyroid gland) affects 5–10% of women of childbearing age.[69] It is the biggest cause of hypothyroidism.[69]

Aetiology

The causes of hypothyroidism include:[67]

● Hashimoto's thyroiditis (an autoimmune disorder)
● Diet low in iodine
● Thyroid surgery or radioactive iodine therapy
● Unidentifiable causes

Causes of hyperthyroidism are:[68]

● Smoking
● High iodine intake (Grave's disease)
● Low iodine intake (nodular goiter)
● Female gender (affects 20 times as many women as men)

Orthodox medical management of thyroid disease

Indications for biochemical tests

Routine thyroid screening is expensive[70] and is not recommended for subfertile patients.[71] However, thyroid investigations are indicated in patients with ovulatory disease or in patients with risk factors for thyroid disease.[71] The risk factors for thyroid disease are outlined in Box 8.1.

Thyroid function tests

If thyroid disease is suspected, then Thyroid Function Tests (TFT) should be performed. This includes testing TSH, free thyroxine (FT4), and free triiodothyronine (FT3) levels. Other thyroid disease markers such as thyroid antibodies may also be tested to identify the cause of thyroid dysfunction, for example, an autoimmune disease.[70] Thyroid tests' reference ranges are provided in Table 8.4.

Management of patients with hypothyroidism

The first step in the development of hypothyroid disease is when the pituitary gland produces increasing levels of TSH, but the FT4 and FT3 levels remain within the normal range.

Box 8.1 Risk factors necessitating thyroid testing

Risk factors for thyroid disease

Women aged >30 years[73]
Family history of thyroid disease or autoimmune thyroid disease[73]
Presence of goitre[73]
Patients with thyroid antibodies, primarily thyroid peroxidase antibodies[73]
Patients with type 1 diabetes mellitus or other autoimmune diseases[70,73]
History of postpartum thyroiditis[70]
Women with subfertility,[73] especially anovulatory type
Women who previously miscarried or had preterm delivery[73]
History of head or neck irradiation or prior thyroid surgery[70,73]
Patients living in an area with iodine deficiency[73]
Patients with clinical signs and symptoms of hypothyroidism:[73]
- Fatigue, tiredness
- Weight gain
- Constipation
- Irregular periods
- Low libido
- Hair loss
- Brittle hair and nails
- Dry, itchy skin
- Difficulty learning and remembering

Patients with clinical signs and symptoms of hyperthyroidism:[68]
- Irritability
- Heat intolerance and excessive sweating
- Palpitations
- Weight loss with increased appetite
- Increased bowel frequency
- Tachycardia
- Fine tremors
- Warm and moist skin
- Muscle weakness
- Eyelid retraction or lag

Table 8.4 Thyroid tests' reference ranges

Hormones	Normal reference ranges[a]	Notes
Thyroid Stimulating Hormone (TSH)	0.4–4.5 mU/L[70]	New emerging consensus: 0.4–2.5 mIU/L[72] The American Thyroid Association guidelines recommend that women with a history of infertility or miscarriages should have a TSH <2.5 mU/L[73]
Free thyroxine (FT4)	9.0–25 pmol/L[70]	
Total thyroxine (TT4)	60–160 nmol/L[70]	
Free triiodothyronine (FT3)	3.5–7.8 pmol/L[70]	
Total triiodothyronine (TT3)	1.2–2.6 nmol/L[70]	
Thyroid peroxidase antibody (TPOAb)	0–35 IU/mL[74,75]	
Thyroglobulin antibody (TgAb)	0–40 IU/mL[74,75]	

[a] For exact values, check the laboratory report because reference ranges vary among different laboratories.

This presentation is referred to as subclinical hypothyroidism, and patients are usually asymptomatic.[70]

Overt hypothyroidism is diagnosed when the thyroid gland produces progressively less FT4, despite increasing levels of TSH. At this stage, patients can become symptomatic and require medical treatment.[70]

Thyroid peroxidase (TPOAb) and thyroglobulin (TgAb) antibody levels confirm an autoimmune origin of thyroid disease.[73] Universal screening for antithyroid antibodies is not currently recommended.[70,73] Women with elevated thyroid antibodies should have their TSH levels screened before pregnancy and also during the first and second trimesters of pregnancy because they are at an increased risk of developing hypothyroidism during pregnancy.[73]

The British Thyroid Association recommends the following patient management pathway (see Table 8.4 for thyroid hormone reference ranges)[70]:

- Patients with overt hypothyroidism (TSH >10 mU/L and low FT4) should be treated with thyroxine medication.
- Patients with subclinical hypothyroidism (TSH >10 mU/L and normal FT4) should be retested 3–6 months later. If the TSH level is still raised at that time, they should be treated with thyroxine medication.
- Patients with TSH levels >4.5 mU/L and normal FT4 should have their thyroid antibodies tested:
  - If antibodies are raised, these patients should have their TSH retested annually or earlier if patients develop symptoms of thyroid disease.
  - If antibodies are normal, these patients should have their TSH retested every 3 years.

The British Thyroid Association recommends that patients who are pregnant, who are planning to become pregnant, or have a goiter and TSH levels >4.5 mU/L (irrespective of their antibody status) should be treated with thyroxine medication. The aim of this treatment is to stabilize TSH levels in the low-normal range (0.4–2.0 mU/L) and FT4 levels in the upper normal range. Trimester specific reference ranges should be used when assessing these patients after they conceive.[70]

In its latest guidelines, the American Thyroid Association recommends that if women with risk factors for thyroid disease (including a history of subfertility and/or pregnancy loss) have TSH levels ≥2.5 mU/L on two separate occasions, they should be given a low dose thyroxine treatment.[73]

It should be noted that there is a lack of consensus on what is considered a normal range of TSH. A new consensus is emerging that the current normal reference range for TSH is set too high and should be lowered to 3.0 mU/L,[76] 2.5 mU/L,[72,77] or even 2.0 mU/L[78] because a lower level is more clinically relevant. This opinion is not universally supported.[79]

Management of patients with hyperthyroidism

According to the British Thyroid Association, the diagnosis of hyperthyroidism is confirmed if the TSH level is below the reference range and the level of FT4 is elevated.[70] FT3 should be measured when TSH is low, but FT4 is not elevated. If FT3 is raised, this can indicate mild cases of toxic nodular hyperthyroidism and the early stages of Graves disease. The full British Thyroid Association guidelines review the significance of other combinations of results, which are outside of the scope of this book. Readers who are interested in learning more are advised to refer to the full guidelines.[70]

Treatment of hyperthyroidism depends on the severity and the cause of the hyperthyroidism and may involve thionamides, surgery, or radioiodine treatment.[70]

CLINICAL TIPS

HYPOTHYROIDISM MEDICATION

Certain conditions, foods, medications, and supplements may interfere with absorption of levothyroxine medication. Therefore, patients should be advised to make relevant adjustments, for example, to take multivitamins at different times from the medication. Factors known to affect absorption of thyroid medication include:[80]

- Multivitamins (which contain ferrous sulphate (iron) or calcium carbonate)
- Ferrous sulphate (iron)
- Malabsorption conditions (e.g., celiac disease)
- Diet: ingestion with meal, espresso coffee, high fibre diet, soy

A time gap of 4–6 h is recommended between intake of medication and consumption of such foods and supplements.[81]

Effect of thyroid disease on fertility and pregnancy

Effect on ovarian reserve

Women with subclinical hypothyroidism[82] and/or raised thyroid antibodies[75] have been shown to have significantly lower ovarian reserve irrespective of their age.

Therefore, it may be prudent to refer patients with signs of diminishing ovarian reserve (high FSH levels, low Anti-Müllerian Hormone (AMH) levels, low Antral Follicle Count) for investigation of their thyroid function.

Effect on the menstrual cycle

Untreated hypothyroidism can have a detrimental effect on fertility and can cause anovulation or irregular ovulation.[67] It is also associated with oligomenorrhoea (infrequent or very light menstruation).[83] Any menstrual cycle and/or ovulation irregularities may reduce the chances of conception.

Hyperthyroidism is associated with hypomenorrhoea (scant) and/or polymenorrhoea (very frequent (<21 days) menstruation).[83]

Effect on ART

High oestrogen levels during controlled ovarian stimulation can have an adverse effect on pre-existing thyroid disease.[83]

A lower fertilization rate is often reported in women with hypothyroidism compared with euthyroid women.[84,85]

Raised thyroid antibody levels may adversely affect the rates of clinical pregnancy.[86] A meta-analysis found that treatment with thyroxin improves the clinical pregnancy outcomes in women with subclinical hypothyroidism or autoimmune thyroid disease undergoing ART treatment.[87]

CLINICAL TIPS

HYPOTHYROIDISM MEDICATION AND IVF

High oestrogen levels during controlled ovarian stimulation have been shown to negatively affect thyroid hormones, causing TSH to rise above pregnancy-specific reference range levels even before conception occurs.[88]

Therefore, patients taking thyroxine medication while undergoing controlled ovarian stimulation may need to discuss with their endocrinologist possibly increasing their thyroxine medication while undergoing IVF.

Effect on pregnancy and the foetus

During the first 10–12 weeks' gestation, the baby is completely dependent on the mother's ability to produce adequate thyroid hormones. After this time, the baby is able to produce its own thyroid hormones but is still dependent on its mother taking an adequate amount of iodine.

Untreated hypothyroidism can have a detrimental effect on pregnancy and can:[67]

- Affect the development of an embryo.
- Lead to major and profound complications during pregnancy and postpartum, such as miscarriages, premature birth, and low birth weight.
- Affect the development of the baby's mental capacity.

Untreated hyperthyroidism is associated with:[89]

- Miscarriages
- Pregnancy-induced hypertension
- Prematurity
- Low birth weight
- Intrauterine growth restriction
- Stillbirth
- Thyrotoxic crisis (thyroid storm)
- Maternal congestive heart failure

Because of the severe detrimental effects that thyroid disease can have on conception and pregnancy, all women with subclinical or overt thyroid disease should be monitored very closely during their pregnancy. Their medication levels may need to be adjusted every 4–6 weeks.[89]

In 2012, the American Thyroid Association published guidelines on the diagnosis and management of thyroid disease during pregnancy and postpartum. These guidelines were approved by the ATA Board of Directors and officially endorsed by the American Association of Clinical Endocrinologists (AACE), the British Thyroid Association (BTA), the Endocrine Society of Australia (ESA), the European Association of Nuclear Medicine (EANM), the European Thyroid Association (ETA), the Italian Association of Clinical Endocrinologists (AME), the Korean Thyroid Association (KTA), and the Latin American Thyroid Society (LATS).[73]

There is disagreement in the published literature about whether subclinical or overt hypothyroidism affects pregnancy outcomes. In its latest clinical practice guidelines, the American Thyroid Association states that high-quality evidence supports the view that both subclinical and overt hypothyroidism increase the risk of adverse pregnancy outcomes.[73]

Raised thyroid antibodies have been linked to pregnancy loss.[73] A large meta-analysis found that pregnant women with subclinical hypothyroidism or thyroid antibodies have an increased risk of complications, especially preeclampsia, perinatal mortality, and (recurrent) miscarriage.[90]

Whilst treating overt and subclinical thyroid disease in women who are trying to conceive or are pregnant[70,73] is recommended, there is not enough good-quality evidence to determine if treating euthyroid women with raised thyroid antibodies improves pregnancy outcomes and what treatment is the most effective.[91] Therefore, treatment of euthyroid women with raised thyroid antibodies is only recommended in the research setting.[91]

All thyroid medication crosses the placenta.[83] Therefore, any possible beneficial effects of treatment with thyroxine medication should be balanced with the risk of adverse effects on the foetus.

CLINICAL TIPS

THYROID MEDICATION DOSE AND PREGNANCY

Once pregnant, a woman's physiological demand for thyroid hormones rises immediately. It is therefore recommended that women on levothyroxine medication should independently increase their baseline dose of medication by 30% (or in some cases even more) immediately on biochemical confirmation of pregnancy.[73,89]

Effect on male fertility and reproductive health

Thyroid disease may affect male reproductive functions. However, this has not been extensively investigated. Most of the human studies are small, and the effects observed are not always statistically significant. After reviewing the available evidence, Krassas *et al.* concluded that thyroid disease can affect the male reproductive system in a number of ways:[83]

- Thyroid disease can disrupt the reproductive hormonal balance.
- Thyroid disease can affect sexual function, producing erectile abnormalities, low libido, and premature or delayed ejaculation.
- Hyperthyroidism can affect sperm motility.
- Hypothyroidism can affect sperm morphology.

Lifestyle factors

Iodine is a significant component of the thyroid hormones.[92] Therefore, it is recommended that all women who are attempting to conceive or who are pregnant should take 250 µg of iodine supplement.[73,93,94] They should also eat foods rich in iodine, such as cow's milk, yoghurt, eggs, cheese, white fish, oily fish, shellfish, meat, and poultry.[94]

The role of acupuncture

Referral for investigations

When obtaining patients' medical and infertility history, an acupuncturist needs to be aware of possible clinical signs of thyroid disease and refer patients for investigations, if appropriate.

Treatment with acupuncture

Management of patients with thyroid disease, particularly subfertile patients or patients suffering from miscarriage(s), is complicated by a lack of consensus on what is considered a normal range of TSH. A new consensus is emerging that the current normal reference range for TSH is set too high and

should be lowered to a more clinically relevant level of 3.0 mU/L,[76] 2.5 mU/L,[72,77] or even 2.0 mU/L.[78]

As already mentioned, there is also lack of consensus in the major thyroid medical associations' guidelines about what should be done in cases where women with a history of subfertility have TSH levels >2.0 mU/L but <4.5 mU/L. According to the American Thyroid Association's 2012 Guidelines on the Diagnosis and Management of Thyroid Disease During Pregnancy and Postpartum, these women would benefit from low-dose thyroxine replacement,[73] whereas according to the British Thyroid Association's Guidelines for the Use of Thyroid Function Tests, these TSH levels are of no concern unless they rise to >4.5 mU/L.[70]

This lack of clarity is, to an extent, reflected in the way patients with thyroid test results in this range are medically managed by their doctors. In our experience, there is a wide variation in how patients whose TSH is within this range are managed. Some patients are prescribed thyroxine medication, whereas others are told that they require no treatment.

There is also much variation in how patients with raised thyroid antibodies are managed. Some patients are prescribed thyroxine, some patients are given immunosuppressant therapies, and some patients are not given any medical treatment at all.

For patients with these borderline thyroid hormone levels who are not given any Orthodox medical treatment, acupuncture treatment may be the only way to help reduce the negative effects that their condition may potentially have on their reproductive health.

In those patients who are prescribed thyroid medication, acupuncture may enhance its effectiveness and the patient's response. Table 8.5 provides an overview of common syndromes and pathology associated with hypothyroidism and ART. Table 8.6 provides an overview of common syndromes and pathology associated with hyperthyroidism and ART. Figure 8.4 summarizes how to manage patients with thyroid disease in preparation for ART.

Table 8.5 Overview of TCM syndromes and pathology associated with hypothyroidism	
General manifestations	Fatigue, tiredness, weight gain, constipation, irregular periods, low libido, erectile abnormalities, premature or delayed ejaculation, hair loss, brittle hair and nails, dry itchy skin, difficulty learning and remembering,[73] anovulation or irregular ovulation, oligomenorrhoea (infrequent or very light menstruation)[67,83]
Fertility and ART associations	Low ovarian reserve[75,82] Poor sperm morphology[83] Lower fertilization rates[84,85] Affect on embryo development:[67] an increased embryo 'drop out' rate during embryonic development in the laboratory Failed IVF[86] Miscarriage(s)[67] Premature birth[67] Low birth weight[67]

Table 8.5   Overview of TCM syndromes and pathology associated with hypothyroidism—cont'd

Blood test indication	Raised TSH, low FT4 or Raised TSH, normal FT4 (subclinical)
Outline of TCM pathology, differentiation, and treatment	*Kidney Jing (Essence) Deficiency*[95] Key symptoms: exhaustion,[96,97] low levels of energy,[98] depression,[97] listlessness,[99] hair loss,[99,100] forgetfulness,[101] poor memory,[99] irregular periods,[102] weak sexual activity[99] Pulse: leathery,[103] weak, fine Tongue: pale, may have white coating or be red Acupuncture points: REN4, KID12, KID4 (moxa)
	Qi Deficiency[95,104] Key symptoms: tiredness,[105–107] lassitude,[106] breathlessness,[108] sweating,[105] poor appetite,[106] palpitations[105] Pulse: empty[106] Tongue: normal or pale[106] Acupuncture points: LI18, REN17, REN4, REN12, ST36, LU9, HE5, LI10 (moxa)
	Yang Deficiency[95,104] Key symptoms: tiredness,[104–106] lethargy,[105] overweight, feeling of cold,[99,105] bright white/pale face,[105] cold limbs,[105] aversion to cold,[95] low libido, impotence[99] Pulse: deep-weak[105] Tongue: pale, wet, swollen[105] Acupuncture points: DU4, KID3, BL52, REN17, REN6, HE5, ST11 (moxa)
	Blood/Yin Deficiency[95,104] Key symptoms: poor memory,[105] forgetfulness,[109] brittle nails, dry hair/skin,[110,111] impotence,[112,113] premature ejaculation,[100,114] constipation,[99,107] dizziness,[99,105,111] scant menstruation,[111] infrequent or irregular menstrual cycles,[115,116] hair loss[110] Pulse: fine, choppy[105] Tongue: pale, thin, dry[105] Acupuncture points: HE6, LIV3, REN4, REN12, SP6, ST39, ST9
	Phlegm-Dampness Key symptoms: somnolence,[110] tiredness, muzzy head, dizziness,[117] overweight[110] Pulse: wiry, fine, slippery Tongue: sticky coating or dry[117] Acupuncture points: ST40, ST36, SP9, SP3, ST11 (moxa)
Hashimoto thyroiditis	*Damp-Phlegm, Spleen-Qi Xu, Kidney Yang*[118] Key symptoms: signs and symptoms of hypothyroidism, raised thyroid antibodies, recurrent miscarriage, preeclampsia, perinatal mortality,[90] drooping eyelids, swelling of the face[104] Acupuncture points: REN4, REN22, REN23, LI18, HE7, ST40, SP3, KID3, ST36 (moxa)

Table 8.6 Overview of TCM syndromes and pathology associated with hyperthyroidism

General manifestations	Irritability, heat intolerance, excessive sweating, palpitations, tachycardia, fine tremors, warm and moist skin, weight loss with increased appetite, increased bowel movements, oligomenorrhoea, eyelid retraction or lag[68]
Fertility and ART associations	Poor sperm motility[83] Miscarriage(s)[89] Pregnancy-induced hypertension[89] Premature birth[89] Low birth weight[89] Intrauterine growth restriction[89] Stillbirth[89] Maternal congestive heart failure[89] Thyroid storm[89]

Continued

Table 8.6 Overview of TCM syndromes and pathology associated with hyperthyroidism—cont'd

Blood test indication	Low TSH, raised FT4
Outline of TCM pathology, differentiation, and treatment	*Yin Deficiency with Empty-Heat/Fire*[119,120] Key symptoms: scant menstrual flow, infrequent menstruation, 'menstrual block',[116] palpitations,[115] tachycardia,[115] nervousness, insomnia,[120] fine tremors, feeling warm, night sweats,[109,115,116] weight loss,[121] eye distension,[119] eye lag Pulse: rapid[99,120] Tongue: red, peeled[99] Acupuncture points: BL15, BL18, BL17, BL23, KID6, KID2, LIV8
	Phlegm-Heat/Fire[119,120] Key symptoms: eye retraction,[120,122] eye lag, vexation, palpitations, sweating,[122,123] nodular[119] goitre[120,123] Pulse: rapid, slippery, wiry Tongue: sticky yellow coating[122] Acupuncture points: P5, ST40, HE8, HE7, ST44, LI11
	Fire[119] Key symptoms: vexation, agitation, quick temper, heat intolerance,[109,116,124,125] eye distension, eyelid retraction, increased bowel frequency,[119] sweating, increased appetite, weight loss,[110] insomnia[119] Pulse: rapid Tongue: red Acupuncture points: P8, HE9, LIV2, ST44, LI11, SI4

Management during pregnancy

Once a woman conceives, her thyroid hormones are affected by the developing pregnancy. Therefore, patients who have overt, subclinical, or autoimmune thyroid disease must be very closely supervised, both by acupuncturists and by their endocrinologist. If necessary, acupuncturists should re-refer patients.

 Case study

Subclinical Thyroid Disease and IVF

Sandra, who was 34 years old, presented for acupuncture treatment in preparation for and during her second round of IVF. In her first cycle of IVF, she had two good-quality blastocysts transferred. Sandra began to bleed on the 11th day following egg retrieval, and her pregnancy test was negative.

When reviewing her test results, I noticed that her TSH level was 2.68 mU/L and FT4 was 11.9 pmol/L (the lower end of the normal range). On further questioning, Sandra revealed that her mother had thyroid disease. She also reported feeling tired; needing to use a blanket in the evenings because she felt very cold; and having irregular menstrual cycles, low libido, and hair loss.

In view of Sandra's history of infertility, her symptomatology, her slightly elevated TSH level, and her family history of thyroid disease, I referred her to an endocrinologist with a special interest in infertility. Sandra underwent further thyroid investigations. Her TSH level was even more elevated (4.7 mU/L), and her thyroid peroxidase antibodies were also elevated. Sandra was prescribed 75 μg of thyroxine per day. When reviewed a month later, her TSH was 1.4 mU/L, and she was given the go-ahead for her second IVF cycle.

In the meantime, she was receiving weekly acupuncture treatment. Her main TCM syndromes were Spleen Yang Deficiency and Phlegm. Acupuncture points prescription included SP3, SP6, SP9, ST36, ST40, and ST29.

Sandra underwent her second cycle of IVF. She had two top-grade blastocysts transferred, and two blastocysts were frozen. She conceived and successfully carried to full term. Sandra delivered a healthy baby girl naturally.

This case is a good example of how important it is that acupuncturists check all test results and, if required, refer patients for a second opinion. An integrated approach to subfertility care almost certainly made a difference to the outcome of this patient's second IVF treatment cycle.

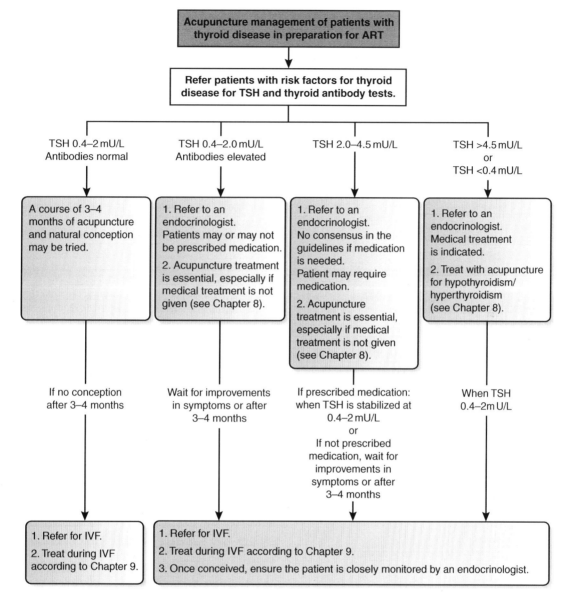

Figure 8.4 Acupuncture management of patients with thyroid disease in preparation for ART.

ENDOMETRIOSIS

Overview

Endometriosis is defined as the presence of endometrial glands or stroma outside the uterus.[126] It is an oestrogen-dependent disease that commonly affects women of childbearing age.[126] The endometrial tissue is typically found (in decreasing order of prevalence) on the ovaries, anterior/posterior cul-de-sac, broad ligaments and uterosacral ligaments, uterus, fallopian tubes, sigmoid colon, and appendix.[127] Endometrial tissue has also been found in the upper abdomen, peripheral and axial skeleton, lungs, diaphragm, and central nervous system.[127] The ovaries are affected by the formation of endometriomas ('chocolate cysts'), which can range from 1 to 8 mm in diameter.[128]

There are many hypotheses to explain endometriosis. The most accepted explanation is that endometriosis is caused by retrograde menstruation.[127,128] This may be exacerbated by a compromised immune system that fails to clear the lesions.[127,129] Distal locations could result from lymphatic or haematogenous spread or metaplastic transformation.[127,129]

Risk factors

Risk factors for endometriosis include:

- Low BMI[130–133]
- Alcohol use[130,131]
- Smoking[130,131]
- Low vitamin D levels[134]
- Diet low in dairy[134]
- Genetic predisposition[135]
- African American ethnicity[130,131]
- Early or late menarche[136]

Signs and symptoms

Patients may be completely asymptomatic or have a wide range of signs and symptoms.[137] Medical history and clinical signs suggestive of endometriosis include:

- Dysmenorrhoea (severely painful menstruation)[130,138]
- Lower abdominal pain[138] or bloating[139]
- Lethargy[139]
- Cyclic or chronic pelvic pain[130,138]
- Constipation or diarrhoea[139]
- Low back pain[138,139]
- Dyspareunia (painful intercourse)[130,138]
- Dyschezia (pain on defecation)[138]
- Pain on micturition (urination)[138]
- Pain on exercise[138]
- Loin pain[138]
- A fixed retroverted uterus[130]
- An adnexal mass[130]
- Uterosacral ligament nodularity, thickening, or tenderness (on vaginal or rectal examination by a doctor)[130]
- Endometrioma(s) visualized on ultrasound examination[130]

If the endometrial tissue affects the bladder, a patient may experience urinary symptoms such as frequent or painful urination.[140] If the bowel is affected, there may be alteration of bowel habits.[141] The symptoms that are experienced are usually cyclical in their pattern.

Pregnancy may reduce the severity of endometriosis, but symptoms usually return some time after pregnancy.[142]

Diagnosis and staging

The only way to confirm the diagnosis of endometriosis is by laparoscopy and histological evaluation.[130] Endometrial lesions can be red, pigmented, or white. White lesions are more difficult to examine visually.[128] Therefore, if the diagnosis is not apparent on visual inspection during surgery, then histological evaluation is necessary.[128,130] However, as with any surgery, the risks of surgery must be balanced with any possible benefits to be gained by confirming or excluding endometriosis. For example, if a woman who is trying to conceive is suspected to have endometriosis and her husband's sperm parameters are poor, this couple should be referred for IVF because there is no benefit to be gained from confirmation of an endometriosis diagnosis.

Serum levels of cancer antigen 125 can be raised in patients with endometriosis, but because of poor sensitivity and specificity, this should not be used as a diagnostic tool.[128] Other biomarkers of endometriosis are currently under investigation.[143]

Endometriosis can be staged according to the ASRM classification:[142]

- Stage I: minimal
- Stage II: mild
- Stage III: moderate
- Stage IV: severe

The classification depends on the location, severity, and depth of endometrial implants, and the presence and severity of adhesions and/or endometriomas. Minimal or mild endometriosis is characterized by superficial lesions and mild adhesions. Moderate to severe endometriosis is characterized by the presence of endometriomas and more severe adhesions.[142]

The Endometriosis Fertility Index (EFI) is a new validated tool that has recently been developed to predict pregnancy rates in patients with confirmed endometriosis who may want to attempt a natural conception; use of the EFI may help to determine which patients may benefit from ART treatment.[144]

Effect on fertility and reproductive health

Approximately 25–50% of subfertile women have endometriosis, and 30–50% of women with endometriosis are subfertile.[130,131] Though endometriosis is associated with subfertility, the link has not been conclusively proven, and the causal relationship has not been clearly established.[130] However, it is well established that endometriosis can cause physiological changes in the body that may compromise fertility.[130]

The ASRM reviewed the evidence on the possible mechanisms of how endometriosis could affect fertility. Several mechanisms have been proposed although it should be noted that none of these mechanisms have been proven. These postulated mechanisms include:[130]

- Distorted pelvis anatomy: the presence of endometriosis could lead to the formation of adhesions, fibrosis, and scarring that may distort the pelvic cavity and lead to compromised functioning of reproductive anatomy. The transportation function of the fallopian tubes has also been shown to be compromised in women with endometriosis although more research is necessary to confirm this.

- Altered peritoneal function: women with endometriosis have been shown to have an increased volume of peritoneal fluid and elevated inflammatory markers. This may raise the possibility that endometriosis is either caused by or results in systemic inflammation.
- Hormonal and menstrual cycle abnormalities: women with endometriosis may have menstrual cycle abnormalities such as an abnormally long follicular phase (including low oestrogen levels) and luteal phase dysfunction (including low progesterone levels). They may also have abnormal follicular growth, unruptured follicle syndrome, and premature and/or multiple LH surges.
- Impaired embryo implantation: this may be caused by the lack of certain molecules or enzymes in the endometrium of women with endometriosis, but more research is needed to investigate this further. Women with endometriosis also have increased antibodies to endometrial antigens, which can affect endometrial receptivity and embryo implantation.
- Compromised egg and embryo quality: embryos derived from women with endometriosis appear to develop more slowly. Donor embryos obtained from women with endometriosis have lower implantation rates, whereas donor embryos from women without endometriosis have normal implantation rates even if they are transferred into women with endometriosis. This suggests that the faulty implantation is caused by embryo quality.

There is also growing evidence that endometriomas adversely affect ovarian reserve.[145]

Orthodox medical treatment

Endometriosis treatment options include:
- Expectant management (close monitoring)[127]
- Medical treatment[127,128]
  - Nonsteroidal anti-inflammatory drugs
  - Combination oral contraceptives
  - Progestins (oral, parenteral, implants, intrauterine devices)
  - GnRH agonists
  - Danazol
  - Aromatase inhibitors
- Surgical treatment[127,128]
  - Laparoscopy with surgical excision of lesions
  - Laparotomy with surgical excision of lesions
  - Hysterectomy with ovarian conservation
  - Hysterectomy with removal of ovaries
- ART treatment (to assist with conception)[127]

The choice of endometriosis treatment depends on the goal of the treatment. In subfertile patients, the aim of the treatment is to reduce the negative effects that endometriosis could have on a woman's fertility and ability to conceive (for example, the aim would be to reduce endometrial tissue implants and restore normal pelvis anatomy). Therefore, the treatment options appropriate for women not planning pregnancy might not be equally suitable for women actively trying to conceive.

Expectant management

Expectant management may be appropriate for patients with mild to moderate disease. However, it may lead to a delay in other, more effective treatment methods, such as IVF.[127] Expectant management should only be considered for younger patients with good ovarian reserve.[130] For older patients (>35 years of age), more aggressive treatments, such as IVF, should be considered.[130]

The newly developed EFI tool may help to identify those patients who are least likely to benefit from expectant management.[144]

Medical treatment

As described earlier, endometriosis is an oestrogen-dependent disorder.[127] Medical treatment aims to reduce oestrogen production; this suppresses ovulation, thus rending women infertile while on such medication.[130] A 2007 Cochrane review found that ovulation-suppressing agents (danazol, progestins, oral contraceptives, and GnRH agonists) produced no beneficial effect in infertile women and delayed live births.[146]

However, pretreatment with GnRH agonists may improve IVF outcomes. A 2006 Cochrane review found that long-term (3–6 months) GnRH agonist treatment in preparation for IVF or ICSI increased the chances of pregnancy fourfold.[147] Pretreatment with oral contraceptives for 6–8 weeks before ART also improves outcomes.[148] Data is inconclusive about whether pretreatment with a GnRH agonist improves outcomes in patients with endometriomas.[127]

In summary, prolonged therapy with a GnRH agonist or contraceptive agents should be considered before ART but should not be administered to assist with natural conception.

Surgical treatment

The benefits of surgery for endometriosis include restoration of pelvic anatomy and removal of endometriotic implants and endometriomas, with a resulting decrease in inflammation.[127] It is well established that laparoscopic surgical removal of endometriosis is effective in improving fertility in patients with stage I/II endometriosis.[149] The ASRM also recommends conservative surgery in subfertile women with stage III/IV endometriosis.[130] If conception does not occur after surgery, additional surgeries will not offer any additional benefits, and these patients should be referred for ART treatment.[130]

A 2008 Cochrane review found that surgical removal of endometriomas is likely to increase chances of natural conception.[150] However, it is not clear if the surgical removal of endometriomas improves IVF outcomes.[130,151] The ASRM recommends that only the endometriomas that are >4 cm in diameter should be surgically removed before IVF to improve access to follicles and possibly improve response to ovarian stimulation.[130] Resection (rather than ablation or drainage) is the preferred surgical management of endometriomas.[130]

Removal of endometriomas may result in damage to ovarian tissue and reduce ovarian reserve.[152] Therefore, any beneficial effects of such surgery need to be carefully balanced against the risk of ovarian damage. A 2004 Cochrane review found that suppression with a GnRH agonist prior to surgery may decrease the size of endometriotic implants and, therefore, reduce the size of the ovarian tissue that needs to be surgically removed.[153]

ART treatment

There is a consensus that a stimulated Intrauterine Insemination (IUI) is an effective treatment option in women with mild to moderate endometriosis.[126,149] However, IVF is preferable in patients with severe endometriosis.[149]

Endometriosis may affect IVF outcomes. A 2013 meta-analysis of 27 studies and 8984 women undergoing IVF concluded that the presence of severe endometriosis (stage III/IV) is significantly associated with poor implantation and pregnancy rates. There was also a nonsignificant trend of reduced live birth rates. Mild endometriosis (stage I/II) did not appear to have detrimental effects.[154]

As mentioned earlier, long-term pretreatment with a GnRH agonist or oral contraceptives may improve IVF outcomes.[147,148] The ICSI fertilization method has been shown to result in better fertilization rates, a higher mean number of embryos, and lower rates of total fertilization failure or abnormal fertilization.[155]

The role of acupuncture

Referral

Up to one in every two subfertile patients who consult fertility acupuncturists may have endometriosis. Some of these patients may not be aware that they have the disorder. Therefore, acupuncturists need to be hypervigilant about screening patients for symptoms of endometriosis. This is particularly important because these patients can be guided to seek medical treatment if the acupuncturist suspects they have severe endometriosis.

If severe endometriosis is suspected, these patients should be referred for IVF if they are not already

undergoing ART treatment. Patients with mild symptoms may also benefit from an immediate referral if they are over the age of 35 or have evidence of reduced ovarian reserve. Younger patients with good ovarian reserve may benefit from a trial of acupuncture treatment to help them conceive naturally.

All patients with severe endometriosis (stage III/IV) will benefit from long-term pretreatment with a GnRH agonist, and patients with endometriomas >4 cm may benefit from surgery prior to IVF. The acupuncturists' role is to refer the affected patients.

Figure 8.5 summarizes how to manage patients with endometriosis in preparation for ART.

Treatment with acupuncture

In the authors' opinion, acupuncture may improve ART outcomes in patients with endometriosis by optimizing the quality of the eggs and the embryos, improving endometrial receptivity, and reducing inflammation. Acupuncturists should aim to reduce the severity of the underlying TCM pathology.

In TCM, chronic pelvic pain is associated with Blood Stasis, Damp-Heat, and Kidney Deficiency.[124,156] Cold or Heat may also cause pain. Table 8.7 provides the differential diagnosis and treatment with acupuncture. The section 'The importance of menstrual cycle regulation' provides detailed algorithms that may be useful in endometriosis patients suffering with painful periods and/or other menstrual abnormalities. Regulating the menstrual cycle can help to rectify Qi and Blood dysfunction, facilitate the flow of Qi and Blood in the Uterus, and promote fertility.

!	Red flag

Acute pelvic pain

Patients with acute pelvic pain should be referred immediately to their GP to exclude dangerous pathology – for example, an infection, appendicitis, or ovarian torsion.

	Case study

Stage IV Endometriosis

Kelly presented for acupuncture treatment to help prepare her for her first IVF cycle. She was 33 years old and suffered from very severe stage IV endometriosis, which affected her uterus, cervix, bladder, and bowels and caused extensive anatomical pelvic distortion, including scarring and adhesions. In the past, she also had endometriomas.

Case study—cont'd

The medical treatment of her endometriosis included three surgeries and a 6-month course of Zoladex to suppress her menstrual cycles. Her AMH was 3.5 pmol/L, which is very low for her age, possibly a result of damaged ovarian tissues caused by her several surgical procedures.

Manifestations

- Lower backache
- Feeling very cold, especially hands and feet
- Very tired
- Frequent urination
- Very loose urgent bowel motion, painful during periods
- Menstruation: severe abdominal pain that spreads into the upper legs and that requires strong painkillers, very heavy bleeding, dark clots (small and large)
- Premenstrual symptoms (sore breasts, tearful, irritable)
- Tongue: very pale
- Pulse: tight on all positions

TCM Syndromes

- Liver Qi Stagnation and Blood Stasis
- Cold in the Uterus
- Kidney Yang Deficiency
- Blood Deficiency

Basic Acupuncture Prescription

SP4+P6, SP10, SP6, SP8, ST36, ST28, ST29, and KID7

Kelly received seven acupuncture treatments during the preparation phase. Because Kelly's ovarian reserve was so poor, she needed a lot of acupuncture support during IVF. She had four acupuncture treatment sessions during the stimulation phase (including EA). As predicted, her ovarian response to stimulation was not very good. Kelly produced three eggs, of which two fertilized. One top-grade embryo was transferred on day 2, and the other embryo, also top-grade, was frozen. Kelly's pregnancy test was positive. Her pregnancy was uneventful and she had a healthy baby girl.

Despite severe endometriosis that affected Kelly's ovarian reserve and reproductive tract function, she conceived after only one IVF cycle. She did not produce many eggs, but her embryos were good quality, which may have been a result of the influence of acupuncture treatment.

UNEXPLAINED SUBFERTILITY

Overview

In 8–20% of infertile couples, no medical cause of subfertility will be identified,[178,179] and they will be diagnosed with unexplained infertility. The diagnosis is problematic. For example, some couples may have subtle abnormalities in the reproductive system that the standard infertility investigations may fail to identify.[180]

The diagnosis also depends on what is included in the investigations. For example, thyroid disease may cause infertility. However, routine thyroid investigations are not currently recommended. Therefore, a couple with a diagnosis of unexplained infertility may in fact be suffering from infertility caused by thyroid disease.

Orthodox medical management

Treatment options include expectant management, natural IUI, or IUI with ovarian stimulation and IVF. Evidence suggests that there is no significant difference in live birth rates between these different treatment options.[181] Therefore, IVF should only be considered if other treatments fail.[181]

TCM management

Couples with no medical causes of infertility may have identifiable TCM syndromes of disharmony. Addressing these syndromes with acupuncture may potentially result in spontaneous pregnancies. Therefore, careful TCM diagnosis and individualized treatment is essential (see Chapter 5).

Additionally, acupuncturists may need to review the results of conventional medical tests and investigations. A referral for further tests may be necessary. For example, if any test results are borderline, or if an acupuncturist suspects a medical cause or disease, but the appropriate tests have not been carried out to exclude the suspected cause or disease, a patient should be referred to his or her doctor for further investigations (see Chapter 4).

Modifiable lifestyle factor(s) may cause infertility. For example, a couple may not be aware of the importance of frequent and well-timed intercourse. Therefore, it is essential that lifestyle factors are reviewed in all patients but especially in patients with unexplained infertility (see Chapter 7).

SECONDARY SUBFERTILITY

Overview

Secondary infertility refers to an inability to conceive after successful live birth(s). It is estimated to affect about 10% of couples.[182] It can affect the female, male, or both partners. If one of the partners had previously had a child with a different partner, he or she may have developed secondary subfertility subsequent to that pregnancy.

In general, the causes of secondary infertility are the same as for primary infertility. However, some factors may be more relevant.

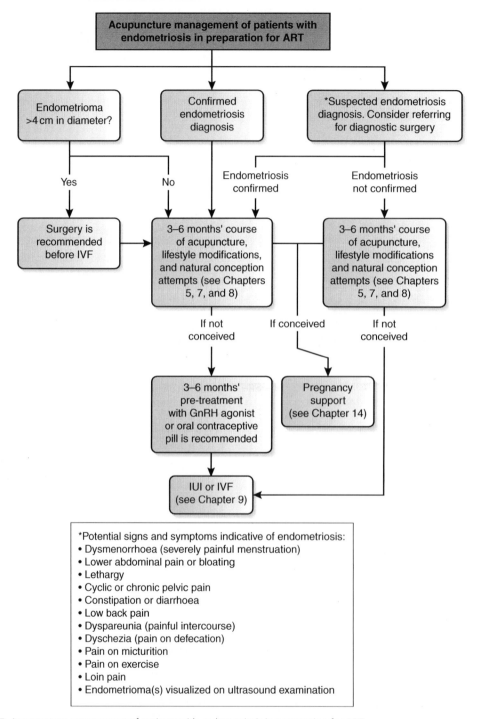

Figure 8.5 Acupuncture management of patients with endometriosis in preparation for ART.

Table 8.7 Common TCM syndromes in patients with endometriosis and their treatment in preparation for ART

Common TCM syndromes	Liver Blood Stasis[15,124,156–158] and Liver Qi Stagnation[159,160]	Kidney Deficiency[124,156]	Damp-Heat[124,156,157]	Cold and Blood Stasis[160]	Heat[157] and Blood Stasis[160]
Pain outside of menstruation	*Stasis*: fixed, stabbing,[124,156] aggravated by pressure[124] *Stagnation*: not fixed, intermittent,[156] aggravated by emotions[161]	Constant, more severe when tired	Intermittent, aggravated by pressure,[162] pelvic/sacrum heaviness[163]	Constant,[164] improves with heat,[160,164] aggravated by cold[156,164]	Intermittent[156] with a feeling of heat[160]
Pain during menstruation	*Stasis*: severe,[163] sharp, can begin just before menstruation[165] *Stagnation*: distension in lower abdomen and breasts[161]	Consistently dull and mild,[161,166] relieved by pressure and warmth[161]	Heavy sensation,[167] continuous[163]	Severe and cramping[163]	Dull, mild discomfort[166]
Mid-cycle and luteal phase	Mid-cycle pain[163] Premenstrual spotting[125]	Mid-cycle pain[168] Premenstrual spotting[125]	Mid-cycle pain[169] Premenstrual spotting[163]		Premenstrual spotting[125]
Menstrual cycle irregularities	Short[163] or late[162]	Short or possibly late[162,163]		Late cycles[163]	Early cycles[169]
Vaginal discharges (infections must be excluded)		Profuse, dilute, white, no odour[169]	White, yellow, greenish, reddish-white, curdled, sticky, thick, offensive leathery odour[169,170]	Watery, white offensive fishy odour[169]	Toxic-Heat causes profuse yellow discharge with an offensive, leathery odour[169]
Other	Abdominal masses may be hard and immovable or movable and 'come and go'[170] Lower back pain improves with exercise, worse with inactivity[171] Painful intercourse[170]	Late menarche[169] Chronic lower back pain[171]	Painful intercourse[170]	Aversion to cold[160,164]	Early menarche[169] Painful intercourse[170]
Urination (sinister causes of urinary symptoms must be excluded)	Abdominal pain and distension before urination, 'disinhibited' urination with urgency,[124] may be scant amount[172]	Dull pain after urination, frequent urination,[124,172] dribbling of urine or incontinence[172]	Abdominal pain and distension, 'constrained'[124] burning urination,[172] dark and turbid colour, urgent frequent but scant amount, may have blood in urine[172]	Pale and copious urine[172]	Reddish or dark urine,[156] painful or burning urination, incontinence[172]

Continued

Table 8.7 Common TCM syndromes in patients with endometriosis and their treatment in preparation for ART—cont'd

Common TCM syndromes	Liver Blood Stasis[15,124,156–158] and Liver Qi Stagnation[159,160]	Kidney Deficiency[124,156]	Damp-Heat[124,156,157]	Cold and Blood Stasis[160]	Heat[157] and Blood Stasis[160]
Stools (sinister causes of rectal bleeding must be excluded)	Constipation with small stools or alternation of diarrhoea and constipation, may have blood in stools[173]	Chronic loose stools or chronic constipation[173]	Diarrhoea, foul smelling, mucus, blood in stools,[173] pain relieved by defecation[173]	Bouts of pain with diarrhoea[164] or constipation without dry stools, spastic abdominal pain[173]	Constipation[160] or diarrhoea,[156] may have blood in stools[173]
Pulse	Choppy, firm, wiry[160]	Leathery, weak, deep, fine, slow	Slippery, soft, rapid,[124] or surging[162]	Slow,[164] tight[156,164]	Rapid, surging[156]
Tongue	Purple[124] or purple areas, bruised appearance[160] or dark red	Pale, may have white coating, be swollen, and/or have a wet or a red tongue body	Thick greasy yellow coating[162]	Blue, purple-blue, white coating[160]	Red tongue, yellow coating[156]
Treatment principles	Alleviate pain Eliminate Blood Stasis Unblock Qi and Blood flow Benefit the Uterus and promote fertility	Alleviate pain Tonify and nourish the Kidney, warm the Kidney Benefit the Uterus and promote fertility	Alleviate pain Transform Damp-Heat Benefit the Uterus and promote fertility	Alleviate pain Warm Cold	Alleviate pain Clear Fire and Cool Blood
Acupuncture points appropriate for all syndromes	<ul><li>SP4 + P6: Opens the Chong Mai (Penetrating Vessel),[52] eliminates Blood Stasis, reduces pain, regulates Blood in the Uterus, nourishes Blood, benefits Jing (Essence), regulates Qi[56]</li><li>SP6: Tonifies the Kidney and regulates and nourishes the Liver, alleviates pain, resolves mid-cycle spotting,[52] helps reduce pain on intercourse, benefits the Bladder, resolves masses, and promotes fertility[52]</li><li>REN4: Tonifies the Kidney, Yuan (Original) Qi[61,174] benefits Jing (Essence),[61] Qi and Blood, Yin and Yang,[61,174] and benefits the Uterus and assists conception[61]</li><li>KID5: Alleviates pain, resolves Blood disorders, regulates Qi and Blood, benefits the Kidney, and regulates the Ren (Conception) and Chong (Penetrating) Mai (Vessels)[53]</li><li>ST30: Regulates Qi in the Uterus and Lower Jiao, regulates the Chong Mai (Penetrating Vessel), disperses Stagnation and alleviates pain, resolves masses, and promotes fertility[58]</li><li>SP8: Alleviates pain and tonifies Jing (Essence)[52]</li><li>ST26: Regulates Qi and alleviates pain[58]</li><li>REN3: Transforms Damp-Heat, alleviates pain, reduces pain of the cervix (tenderness of the posterior vaginal fornix), resolves spotting, abdominal masses, vaginal discharge, eliminates Stagnation, benefits the Uterus, reinforces Yang-Qi,[61] and promotes fertility</li><li>LIV5: Transforms Damp-Heat from the Lower Jiao, alleviates pain, resolves vaginal discharge, regulates Liver Qi, regulates dysfunction of Qi and Blood Stasis,[62] promotes fertility, benefits the Uterus, and eases pain during intercourse</li><li>LIV3: Regulates the Lower Jiao and alleviates pain[62]</li></ul>				

Table 8.7 Common TCM syndromes in patients with endometriosis and their treatment in preparation for ART—cont'd

Common TCM syndromes	Liver Blood Stasis[15,124,156–158] and Liver Qi Stagnation[159,160]	Kidney Deficiency[124,156]	Damp-Heat[124,156,157]	Cold and Blood Stasis[160]	Heat[157] and Blood Stasis[160]
Acupuncture points for individual syndromes	**KID14**: Regulates Qi and moves Blood Stasis, resolves destructive Blood, alleviates pain, rectifies constipation or diarrhoea, benefits the Uterus, and promotes fertility[53] **KID18+KID19**: Alleviates stabbing pain, regulates the Lower Jiao, eliminates Blood Stasis, redirects proper Qi and Blood movement, resolves destructive Blood, benefits the Uterus and abdomen, and promotes fertility[53] **ST29**: Warms the Uterus invigorating Blood, resolves Uterine masses, restores the function of the Uterus, promotes fertility,[58] and eases pain on intercourse **ST28**: Regulates the Lower Jiao, dispels Stagnation, alleviates pain and constipation, and benefits the Bladder and Uterus promoting fertility[58] **LIV14+LIV3**: Spreads and nourishes Qi, invigorates Blood, and disperses masses[62] Moxibustion is indicated	**REN2**: Alleviates pain, regulates the Lower Jiao, invigorates and warms the Kidney, tonifies deficiency of all Zang organs, resolves vaginal discharge,[61] eases pain on intercourse, and promotes fertility **KID12+KID13**: Tonifies the Kidney, regulates the Ren and Chong Mai (Conception and Penetrating Vessels) and regulates the Uterus and Lower Jiao[53] **KID3**: Alleviates pain, benefits the Kidney, with moxibustion tonifies Qi and Blood and Jing (Essence),[174] and regulates the Chong and Ren Mai (Penetrating and Conception Vessels) and the bowels[53] The Baliao **BL31– BL34**: Resolves painful urination and diarrhoea, painful periods, vaginal discharge, lower back pain, supplements the Kidney, promotes fertility,[175] and eases pain on intercourse **DU4**: Supplements the Kidney, strengthens Ming Men (Fire of Life), tonifies Kidney	**GB26+GB34**: Alleviates pain, transforms Damp-Heat, drains Damp, regulates the menstrual cycle, resolves vaginal discharge, regulates the Chong and Ren Mai (Penetrating and Conception Vessels) and the Uterus, promotes fertility, and benefits the Kidney[59] **ST25**: Alleviates pain, transforms Damp-Heat, resolves Uterine masses, vaginal discharge, diarrhoea, and promotes fertility[58] **LIV8**: Alleviates pain, transforms Damp-Heat from Lower Jiao, benefits the Uterus, resolves diarrhoea, and promotes fertility[62] and conception **KID10**: Alleviates pain, clears Damp-Heat from the Lower Jiao, modifies bleeding, benefits the Kidney and Bladder, resolves vaginal discharge, and	**REN6**: Strengthens Yang, warms Cold in the Lower Jiao, regulates Qi and harmonizes Blood, reduces pain during the period, and promotes fertility[61] **REN12**: Alleviates pain, regulates Qi, warms Cold[61] **SP15**: Alleviates pain, regulates Qi, and warms Cold[52] **SP4**: Alleviates pain, warms Cold, invigorates Blood, and regulates menses[52] **REN8**: Warms Yang and promotes fertility[61] **ST28**: Eliminates Stagnation of Cold in the Uterus and promotes fertility[58] **ST36**: Alleviates pain and warms	**LIV1+LIV2**: Alleviates pain, clears Fire, regulates Qi, modulates bleeding, regulates the menstrual cycle and the bowels, and benefits the Bladder[62] **SP10**: Alleviates pain, cools Blood, harmonizes menses, regulates the menstrual cycle, benefits the Bladder, and regulates the flow of Blood[52] **KID8**: Alleviates pain, regulates the Ren and Chong Mai (Conception and Penetrating Vessels), clears Heat from the Lower Jiao, modulates bleeding, regulates the menstrual cycle, and rectifies disordered movement of Blood[53] **BL15+BL17+ BL18**: Clears and cools Fire in Blood, harmonizes Blood, and modulates bleeding[175]

Continued

Table 8.7 Common TCM syndromes in patients with endometriosis and their treatment in preparation for ART—cont'd

Common TCM syndromes	Liver Blood Stasis[15,124,156–158] and Liver Qi Stagnation[159,160]	Kidney Deficiency[124,156]	Damp-Heat[124,156,157]	Cold and Blood Stasis[160]	Heat[157] and Blood Stasis[160]
		Yang, regulates the Du Mai (Governing Vessel), benefits the Uterus[176] and lower back, and promotes fertility and conception **BL23**: Reinforces Kidney Jing (Essence) and Yin and Yang, benefits the Uterus, resolves vaginal discharge, benefits the back,[175] warms the Uterus, invigorates Qi and Blood, eases pain on intercourse, and promotes fertility Moxibustion is indicated	facilitates conception[53] **ST36**: Transforms Damp, tonifies Qi[58] **SP9**: Alleviates pain, regulates the Spleen, resolves Damp, regulates the bowels, and resolves vaginal discharge[52]	Cold[177] **DU3+DU4**: Regulates menses, warms Cold, tonifies Jing (Essence) and Qi and Yang, and promotes fertility[177] **KID2**: Warms Cold, tonifies Jing (Essence) and Yang, and regulates the menstrual cycle[53] Moxibustion is indicated	

Notes: Consider TCM combined patterns and syndrome staging (i.e., early, mild, or advanced). Examine pathology and physiology and incorporate into treatment principles.

- Uterine factor: a history of caesarean sections may increase the risk of secondary infertility caused by uterine scarring.[183] Uterine infections following delivery may cause scarring in the uterus and/or fallopian tubes.
- Genetic issues: it is important to enquire if a previous pregnancy was achieved with the same partner or a different partner. If a different partner, it is important to exclude genetic incompatibility issues by referring for karyotyping tests.
- Immune issues: some women may develop immune issues subsequent to a successful delivery.[184]
- Age: it might take longer to conceive another child because of an age-related decline in fertility.
- Menstrual cycle irregularities: did the menstrual cycle return to normal following the previous pregnancy? If not, it may be prudent to refer the patient for hormonal investigations, such as progesterone, thyroid, and prolactin tests.
- Weight: being over- or underweight can affect fertility. Therefore, it is important to ask if one or both partners' weight has changed since the last pregnancy.

- Intercourse practices: a couple may have less frequent intercourse because of, for example, exhaustion from caring for a young baby or toddler.
- Stress: a couple may find their inability to conceive another child a very stressful experience, especially if their first baby was conceived very quickly.
- Occupational factors: have one or both of the partners changed their occupation(s), and, if so, is the new occupation associated with subfertility?
- Breastfeeding: is the female partner still breastfeeding? If so, this may suppress ovulation.

Orthodox medical management of secondary infertility

The Orthodox medical management of secondary infertility is similar to that of primary infertility. Standard tests are normally undertaken. The management of the couple's infertility depends on the findings and subsequent diagnosis.

Acupuncture management of secondary infertility

Acupuncture management of secondary infertility is also similar to that of primary infertility. Ideally, both male and female partners should be assessed and, if necessary, treated with acupuncture. Chapter 5 discusses TCM syndrome differentiation in great detail.

MALE FACTOR SUBFERTILITY

Overview

Male factor as a single cause of infertility is responsible for 20–30% of infertility cases[178,179,185] and combined male and female factors are estimated to affect 25–40% of couples.[2,178,179]

There have been some suggestions that male infertility is on the rise.[186] However, because of heterogeneous measurement methodology, such as comparing data from different populations and using different methods of sperm analysis, this opinion has been questioned by some.[187]

Medical causes

Various congenital or acquired factors can affect the male reproductive tract at pre-testicular, post-testicular, or directly at the testicular level,[188] leading to:

- A decrease or complete cessation of sperm production
- Sperm blocked from being released
- Sperm not functioning properly

The most common medical causes of poor semen parameters in men include cryptorchidism (13%),[189] varicocele (10%),[189] congenital abnormality of the vas deferens (4%),[189] and endocrine abnormality (2%).[189] In 57% of men with severe oligospermia or azoospermia, no causes are found.[189]

Other medical causes include congenital anatomical defects; genetic abnormalities; infections; cancer treatments (including chemotherapy and radiation); scarring from sexually transmitted diseases, injury, or surgery; vasectomy or failure of vasectomy reversal; retrograde ejaculation; and impotence or erectile dysfunction.[188]

Certain medications can affect sperm production, hormone balance, semen parameters, or erectile issues. Appendix VI provides details of the most common pharmaceutical drugs that are known to affect male reproductive function.

Lifestyle factors

Chapter 7 reviewed the effects of various lifestyle factors on male reproductive function and fertility. These are:

- Heavy use of alcohol
- Use of recreational drugs
- Being overweight
- Smoking
- Exposure to various environmental toxins and heat
- Occupational factors
- Nutritionally poor diet
- Lack of exercise
- Psycho-emotional stress
- Older paternal age

Therefore, it is essential to assess modifiable lifestyle factors in patients with subfertility and, if necessary, make recommendations to patients about what they can do to improve their fertility.

Investigations

The investigations of male factor subfertility should include obtaining a medical and reproductive history, a physical examination, and semen analysis.[185,188] Depending on the initial findings, further advanced tests may be required.[185,188]

Chapter 4 reviews the various male infertility tests and investigations, reference ranges, and their interpretation.

Orthodox medical treatment

Treatment options depend on the cause of subfertility and may include:

- Hormonal treatment
- Surgery
- ART (IVF, ICSI, Intracytoplasmic Morphologically Selected Sperm Injection (IMSI), donor sperm IVF)

Hypogonadotrophic hypogonadism

Hypogonadotrophic hypogonadism is characterized by hyposecretions of LH and FSH. This may be caused by genetic factors or acquired factors. Congenital conditions are associated with delayed puberty, sparse or nearly absent body hair, gynaecomastia, and low testicular volume. Acquired conditions may manifest with low ejaculation volume, beard growth, impaired libido, and asthenia. The diagnosis is confirmed by hormone tests. Acquired hypogonadotrophic hypogonadism could be caused by tumours and, therefore, requires more advanced investigations.[188]

Depending on the cause, treatment with hormonal medication is usually successful and is likely to result in spontaneous conception. Depending on which gene is involved in congenital hypogonadotrophic hypogonadism, genetic counselling may be indicated. Treatment with testosterone may improve the man's reproductive function.[188]

Erectile dysfunction

Erectile dysfunction is a rare cause of infertility. It may be caused by other comorbidities, for example, diabetes or psychological factors. The underlying cause will determine the choice of treatment and may involve IVF (potentially necessitating advanced sperm extraction methods) or psychosexual therapy if the erectile dysfunction is of psychogenic origin.[188]

Retrograde ejaculation

Retrograde ejaculation is confirmed by the absence of spermatozoa in semen but their presence in the urine after ejaculation. IVF is indicated in these patients.[188]

Varicocele

Varicocele is a condition where the blood vessels in the scrotum become distended.[190] Although many men with varicocele have normal fertility, the condition is associated with subfertility. The mechanisms by which varicoceles cause infertility are not well understood.[190] Increased scrotal temperature, causing impaired testicular blood drainage and hypoxia, is one of the proposed aetiologies.[190]

Varicocelectomy is the surgical correction of a varicocele. A 2012 Cochrane review concluded that there is some weak evidence that varicocelectomy may improve chances of natural conception.[190]

Absent vas deferens

Absence of the vas deferens is commonly associated with the CFTR genetic mutation (see Chapter 4). IVF with ICSI and testicular biopsy can allow these men to still father a biological child.[188]

Inflammation

The presence of leucocytes (>1 million/mL) is likely to be caused by inflammation of the accessory glands.[188]

Infections

Infections (most commonly *Ureaplasma urealyticum*, *Enterococcus faecalis*, and *Escherichia coli*) and the resulting production of reactive oxygen radicals can affect sperm motility and fertilizing capacity by activated leucocytes.[188] A course of antibiotic therapy may restore normal fertility. Infections and male factor subfertility are reviewed in Chapter 4.

DNA damage

As described in Chapter 4, sperm DNA damage may lead to subfertility and miscarriages. Supplementation with antioxidants may help to reduce DNA damage (see Chapter 7). Frequent ejaculation may also improve sperm DNA parameters.[191,192]

Genetic factors

The most common genetic factors include karyotype abnormalities, Y chromosome microdeletions, and CFTR gene mutation in Congenital Absence of Vas Deferens (CAVD). Treatment depends on the type of abnormality and may require ART. Genetic counselling about the risks of transmission, health consequences, and prevention may also be required.

Unexplained male factor infertility

In a large number of cases, despite extensive investigations, no cause of male factor subfertility will be found. According to Krausz, it is likely that the vast majority of these cases are caused by as yet unknown genetic issues because only a small fraction of the thousand or more genes involved in spermatogenesis have been adequately investigated by reproductive medicine geneticists.[188]

Effect on conception and ART outcomes

Depending on the cause of male factor subfertility, it may only mildly reduce the chances of natural conception – for example, a varicocele – or it may make natural conception impossible – for example, absence of the vas deferens.

ART treatment, in particular specialist fertilization methods such as ICSI or IMSI, can successfully manage many causes of male factor subfertility. However, even with ICSI or IMSI, male factor may contribute to poor fertilization rates or total fertilization failure and to poor embryo development; it may also be responsible for Repeated Implantation Failure (RIF) and/or miscarriages (see Chapters 10 and 12 for detailed discussions of this). Therefore, it is essential that a subfertile male partner's reproductive health is optimized in preparation for ART treatment.

TCM and male factor infertility

TCM pathophysiology

Jing, Qi, Yin, and Yang

As described in Chapter 3, the creation of an embryo results from the combinations of Yang and Yin energies of the male and female. Healthy sperm is essential for fertilization, the embryo's Qi and its development, a successful pregnancy, and the health of the child. The Yang energy instigates fertilization. Therefore, the assessment of male energy Jing, Qi, Yin, and Yang is required in conjunction with analysis of the semen parameters.

Zang organs

There are four main Zang organs associated with male factor subfertility:

- The Kidney[193]
- The Liver[194]

- The Heart[195]
- The Spleen[195]

The Kidney

The Kidney stores and releases Pre-Natal Jing (Essence).[196,197] Kidney Jing (Essence) is associated with semen and reproductive potential.[97,198] The primary role of the male in reproduction is the supply of Jing (Essence).[199] A deficiency of Kidney Jing (Essence) can have a detrimental influence on reproductive health.[198] As men age, their Ming Men (Fire of Life) (which is linked with Kidneys and reproduction) declines.[200] Kidney Yang Deficiency can lead to impotence and reduces the quality of sperm.[201]

The Liver

Liver Qi weakness leads to weakness of Tian Gui[97] and the Kidney, affecting sexual energy and sperm.[198] The channels of the Liver are associated with erectile dysfunction.[200]

The Heart

The Heart generates and stores Shen (Spirit). Shen (Spirit) promotes movement and vitality of Jing (Essence), Qi, and Blood by invigorating and circulating them around the body. Shen (Spirit) is acquired when the body, Heart, and Mind are settled, calm, and 'properly aligned'.[202] The 'Mind directs Jing' (Essence), and Kidney Jing (Essence), this in turn, provides the 'material basis for the Mind'.[203] Therefore, male fertility depends on a good relationship between the Heart and the Kidney.

Stress can adversely affect reproductive health[97] because stress and mental strain consume Kidney Jing (Essence) and affect the Shen (Spirit) and the Mind. Overwork, fear,[198] too much thinking, desire, and anger can negatively affect the Heart. Therefore, it is essential that men keep their body, Shen (Spirit), and Mind in good order.[97]

It is common in fertility acupuncture practice to see the Shen (Spirit) and Mind of male patients affected by stress (for example, work-related stress or stress caused by subfertility or IVF failure). Therefore, regulating the Heart and Shen (Spirit) and, through this, conserving the Kidney Jing (Essence), preserves fertility.

INTERESTING FACTS

THE HEART AND STRESS IN MALE FERTILITY

Psychological stress lowers sperm concentration and progressive motility and increases abnormal forms.[204] In TCM, psychological stress is often associated with Heart pathology. Interestingly, the medieval Chinese physician Sun Simiao made an observation that the Heart was associated with subfertility in men.[195]

The Stomach and Spleen

The Stomach and Spleen are involved in the production of Post-Natal Jing (Essence),[198] which supplements Pre-Natal Jing (Essence). The Spleen is also involved in the production of Qi and Blood through its connection with the Liver, Heart, and Kidney. Weakness in the Stomach or Spleen will therefore affect Jing (Essence) and Qi and Blood, all of which are important for fertility.

Pathogenic factors

Pathogenic factors such as Cold, Damp, Heat, Fire, and Phlegm may damage the production and function of sperm.

Sperm parameters and TCM associations

Contemporary TCM authors have noted TCM syndromes and pathogenic factors commonly seen in male factor infertility patients and their associations with Orthodox medical aetiology and sperm abnormalities (Table 8.8).

Treatment with acupuncture

A general treatment principle for male factor subfertility is to reinforce the Kidney,[200,201,207] balance Yin and Yang,[97,198] and tonify and promote Qi and Blood circulation[193,200,201] (Table 8.9). For differential diagnosis of syndromes, refer to Chapter 5.

Research on acupuncture and male subfertility

Crimmel *et al.* reviewed the research on the treatment of male infertility and erectile dysfunction with TCM and acupuncture. Studies included in the review varied in design, and the methodology in most studies was poor. Nonetheless, the authors described the results as 'limited but promising'. Studies suggest that acupuncture treatment can improve ejaculatory dysfunction, erectile dysfunction, sperm concentration, motility, forward-progressive motility, sperm vitality, and total motile count. This may be achieved because acupuncture increases testosterone levels.[200]

In a more recent review, Huang *et al.* reported similar findings. In addition, the authors state that acupuncture treatment may increase IVF fertilization rates.[211]

Clinical perspective

Importance of treating men

As already mentioned, male factor subfertility is involved in at least 50% of subfertility cases. Yet, in fertility acupuncture practice, we see many more women than men. The significance of male factor subfertility was observed even in

Table 8.8 TCM syndromes and pathogenic factors in male factor subfertility and their Orthodox medical associations

Syndromes/ pathogenic factors	Orthodox medical associations
Kidney Jing (Essence) and/or Qi Deficiency[194,195,200,205–208]	Testicular failure, anatomic/congenital factors,[208] issues with spermatogenesis, poor morphology and motility,[200] absence of sperm in the ejaculate, low sperm count, impotence[15]
Kidney Yang and/or Ming Men (Fire of Life) Deficiency[194,201,205,207–209]	Poor motility,[210] low sperm count, poor morphology[201,207]
Kidney Yin Deficiency[200,201,207] and Liver Yin Deficiency[205,209]	Congenital factors, pituitary factors, issues with spermatogenesis, poor morphology,[194,200,201,210] poor motility,[201,207,209,210] low sperm count[194,201]
Qi[199] and Blood Deficiency[201]	Low count,[201] other sperm parameters may also be affected
Damp-Heat in Lower Jiao[15,194,200,201,205,207,209]	Sexually transmitted diseases,[194] immunological subfertility,[15] infections,[207] inflammation, low sperm count, high rate of dead sperm, incomplete liquefaction of sperm,[201] varicocele, cryptorchidism[200]
Phlegm[194,201] or Damp[194,200,208]	Postinfection, low sperm count, poor morphology and motility, absence of sperm in the ejaculate[201]
Blood Stasis[194,201]	Varicocele, cryptorchidism,[200] postsurgery, low sperm count,[201,207] poor motility[201]
Cold[194,201,208]	Any semen parameters may be affected
Qi Stagnation,[194] Fire,[205,209] or Heat[194,200,207]	Any semen parameters may be affected

Table 8.9 TCM syndromes and acupuncture treatment of male factor subfertility in preparation for ART

Syndromes	Acupuncture points
Generic treatment principle	Benefit Jing (Essence) and promote fertility KID12, REN4, ST30, SP6, LIV3, ST36, HE7, KID3, SP8, BL23+BL52 Moxibustion is indicated (except in Heat or Fire pathology)
Kidney Jing (Essence) Deficiency	Tonify Jing (Essence) REN4 (moxibustion is indicated), LIV3, ST27, ST36, SP6, HE5, SP8, BL23+BL52, KID3
Kidney Yang Deficiency	Tonify Yang REN6, REN8, GB25, DU4, BL23+BL52, LIV3, ST36 Moxibustion is indicated
Kidney Yin Deficiency	Enrich Yin KID6, ST27, SP6, ST36, LIV3, KID3, HE6, SP8
Qi and Blood Deficiency	Tonify and facilitate Qi and Blood flow SP6, ST30, LIV1, ST36, LIV3, HE7, KID3, REN17 Moxibustion is indicated
Damp-Heat	Drain Damp and resolve Heat KID10, LIV8, SP6, DU3, BL23, SP9, LIV5, GB34
Blood Stasis	Eliminate Blood Stasis BL17, BL18, BL15, BL23, LIV3, SP4+P6, SP10
Cold	Warm Cold ST29, ST27, REN4, ST36, REN8, DU4, LI4, KID2 Moxibustion is indicated
Phlegm-Damp	Resolve Phlegm-Damp ST40, ST36, REN9, LIV3, KID13, SP9, ST36, REN3, SP3, SP8 Moxibustion is indicated
Qi Stagnation	Regulate Qi and Blood LIV3, P6, P5, HE7, ST36, LIV8, REN17
Heat/Fire	Clear Heat/Fire P7, LIV2, SP10, LI11, BL18, BL15, BL17, BL21, BL23

the classical TCM literature, with men routinely treated for male factor subfertility.[195,199]

Length of treatment

Spermatogenesis takes about 3 months. Therefore, it is important to treat a male partner for at least 3 months before an improvement in semen parameters can be expected.

Lifestyle factors

It is important that male patients are given evidence-based lifestyle advice and monitored to ensure that the advice is being followed. The effectiveness of acupuncture treatment otherwise could be reduced.

Other markers of male fertility

Semen parameters are not the only measure of male fertility because men with poor semen parameters can still achieve a pregnancy. Other aspects, such as the DNA quality of the sperm, are also important but are not routinely measured because of the high costs of DNA fragmentation tests. In some cases, acupuncture may not achieve a significant change in semen parameters, but it may still increase the chance of pregnancy by improving the genetic quality of sperm and the resulting embryo. Therefore, acupuncturists should use other methods of monitoring progress in response to acupuncture treatment, such as changes in the pulse and tongue and improvement of syndrome signs and symptoms.

Men are usually presumed to be fertile if their semen parameters are normal. However, according to the ASRM, male factor infertility may be present even when the semen analysis is normal.[185] If their DNA fragmentation index were tested, it could indicate in some instances potentially significant infertility. Therefore, there may be value in assessing all male partners from a TCM perspective, and, if TCM pathology is identified, acupuncture treatment should be recommended. Furthermore, in the authors' opinion, all men should be given preconception evidence-based lifestyle advice even if semen parameters are normal (with exceptions in cases where frozen embryos and/or sperm or donor sperm is used). Figure 8.6 summarizes how to manage patients with reversible causes of male factor subfertility.

 Case study

Male Factor Subfertility: Simple to Treat, More Difficult to Manage

Frances and Martin began trying for a baby when they were both 21 years old. After 5 years of trying unsuccessfully, they were referred for further investigations. Frances had irregular menstrual cycles; Martin's sperm count was low (6 million sperm) with very poor motility and morphology. They were advised that they had a 5% chance of conceiving naturally, but IVF/ICSI would be a good alternative option.

First IVF Cycle

Frances began acupuncture treatment 3 months before their first ICSI cycle. Martin did not, partly for financial reasons, partly because he was not keen on the needles, and partly because he hoped that the ICSI technique would overcome his subfertility. During that cycle, 14 eggs were retrieved, of which 12 were mature with seven fertilized by ICSI. Only one medium-quality blastocyst survived and was transferred. This resulted in the birth of their son.

Second IVF Cycle

They decided to try for a sibling 2 years later. Again, Frances had acupuncture, but this time she began the treatment when she was already on downregulation medication. She had over 20 follicles, but only four eggs were retrieved. One egg was mature and fertilized by ICSI. A poor-grade embryo was transferred on day 3. Francis conceived but suffered a preclinical miscarriage.

Review Post Second IVF Cycle

We discussed the importance of preparatory acupuncture in order to allow sufficient time for any underlying pathology to be addressed and lifestyle modifications to be made. I also recommended that Martin have acupuncture in preparation for their next IVF cycle.

Third IVF Cycle

This time both Frances and Martin began acupuncture treatment 3 months in advance. Martin was diagnosed with Qi and Blood Deficiency and received 10 acupuncture sessions. Points used were HE7, ST36, KID3, DU20, and LIV3.

This time, 15 eggs were retrieved, 12 were mature, but only three were fertilized by ICSI (despite Martin's sperm count on the day of fertilization being the best yet, at 19 million). Two medium-grade embryos were transferred on day 2. The treatment was successful, and, in a scan at 6 weeks, a healthy foetal heartbeat was observed (although Frances developed late onset OHSS, which was successfully managed with acupuncture.)

Discussion

This case emphasizes several points:

♦ In couples with both male and female factor subfertility, women are more likely than their partners to present for acupuncture.

♦ Having acupuncture during the preparatory phase is very important.

♦ ICSI is a powerful fertilization technique in male factor subfertility cases. However, in some cases, it can still result in a poor fertilization rate.

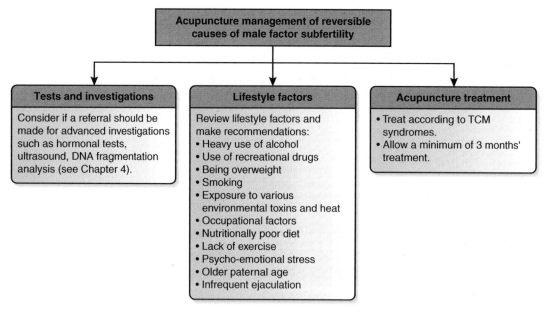

Figure 8.6 Algorithm of acupuncture management of reversible causes of male factor subfertility.

REGULATING THE MENSTRUAL CYCLE WITH ACUPUNCTURE

The importance of menstrual cycle regulation

Menstrual cycle characteristics such as total cycle length and duration of the menstrual bleed may influence fecundity. A cycle length of 30–31 days and a menstrual bleed of 4–5 days are the best for successful conception. For example, a year-long study of 470 women found:[212]

- Most fertile cycles were 30–31 days long, with longer or shorter cycles less likely to result in conception.
- If conception occurred in the shorter or longer cycles, this was more likely to result in miscarriages.
- Cycles with a menstrual bleed of ≤4 days were less fertile.
- Conceptions occurring in cycles with a menstrual bleed of ≥5 days were less likely to result in miscarriages.

Menstrual cycle characteristics have also been shown to influence the outcomes of assisted reproductive treatments. A prospective study of 6271 IVF/ICSI treatment cycles showed a direct significant relationship between mean cycle length and implantation, response to ovarian stimulation, pregnancy and live birth rates, even after adjusting for women's age, with live birth rates almost double in women with cycle length >34 days compared with women with cycle length <26 days.[213] Another study found that

women with shorter cycles had fewer aspirated follicles than women with longer cycles (21–35 days).[214]

Therefore, the use of acupuncture to help regulate the menstrual cycle is likely to assist a woman to successfully conceive, particularly as a fundamental part of the preparation for ART.

INTERESTING FACTS

IMPORTANCE OF MENSTRUAL CYCLE REGULATION IN CLASSICAL TCM

The importance of the menstrual cycle regulation was recognized as far back as the Qing dynasty. Liu Yi-ren, a physician from the Qing dynasty, stated that it is necessary to discuss the menstrual cycle with a female patient.[215]

Principles of regulating the menstrual cycle

As discussed in Chapter 2, the menstrual cycle is divided into four phases: follicular (menses), follicular (postmenses), ovulation, and premenstrual (luteal) phases. It is important to treat patients during every phase of the menstrual cycle as the treatment during one phase will influence the next phase.

Accurately assessing the intercycle activity and the appearance and amount of the menses can help the acupuncturist ascertain the severity of a patient's menstrual cycle abnormalities. This includes the assessment of:[216]

- Activity: arriving early, late, or irregularly (sometimes early, sometimes late), stop-starting flow or prolonged flow
- Amount: scant amount or heavy
- Colour: pale, purple, or bright red
- Consistency: clotted, thin, or thick

The assessment of menses can also provide further diagnostic details regarding the health of the Zangfu organs, Extraordinary Vessels, and the Uterus. Assessment of the menstrual cycle can also help identify the presence of Heat/Fire, Stagnation, Blood Stasis, Phlegm-Damp, and/or Cold.

The next sections provide information about what is considered a regular menstrual cycle and common pathologies during each phase of the menstrual cycle. We would caution against interpreting this information too rigidly. For example:

- A cycle of 25 days may be normal in some women. But, in a subfertile woman, particularly if she is of advanced reproductive age, it can signify Blood, Qi, and Kidney Jing (Essence) Deficiency. Cycle length changes with age, gradually reducing to 27 days in women aged 44 or older.[217]
- It is not generally considered abnormal if a cycle is delayed by a few days. However, this may be caused by the effect of stress on Qi and Blood and can represent subtle pathology. The overall picture should be considered when deciding what is normal and what is not.
- Quoted 'normal' ranges should not discourage the identification of early and minor pathology. As Fu Qing-Zhu recommended, there is often underlying pathology that needs to be assessed and considered before concluding what is or is not normal.[166]

Often menstrual pathology is complex. When assessing menstrual cycle irregularities, it is important to remember that more than one syndrome may be implicated, and these syndromes may combine and exacerbate each other. For example, a woman may have small and big clots or a pattern of mixed heavy and light period.[166]

Regulating the menstrual cycle promotes Yin Yang and provides the means for good-quality eggs and a better hormonal response to stimulation, thus optimizing a woman's chances of conception, embryo vitality, and pregnancy. As described in Chapter 2, follicles develop continually and, therefore, the opportunity to nourish Kidney Jing (Essence) and Yin for the purpose of improving the ovarian reserve also presents continually. There is no need to wait until after the period or until the mid-cycle to nourish Jing (Essence) or Yin. In fact, Kidney Jing (Essence) empowers Tian Gui, which, in turn, supplements and facilitates the Chong (Penetrating) and Ren (Conception) Mai (Vessels) to coordinate Qi and Blood and menses.

Regularity of the menstrual cycle

In TCM, a healthy menstrual cycle is considered to be 28–30 days.[97,218,219] In TCM, the menstrual cycle can be categorized according to its regularity:

- An irregular cycle: more than 7 days variability.[167]
- Early cycle: up to 7,[167] 8,[156] 9,[220] or, in extreme cases, 10 days early.[167]
- Late cycle: 7,[167] 8,[162] or 9[221] days late.
- Extremely late cycle: 50 days[221] to 3–5 months.[167]

Some authors state that irregularities must occur for 2–3 months before a diagnosis can be made.[167,220]

Figure 8.7 outlines principles for regulating the menstrual cycle.

Follicular phase (menses day 1–5)

Ideally, menses should last for about 5 days, the blood loss should not be too scant or too heavy, there should be no pain or clots, and blood should be red.

Common symptomatology experienced by women during menses is pain. The TCM differential diagnosis of pain includes:

- Liver Qi Stagnation and Blood Stasis
  - Distension
  - Severe stabbing pain
  - Worse with pressure
- Cold-Damp Yang Deficiency
  - Severe cramping
  - Better with warmth
- Liver and Kidney Yin Deficiency
  - Dull/mild pain
- Damp-Heat
  - Heavy sensation
  - Steady pain
- Heat
  - Dull/mild
  - Uncomfortable pain
- Kidney Yang and Blood Deficiency
  - Dull/mild
  - Constant pain

Figure 8.8 summarizes how to regulate this phase of the menstrual cycle.

Follicular phase (postmenstrual: days 5–14) or during stimulation

The menstrual bleeding should stop on day 5, and the rest of the follicular phase should be pain free and uneventful.[122,226] Figure 8.9 summarizes treatment principles during this phase.

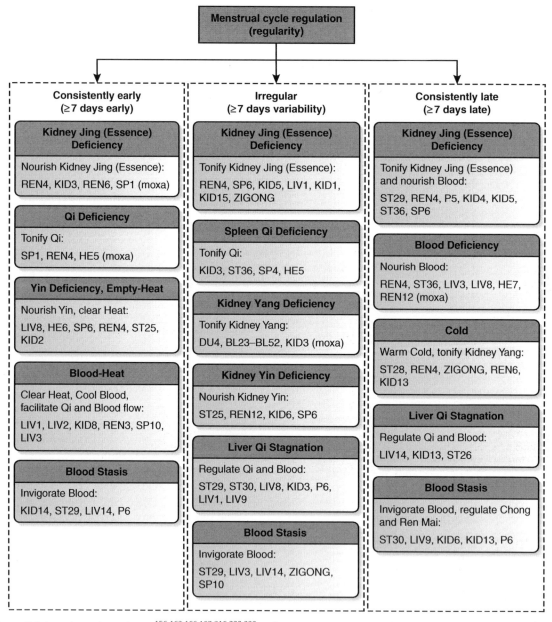

Figure 8.7 Irregular cycle syndromes[156,162,166,167,216,222,223] and acupuncture treatment.

Ovulation (days 14–16) or before egg retrieval

The most common abnormalities during the ovulation phase of the menstrual cycle are spotting and/or ovulation pain. Treatment principles during this stage are outlined in Figure 8.10.

  Red flag

Mid-cycle spotting or bleeding

Bleeding or spotting outside of the menses is considered to be a red flag and, as such, should be investigated by a gynaecologist in order to exclude sinister causes of bleeding.

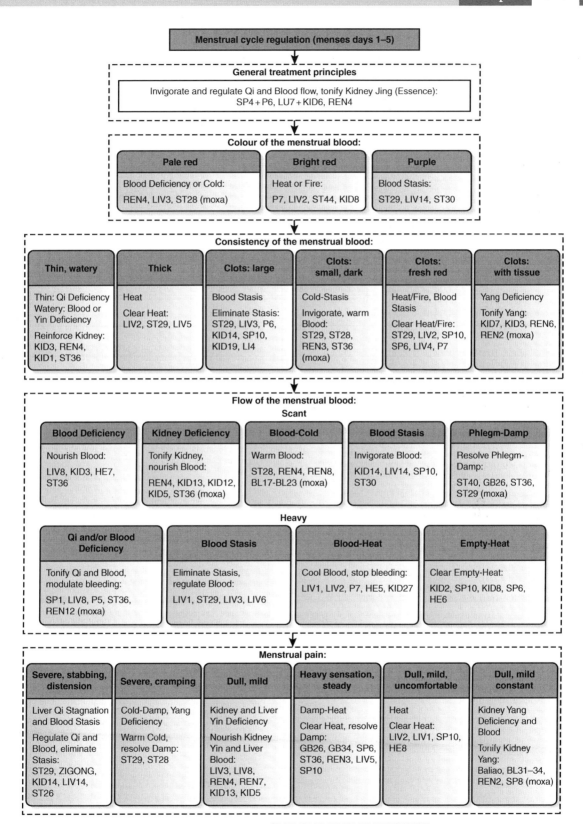

Figure 8.8 Menstrual cycle irregularities (menses: days 1–5)[98,122,124,162,166,167,175,216,222,224,225] and acupuncture treatment.

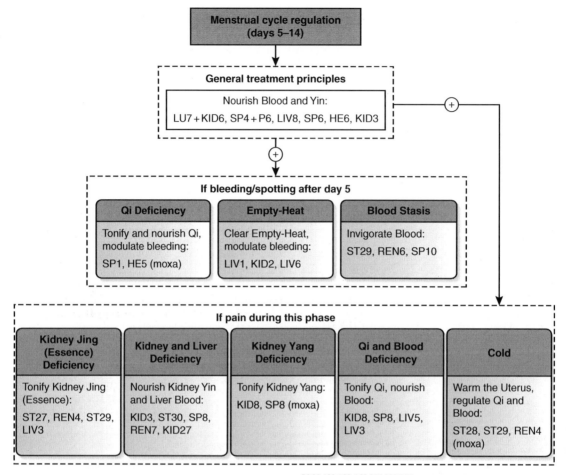

Figure 8.9 Menstrual cycle irregularities (follicular phase: days 5–14)[56,98,122,166–168,216,222,225] and acupuncture treatment.

Luteal phase (days 16–28)

Common symptomatology experienced by women during the luteal phase is emotional tension. The TCM differential diagnosis of emotional tension includes:

- Liver Qi Stagnation
  - Mild irritability[228]
  - Tension, moodiness[228]
  - Clumsiness[228]
  - Depression, crying[167]
- Phlegm-Heat/Fire
  - Pronounced agitation[228]
  - Distorted mood change and perception
  - Depression[228]
- Liver and Kidney Yin Deficiency
  - Depression, crying
  - Irritability[228]
  - Restlessness
- Blood-Heat

- Anger
- Aggressiveness
- Excessive emotionality

It is important to remember that during this phase an embryo could be trying to implant; therefore, care should be taken to use safe acupuncture points to assist with conception. If a patient develops bleeding, this could indicate a very early threatened miscarriage.

The TCM differential diagnosis for bleeding during the luteal phase includes:[116,125,161,165,229]

- Blood-Heat, Qi Stagnation, and Heat/Fire
  - Sudden onset
  - Profuse or scant flow
  - Red, thick, and/or sticky flow
- Yin Deficiency, Empty-Heat/Fire
  - Sudden onset
  - Scant dribbling
  - Fresh red, thick, and/or sticky consistency

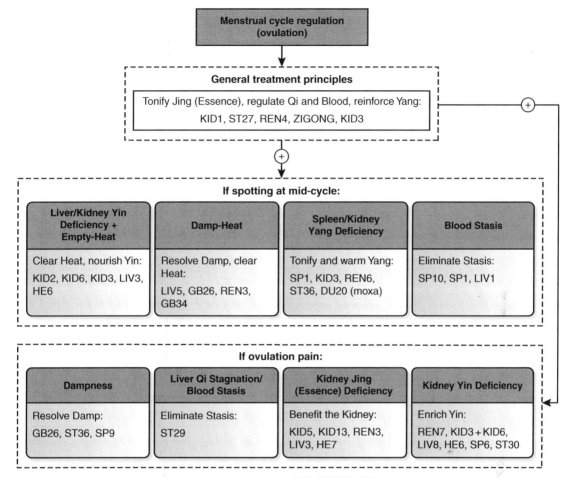

Figure 8.10 Menstrual cycle irregularities (ovulation: days 14–16)[56,98,167,168,222,227] and acupuncture treatment.

- Qi Deficiency
  - Profuse or dribbling flow
  - Pale red, thin consistency
- Liver and Kidney Yin Deficiency
  - Sudden onset
  - Bright-red flow
- Blood Stasis
  - Scant or heavy flow (or mixed)
  - Or dribbling flow (or mixed)
  - Dark red flow, thick and/or clotted consistency
- Qi 'Depression' Stagnation
  - Sudden profuse bleeding
  - Purplish, clotted menses

Figure 8.11 outlines common syndromes that manifest during the luteal phase and the TCM acupuncture treatments for them.

TREATMENT PLANNING: SETTING REALISTIC GOALS

When treating ART patients, the majority of the patients will need to be supported through four stages:

- The initial case intake or case review
- The preparation stage
- ART treatment stage
- Pregnancy support (if the treatment is successful)

Figure 8.12 provides a treatment planning algorithm that integrates conventional Orthodox medical management diagnosis, the patients' adoption and compliance with lifestyle factors, and their ART history along with their TCM acupuncture management.

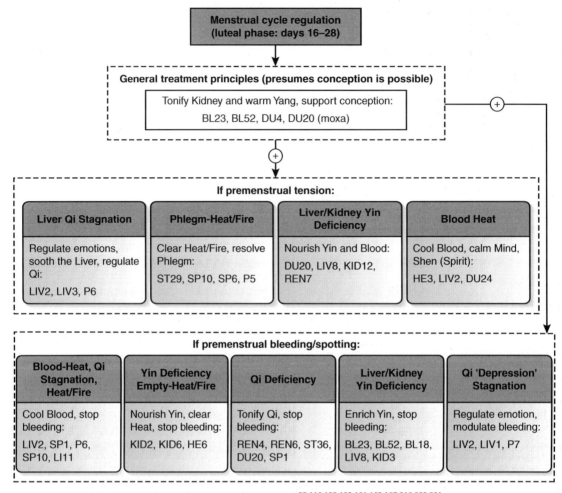

Figure 8.11 Menstrual cycle irregularities (luteal phase: days 16–28)[98,116,122,125,161,165,167,216,230,231] and acupuncture treatment.

Case intake stage (or review stage)

This stage relates to when patients initially present for treatment. The steps outlined here can also be used in cases where previous ART treatment has failed and patients re-present for a new treatment cycle.

Medical history and diagnosis

All the medical details (such as any medical diagnoses, tests and investigations, etc.) should be reviewed. If an additional medical diagnosis is suspected, patients should be referred for further investigations. For example, if a woman is suspected to suffer from thyroid disease, she should be referred for TFTs because, if left untreated, this disease may potentially cause IVF and/or pregnancy to fail.

Lifestyle factors

A full review of lifestyle factors in both partners (such as weight, smoking, alcohol intake, diet and supplements, etc.) should be undertaken and recommendations on how to modify these (if necessary) should be provided.

Previous ART treatment history

If applicable, a full review of any previous ART treatment cycles should be carried out and corrective or preventative measures should be planned for the stages that did not go well or where complications occurred. For example, if the fertilization rate was low, then the possible reasons why this happened should be looked into and, if possible, steps should be taken to improve the fertilization rate for the next round of treatment.

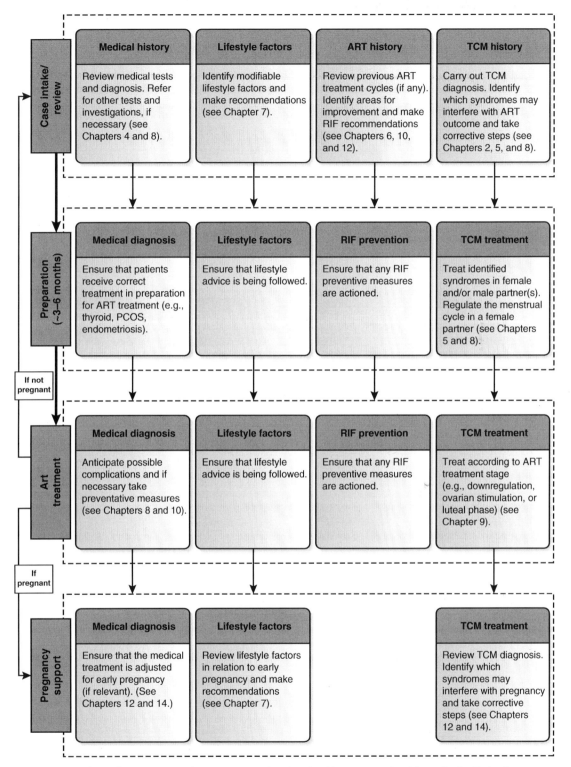

Figure 8.12 Orthodox and TCM integrated ART treatment planning algorithm. ART, Assisted Reproductive Technology; RIF, Repeated Implantation Failure; TCM, Traditional Chinese Medicine.

TCM history

A full TCM diagnostic triage should be undertaken, ideally in both male and female partners.

Preparation stage

The preparation stage is very important because it takes time for any lifestyle modifications and Orthodox and TCM treatments to influence a patient's constitution. Three months of weekly treatments is a recommended time frame for most patients. However, some patients present very close to their treatment cycle, leaving very little time for preparation. Several options are available in these cases:

- In complex cases that require major lifestyle modifications and/or Orthodox or TCM treatment, it may be prudent to recommend delaying ART treatment. In the authors' experience, this option may not be favoured by some patients because they may have already made plans for the treatment – for example, booked time off work. Patients also dislike the idea of delaying the treatment. However, many understand the reasons and are happy to follow such advice.
- Alternatively, more frequent acupuncture treatment should be recommended (for example, instead of weekly sessions, acupuncture should be carried out every 3–4 days). It is suggested that acupuncture treatment in the management of patients is dose dependent.[232–234] Therefore, potentially similar treatment outcomes may be achieved in 1 month compared with 3 months of acupuncture treatment if the same number of treatment sessions are administered.
- In simple cases where no major pathologies are present and no major lifestyle modifications are necessary, it is in our opinion acceptable to go straight to the ART treatment stage.

Medical diagnosis

In patients with subfertility-related medical conditions, it is important to ensure they are receiving correct treatment for them. For example, if a woman has been diagnosed with hypothyroidism, it is important to check that that she is taking her medication.

Lifestyle factors

It is important to check that patients have understood and are following the appropriate lifestyle advice.

Repeated Implantation Failure prevention

If a patient has previously undergone ART treatment and areas for improvement have been identified during the review process, then the patient should be assisted in taking steps to prevent similar issues or complications arising in the next treatment cycle. For example, if the patient's response to ovarian stimulation was poor, she may need to speak to her consultant about changing her IVF treatment protocol or increasing the dose of medication.

TCM treatment

During the preparation stage, acupuncture treatment should focus on reducing the severity of TCM syndromes identified in either or both partners. In female patients, it is important to regulate their menstrual cycles in preparation for ART treatment (see the section 'The importance of menstrual cycle regulation').

ART treatment stage

This stage usually begins when patients start their ART treatment medication and lasts until the pregnancy test date. If the ART treatment cycle is not controlled with medication, then the ART treatment stage starts with day 1 of the menstrual cycle during which the eggs will be retrieved and/or embryos transferred.

Medical diagnosis

By this stage, any underlying medical comorbidities that may have an effect on ART outcomes should be well controlled. However, in some cases (for example, in patients with thyroid disease) medication may need to be altered during this stage. Some medical conditions are associated with complications; therefore, fertility acupuncturists should take a prophylactic approach to the treatment of such patients. For example, women diagnosed with reduced ovarian reserve are likely to respond poorly to ovarian stimulation. Therefore, the frequency of acupuncture treatment in such patients may need to be increased in order to improve the ovarian response.

Lifestyle factors

Just as in the preparation phase, patients should be encouraged to continue their lifestyle modifications.

RIF prevention

By this stage, all RIF preventative measures should be in place. However, it may be prudent to review each case to ensure that nothing has been omitted from the management protocol.

TCM treatment

Acupuncture treatment should be based partly on the syndromes identified at the original case intake, partly on any new syndromes that develop, and partly according to the patient's staging in the ART treatment process. Acupuncture treatment frequency will depend on the ART protocol, the patient's response to medication, and the patient's need for emotional support (see Chapter 9).

Pregnancy support

In those patients who conceive, the focus should now change to pregnancy-supporting treatment.

Medical diagnosis

The treatment of some medical conditions may need to be adjusted during pregnancy. It is important that patients for whom this may be relevant have a full review of their treatment.

Lifestyle factors

Female patients need to continue making lifestyle modifications.

RIF prevention

Some RIF treatments may need to be continued during pregnancy. For example, patients who need reproductive immunology treatment in order to prevent implantation failure often need to continue their treatments.

TCM treatment

Acupuncture treatment focus should now change to supporting early pregnancy. A patient should be monitored in case new syndromes become evident.

With patients who do not successfully conceive, a full review should be undertaken. Then the treatment cycle will begin again. Some patients may decide not to continue with any further treatment.

SUMMARY

Tubal factor infertility

Tubal factor infertility does not negatively influence IVF outcomes unless patients have hydrosalpinges. These patients would benefit from surgical removal of the affected fallopian tube(s) prior to undergoing IVF. Furthermore, patients with mild tubal pathology may still conceive in a natural cycle, and, therefore, a course of acupuncture treatment and natural conception attempts is justifiable in cases where there are no other indications for IVF.

Anovulation

Women with WHO grade I or II anovulation (including patients with PCOS) can benefit from acupuncture treatment to help them re-establish ovulatory cycles. Lifestyle modifications (for example, weight loss or gain) are also an important part of the management of these patients. If these patients fail to re-establish ovulatory cycles or if they do not conceive, the first-line treatment in these cases is ovulation induction with CC. Acupuncture treatment may help to enhance the effectiveness of CC.

Patients with WHO grade III anovulation will need donor egg IVF. Treating these patients with acupuncture in preparation for and during IVF is recommended.

Thyroid disease

In the authors' experience, TFTs are often omitted when patients are investigated for infertility. This is often the case even in patients with risk factors for thyroid disease. There is significant disagreement within the medical profession on what constitutes a normal range of hormone levels and how to manage patients with subclinical thyroid disease. Untreated thyroid disease (overt and subclinical) can have a detrimental effect on fertility and pregnancy and may reduce IVF success rates. Therefore, acupuncturists must screen all patients for risk factors of thyroid disease and, if necessary, refer for thyroid investigations.

Endometriosis

Endometriosis is strongly associated with subfertility and can adversely affect the outcome of ART treatment. However, patients with both mild and severe endometriosis (without serious anatomical pathology) may still conceive naturally. Therefore, a course of acupuncture treatment and natural conception attempts is justifiable in cases where there are no other indications for IVF. If patients fail to conceive naturally, they may benefit from pretreatment with a GnRH agonist prior to undergoing IVF. The acupuncturist's role is to ensure that patients are informed about GnRH agonist treatment.

Endometriomas that are >4 cm in diameter may compromise a patient's response to ovarian stimulation and, therefore, should be surgically removed before IVF.

Male factor subfertility

At least 50% of subfertile couples will be affected by male factor subfertility. Therefore, it is essential that male partners with evidence of male factor subfertility are encouraged to have a course of acupuncture treatment. It is important to treat them for a minimum of 3 months because that is how long it takes to produce mature sperm.

Menstrual cycle

Research shows that menstrual cycle characteristics such as cycle length, regularity, number of days of menstrual bleed can have an adverse effect on conception, miscarriage rates and IVF outcome. The importance of menstrual cycle regulation was discussed in Classical TCM as far back as the Eastern Han Dynasty. Therefore, when treating a female patient in preparation for ART, the menstrual cycle should be assessed and if necessary treatment and management should be individualized based on identified syndromes and include acupuncture points that will help to regulate the cycle.

REFERENCES

1. Hull MG, Glazener CM, Kelly NJ, et al. Population study of causes, treatment, and outcome of infertility. Br Med J (Clin Res Ed) 1985;291:1693–7.

2. Wilkes S, Chinn DJ, Murdoch A, et al. Epidemiology and management of infertility: a population-based study in UK primary care. Fam Pract 2009;26:269–74.

3. National Collaborating Centre for Women's and Children's Health, Commissioned by the National Institute for Health and Clinical Excellence. Introduction. In: Fertility: assessment and treatment for people with fertility problems. NICE clinical guideline. 2nd ed. London: The Royal College of Obstetricians and Gynaecologists; 2013. p. 47–9 [chapter 2].

4. Harris-Glocker M, McLaren JF. Role of female pelvic anatomy in infertility. Clin Anat 2013;26:89–96.

5. Collins JA. Evidence-based infertility: evaluation of the female partner. Int Congr Ser 2004;1266:57–62.

6. Dessole S, Meloni GB, Capobianco G, et al. A second hysterosalpingography reduces the use of selective technique for treatment of a proximal tubal obstruction. Fertil Steril 2000;73:1037–9.

7. Evers JLH, Land JA, Mol BW. Evidence-based medicine for diagnostic questions. Semin Reprod Med 2003;21:009–16.

8. Luttjeboer F, Harada T, Hughes E, et al. Tubal flushing for subfertility. Cochrane Database Syst Rev 2007; (3):CD003718.

9. National Collaborating Centre for Women's and Children's Health, Commissioned by the National Institute for Health and Clinical Excellence. Tubal and uterine surgery. In: Fertility: assessment and treatment for people with fertility problems. NICE clinical guideline. 2nd ed. London: The Royal College of Obstetricians and Gynaecologists; 2013. p. 183–7 [chapter 9].

10. Practice Committee of the American Society for Reproductive Medicine. Committee opinion: role of tubal surgery in the era of assisted reproductive technology. Fertil Steril 2012;97:539–45.

11. Strandell A. The influence of hydrosalpinx on IVF and embryo transfer: a review. Hum Reprod Update 2000;6:387–95.

12. Johnson N, van Voorst S, Sowter MC, et al. Surgical treatment for tubal disease in women due to undergo in vitro fertilisation. Cochrane Database Syst Rev 2010; (1):CD002125.

13. Maughan TA, Zhai X. The acupuncture treatment of female infertility – with particular reference to egg quality and endometrial receptiveness. J Chin Med 2012;98:13–21.

14. Maciocia G. Infertility. In: Obstetrics and gynecology in Chinese medicine. 2nd ed. Edinburgh: Elsevier Health Sciences; 2011. p. 685–734 [chapter 57].

15. Xu X, Yin H, Tang D, et al. Application of Traditional Chinese Medicine in the treatment of infertility. Hum Fertil 2003;6:161–8.

16. Lyttleton J. Blockage of the fallopian tubes. In: Treatment of infertility with Chinese medicine. 2nd ed. London: Churchill Livingstone/Elsevier; 2013. p. 233–49 [chapter 6].

17. Ying-qiu C, Li Z. Treatment of tubal inflammatory obstruction mainly by thunder-fire moxibustion: a report of 54 cases. J Acupunct Tuina Sci 2005;3:18–9.

18. Magarelli PC, Cridennda D, Cohen M. The demographics of acupuncture's impact on IVF outcomes: infertility diagnosis and SART/CDC age groups. Fertil Steril 2007;87:S10–1.

19. Madaschi C, Braga DPAF, de Figueira RCS, et al. Effect of acupuncture on assisted reproduction treatment outcomes. Acupunct Med 2010;28:180–4.

20. Broekmans F. The initial fertility assessment: a medical check-up of the couple experiencing difficulties conceiving. In: de Haan N, Spelt M, Gobel R, editors. Reproductive medicine: a textbook for paramedics. Amsterdam: Elsevier Gezondheidszorg; 2010. p. 21–39 [chapter 1].

21. Practice Committee of the American Society for Reproductive Medicine. Use of clomiphene citrate in women. Fertil Steril 2006;86: S187–93.

22. Kerin JF, Liu JH, Phillipou G, et al. Evidence for a hypothalamic site of action of clomiphene citrate in women. J Clin Endocrinol Metab 1985;61:265–8.

23. Kettel LM, Roseff SJ, Berga SL, et al. Hypothalamic-pituitary-ovarian response to clomiphene citrate in women with polycystic ovary syndrome. Fertil Steril 1993;59:532–8.

24. MD024. Female infertility pharmacotherapy – stimulation protocols. ASRM Learning Course Notes; 2010.

25. The Rotterdam ESHRE/ASRM-sponsored PCOS consensus workshop group. Revised 2003 consensus on diagnostic criteria and long-term health risks related to

polycystic ovary syndrome (PCOS). Hum Reprod 2004;19:41–7.

26. Fauser BC, Tarlatzis BC, Rebar RW, et al. Consensus on women's health aspects of polycystic ovary syndrome (PCOS): the Amsterdam ESHRE/ASRM-sponsored 3rd PCOS consensus workshop group. Fertil Steril 2012;97:28–38.e25.

27. Tehrani FR, Solaymani-Dodaran M, Hedayati M, et al. Is polycystic ovary syndrome an exception for reproductive aging? Hum Reprod 2010;25:1775–81.

28. Cocksedge KA, Li TC, Saravelos SH, et al. A reappraisal of the role of polycystic ovary syndrome in recurrent miscarriage. Reprod Biomed Online 2008;17:151–60.

29. Rittenberg V, Seshadri S, Sunkara SK, et al. Effect of body mass index on IVF treatment outcome: an updated systematic review and meta-analysis. Reprod Biomed Online 2011;23:421–39.

30. Thatcher SS, Jackson EM. Pregnancy outcome in infertile patients with polycystic ovary syndrome who were treated with metformin. Fertil Steril 2006;85:1002–9.

31. Barnhart KT. Epidemiology of male and female reproductive disorders and impact on fertility regulation and population growth. Fertil Steril 2011;95:2200–3.

32. Farrell K, Antoni MH. Insulin resistance, obesity, inflammation, and depression in polycystic ovary syndrome: biobehavioral mechanisms and interventions. Fertil Steril 2010;94:1565–74.

33. Thessaloniki ESHRE/ASRM-Sponsored PCOS Consensus Workshop Group. Consensus on infertility treatment related to polycystic ovary syndrome. Fertil Steril 2008;89:505–22.

34. Moran LJ, Ko H, Misso M, et al. Dietary composition in the treatment of polycystic ovary syndrome: a systematic review to inform evidence-based guidelines. Hum Reprod Update 2013;19:432, first published online 31 May, 2013.

35. Onalan G, Pabuçcu R, Goktolga U, et al. Metformin treatment in patients with polycystic ovary syndrome undergoing in vitro fertilization: a prospective randomized trial. Fertil Steril 2005;84:798–801.

36. Heijnen EM, Eijkemans MJ, Hughes EG, et al. A meta-analysis of outcomes of conventional IVF in women with polycystic ovary syndrome. Hum Reprod Update 2006;12:13–21.

37. Practice Committee of American Society for Reproductive Medicine. Obesity and reproduction: an educational bulletin. Fertil Steril 2008;90:S21–9.

38. Swanton A, Storey L, McVeigh E, et al. IVF outcome in women with PCOS, PCO and normal ovarian morphology. Eur J Obstet Gynecol Reprod Biol 2010;149:68–71.

39. Huang JY, Rosenwaks Z. In vitro fertilisation treatment and factors affecting success. Best Pract Res Clin Obstet Gynaecol 2012;26:777–88.

40. Tummon I, Gavrilova-Jordan L, Allemand MC, et al. Polycystic ovaries and ovarian hyperstimulation syndrome: a systematic review*. Acta Obstet Gynecol Scand 2005;84:611–6.

41. Junk SM, Yeap D. Improved implantation and ongoing pregnancy rates after single-embryo transfer with an optimized protocol for in vitro oocyte maturation in women with polycystic ovaries and polycystic ovary syndrome. Fertil Steril 2012;98:888–92.

42. Thomson RL, Spedding S, Buckley JD. Vitamin D in the aetiology and management of polycystic ovary syndrome. Clin Endocrinol (Oxf) 2012;77:343–50.

43. Lerchbaum E, Obermayer-Pietsch B. Vitamin D and fertility: a systematic review. Eur J Endocrinol 2012;166:765–78.

44. Lim DC, Chen W, Cheng LN, et al. Acupuncture for polycystic ovarian syndrome. Cochrane Database Syst Rev 2011;(8):CD007689.

45. Lim CE, Wong WS. Current evidence of acupuncture on polycystic ovarian syndrome. Gynecol Endocrinol 2010;26:473–8.

46. Cui W, Li J, Sun W, et al. Effect of electroacupuncture on oocyte quality and pregnancy for patients with PCOS undergoing in vitro fertilization and embryo transfervitro fertilization and embryo transfer. Zhongguo Zhen Jiu 2011;31:687–91.

47. Rashidi BH, Tehrani ES, Hamedani NA, et al. Effects of acupuncture on the outcome of in vitro fertilisation and intracytoplasmic sperm injection in women with polycystic ovarian syndrome. Acupunct Med 2013;31:151–6.

48. Stener-Victorin E, Waldenström U, Tägnfors U, et al. Effects of electro-acupuncture on anovulation in women with polycystic ovary syndrome. Acta Obstet Gynecol Scand 2000;79:180–8.

49. Maciocia G. Abdominal masses: ovarian cysts, polycystic ovary disease, cervical dysplasia. In: Obstetrics and gynecology in Chinese medicine. New York: Churchill Livingstone; 1998. p. 791–816 [chapter 60].

50. Lyttleton J. Gynaecological disorders which can cause infertility. In: Treatment of infertility with Chinese medicine. London: Churchill Livingstone; 2004. p. 165–234 [chapter 5].

51. Jiang D. TCM treatment of polycystic ovary and PCOS. J Assoc Tradit Chin Med (UK) 2010;17:11–4.

52. Deadman P, Al-Khafaji M, Baker K. The Spleen channel. In: A manual of acupuncture. England: Journal of Chinese Medicine Publications; 1998. p. 175–206.

53. Deadman P, Al-Khafaji M, Baker K. The Kidney channel. In: A manual of acupuncture. England: Journal of Chinese Medicine Publications; 1998. p. 329–64.

54. Deadman P, Al-Khafaji M, Baker K. The Lung channel. In: A manual of acupuncture. England: Journal of Chinese Medicine Publications; 1998. p. 71–92.

55. Maciocia G. Women's pathology. In: Obstetrics and gynecology in Chinese medicine. New York: Churchill Livingstone; 1998. p. 31–49 [chapter 3].

56. Maciocia G. Women's physiology. In: Obstetrics and gynecology in Chinese medicine. New York: Churchill Livingstone; 1998. p. 7–29 [chapter 2].

57. Deadman P, Al-Khafaji M, Baker K. The extraordinary points. In: A manual of acupuncture. England: Journal of Chinese Medicine Publications; 1998. p. 563–86.

58. Deadman P, Al-Khafaji M, Baker K. The Stomach channel. In: A manual of acupuncture. England: Journal of Chinese Medicine Publications; 1998. p. 123–74.

59. Deadman P, Al-Khafaji M, Baker K. The Gallbladder channel. In: A manual of acupuncture. England: Journal of Chinese Medicine Publications; 1998. p. 415–66.

60. Deadman P, Al-Khafaji M, Baker K. The Pericardium channel. In: A manual of acupuncture. England: Journal of Chinese Medicine Publications; 1998. p. 365–84.

61. Deadman P, Al-Khafaji M, Baker K. The conception vessel. In: A manual of acupuncture. England: Journal of Chinese Medicine Publications; 1998. p. 493–526.

62. Deadman P, Al-Khafaji M, Baker K. The Liver channel. In: A manual of acupuncture. England: Journal of Chinese Medicine Publications; 1998. p. 467–92.

63. Stener-Victorin E, Jedel E, Janson PO, et al. Low-frequency electroacupuncture and physical exercise decrease high muscle sympathetic nerve activity in polycystic ovary syndrome. Am J Physiol Regul Integr Comp Physiol 2009;297:R387–95.

64. Gamus D. Electro-acupuncture in polycystic ovary syndrome: a potent placebo or a new promising treatment? Focus Altern Complement Ther 2011;16:229–30.

65. Johansson J, Redman L, Veldhuis PP, et al. Acupuncture for ovulation induction in polycystic ovary syndrome: a randomized controlled trial. Am J Physiol Endocrinol Metab 2013;204: E934–43.

66. Lu HC. Five sounds and five flavours. In: A complete translation of the Yellow Emperor's classics of internal medicine and the difficult classic (Nei-Jing and Nan-Jing). Vancouver: International College of Traditional Chinese Medicine; 2004. p. 546–8, Section three: Spiritual pivot [Ling Shu] [chapter 65].

67. ASRM. Hypothyroidism. Available from: http://www. reproductivefacts.org/ Hypothyroidism_factsheet/ [accessed 26 July 2013].

68. Nygaard B. Hyperthyroidism (primary). Clin Evid (Online) 2010;2010:0611.

69. Konova E. The role of NK cells in the autoimmune thyroid disease-associated pregnancy loss. Clin Rev Allergy Immunol 2010;39:176–84.

70. The Association for Clinical Biochemistry (ACB), The British Thyroid Association (BTA), The British Thyroid Foundation (BTF). UK guidelines for the use of thyroid function tests. Report of the The Association for Clinical Biochemistry (ACB), The British Thyroid Association (BTA) and The British Thyroid Foundation (BTF). British Thyroid Association, London; 2006.

71. National Collaborating Centre for Women's and Children's Health, Commissioned by the National Institute for Health and Clinical Excellence. Guideline summary. In: Fertility: assessment and treatment for people with fertility problems. NICE clinical guideline. 2nd ed. London: The Royal College of Obstetricians and Gynaecologists; 2013. p. 1–46 [chapter 1].

72. The Practice Committee of the American Society for Reproductive Medicine. Evaluation and treatment of recurrent pregnancy loss: a committee opinion. Fertil Steril 2012;98:1103–11.

73. De Groot L, Abalovich M, Alexander EK, et al. Management of thyroid dysfunction during pregnancy and postpartum: an Endocrine Society clinical practice guideline. J Clin Endocrinol Metab 2012;97:2543–65.

74. Reh A, Chaudhry S, Mendelsohn F, et al. Effect of autoimmune thyroid disease in older euthyroid infertile woman during the first 35 days of an IVF cycle. Fertil Steril 2011;95:1178–81.

75. Revelli A, Casano S, Piane LD, et al. A retrospective study on IVF outcome in euthyroid patients with anti-thyroid antibodies: effects of levothyroxine, acetyl-salicylic acid and prednisolone adjuvant treatments. Reprod Biol Endocrinol 2009;7:137.

76. Spencer CA, Hollowell JG, Kazarosyan M, et al. National health and nutrition examination survey III thyroid-stimulating hormone (TSH)-thyroperoxidase antibody relationships demonstrate that TSH upper reference limits may be skewed by occult thyroid dysfunction. J Clin Endocrinol Metab 2007;92:4236–40.

77. Negro R, Schwartz A, Gismondi R, et al. Increased pregnancy loss rate in thyroid antibody negative women with TSH levels between 2.5 and 5.0 in the first trimester of pregnancy. J Clin Endocrinol Metab 2010;95:E44–8.

78. Wartofsky L, Dickey RA. The evidence for a narrower thyrotropin reference range is compelling. J Clin Endocrinol Metab 2005;90:5483–8.

79. Brabant G, Beck-Peccoz P, Jarzab B, et al. Is there a need to redefine the upper normal limit of TSH? Eur J Endocrinol 2006;154:633–7.

80. Garber JR, Cobin RH, Gharib H, et al. Clinical practice guidelines for hypothyroidism in adults: cosponsored by the American Association of Clinical Endocrinologists and the American Thyroid Association. Endocr Pract 2012;18:988–1028.

81. Khandelwal D, Tandon N. Overt and subclinical hypothyroidism: who to treat and how. Drugs 2012;72:17–33.

82. Michalakis KG, Mesen TB, Brayboy LM, et al. Subclinical elevations of thyroid-stimulating hormone and assisted reproductive technology outcomes. Fertil Steril 2011;95:2634–7.

83. Krassas GE, Poppe K, Glinoer D. Thyroid function and human reproductive health. Endocr Rev 2010;31:702–55.

84. Scoccia B, Demir H, Kang Y, et al. In vitro fertilization pregnancy rates in levothyroxine-treated women with hypothyroidism compared to women without thyroid dysfunction disorders. Thyroid 2012;22:631–6.

85. Cramer DW, Sluss PM, Powers RD, et al. Serum prolactin and TSH in an in vitro fertilization population: is

there a link between fertilization and thyroid function? J Assist Reprod Genet 2003;20:210–5.

86. Kilic S, Tasdemir N, Yilmaz N, et al. The effect of anti-thyroid antibodies on endometrial volume, embryo grade and IVF outcome. Gynecol Endocrinol 2008;24:649–55.

87. Velkeniers B, Van Meerhaeghe A, Poppe K, et al. Levothyroxine treatment and pregnancy outcome in women with subclinical hypothyroidism undergoing assisted reproduction technologies: systematic review and meta-analysis of RCTs. Hum Reprod Update 2013;19:251–8.

88. Gracia CR, Morse CB, Chan G, et al. Thyroid function during controlled ovarian hyperstimulation as part of in vitro fertilization. Fertil Steril 2012;97:585–91.

89. Stagnaro-Green A, Abalovich M, Alexander E, et al. Guidelines of the American Thyroid Association for the diagnosis and management of thyroid disease during pregnancy and postpartum. Thyroid 2011;21:1081–125.

90. van den Boogaard E, Vissenberg R, Land JA, et al. Significance of (sub) clinical thyroid dysfunction and thyroid autoimmunity before conception and in early pregnancy: a systematic review. Hum Reprod Update 2011;17:605–19.

91. Vissenberg R, van den Boogaard E, van Wely M, et al. Treatment of thyroid disorders before conception and in early pregnancy: a systematic review. Hum Reprod Update 2012;18:360–73.

92. WHO. Iodine deficiency, health consequences, assessment and control. In: Andersson M, de Benoist B, Darnton-Hill I, Delange F, editors. Iodine deficiency in Europe: a continuing public health problem. Geneva: WHO Press; 2007. p. 8–19.

93. Anderson K, Nisenblat V, Norman R. Lifestyle factors in people seeking infertility treatment – a review. Aust N Z J Obstet Gynaecol 2010;50:8–20.

94. The British Dietetic Association. Food fact sheet. Iodine. Available from: http://www.bda.uk.com/foodfacts/Iodine.pdf [accessed 10 June 2013].

95. Chunxiang T. How to give TCM differential treatment for hypothyroidism? J Tradit Chin Med 2008;28:231–2.

96. Liu F. Medical essays. In: The Essence of Liu Feng-Wu's gynecology. 1st ed. Boulder: Blue Poppy Press; 1998. p. 13–9, Section 2. A talk on the Kidneys [chapter 1].

97. Unschuld PU, Tessenow H, Jinsheng Z. Discourse on the true [Qi endowed by] Heaven in high antiquity. Huang Di Nei Jing Su Wen, vol. 1. Berkeley: University of California Press; 2011. p. 29–44 [chapter 1].

98. Lyttleton J. Diagnosis and treatment of female infertility. In: Treatment of infertility with Chinese medicine. London: Churchill Livingstone; 2004. p. 83–164 [chapter 4].

99. Maciocia G. Kidney patterns. In: The foundations of Chinese medicine: a comprehensive text for acupuncturists and herbalists. Edinburgh, NY: Churchill Livingstone; 1989. p. 249–63 [chapter 25].

100. Lu HC. Kidneys. In: Syndromes in Traditional Chinese Medicine. Marston: CreateSpace Independent Publishing Platform; 2013. p. 328–54 [chapter 30].

101. Unschuld PU, Tessenow H, Jinsheng Z. The generation and completion of the five depots. Huang Di Nei Jing Su Wen, vol. 1. Berkeley: University of California Press; 2011. p. 185–201 [chapter 10].

102. Rochat de la Vallee E. Infertility. In: Root C, editor. The essential women, female health and fertility in Chinese classical texts. Norfolk: Monkey Press; 2007. p. 72–83.

103. Li Shi Zhen. The twenty-seven pulse states. In: Seifert GM, editor. Hoc Ku Huynh, translator. Pulse diagnosis. Brookline: Paradigm Press; 1985. p. 61–101 [chapter 11].

104. Pi'an S. Hashimoto's thyroiditis. In: Ward T, (editor). Shen's textbook on the management of autoimmune diseases with Chinese medicine. Barnet, Herts, UK: Donica Publishing Ltd; 2012. p. 531–54 [chapter 19].

105. Maciocia G. Heart patterns. In: The foundations of Chinese medicine: a comprehensive text for

acupuncturists and herbalists. Edinburgh, NY: Churchill Livingstone; 1989. p. 201–13 [chapter 21].

106. Maciocia G. Spleen patterns. In: The foundations of Chinese medicine: a comprehensive text for acupuncturists and herbalists. Edinburgh, NY: Churchill Livingstone; 1989. p. 241–8 [chapter 24].

107. Maciocia G. Stomach patterns. In: The foundations of Chinese medicine: a comprehensive text for acupuncturists and herbalists. Edinburgh, NY: Churchill Livingstone; 1989. p. 265–72 [chapter 26].

108. Maciocia G. Lung patterns. In: The foundations of Chinese medicine: a comprehensive text for acupuncturists and herbalists. Edinburgh, NY: Churchill Livingstone; 1989. p. 231–40 [chapter 23].

109. Wiseman N, Feng Y. H. A practical dictionary of Chinese medicine. 2nd ed. Brookline, MA: Paradigm Publications; 1998, p. 251–94.

110. Hua Tuo. Book one. In: Flaws B, editor. Yang S, translator. Master Hua's classic of the central viscera: a translation of Hua Tuo's Zhong Zang Jing. Boulder, CO: Blue Poppy Press; 1993. p. 1–92.

111. Maciocia G. Liver patterns. In: The foundations of Chinese medicine: a comprehensive text for acupuncturists and herbalists. Edinburgh, NY: Churchill Livingstone; 1989. p. 215–29 [chapter 22].

112. Lu HC. Various types of energy. In: A complete translation of the Yellow Emperor's classics of internal medicine and the difficult classic (Nei-Jing and Nan-Jing). Vancouver: International College of Traditional Chinese Medicine; 2004. p. 489–90, Section three: Spiritual pivot [Ling Shu] [chapter 30].

113. Soszka S. Liver and Gallbladder based erectile dysfunction: treatment by Chinese medicine (part one). J Chin Med 2002;68:5–14.

114. Ross J. Shen (Kidneys) and Pang Guang Bladder. In: Zang Fu, the organ systems of traditional

Chinese medicine: functions, interrelationships and patterns of disharmony in theory and practice. 2nd ed. Edinburgh: Churchill Livingstone; 1985. p. 65–82, Part 2 [chapter 7].

115. Wiseman N, Feng Y. K. A practical dictionary of Chinese medicine. 2nd ed. Brookline, MA: Paradigm Publications; 1998, p. 324–37.

116. Wiseman N, Feng Y. L. A practical dictionary of Chinese medicine. 2nd ed. Brookline, Mass: Paradigm Publications; 1998, p. 338–81.

117. Maciocia G. Identification according to pathogenic factors. In: The foundations of Chinese medicine: a comprehensive text for acupuncturists and herbalists. Edinburgh, NY: Churchill Livingstone; 1989. p. 293–302 [chapter 32].

118. Maciocia online: the treatment of autoimmune diseases with Chinese medicine – part 1. Available from: http://maciociaonline.blogspot.co.uk/2013/01/the-treatment-of-autoimmune-diseases.html [accessed 18 January 2013].

119. Wei Z. The differentiation and TCM treatment of hyperthyroidism. J Chin Med 1998;57:30–2.

120. Appleyard I. The treatment of hyperthyroidism by acupuncture. J Chin Med 2006;81:5–10.

121. Maciocia G. Body. In: Diagnosis in Chinese medicine: a comprehensive guide. Edinburgh: Elsevier; 2004. p. 709–15 [chapter 68].

122. Wiseman N, Feng Y. P. A practical dictionary of Chinese medicine. 2nd ed. Brookline, MA: Paradigm Publications; 1998, p. 423–74.

123. Canruo S. The treatment of thyroid diseases by acupuncture. J Chin Med 1987;23:29–34.

124. Wiseman N, Feng Y. S. A practical dictionary of Chinese medicine. 2nd ed. Brookline, MA: Paradigm Publications; 1998, p. 511–601.

125. Wiseman N, Feng Y. F. A practical dictionary of Chinese medicine. 2nd ed. Brookline, MA: Paradigm Publications; 1998, p. 193–233.

126. Koch J, Rowan K, Rombauts L, et al. Endometriosis and infertility – a consensus statement from ACCEPT (Australasian CREI Consensus Expert Panel on Trial evidence).

Aust N Z J Obstet Gynaecol 2012;52:513–22.

127. Macer ML, Taylor HS. Endometriosis and infertility: a review of the pathogenesis and treatment of endometriosis-associated infertility. Obstet Gynecol Clin North Am 2012;39:535–49.

128. Bedaiwy MA, Liu J. Pathophysiology, diagnosis, and surgical management of endometriosis: a chronic disease. SRM 2010;8:4–8.

129. Giudice LC. Clinical practice. Endometriosis. N Engl J Med 2010;362:2389–98.

130. The Practice Committee of the American Society for Reproductive Medicine. Endometriosis and infertility: a committee opinion. Fertil Steril 2012;98:591–8.

131. Missmer SA, Hankinson SE, Spiegelman D, et al. Incidence of laparoscopically confirmed endometriosis by demographic, anthropometric, and lifestyle factors. Am J Epidemiol 2004;160:784–96.

132. Shah DK, Correia KF, Vitonis AF, et al. Body size and endometriosis: results from 20 years of follow-up within the nurses' health study II prospective cohort. Hum Reprod 2013;28:1783–92.

133. Hediger ML, Hartnett HJ, Louis GM. Association of endometriosis with body size and figure. Fertil Steril 2005;84:1366–74.

134. Harris HR, Chavarro JE, Malspeis S, et al. Dairy-Food, calcium, magnesium, and vitamin D intake and endometriosis: a prospective cohort study. Am J Epidemiol 2013;177:420–30.

135. Dalsgaard T, Hjordt Hansen V, Hartwell D, et al. Reproductive prognosis in daughters of women with and without endometriosis. Hum Reprod 2013;28:2284–8.

136. Farquhar C. Endometriosis. BMJ 2007;334:249–53.

137. Senapati S, Barnhart K. Managing endometriosis-associated infertility. Clin Obstet Gynecol 2011;54:720–6.

138. Prentice A. Regular review: endometriosis. BMJ 2001;323:93–5.

139. Engemise S, Gordon C, Konje JC. Endometriosis. BMJ 2010;340: c2168.

140. Tirlapur SA, Kuhrt K, Chaliha C, et al. The 'evil twin syndrome' in chronic pelvic pain: a systematic review of prevalence studies of bladder pain syndrome and endometriosis. Int J Surg 2013;11:233–7.

141. Cameron IC, Rogers S, Collins MC, et al. Intestinal endometriosis: presentation, investigation, and surgical management. Int J Colorectal Dis 1995;10:83–6.

142. ASRM patient fact sheet: endometriosis. Available from: http://www.asrm.org/Endometriosis_booklet/ [accessed 9 August 2013].

143. Fassbender A, Vodolazkaia A, Saunders P, et al. Biomarkers of endometriosis. Fertil Steril 2013;99:1135–45.

144. Adamson GD, Pasta DJ. Endometriosis fertility index: the new, validated endometriosis staging system. Fertil Steril 2010;94:1609–15.

145. Uncu G, Kasapoglu I, Ozerkan K, et al. Prospective assessment of the impact of endometriomas and their removal on ovarian reserve and determinants of the rate of decline in ovarian reserve. Hum Reprod 2013;28:2140–5.

146. Hughes E, Brown J, Collins JJ, et al. Ovulation suppression for endometriosis. Cochrane Database Syst Rev 2007;(3):CD000155.

147. Sallam HN, Garcia-Velasco JA, Dias S, et al. Long-term pituitary down-regulation before in vitro fertilization (IVF) for women with endometriosis. Cochrane Database Syst Rev 2006;(1):CD004635.

148. de Ziegler D, Gayet V, Aubriot FX, et al. Use of oral contraceptives in women with endometriosis before assisted reproduction treatment improves outcomes. Fertil Steril 2010;94:2796–9.

149. Johnson NP, Hummelshoj L, for the World Endometriosis Society Montpellier Consortium. Consensus on current management of endometriosis. Hum Reprod 2013;28:1552–68.

150. Hart RJ, Hickey M, Maouris P, et al. Excisional surgery versus ablative

surgery for ovarian endometriomata. Cochrane Database Syst Rev 2008;(2): CD004992.

151. Surrey ES. Endometriosis and assisted reproductive technologies: maximizing outcomes. Semin Reprod Med 2013;31:154–63.

152. Somigliana E, Berlanda N, Benaglia L, et al. Surgical excision of endometriomas and ovarian reserve: a systematic review on serum anti-Müllerian hormone level modifications. Fertil Steril 2012;98:1531–8.

153. Yap C, Furness S, Farquhar C. Pre and post operative medical therapy for endometriosis surgery. Cochrane Database Syst Rev 2004;(3): CD003678.

154. Harb H, Gallos I, Chu J, et al. The effect of endometriosis on in vitro fertilisation outcome: a systematic review and meta-analysis. BJOG 2013;120:1308–20.

155. Komsky-Elbaz A, Raziel A, Friedler S, et al. Conventional IVF versus ICSI in sibling oocytes from couples with endometriosis and normozoospermic semen. J Assist Reprod Genet 2013;30:251–7.

156. Wiseman N, Feng Y. A practical dictionary of Chinese medicine. 2nd ed. Brookline, MA: Paradigm Publications; 1998, p. 1–13.

157. Zhou J, Qu F. Treating gynaecological disorders with traditional Chinese medicine: a review. Afr J Tradit Complement Altern Med 2009;6:494–517.

158. Wang D, Wang Z, Yu C. Endometriosis treated by the method of resolving blood stasis to eliminate obstruction in the lower-Jiao. J Tradit Chin Med 1998;18:7–11.

159. Yu F, Tian X. Clinical observation on treatment of endometriosis with acupuncture plus herbs. J Acupunct Tuina Sci 2005;3:48–51.

160. Jiang H, Shen Y, Wang XG. Current progress of Chinese medicinal treatment of endometriosis. Chin J Integr Med 2010;16:283–8.

161. Wiseman N, Feng Y. Q. A practical dictionary of Chinese medicine. 2nd ed. Brookline, MA: Paradigm Publications; 1998, p. 475–91.

162. Wiseman N, Feng Y. D. A practical dictionary of Chinese medicine.

2nd ed. Brookline, MA: Paradigm Publications; 1998, p. 108–65.

163. Maciocia G. Menstrual symptoms. In: Diagnosis in Chinese medicine: a comprehensive guide. Edinburgh: Elsevier; 2004. p. 826–30 [chapter 84].

164. Wiseman N, Feng Y. C. A practical dictionary of Chinese medicine. 2nd ed. Brookline, MA: Paradigm Publications; 1998, p. 53–107.

165. Wiseman N, Feng Y. B. A practical dictionary of Chinese medicine. 2nd ed. Brookline, MA: Paradigm Publications; 1998, p. 14–52.

166. Fu Qing-zhu. Tiao Jing regulating the menses. In: Flaws B, editor. Yang S, Liu D, translators. Fu Qing-Zhu's gynecology. 2nd ed. Chelsea: Blue Poppy Press; 1992. p. 29–54, Part 1 [chapter 1].

167. Tan Y, Qi C, Zhang Q, et al. Menstrual diseases. In: Gynecology of Traditional Chinese Medicine, Chinese-English bilingual textbooks for international students of Chinese TCM institutions. China: People's Medical Publishing House; 2007. p. 211–308 [chapter 7].

168. Maciocia G. Bleeding between periods. In: Obstetrics and gynecology in Chinese medicine. 2nd ed. Edinburgh: Elsevier Health Sciences; 2011. p. 285–95 [chapter 15].

169. Maciocia G. Women's symptoms. In: Diagnosis in Chinese medicine: a comprehensive guide. Edinburgh: Elsevier; 2004. p. 395–409 [chapter 46].

170. Maciocia G. Miscellaneous gynecological symptoms. In: Diagnosis in Chinese medicine: a comprehensive guide. Edinburgh: Elsevier; 2004. p. 854–60 [chapter 89].

171. Maciocia G. Lower back. In: Diagnosis in Chinese medicine: a comprehensive guide. Edinburgh: Elsevier; 2004. p. 703–8 [chapter 67].

172. Maciocia G. Urination. In: Diagnosis in Chinese medicine: a comprehensive guide. Edinburgh: Elsevier; 2004. p. 753–9 [chapter 73].

173. Maciocia G. Defecation. In: Diagnosis in Chinese medicine: a comprehensive guide. Edinburgh:

Elsevier; 2004. p. 747–52 [chapter 72].

174. Lade A. Point images and function. In: Acupuncture points: images and functions. Seattle, WA: Eastland Press; 1989. p. 27–309 [chapter 3].

175. Deadman P, Al-Khafaji M, Baker K. The Bladder channel. In: A manual of acupuncture. England: Journal of Chinese Medicine Publications; 1998. p. 249–328.

176. Shizhen L. Governor Vessel (Du Mai). In: Mayor D, (editor). Clinical application of commonly used acupuncture points. St. Albans, Herts: Donica Publishing, Ltd; 2007. p. 863–919 [chapter 15].

177. Lade A. Point classification. In: Acupuncture points: images and functions. Seattle, WA: Eastland Press; 1989. p. 7–26 [chapter 2].

178. ESHRE ART fact sheet. Available from: http://www.eshre.eu/ESHRE/English/Guidelines-Legal/ART-fact-sheet/page.aspx/1061 [accessed 13 December 2012].

179. Thonneau P, Marchand S, Tallec A, et al. Incidence and main causes of infertility in a resident population (1 850 000) of three French regions (1988–1989)*. Hum Reprod 1991;6:811–6.

180. Kamath MS, Bhattacharya S. Demographics of infertility and management of unexplained infertility. Best Pract Res Clin Obstet Gynaecol 2012;26:729–38.

181. Pandian Z, Bhattacharya S. IVF for unexplained infertility. Hum Reprod Update 2013;19:431.

182. Mascarenhas MN, Flaxman SR, Boerma T, et al. National, regional, and global trends in infertility prevalence since 1990: a systematic analysis of 277 health surveys. PLoS Med 2012;9:e1001356.

183. Gurol-Urganci I, Bou-Antoun S, Lim CP, et al. Impact of caesarean section on subsequent fertility: a systematic review and meta-analysis. Hum Reprod 2013;28:1943–52.

184. Beer AE, Kantecki J, Reed J. Category 5 immune problems – part one. In: Is your body baby-friendly: "unexplained" infertility, miscarriage and IVF failure explained. Houston, TX: AJR Pub.; 2006. p. 69–90.

185. Practice Committee of American Society for Reproductive Medicine. Diagnostic evaluation of the infertile male: a committee opinion. Fertil Steril 2012;98:294–301.

186. Carlsen E, Giwercman A, Keiding N, et al. Evidence for decreasing quality of semen during past 50 years. BMJ 1992;305:609–13.

187. Merzenich H, Zeeb H, Blettner M. Decreasing sperm quality: a global problem? BMC Public Health 2010;10:24.

188. Krausz C. Male infertility: pathogenesis and clinical diagnosis. Best Pract Res Clin Endocrinol Metab 2011;25:271–85.

189. ESHRE Capri Workshop Group. Diagnosis and management of the infertile couple: missing information. Hum Reprod Update 2004;10:295–307.

190. Kroese AC, de Lange NM, Collins J, et al. Surgery or embolization for varicoceles in subfertile men. Cochrane Database Syst Rev 2012;10, CD000479.

191. Elzanaty S, Malm J, Giwercman A. Duration of sexual abstinence: epididymal and accessory sex gland secretions and their relationship to sperm motility. Hum Reprod 2005;20:221–5.

192. Levitas E, Lunenfeld E, Weiss N, et al. Relationship between the duration of sexual abstinence and semen quality: analysis of 9,489 semen samples. Fertil Steril 2005;83:1680–6.

193. He J, Li D, He Y, et al. Acupuncture-moxibustion therapy for infertility due to sperm abnormality. J Acupunct Tuina Sci 2011;9:215–8.

194. Deadman P. The treatment of male subfertility with acupuncture. J Chin Med 2008;88:5–16.

195. Sun Si-Miao. Translation. In: Wilms S, translator. Bèi Jí Qian Jin Yào Fang. Essential prescriptions worth a thousand in gold for every emergency. 3 Volumes on gynecology, vol. 2. Portland: The Chinese Medicine Database; 2007. p. 52–216 [chapter 2].

196. Larre C, Rochat de la Vallee E. The power to arouse. In: Root C, editor. The Kidney. 2nd ed. Norfolk: Biddles; 1989. p. 47–9, Su Wen [chapter 8].

197. Larre C, Rochat de la Vallee E. The power to store. In: Root C, editor. The Kidney. 2nd ed. Norfolk: Biddles; 1989. p. 51–4, Su Wen [chapter 9].

198. Lu HC. On the heavenly truth. In: A complete translation of the Yellow Emperor's classics of internal medicine and the difficult classic (Nei-Jing and Nan-Jing). Vancouver: International College of Traditional Chinese Medicine; 2004. p. 65–72, Section two: Essential questions [Su Wen] [chapter 1].

199. Sun Si-Miao. Prolegomena. In: Wilms S, translator. Bèi Jí Qian Jin Yào Fang. Essential prescriptions worth a thousand in gold for every emergency. 3 Volumes on gynecology. Portland: The Chinese Medicine Database; 2007. p. 4–50 [chapter 1].

200. Crimmel AS, Conner CS, Monga M. Withered Yang: a review of traditional Chinese medical treatment of male infertility and erectile dysfunction. J Androl 2001;22:173–82.

201. Dou Z. Eight TCM, treatment methods for male infertility caused by sperm disorders. J Assoc Tradit Chin Med 2008;15:17–20.

202. Kirkland R. Varieties of Taoism in ancient China: a preliminary comparison of themes in the Nei Yehand other Taoist classics. Available from: http://www.optim.ee/mati/Taoism/VARIETIES.pdf.

203. Maciocia G. Yin organ interrelationships. In: The foundations of Chinese medicine: a comprehensive text for acupuncturists and herbalists. Edinburgh, NY: Churchill Livingstone; 1989. p. 105–10 [chapter 12].

204. Li Y, Lin H, Li Y, et al. Association between socio-psycho-behavioral factors and male semen quality: systematic review and meta-analyses. Fertil Steril 2011;95:116–23.

205. Jiasheng Z. The acupuncture treatment of 248 cases of male infertility. J Chin Med 1987;25:28–30.

206. Ming-hua P. Treatment of oligospermia by acupuncture in 39 cases. J Acupunct Tuina Sci 2005;3:8–9.

207. Lyttleton J. Male infertility. In: Treatment of infertility with Chinese medicine. London: Churchill Livingstone; 2004. p. 255–76 [chapter 7].

208. Bo W, Guoan L, Weidong S, et al. Therapeutic efficacy observation on combined acupuncture and herbal formula for male sterility. J Acupunct Tuina Sci 2011;9:211–4.

209. Sheng ZJ. Male infertility. Clinical treatments of 248 cases. EJOM 2000;3:25–6.

210. Zhen-bei Y. Treatment of male sterility by acupuncture: a report of 34 cases. J Acupunct Tuina Sci 2005;3:6–7.

211. Huang DM, Huang GY, Lu FE, et al. Acupuncture for infertility: is it an effective therapy? Chin J Integr Med 2011;17:386–95.

212. Small CM, Manatunga AK, Klein M, et al. Menstrual cycle characteristics. Epidemiology 2006;17:52–60.

213. Brodin T, Bergh T, Berglund L, et al. Menstrual cycle length is an age-independent marker of female fertility: results from 6271 treatment cycles of in vitro fertilization. Fertil Steril 2008;90:1656–61.

214. Popovic-Todorovic B. A prospective study of predictive factors of ovarian response in 'standard' IVF/ICSI patients treated with recombinant FSH. A suggestion for a recombinant FSH dosage normogram. Hum Reprod 2003;18:781–7.

215. Liu Y. The necessity of rational enquiry. In: The heart transmission of medicine. Boulder: Blue Poppy Press; 1997. p. 9–10 [chapter 5].

216. Wiseman N, Feng Y. M. A practical dictionary of Chinese medicine. 2nd ed. Brookline, MA: Paradigm Publications; 1998. p. 382–404.

217. Harlow SD, Lin X, Ho MJ. Analysis of menstrual diary data across the reproductive life span applicability of the bipartite model approach and the importance of within-woman variance. J Clin Epidemiol 2000;53:722–33.

218. Furth C. Nourishing life: Ming bodies of generation and longevity. In: A flourishing Yin: gender in China's medical history, 960–1665. California and Los Angeles: University of California Press; 1999. p. 187–223 [chapter 6].

219. Wu YL. Notes. In: Reproducing women: medicine, metaphor, and

childbirth in late imperial China. Berkeley: University of California Press; 2010. p. 237–309.

220. Maciocia G. Early periods. In: Obstetrics and gynecology in Chinese medicine. 2nd ed. Edinburgh: Elsevier Health Sciences; 2011. p. 201–11 [chapter 8].

221. Maciocia G. Late periods. In: Obstetrics and gynecology in Chinese medicine. 2nd ed. Edinburgh: Elsevier Health Sciences; 2011. p. 211–25 [chapter 9].

222. Liu F. Medical essays. In: The Essence of Liu Feng-Wu's gynecology. 1st ed. Boulder: Blue Poppy Press; 1998. p. 45–60. The treatment of Blood patterns in gynecology as learned through practice. Section 5 [chapter 1].

223. Maciocia G. Irregular periods. In: Obstetrics and gynecology in Chinese Medicine. 2nd ed. Edinburgh: Elsevier Health Sciences; 2011. p. 225–31 [chapter 10].

224. Guicheng X. Discussion of the menstrual cycle. The cycle-regulating treatment. J Chin Med 2001;67:30–3.

225. Maciocia G. Painful periods. In: Obstetrics and gynecology in Chinese medicine. 2nd ed. Edinburgh: Elsevier Health Sciences; 2011. p. 255–85 [chapter 14].

226. Maciocia G. Long periods. In: Obstetrics and gynecology in Chinese medicine. 2nd ed. Edinburgh: Elsevier Health Sciences; 2011. p. 249–55 [chapter 13].

227. Maciocia G. Diagnosis. In: Obstetrics and gynecology in Chinese medicine. 2nd ed. Edinburgh: Elsevier Health Sciences; 2011. p. 97–110 [chapter 5].

228. Maciocia G. Pre-menstrual syndrome. In: Obstetrics and gynecology in Chinese medicine. 2nd ed. New York: Churchill Livingstone; 1998. p. 339–58 [chapter 18].

229. Maciocia G. Flooding and trickling. In: Obstetrics and gynecology in Chinese medicine. New York: Churchill Livingstone; 1998. p. 303–38 [chapter 17].

230. Maciocia G. Pre-menstrual syndrome. In: Obstetrics and

gynecology in Chinese medicine. 2nd ed. Edinburgh: Elsevier Health Sciences; 2011. p. 357–79 [chapter 18].

231. Maciocia G. Flooding and trickling. In: Obstetrics and gynecology in Chinese medicine. Edinburgh: Elsevier Health Sciences; 2011. p. 319–57 [chapter 17].

232. Magarelli PC, Cohen M, Cridennda DK. Proposed mechanism of action of acupuncture on IVF outcomes. Fertil Steril 2006;86:S174–5.

233. Langevin HM, Wayne PM, Macpherson H, et al. Paradoxes in acupuncture research: strategies for moving forward. Evid Based Complement Alternat Med 2011;2011:180805.

234. White A, Cummings M, Barlas P, et al. Defining an adequate dose of acupuncture using a neurophysiological approach – a narrative review of the literature. Acupunct Med 2008;26:111–20.

Chapter | 9 |

Acupuncture during ART

Chapter 6 introduced different types of Assisted Reproductive Technology (ART) treatments and techniques and explained how pharmacological drugs are used in manipulating reproductive hormones. This chapter builds on that knowledge. It provides detailed information about each type of ART treatment and recommends an acupuncture treatment protocol that can be used alongside ART.

TREATMENT DURING IVF

In Vitro Fertilization (IVF) is an ART procedure that involves fertilization of an egg by sperm in a laboratory dish.[1] It is usually divided into several stages:

- Pretreatment (also referred to as suppression or downregulation)
- Ovarian stimulation
- Final egg maturation (or trigger)
- Egg retrieval
- Fertilization of the eggs in the laboratory (*in vitro*)
- Culturing of embryos
- Embryo transfer
- Luteal phase (often referred to by patients as the 'two-week wait')

Pretreatment phase (suppression or downregulation)

Orthodox medical protocol

What happens during the pretreatment phase depends on the protocol used. There are two main IVF protocols: Gonadotrophin Releasing Hormone (GnRH) agonist and GnRH antagonist (although other protocols are sometimes used). GnRH agonists or antagonists are administered to block the release of Follicle Stimulating Hormone (FSH) and Luteinizing Hormone (LH) by the pituitary gland. As a result, follicular growth is inhibited, preventing premature LH surge and spontaneous ovulation and allowing for the availability of more homogenous-sized follicles for recruitment.[2]

GnRH agonist

The GnRH agonist mode of action is to stimulate the pituitary gland to produce more LH and FSH, which causes an increase in oestrogen levels (flare-up). After approximately 10 days, pituitary suppression is achieved by exhaustion of the gonadotrophic pituitary cells resulting in the decline of FSH, LH, and oestrogen comparable to menopause.[2] Gonadotrophin ovarian stimulation begins once adequate pituitary suppression is confirmed by baseline evaluation.[3]

There are two types of GnRH agonist protocols: the long protocol and the short protocol. The long protocol usually commences in the mid-luteal phase of the pretreatment cycle[3,4] although it may begin up to 4 weeks before ovarian stimulation.[2] This phase is sometimes referred to as the 'downregulation' or 'suppression' phase.

In the short agonist protocol, a GnRH agonist is usually administered from day 2 or 3 of the menstrual cycle once the baseline evaluation confirms a thin endometrium and 'quiet' ovaries.[5,6]

Common preparations of GnRH agonist medications include buserelin (Suprefact®) as a subcutaneous injection and nafarelin (Synarel®) as a nasal spray.

GnRH antagonist

The GnRH antagonist is usually started on day 5 or 6 of gonadotrophin stimulation.[2] With the antagonist protocol, there is no 'downregulation'. A GnRH antagonist binds to and blocks GnRH receptors on the pituitary gland, and the suppression effect is instant.[2]

Common preparations of GnRH antagonists include cetrorelix (Cetrotide®) and ganirelix (Orgalutran®), which are both administered as subcutaneous injections.

In our experience, the GnRH agonist long protocol is used more frequently. This may be because the antagonist protocol is less practical logistically because fertility clinics are unable to conveniently schedule or programme the treatment cycle. It may also be because older research suggested better pregnancy rates with the agonist protocol. However, a 2011 Cochrane review concluded that pregnancy rates are similar for both GnRH antagonist and agonist protocols.[7] Another Cochrane review concluded that, in poor responders, the GnRH agonist long protocol resulted in fewer eggs when compared to the shorter GnRH agonist protocol or the GnRH antagonist protocol.[8]

Table 9.1 summarizes the key differences between the GnRH agonist and antagonist analogues.

CLINICAL TIPS

IVF TREATMENT PROTOCOL

Ask your patient to provide you with a copy of her IVF treatment protocol. This will help you to more accurately plan your acupuncture treatment.

Baseline evaluation

A baseline evaluation is used to ensure the woman can go ahead with ovarian stimulation. Evaluation is done in all protocols, but the intra-protocol timing is slightly different[2]:

- In the agonist long protocol, a baseline evaluation is usually undertaken after 14 days of administering medication.[2]
- In the agonist short protocol and in the antagonist protocol, it is usually done in the first few days of the treatment cycle.[2,5,6]

The baseline evaluation involves a transvaginal scan to check the ovaries for cysts and to measure the thickness of the uterine lining. Oestrogen levels in the blood are also checked. Some clinics monitor the level of other hormones (for example, FSH and/or progesterone). Ovarian stimulation cannot be initiated if there are ovarian cysts >25 mm, if the endometrium is too thick, or if the oestrogen level is $\geq$370 pmol/L (100 pg/mL).[6]

If the baseline evaluation shows that the woman has not fully downregulated, the GnRH agonist may be administered for longer, the dose may be increased, or the treatment cycle may be cancelled.

If appropriate downregulation of the pituitary gland and ovarian suppression have been achieved, there are no large cysts, and oestrogen levels are low, the patient is advised to start ovarian stimulation with gonadotrophins. The GnRH agonist is continued (usually at half dose) until hCG administration, or the GnRH antagonist is initiated on day 5 or 6 of ovarian stimulation.[2] Table 9.2 summarizes the events during the pretreatment phase.

TCM protocol

Acupuncture treatment during the pretreatment cycle depends on the protocol used. If the long GnRH agonist

Table 9.1 Comparison of GnRH agonist and GnRH antagonist analogues

	Agonist	Antagonist
Mode of action	After 10 days the pituitary store of gonadotrophins is depleted. The pituitary is desensitized	Immediately binds to and blocks GnRH receptors on the pituitary gland[2]
When their administration begins	Usually on day 21 of pretreatment cycle. But can be up to 4 weeks before the treatment cycle, or on day 1 of the treatment cycle ('short protocol')[2]	Day 5 or 6 of ovarian stimulation[2]
Disadvantages	The long protocol is associated with the development of ovarian cysts and symptoms such as headaches and hot flushes that result from oestrogen deficiency[4] Increased risk of OHSS[7]	Limited programming of cycles and consequently increased rate of weekend egg retrievals.[9] This is because the stimulation starts on days 2 or 3 of menstrual cycle and this is an unpredictable event.[9] One way to avoid this is to use the oral contraceptive pill in the menstrual cycle before the start of the stimulation phase.[9] However, a meta-analysis found that pretreatment with oral contraceptive pill significantly reduced rates of ongoing pregnancy.[9,10] Pretreatment with oestrogen is another method of programming the GnRH-antagonist cycles to tie in with the fertility clinics logistical needs[9]

Table 9.2 Summary of pretreatment phase: suppression with GnRH analogues

What happens	Ovarian activity is suppressed by medication	
Why it is done	Prevents premature LH surge and spontaneous ovulation	
Medication	*Agonist protocol* buserelin (Suprefact®) nafarelin (Synarel®)	*Antagonist protocol* cetrorelix (Cetrotide®) ganirelix (Orgalutran®)
How it is achieved	GnRH agonist initially causes hypersecretion of FSH and LH and elevated oestrogen levels. After 10 days the reserves of FSH and LH become depleted and the cycle is suppressed	GnRH antagonist binds to the pituitary receptors and instantly blocks LH production
Monitoring	Baseline ultrasound scan is done after approximately 14 days of administering GnRH agonist (if long protocol) or on cycle days 1–3 if short protocol[2]	Baseline ultrasound scan is done on treatment cycle days 1–3[2]

protocol is used with the purpose of suppressing gonadotrophin secretions by the pituitary, or if the GnRH antagonist is used together with pretreatment medication (for example, a contraceptive pill), acupuncture treatment aims to:

- Treat the adverse effects of medication, which for the GnRH agonist tend to be quite severe because they induce low oestrogen levels; this may cause hot flashes, perspiration, headaches, mood fluctuations, insomnia, nervousness, sore breasts, and fatigue.[2]
- Support the patient emotionally.
- Continue to address any underlying TCM pathology.

If the short GnRH agonist or GnRH antagonist (without pretreatment medication) protocols are used, then acupuncture potentially plays a greater role. As described in Chapter 2, at the end of the luteal phase of every menstrual cycle (days 23–28), several antral follicles are selected ('recruited') to continue developing. Their subsequent development depends on high levels of gonadotrophins, in particular FSH and LH.[11] Acupuncture may improve follicular recruitment and development by improving the blood supply and, therefore, the delivery of these hormones to the ovary and follicles.[12,13] Acupuncture may also increase FSH and LH secretions.[14]

With the short GnRH agonist or GnRH antagonist (without pretreatment medication) protocols, acupuncture during the pretreatment cycle aims to:

- Regulate the menstrual cycle to ensure that ovarian stimulation can be started on schedule.
- Assist with follicular recruitment in the late luteal phase to maximize the number of antral follicles available for ovarian stimulation.
- Support the patient emotionally.
- Continue to address any underlying TCM pathology.

Tables 9.3 and 9.4 summarize acupuncture treatment protocols during the pretreatment phase.

CLINICAL TIPS

PULSE DURING DOWNREGULATION

The pulse may alter and become weak during the later stages of the downregulation phase as a result of pituitary suppression. This may be benign and is not a cause for concern.

Ovarian stimulation phase

Orthodox medical protocol

In a natural cycle, because of the limited production of FSH, only one or rarely two eggs are released from the ovary. The rest of the follicles recruited in that cycle become atretic. During the ovarian stimulation phase of IVF, women inject large doses of gonadotrophin hormones. Gonadotrophins are FSH- and/or LH-containing compounds that are used to stimulate ovarian follicular development. They function in a similar way to natural FSH, but the dose used in IVF is much higher. This allows the recruitment of more ovarian follicles by rescuing them from atresia and helping them to grow and develop.[30] The greater the number of developing follicles, the higher the yield of eggs and, therefore, the greater the probability of more embryos being created. This, in turn, increases the likelihood of a successful outcome.

While maximizing egg yield is important, the risk of ovarian hyperstimulation syndrome (OHSS) should be minimized.[31] Therefore, the prescribed dose of FSH medication is usually decided based on each patient's individual circumstances.[4] For example, the patient's age, her ovarian reserve, the number of risk factors for OHSS, any history of poor response to stimulation, and the patient's weight are all factors to be considered. The standard dose of

Table 9.3 Pretreatment phase acupuncture protocol

To be used in:
- Long GnRH agonist protocol
- GnRH antagonist protocol (with pretreatment medication)

When to provide acupuncture treatment		Up to 4 weeks before the ovarian stimulation begins. But more commonly beginning on day 21 of the pretreatment cycle
Timing and frequency		Treat once a week until the start of ovarian stimulation
Needling method and techniques		Manual acupuncture is usually adequate. Some acupuncturists recommend not using any abdominal points to avoid thickening the endometrial lining.[15] Our experience is that abdominal points do not normally interfere with the pituitary suppression and do not usually cause the endometrium to thicken
Main points prescription		Nourish Yin, clear Heat, regulate Qi,[16] Blood, emotion, and harmonize the Liver: LIV3,[16,17] P6,[18] SP6,[16] SP10,[16,19] YINTANG
TCM acupuncture treatment modifications	Headaches	GB20,[20] LI4[16,21]
	Hot flashes	KID6, KID2, KID1,[22] HE6[23]
	Insomnia	HE7,[23] P7,[18] ANMIAN[24]
	Fatigue	ST36,[16,25] HUANMEN[24]

Table 9.4 Pretreatment phase acupuncture protocol

To be used in:
- Short GnRH agonist protocol
- GnRH antagonist protocol (without pretreatment medication)
- Natural (unsuppressed) pretreatment cycle

When to provide acupuncture treatment	Menstrual cycle before the ovarian stimulation begins
Timing and frequency	Weekly sessions during the first 3 weeks of the pretreatment cycle
	Twice weekly during the last week of the pretreatment cycle (when the process of follicular recruitment begins)
Needling method and techniques	Manual acupuncture is usually adequate during the first 3 weeks. Abdominal points are essential during the late luteal phase when the follicular recruitment begins. Electroacupuncture and a heat lamp may be used during this phase
Main points prescription	*Pretreatment cycle days 1–5 (menses)*: invigorate, regulate Qi and Blood, tonify Kidney Jing (Essence): SP4 + P6,[26] LU7 + KID6,[27] REN4[28]
	Pretreatment cycle days 5–14: nourish Blood and Yin: SP4 + P6,[26] LIV8,[17] SP6,[19] HE6,[23] KID3,[22] LU7 + KID6[27]
	Pretreatment cycle days 14–16 (ovulation): tonify Jing (Essence), regulate Qi and Blood, reinforce Yang: KID1,[22] ST27,[25] REN4,[28] KID3,[22] ZIGONG[24]
	Pretreatment cycle day 16 until ovarian stimulation begins: Smith et al. consensus on acupuncture points useful during ovarian stimulation.[29] Using these points during the late luteal phase of the pre-treatment cycle may help with follicular recruitment: SP4 + P6, LU7 + KID6, ZIGONG, REN4, ST36, SP6, ST29

stimulation is between 150 and 300 IU of FSH per day.[32] In patients at risk of poor response, the starting dose of FSH may need to be between 300 and 450 IU/day.[32] Doses higher than this are ineffective.[32,33]

There are three types of gonadotrophins:[34]

- Urinary extracts: Human Menopausal Gonadotrophins or hMG (menotrophin), usually contains FSH and LH (ratio 1:1). Common preparations are Merional® and Menopur®.
- Purified urinary FSH extracts or FSH-P (urofollitropin). A common preparation is Fostimon®.
- Recombinant synthetic hormone or rFSH (follitropin). A common preparation is Gonal-F®.

A 2011 Cochrane review evaluated the effectiveness of different gonadotrophin formulations and concluded that there is no significant difference between various preparations. Therefore, the choice of gonadotrophin medication should be based on availability and cost.[35]

During the ovarian stimulation phase, patients continue taking GnRH analogues (agonist or antagonist) in order to stop premature LH surge and spontaneous ovulation.

Patient monitoring

Follicular and endometrial development is monitored by transvaginal ultrasound. Monitoring usually begins on days 5–7 of the ovarian stimulation stage. Many clinics also check serum oestrogen levels. The monitoring may start earlier in patients at risk of OHSS or poor ovarian response. Typically, the scan is repeated every 1–3 days. Patients' response to stimulation medication is monitored; if necessary, their dose of medication is adjusted. Monitoring also helps ART consultants decide when the patient is ready for egg retrieval.

Follicular growth

A review by Baerwald et al. established that during ovarian stimulation cycles ovulatory follicles' mean growth rate is 1.64 ± 0.02 mm/day.[36] Interestingly, anovulatory follicles grow at the slightly faster rate of 1.85 ± 0.04 mm/day,[36] which is a little faster compared to a natural cycle (1.48 ± 0.10 mm for ovulatory and 1.41 ± 0.06 mm for anovulatory follicles).[36] Thus, it is undesirable for follicles to develop too quickly or too slowly. It is also better if follicles are homogenous (similar) in size.[37] Chapter 10 discusses how to manage patients with poor responses to ovarian stimulation and Chapter 11 discusses how to manage patients with OHSS.

Oestrogen levels

Each mature egg produces approximately 600–800 pmol/L (163–218 pg/mL) of oestrogen.[2,38] Peak serum oestrogen levels of >9000 pmol/L (2500 pg/mL) are associated with a high risk of developing OHSS.[39]

Endometrial development

For the embryo to be able to implant, the endometrial lining needs to be of appropriate thickness and receptive to the embryo. The thickness of the endometrial lining during the late follicular phase needs to be at least 6–8 mm[40] and can be up to 16–17 mm or, in some instances, even thicker.[41,42] The lining also needs to be trilaminar (triple layer) in appearance (Figure 9.1).

Implantation, clinical, and ongoing pregnancy rates are significantly increased if the endometrial lining is greater than 9–10 mm.[41,43,44] Clinical pregnancy and live birth rates increase linearly with increasing thickness of the endometrium even after adjusting for age and embryo

Figure 9.1 Endometrial lining showing three layers (trilaminar appearance).

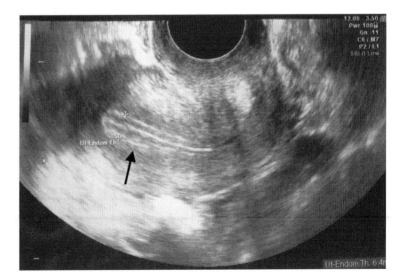

Table 9.5 Summary of ovarian stimulation phase

What happens	Follicular recruitment and growth is stimulated by gonadotrophin medication
Why it is done	To increase the yield of eggs
Medication	Menotrophin (Merional®), urofollitropin (Fostimon®), follitropin (Gonal-F®) 150 to 450 IU (usually injected subcutaneously in the abdomen)
How it is achieved	Gonadotrophins injected during this phase work exactly the same way as natural FSH, but the dosages are much higher, which results in more eggs being produced
Monitoring	Follicular and endometrial development and serum oestrogen levels are monitored by transvaginal scans and blood tests. Monitoring normally starts around day 5–7 of ovarian stimulation, and is then repeated every 1–3 days

quality.[41,42] There does not appear to be an upper limit to endometrial thickness, with a lining >14 mm thick not associated with adverse outcomes.[45,46] Chapter 2 described in detail how the endometrial lining develops, and Chapter 10 discusses how to manage patients with a thin endometrial lining. Table 9.5 summarizes what happens during the ovarian stimulation phase.

TCM protocol

In their consensus paper, Smith *et al.* attempted to establish an agreement amongst 17 TCM recognized experts in the field of acupuncture and ART on how best to manage women who are undergoing ART treatment. Amongst 17 experts, 16 of them agreed that it is important to treat women during the ovarian stimulation phase.[29]

A 2012 meta-analysis found that acupuncture during IVF significantly increases clinical pregnancy rates and live birth rates. The effect is more significant if acupuncture is administered during the ovarian stimulation phase and not just at embryo transfer.[47]

Acupuncture during ovarian stimulation may help to increase the number of retrieved eggs[48] and increase endometrial thickness.[49–51] A recently published randomized controlled trial (RCT) showed that patients who received acupuncture treatment during the stimulation phase of an IVF cycle had a significantly thicker endometrial lining compared to the control and sham groups (10.3 mm vs. 8.7 mm vs. 8.5 mm, respectively). They also had a statistically significant greater number of retrieved eggs (8 vs. 6 vs. 6, respectively).[48]

It is important to administer the first acupuncture session within the first 3 days of starting ovarian stimulation medication, with the aim of enhancing follicular recruitment and follicular synchronicity, which research shows is vital for IVF outcomes.[37] Subsequently, the acupuncture treatment frequency depends on each patient's individual response to stimulation.

Acupuncturists need to regularly evaluate a patient's response. This can be achieved by asking patients to bring their test results, such as:

- The results of ultrasound scans: the number and size of follicles and the thickness and quality of the endometrium
- Oestrogen level results

Collecting this information will also help with the IVF audit should the treatment not succeed (see Chapter 12).

Based on the findings, acupuncture treatment may need to be modified accordingly. Table 9.6 provides a basic acupuncture treatment protocol and guidance on how to modify it.

Table 9.6 Ovarian stimulation phase acupuncture protocol and modifications

Timing and frequency	*Session 1*: ideally between days 1–3 from the commencement of stimulation medication in order to assist with the recruitment of follicles
	Subsequent sessions: twice weekly to every other day until the trigger injection[29]
Needling method and techniques	Manual and electroacupuncture; needling duration 25–30 min; obtain de qi, individualize points prescription.[29] Moxa or a heat lamp on the lower abdomen can be used
	Tonification method: deficient syndrome(s)
	Even or reduction method: excess syndrome(s)
Main points prescription	Smith *et al.* Delphi consensus (in the order of importance):[29] Innervation areas close to ovaries and uterus, SP4+P6, LU7+KID6, ZIGONG, REN4, ST36, SP6, ST29, REN3, REN6, KID3, BL23, YINTANG

Table 9.6 Ovarian stimulation phase acupuncture protocol and modifications—cont'd

TCM acupuncture treatment modifications (also see Chapter 5)	Qi Stagnation	Regulate Qi: LIV3,[17] P6,[18] ST30,[25] HE5[23]
	Blood Stasis	Invigorate Blood, move Stasis: SP10,[19] SP8,[19] KID14[22]
	Heat/Fire	Drain Heat/Fire: LIV2,[17] P7,[18] SJ5[52]
	Cold	Warm Cold: ST28,[25] REN8 moxa[28]
	Blood Deficiency	Nourish and regulate Blood: LIV8,[17] ST25,[25] HE6[23]
	Qi Deficiency	Tonify and regulate Qi: ST27,[25] LU9,[53] SP3[19]
	Kidney Jing (Essence) Deficiency	Tonify and regulate the Kidneys: KID12,[22] ST27,[25] BL52[54] moxa
	Kidney Yang Deficiency	Tonify Yang: KID2,[22] DU4[55] moxa
	Shen (Spirit) Disturbed	Calm the Shen (Spirit): HE5,[23] HE6,[23] DU24[55]
	Kidney Yin Deficiency	Regulate the Kidneys and enrich Yin: KID1,[22] HE7[23]
Orthodox medical conditions modifications	Advanced reproductive age, low ovarian reserve, poor response to ovarian stimulation	Reinforce and tonify Kidney Jing (Essence), enrich and nourish Yin and Blood, regulate Qi: ST27, KID12, KID13, HE6
		Treatments need to be more frequent, every 2–3 days (also see Chapter 10)
	Thin uterine lining	Enrich Yin, nourish, and regulate Blood: BL23,[54] BL17,[54] BL18,[54] HE7[23] moxa (also see Chapter 10)
	OHSS, high oestrogen levels	Regulate fluids, Qi, and Blood: REN9,[28] SP9, SP7,[19] LIV5[17] (also see Chapter 11)
	PCOS	Drain Dampness, benefit the Uterus: GB26,[20] ST28,[25] TITUO (also see Chapter 8)
	Hypothyroidism	Tonify and regulate Qi and Yang: KID4,[22] REN17,[28] SP3,[19] BL20[54] moxa (also see Chapter 8)
	Hyperthyroidism	Clear Heat/Fire, nourish and regulate Blood: BL21,[54] BL15,[54] BL17,[54] BL18[54] (also see Chapter 8)
	Endometriosis	Regulate the Chong and Ren Mai (Penetrating and Conception Vessels), Qi and Blood: KID5,[22] ST26,[25] REN2,[28] LIV14, LIV1[17] (also see Chapter 8)
	Reproductive immune issues	Regulate the Chong and Ren Mai (Penetrating and Conception Vessels), harmonize, tonify, regulate, and nourish Qi, Blood, and Yin: SP4, LU7, SP6, ST36, REN4, LIV3, SP10 (also see Chapter 12)
	Thrombophilia and other clotting conditions	Eliminate Blood-Stasis, regulate Blood, clear Heat: KID14,[22] LIV14,[17] SP10[19] (also see Chapter 12)
Lifestyle advice	Practise positive visualization, meditation, yoga, tai chi, keep warm[29]	
	Eat a balanced diet according to identified TCM syndromes	
	Other lifestyle advice may be applicable in individual patients (see Chapter 7)	

In couples with male factor infertility, it is very important to continue treating the male partner until the day of egg retrieval (see Chapter 8).

Final egg maturation and ovulation induction

Orthodox medical protocol

A woman is deemed ready for egg retrieval when the leading follicle reaches 15–20 mm in diameter.[2,6] ART clinics vary in their choice of ideal leading follicle size. Once a woman is considered ready, she injects the Human Chorionic Gonadotrophin (hCG) trigger medication (5000–10,000 IU of hCG intramuscularly or subcutaneously or 250 μg of recombinant hCG subcutaneously).[6] hCG mimics the action of LH[2] and induces final follicular maturation (progression of the immature oocyte (egg) at prophase I through meiotic maturation to metaphase II).[56]

The injection is usually done 36 h before the egg retrieval procedure. The timing of the trigger injection and egg retrieval procedure is very important. If the eggs are not retrieved on time, the follicles may rupture, and a woman may ovulate spontaneously 38–40 h after the trigger injection. This is because the downregulation medication, which prevents spontaneous ovulation, is usually discontinued on the day of the trigger injection.[2] Table 9.7 summarizes what happens at this stage of IVF.

Table 9.7 Summary of final egg maturation and ovulation induction phase	
What happens	High dosage of hCG induces the final egg maturation
	In some cases other preparations may be used to trigger ovulation (for example, GnRH agonist can be used instead of hCG in patients at risk of OHSS)[57–60]
Why is it done	To facilitate final follicular and egg maturation in preparation for egg retrieval and subsequent fertilization
Medication	5000–10,000 IU of hCG intramuscularly or subcutaneously (for example, Pregnyl®) or 250 μg of recombinant hCG subcutaneously (for example, Ovitrelle®)
How it is achieved	hCG trigger medication mimics the action of LH and initiates the final egg maturation process
Monitoring	Follicles are monitored by ultrasound. Trigger injection is scheduled when the leading follicle is 15–20 mm in diameter

TCM protocol

In the authors' experience, administering acupuncture treatment between the trigger injection and the egg retrieval procedure helps with the final egg maturation, potentially resulting in more mature eggs being retrieved. This approach has been advocated by some other authors.[13,29] There is a potential explanation as to why more eggs may be retrieved.

- Once a woman self-administers her trigger medication, this forces additional follicular growth and maturation of the eggs. Before the LH surge (or hCG trigger), the granulosa wall of the follicles is avascular. After the LH surge and some time before ovulation, it becomes invaded by blood vessels.[61] Good follicular vascularization on the day of the hCG trigger[62] and 36 h after the hCG trigger[63] has been associated with higher pregnancy rates following controlled ovarian stimulation.
- Limited human and animal research shows that acupuncture improves utero-ovarian blood flow[50,51,64,65] and, therefore, may improve blood supply and hormone and nutrient delivery to these follicles. Based on this research, one of the world's leading experts on folliculogenesis, Alain Gougeon, believes that acupuncture treatment delivered precisely between the LH surge and ovulation could potentially reinforce the natural increase of ovarian vascularization induced by the LH surge (A. Gougeon, personal communication). Gougeon also thinks that this could be especially pertinent in older women.
- As hCG trigger medication mimics the action of LH, a similar response is likely if acupuncture treatment is administered between the trigger injection and egg retrieval.

Not all patients need acupuncture treatment during this phase. We would recommend acupuncture treatment for patients who have several intermediate-sized follicles (12–15 mm in diameter). Table 9.8 summarizes the acupuncture treatment protocol for final egg maturation.

Egg retrieval

Orthodox medical protocol

Egg retrieval is done as an outpatient procedure. The patient may be placed under sedation, may have a local anaesthetic, or may undergo light general anaesthesia. An ultrasound probe is attached to the needle, then inserted through the vaginal wall and used to puncture and vacuum-aspirate each follicle. The fluid is then aspirated into a test tube.[2] Patients are usually discharged after a few hours.

The aspirated fluid is emptied into several Petri dishes to reduce the risk of accidental damage to the eggs in any one Petri dish. The fluid contents are then examined under a microscope.[2] Retrieved eggs are then scored, depending on their maturity and are classified as immature, mature,

Table 9.8 Acupuncture final egg maturation protocol (optional)	
Timing and frequency	One treatment session on the day between the trigger injection and egg retrieval
	If logistically impractical to administer treatment at this time (for example, because this day is on a weekend day), then: • Do the treatment on the day of trigger injection or • Apply semi-permanent needles during the last acupuncture session before the trigger injection and ask the patient to remove them before egg retrieval
Needling method and techniques	Electroacupuncture and a heat lamp are useful adjuncts
Main points prescription	SP4 + P6, ZIGONG (EA), ST29 (EA), SP10, SP6, ST36, LIV8, REN4, HE5, YINTANG

Table 9.9 Summary of egg retrieval protocol	
What happens	Follicles are aspirated under vaginal ultrasound guidance. Aspirated fluid is examined for presence of eggs
Medication	Sedation, general anaesthetic, or paracervical block. Gas and air can also be used
	Antibiotics are given afterwards to reduce the risk of post-surgical infection
Monitoring	Patient is normally discharged home after a few hours, unless there are complications

overripe, atretic, luteinized, or with fractured zona.[66] It is important to note that no consensus exists in the field of ART medicine about egg scoring, and, therefore, it is a very subjective scoring process.[66] Eggs are considered mature if they are in metaphase II (the second phase of maturation), and the first polar body has been discharged.[66] Immature eggs can potentially be matured in the laboratory using *In Vitro* Maturation (IVM).

If fresh sperm is used for fertilization of the eggs, which is the situation in the vast majority of procedures, then the sperm sample is collected on the same day by masturbation or via assisted sperm retrieval methods (see Chapter 6). The spermatozoa are then removed from the seminal fluid.[2]

Table 9.9 summarizes what happens during the egg retrieval procedure.

TCM protocol

Research suggests that acupuncture can be used as an effective pain-relieving method during the egg retrieval procedure.[67-69] However, in our experience, provision of acupuncture pain relief may be difficult to achieve because many ART clinics prefer to use conventional methods of pain relief.

In cases where acupuncture analgesia during egg retrieval can be used, acupuncturists should consider a treatment protocol by Sator-Katzenschlager and colleagues that has been shown to produce significant pain relief. In this RCT study, pain levels were significantly lower during and after the egg retrieval procedure in a group that received auricular electroacupuncture compared to pain levels in a group that received manual auricular acupuncture or a group that received no acupuncture.[68] Table 9.10 provides a description of the auricular electroacupuncture protocol.

Other acupuncture protocols have been used and have shown faster recovery times in patients who received electroacupuncture.[70,71]

In vitro fertilization

If the eggs are fertilized by a conventional IVF method, they are placed in a culture dish with a large number of motile sperm (50,000–100,000 per mL). Sperm then attempt to fertilize the egg in a similar manner as would happen in natural or *in vivo* fertilization.[2]

In Intracytoplasmic Sperm Injection (ICSI), one sperm is injected directly into each egg. Before a sperm is injected, it needs to be immobilized by removing its tail. With this technique, it is not necessary for sperm to undergo capacitation and the subsequent acrosome reaction (which is required for *in vivo* fertilization).[2] A variant of ICSI called

Table 9.10 Acupuncture analgesia for egg retrieval procedure	
Acupuncture protocol[68]	• Acupuncture needles (27 gauge, 3 mm length) inserted in auricular points 57 (Uterus), 55 (Shenmen), and 29 (Cushion/Occiput) on the dominant side • Needles are then covered by adhesive tape and connected to a miniature stimulator worn behind the ear (P-Stim™, Biegler GmbH) • Electroacupuncture stimulation: continuous low frequency with constant current of 1 Hz biphasic, 2 mA applied half an hour before egg retrieval procedure and finishing 1 h after the procedure

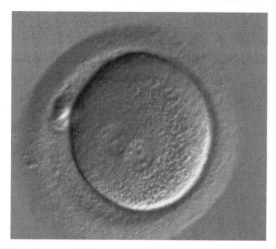

Figure 9.2 Fertilized egg showing two pronuclei.
Courtesy of Mr A. Gorgy at The Fertility and Gynaecology Academy and City Fertility, London, UK.

Intracytoplasmic Morphologically Selected Sperm Injection (IMSI) may also be used. Chapter 6 discusses indications for ICSI and IMSI fertilization methods.

The presence of two centrally positioned pronuclei with clearly defined membranes and two polar bodies 17 h (in IVF) and 18 h (in ICSI) after insemination confirms fertilization (Figure 9.2).[72]

About 60–70% of retrieved eggs are normally fertilized. The rates of fertilization are similar in IVF and ICSI.[73] If the pronuclei cannot be seen, it could be because either the eggs failed to fertilize or fertilization was delayed. In rare cases, none of the retrieved eggs are fertilized. Chapter 10 discusses in detail low fertilization rates and total fertilization failure. Table 9.11 summarizes the fertilization process.

The day after egg retrieval patients usually receive a telephone call from the ART unit to inform them how many of their eggs were successfully fertilized. For most

patients, waiting for this telephone call is a very anxiety-inducing period.

Embryo culture period (day after egg retrieval to day before embryo transfer)

Orthodox medical protocol

The created embryos continue dividing for up to 5 days. During their development, they are kept in a very stringently controlled culture medium. Specific components of culture media vary significantly amongst different laboratories and clinics. The components of the culture media may potentially influence the treatment outcome (see the section on repeated implantation failure in Chapter 12).

Developing embryos are very sensitive to temperature and pH environmental variations, and these conditions need to be continually monitored. Most culture media also contain antibiotics so that bacteria introduced during egg pick up or with sperm are eliminated.[74]

Embryologists monitor embryonic development and make the decision as to when the embryo transfer should be done. Their decision is based on the number and grading of embryos (embryo grading is discussed in Chapter 6). In rare cases, embryo transfer may be cancelled, for example, if a patient experiences severe OHSS. In this circumstance, all embryos are frozen. A cycle may also be cancelled if none of the embryos survive.

Many ART clinics are now using advanced incubation systems (sometimes referred to as embryoscopes) that provide stable environments for embryos. Embryoscopes also incorporate time-lapse imaging and monitoring of the developing embryos. The advantages of these technological systems are that embryos are handled less, and the time-lapse imaging provides the embryologist with the embryo development information he or she might not otherwise have. This improves clinical decision making about which embryos should be transferred.[75]

The embryos can be transferred on days 2, 3, or 5 after egg retrieval. The advantages and disadvantages of transferring on different days are extensively discussed in the section on repeated implantation failure in Chapter 12.

The period during which embryo culturing occurs is extremely stressful for most patients, especially if they do not have many embryos. Some clinics have a policy that an embryologist will telephone the patients on a regular basis to update them on their embryos' development. Other clinics do not have such procedures, and this, in our experience, often increases patients' anxiety and stress levels.

TCM protocol

In our experience, patients do not usually need acupuncture treatment during this phase. The only exception to this is if they develop signs of OHSS. Chapter 11 discusses OHSS in detail.

Table 9.11 Summary of *in vitro* fertilization phase	
Timing	On the day of egg retrieval
What happens	Retrieved eggs are fertilized using the following methods: • Conventional IVF: in a Petri dish • ICSI/IMSI: a single sperm is injected directly into an egg
Why it is done	To create embryos
Monitoring	On the day after egg retrieval, eggs are checked for signs of fertilization: two pronuclei and two polar bodies[73]

Embryo transfer

Orthodox medical protocol

Embryos can be transferred into the uterus at the cleavage stage (day 2 or 3 after egg retrieval) or at the blastocyst stage (day 5 or 6 after egg retrieval).[76]

The embryo transfer procedure is relatively simple and is usually pain free although occasionally sedation or general anaesthesia may be required (for example, in cases of cervical stenosis). A partner or a family member may accompany the woman. The patient is asked to have a full bladder. The patient lies on her back (sometimes with her legs in stirrups), and the doctor uses a speculum to expose the cervix. The cervix may be cleaned with sterile solution or culture medium. The embryologist will load the embryo(s) into a fine, soft catheter for the doctor or nurse to transfer through the vagina and cervix into the womb. Clinicians will have different preferences as to exactly where in the uterus they transfer the embryos. Most aim to place the embryo(s) 1–1.5 cm under the uterine fundus. Some doctors use an abdominal or transvaginal ultrasound to help to position the embryo(s) in the uterus. Using an ultrasound-assisted approach has been shown to increase IVF success rates.[77,78]

The catheter is then removed and checked under the microscope to ensure the embryo(s) have been transferred. The transfer process can take around 15 min. When the embryo transfer is completed, the patient may be left to rest for 15–20 min, although not all clinics recommend this recovery period.

Often couples are given a photograph of the embryos or shown the embryos that will be transferred on a screen before they are loaded into a catheter. If an ultrasound is used, patients and their partners may be given the opportunity to watch the transfer as it progresses. A white dot is seen on the screen once the embryos have been discharged into the uterus. This dot is an air bubble, which is loaded inside the catheter before the embryos and helps the clinician see exactly where the embryo(s) have been placed.

Occasionally, there may be difficulties during the embryo transfer – for example, embryos may become stuck in the catheter, the cervix may be too tight for the catheter to be inserted, or the woman may be too uncomfortable. Difficult transfers have been shown to reduce the IVF success rate.[79–81] Chapter 10 discusses difficult embryo transfers in greater detail. Any surplus embryos can be cryopreserved (frozen) to be used in future Frozen Embryo Transfer (FET) cycles. In some countries, freezing embryos is illegal.

The day of the embryo transfer can have a great emotional impact on a couple. On the morning of the embryo transfer day, many couples worry that the embryo(s) will not 'make it'. They may also be very anxious about arriving at the ART clinic on time, especially if the clinic is some distance away from them. Some women worry about the embryo transfer procedure and possible discomfort. When the embryo(s) are transferred, this can be a very moving experience for the couple, a climax of emotions about and involving everything they have been through to get this far. A woman usually feels very protective of her precious cargo, and many women believe themselves to be pregnant until proven otherwise.

INTERESTING FACTS

BED REST OR NO BED REST FOLLOWING EMBRYO TRANSFER?

Women often worry that the embryos will fall out after the embryo transfer. In the past, many clinics would leave women to rest in a horizontal position for 30 min or even longer after the transfer. Some clinics still do so.

However, research shows that, in 94% of cases, there is no movement of embryos on standing immediately after the embryo transfer; in 4% of cases, there is <1 cm movement; and, in only 2% of cases, there is >4 cm movement.[82]

TCM protocol

Acupuncture treatment around the time of embryo transfer has been shown to increase pregnancy rates[83–86] although not all studies demonstrate this effect.[87–90]

Many studies use the points prescription based on the Paulus et al.[84] study, in most cases without adequate acupuncture treatment during the other stages of IVF (see section 'Critique of acupuncture and IVF research'). However, the Paulus protocol does appear to be helpful and is preferred by patients who learn of it from the Internet. The Paulus protocol treatment on the day of embryo transfer can be individualized based on a patient's TCM diagnosis. Table 9.12 summarizes acupuncture treatment protocols that can be used on the embryo transfer day.

We would like to note that there is no need to be too rigid about this treatment protocol. In our experience, treating patients within 24 h of embryo transfer is often just as effective as doing the treatment 25 min before and after the transfer.

Critique of acupuncture and IVF research

Despite there being over 40 published clinical trials on acupuncture and IVF[13] and at least 10 systematic reviews, it is still not clear to what extent acupuncture influences IVF outcomes. Earlier systematic reviews suggested benefits with the use of acupuncture and IVF. More recent reviews (with one exception) do not support this beneficial relationship.

A systematic review and meta-analysis by Manheimer et al. of seven trials (1366 participants) concluded that acupuncture administered at the time of embryo transfer improves live birth rates.[92]

A Cochrane review by Cheong et al. analysed 13 RCTs and concluded that acupuncture performed on the day of embryo transfer significantly increased live birth rates.[14]

A systematic review and meta-analysis by El-Toukhy et al. of 13 trials (2500 participants) found that acupuncture did

Table 9.12 Acupuncture treatment protocols for the use around the time of embryo transfer

Timing	On the day of embryo transfer (day 2, 3, or 5 post egg retrieval). If logistically impractical, the treatment can be carried out within 24 h of the transfer		
Paulus et al. 2002[84]	*Treatment 1: 25 min before embryo transfer*		
	P6, SP8, LIV3, DU20, ST29		
	Left ear: Shenmen (55), Zigong (58)		
	Right ear: Neifenmi (22), Naodian (34)		
	Treatment 2: 25 min after embryo transfer		
	ST36, SP6, SP10, LI4		
	Right ear: Shenmen (55), Zigong (58)		
	Left ear: Neifenmi (22), Naodian (34)		
	Method		
	Strong de qi sensation was obtained during the initial insertion and again 10 min later. Needles were retained for 25 min		
Dieterle et al.[91]	*Treatment 30 min after embryo transfer*		
	REN4, REN6, ST29, P6, SP10, SP8. Herbal seeds placed on ear points Shenmen (55), Zigong (58), Neifenmi (22), Pizhixia (33)		
Omodei et al.[86]	*Treatment 1: 25 min before embryo transfer*		
	YINTANG, LI4, ST36, SP6, LIV3		
	Treatment 2: 25 min after embryo transfer		
	'Shenmen, Uterus, Kidney, and Heart'		
Other acupuncture prescriptions	Before transfer (2- or 3-day-old embryos)	Empiric prescription	SP4 + P6, LIV3, LI4, REN4, SP6, ST36, SP10, ZIGONG, ST29, YINTANG
		Blood Deficiency	Add BL17, BL15, BL18, BL23 moxa
		Kidney Yang Deficiency	Add KID3, REN12, KID7 moxa
		Blood Stasis	Add SP8
		Dampness	Add SP9, ST28, REN3, LIV5, BL20, SP3 moxa
		Heat/Fire	Add LIV2, LIV4, ST45, SJ5
	After transfer (2- or 3-day-old embryos)	Empiric prescription	REN4, REN6, KID7, ST36, DU20
		Blood Deficiency	Add LIV8, P6, HE6
		Kidney Yang Deficiency	Add DU4, BL23, BL52 moxa
		Dampness	Add BL20, SP5 moxa
		Blood-Stasis	Add SP10
		Heat/Fire	Add LI11, P7, KID8
	After transfer (day 5 blastocyst transfer)	Empiric prescription	REN12, REN6, DU20, HE5

not have a significant effect on clinical or live birth rates.[93] The authors updated their results in 2009 after publication of another RCT and confirmed their original findings.[94]

A systematic review and meta-analysis by Qu et al. of 17 trials found no evidence of significant benefit with the use of acupuncture during IVF or ICSI.[95]

A systematic review and meta-analysis by Zheng et al. of 24 trials (5807 participants) found that acupuncture significantly improved clinical pregnancy rates but not live birth rates. When the authors excluded studies that used the Streitberger sham needle, acupuncture was shown to have a statistically significant influence on live birth rates, especially if, in addition to acupuncture at embryo transfer, acupuncture was also administered during the ovarian stimulation phase and egg retrieval.[47]

A systematic review and meta-analysis by Manheimer et al. of 16 trials (4021) participants found that acupuncture offers no benefit for IVF.[96]

An updated Cochrane review by Cheong et al. after analysis of 20 RCTs concluded that acupuncture had no effect on live birth rates.[97]

The reason why the reviews produce such mixed results might be in part caused by the different inclusion and exclusion criteria they used for selecting trials for analysis. Another reason is the methodological limitations of many trials.[98] In this section, we outline some of the issues with the research on acupuncture treatment and IVF.

Sample size

Most IVF acupuncture studies are relatively small and, therefore, may be underpowered.[99,100] In their review paper, Meldrum et al. state that in order to achieve more meaningful results, future studies need to recruit at least 996 and potentially as many as 3829 participants for each of the acupuncture and control groups.[99] El-Toukhy and Khalaf state that 2300 women need to be recruited in each arm of future studies investigating the effect of acupuncture on clinical pregnancy rates and an even greater number of women should be recruited for studies using live birth rate as an outcome measure.[101]

Control intervention

Finding a reliable placebo control intervention may affect the outcomes of the studies. Common control interventions in acupuncture studies include using the Streitberger sham needle, needling non-acupoint locations, or needling real acupoints shallowly.[102] None of these options are perfect. In needling non-acupoint locations, it may be difficult to find a nontherapeutic site on the skin that is not near an acupuncture point.[102] Shallow needling is a valid therapeutic acupuncture technique.[102]

The Streitberger needle may not be an inactive control.[103] In two validation trials of the Streitberger sham needle, it was found that these needles elicit the de qi sensation

in many participants; therefore, this needle may not be an inert placebo.[96,104,105]

In their meta-analysis, Zheng et al. found that acupuncture improves clinical pregnancy rates and live birth rates only if the studies that do not use the Streitberger sham needle are included in the analysis. The authors conclude that the Streitberger control may not be inactive.[47] However, some experts feel that removing the Streitberger control is not scientifically valid.[99] Other placebo acupuncture devices are being developed.[102] Perhaps in time these may offer a better control technique.

Individualization of treatment

Most acupuncture studies use fixed protocols.[13] This could be compared to IVF consultants prescribing the same dose of FSH medication to women with good ovarian reserve and women with poor ovarian reserve. In clinical reality, patients are treated on an individual basis.

However, the studies also need to be reproducible[100] and comparable.[95,98] Therefore, fixed detailed (individualized) protocols should be used in future studies,[100] and the Standards for Reporting Interventions in Clinical Trials of Acupuncture (STRICTA) guidelines should be followed when reporting acupuncture intervention.[106]

Outcome measures

Many acupuncture studies report limited outcome measures.[100] For example, some only report implantation rates. All relevant outcome measures should be reported in future IVF studies, including clinical pregnancy, biochemical pregnancy, ongoing pregnancy, implantation rate, live birth rate, and miscarriage rate.[95]

Acupuncture treatment may also potentially have a positive effect on other outcomes such as emotional and physical well-being of patients undergoing IVF treatment, ovarian response to stimulation, total amount of medication used, number of mature eggs retrieved, thickness of the endometrial lining, fertilization rate, embryo grades, and discomfort during the embryo transfer procedure. Based on our interpretation of the literature, we believe that future studies should consider all potential outcome measures.

Dose of acupuncture

The success rates reported in studies may be influenced by the dose of acupuncture treatment.[100] For example, the total number of treatment sessions may be inadequate or the number of acupuncture points used may be insufficient.[13]

El-Toukhy and Khalaf looked for evidence of dose effect of acupuncture in their review paper and failed to find it.[107] However, in our opinion, in the studies evaluated by El-Toukhy and Khalaf that included extra treatment sessions,[83,90,108] there was still undertreatment of patients. For example, in our opinion, treating patients during the pretreatment cycle and during the first few days of ovarian stimulation may help to recruit more follicles, which could potentially lead to better outcomes.

Timing of acupuncture treatment

The majority of studies administered acupuncture around the time of embryo transfer. We are unaware of any acupuncture IVF studies using acupuncture in the 3–6 months' preparation phase preceding IVF. This seems surprising because, ultimately, the outcome of IVF depends on the quality of the eggs,[109,110] sperm,[111–113] and the resulting embryo.[114] Endometrial thickness and uterine receptivity are also highly important for IVF success.[41,43,44]

As Figure 9.3 shows, the timeframe over which the eggs, sperm, and endometrium develop is many months before the embryo transfer day. Administering acupuncture treatment only on the day of embryo transfer (as has been done by most studies) may be considered undertreatment because, by this stage, all key elements essential for a good-quality embryo to develop and likely to influence the outcome are beyond the stage where they can be improved by acupuncture.

The key stages influencing IVF outcome are as follows:

Key influence 1: follicular development (6 months before egg retrieval)

- As described in Chapter 2, ovarian follicles take approximately 1 year to develop from their dormant stage to the ovulatory stage. Follicles larger than 0.08 mm in diameter (otherwise called secondary follicles), at around 190 days or 6 months before ovulation, begin to respond to their environment by acquiring arterioles. The patency and efficiency of the arteriolar supply determines the effectiveness of the delivery of reproductive hormones and nutrition to the follicles. Colour Doppler studies show that the development of follicles is directly correlated with their circulatory supply.[115,116]
- Limited human and animal research shows that acupuncture improves utero-ovarian blood flow[50,51,64,65] and, therefore, may potentially improve circulatory supply and hormone and nutrient delivery to these follicles.
- Consequently, we suggest treating women using TCM acupuncture approaches during these 6 months prior to embryo transfer, which we believe may potentially influence follicular development.

Key influence 2: sperm (3 months before sperm collection)

- Chapter 2 described the process of spermatogenesis, which occurs over a 3-month period. The research on the effect of acupuncture on sperm parameters is limited (see Chapter 8). If acupuncture can exert a positive influence on the process of spermatogenesis and the sperm parameters, which is still unclear, then such an effect can only be achieved by treating men during the 3 months preceding the day of sperm collection.

Key influence 3: recruitment of follicles (late luteal/early follicular phase)

- In response to rising FSH levels, follicular recruitment begins either at the end of the luteal phase[115] (in an unsuppressed cycle) or in the first few days of the stimulation phase at the time when women begin to inject gonadotrophins. We would posit that administering acupuncture treatment at the end of the luteal phase (in unsuppressed cycles) and at the beginning of the follicular or stimulation phase may potentially influence follicular recruitment, resulting in a greater pool of follicles available for stimulation.

Key influence 4: endometrial lining (stimulation phase)

- The endometrium develops during the stimulation phase. Therefore, in order to influence the development of the endometrium, frequent acupuncture treatments should be administered during the stimulation phase. There is preliminary research evidence suggesting that acupuncture may positively influence endometrial development.[48]

Key influence 5: follicular response to gonadotrophin stimulation

- Colour Doppler studies show that follicular development is directly correlated with their blood supply.[115,116] Good-quality blood supply to a follicle during the ovarian stimulation phase has been associated with a greater likelihood of recovering a mature egg,[117,118] higher-grade embryos,[117] and an improved chance of pregnancy.[119,120] Poor blood supply can result in a longer stimulation phase being required and fewer eggs being recruited.[121]
- A limited amount of human and animal research shows that acupuncture improves utero-ovarian blood flow.[50,51,64,65] Improved utero-ovarian blood flow may improve follicular blood perfusion during the stimulation phase.
- More research is necessary to investigate further to what extent acupuncture improves utero-ovarian blood flow. Based on the presently available research findings, we would recommend that women be treated throughout the stimulation phase,[13] which on average lasts for 12 days.[122] Treatments should be administered every 2–4 days.[29]

Key influence 6: final follicular and egg maturation (between ovulation trigger and egg retrieval)

- Before the LH surge, the granulosa wall of the follicles is avascular. After the LH surge and some time before ovulation, it becomes invaded by blood vessels.[61] Good follicular vascularization on the day of the hCG trigger[62] and 36 h after the hCG trigger[63] has been associated with higher pregnancy rates following controlled ovarian stimulation.
- Based on the limited research demonstrating that acupuncture improves ovarian blood flow (see above), one of the world's leading experts on folliculogenesis, Alain Gougeon, believes that if the acupuncture

Timeline of key events leading to successful IVF outcome									
IVF phases	**Preparation phase (3–4 months)**		**Pretreatment phase (up to 4 weeks before stimulation)**				**Stimulation phase (on average 12 days)**		**Luteal phase (the last 2 weeks)**
Time/key events	**Months 6–4**	**Month 3**	**Pretreatment cycle**				**IVF treatment cycle**		
			Week 8	**Week 7**	**Week 6**	**Week 5**	**Week 4**	**Week 3**	**Week 2**	**Week 1**
1 Follicular development	Follicular development takes 12 months. The last 6 months of development may be influenced by acupuncture.									
2 Sperm production		Sperm development takes ~3 months, which may be influenced by acupuncture.								
3 Follicular recruitment						Follicles are recruited during late luteal/early follicular phase. Acupuncture treatment during this time may improve follicular recruitment.			
4 Endometrial development							Endometrium develops during the stimulation phase. Acupuncture during this phase may increase its thickness and quality.		
5 Follicular response to medication							Follicles grow rapidly in response to ovarian stimulation. Acupuncture during this phase may improve ovarian response to stimulation.		
6 Final egg maturation								Acupuncture between hCG trigger and egg retrieval may help with final egg maturation.	
7 Egg retrieval								Acupuncture may reduce pain during egg retrieval procedure.	
8 Embryo transfer									Acupuncture on the day of embryo transfer (2, 3, or 5 post egg retrieval) may be used.
9 Implantation									Acupuncture during implantation window (days 4–8 post egg retrieval) may help with embryo implantation.

Figure 9.3 Timeline of key events leading to successful IVF.

251

treatment is delivered precisely between the LH surge and ovulation, it could potentially reinforce the natural increase of ovarian vascularization induced by the LH surge (A. Gougeon, personal communication). Gougeon also believes that the use of acupuncture at this time could be especially appropriate in the management of older women. Because hCG trigger medication mimics the action of LH, we would hypothesize that a similar response is likely if acupuncture treatment is administered between the trigger injection and egg retrieval.

- Our clinical experience confirms that acupuncture treatment on the day between the trigger injection and egg retrieval appears to greatly affect egg maturation. The value of administration of acupuncture treatment at this stage is supported by other authors.[13,29]

Key influence 7: pain relief during egg retrieval (optional)

- Acupuncture has been shown to be an effective pain relieving method during the egg retrieval procedure,[68] and it may aid with postsurgical recovery.[67,70,71,123] However, there is no evidence that administering acupuncture on the day of egg retrieval influences conception rates.

Key influence 8: embryo transfer (days 2, 3, or 5 after egg retrieval)

- The majority of the published research on acupuncture and IVF has been done to study the effect of administering acupuncture during the embryo transfer phase. The effect of acupuncture on the day of embryo transfer may have a positive influence on IVF outcomes. However, research results are mixed and equivocal (Critique of acupuncture and IVF research).

- It is unclear exactly what the administration of acupuncture treatment on the day of embryo transfer is likely to influence because eggs, sperm, embryos, and the endometrium are already developed. Logically, the only aspects acupuncture may help with on the day of embryo transfer are the reduction of uterine contractions and the reduction of stress levels, provided that a woman does not develop a stress response because of a rigid schedule of acupuncture treatments. It is also possible that acupuncture may modulate a woman's immune response to the embryo.

Key influence 9: implantation and endometrial receptivity (days 4–8 post egg retrieval)

- In controlled ovarian stimulation cycles, the implantation window is in the range of 4–8 days post egg retrieval.[124] Good utero-ovarian blood flow during the peri-implantation period influences conception rates in women undergoing IVF.[125] A delay in achieving adequate uterine perfusion may affect endometrial receptivity.[125] It has been found that good uterine blood supply on the day of hCG administration is associated with conceptions in IVF patients.[126]

- As already discussed, acupuncture has been shown to improve blood supply to the uterus, and acupuncture could therefore potentially influence implantation if administered on days 4–8 after egg retrieval.

In conclusion, treating women only on the day of embryo transfer (as the majority of studies seem to do) fails to maximize the potential benefit acupuncture could offer. In comparison to conventional IVF, the use of acupuncture only on the day of embryo transfer may be compared to carrying out an embryo transfer procedure without adequate ovarian stimulation. The results in both instances may well be suboptimal.

Stress of acupuncture treatment

The other issue with fixed protocols focusing on the day of embryo transfer is that their use could potentially generate an unnecessary stress in patients.

Meldrum et al. in their review paper suggest that in some instances the provision of acupuncture treatment on embryo transfer day can be detrimental rather than beneficial. They suggest examples such as procedurally induced stress caused by strong acupuncture needling technique or a stress response induced on the day of embryo transfer caused by anxiety associated with logistical and practical issues such as travelling to and from an acupuncture clinic for embryo transfer acupuncture protocols to be administered.[99]

Manheimer et al. in their systematic review and meta-analysis hint at a similar opinion, stating 'Although it was not a statistically significant subgroup finding, there was a trend suggesting that acupuncture administered on-site of the IVF clinic had more positive effects than acupuncture administered off-site of the IVF clinic'.[96] The authors, however, did acknowledge that their opinion was based only on the study by Craig et al.[127]

In our opinion too rigid an adherence to the timing of the administration of acupuncture protocols to some patients who may have a tendency to be anxious may indeed cause stress. Other authors also acknowledge the detrimental aspect of trying to adhere to a rigidly applied protocol.[13]

Confounding factors

Many studies fail to control for confounding factors, such as weight, nutrition, alcohol consumption, smoking, and medical factors such as hormonal and ovarian status. Future studies should aim to control for such confounding factors.

What about men?

Male factor contributes to up to 40% of infertility cases.[128] Male factor subfertility may also lead to implantation failure[111–113] and miscarriages.[129,130] Most if not all studies investigating the effect of acupuncture on IVF outcomes treat either a male or a female partner. We are unaware of a single trial where a couple is treated as a unit. It would be interesting to see if treating both partners in preparation for and during IVF would produce better outcomes.

Practical considerations in treating patients on the day of embryo transfer

In many cases, it is difficult to know in advance when the transfer of the embryo will take place, especially if there are not many embryos. Patients get regular telephone calls updating them on how their embryos are developing and when the transfer is likely to take place. In some cases patients are asked to come in for the embryo transfer procedure at very short notice.

Many patients are aware of the embryo transfer acupuncture treatment protocols. Patients often expect their acupuncturist to perform them on demand. Consequently, fertility acupuncturists may need to be available at short notice for the provision of embryo transfer treatments. This poses a practical problem: potentially being on call 7 days a week, 365 days a year. For the acupuncturists specializing in treating patients with fertility issues this means that the busier their fertility practice is, the more likely they are to work on days off (including at the weekend). Planning family and social life therefore often revolves around, and is constrained by, being available to provide 'transfer appointments'.

One way to manage this type of workload is to team up with another acupuncturist who specializes in infertility. The acupuncturists do not need to work in the same clinic, as long as they are a reasonable driving distance away from each other. This should enable the team members to support each other, either on a rota or an *ad hoc* basis.

In embryo transfer acupuncture research studies, treatment is often provided within 25 min or so before and after the embryo transfer. Since publication of Paulus 2002 protocol, there has been a lot of debate within the acupuncture profession about the importance of timing of the provision of acupuncture embryo transfer treatment.

Many expert fertility acupuncturists consider that the timing is not critical, and the embryo transfer acupuncture treatments can be done on the day before or day after the transfer, particularly if being rigid with the timing of the transfer treatment creates an unnecessary stress for patients.[99] One study showed lower pregnancy rates in patients who received acupuncture treatment compared to a control group. The acupuncture patients in this study experienced a stressful journey to and from the acupuncture clinic in order to be treated within 25 min of their embryo transfer, which may have influenced the outcome.[13,127]

Luteal phase (the 'two-week wait')

Orthodox medical protocol

GnRH analogs (agonist and antagonists) that are used in IVF interfere with LH production. This affects progesterone production, which is necessary for adequate luteal phase support. Therefore progesterone supplementation is required because it is important for implantation and to reduce uterine irritability.[6]

The supplementation with progesterone usually begins on the evening after egg retrieval. Progesterone can be administered in the following ways:[6]

- Progesterone in oil (for example, 50 mg IM daily)
- Oral micronized progesterone (for example, 600 mg daily)
- 8% progesterone vaginal gel (for example, 90 mL daily)
- Micronized natural progesterone in vaginal tablets (for example, 300 mg daily)

There is no evidence that any one route of progesterone administration is more effective than any other. Intramuscular administration was found to be more effective in a 2002 meta-analysis,[131] but a 2009 meta-analysis found that outcomes were similar for vaginal and intramuscular progesterone administration.[132]

Alternatively, hCG supplementation may be used. Typically 250 µg of recombinant hCG is administered subcutaneously, or 2500–5000 IU is injected intramuscularly 1 week after the ovulation trigger. Progesterone and hCG luteal support produce similar results, but hCG supplementation significantly increases the risk of OHSS.[6]

Oral oestrogen can be added to progesterone during the luteal phase in GnRH agonist cycles. For example, adding 4 mg of oral oestradiol to progesterone supplementation has been shown to significantly increase the pregnancy and implantation rates and has decreased the miscarriage rate compared with the use of progesterone monotherapy.[133] A 2011 Cochrane review found that there was a significant increase in the clinical pregnancy rate when progesterone was combined with transdermal or oral oestrogen. But no effects were found with vaginal oestrogen administration.[134]

Table 9.13 summarizes what happens during the luteal phase.

> ## CLINICAL TIPS
>
> ### PROGESTERONE SUPPORT
>
> Some ART units withdraw progesterone support after a positive pregnancy test whilst other units continue prescribing progesterone until around 12 weeks' gestation or even later.
>
> In the authors' experience, patients with a diagnosis of Yang Deficiency or a history of a miscarriage associated with Yang Deficiency will benefit from being on luteal support until 12 weeks' gestation. If such support is not provided by the ART clinic, acupuncture and moxibustion to support Yang is essential throughout the first 12 weeks.

Table 9.13 Summary of the luteal phase (the 'two-week wait')	
Timing	The day of egg retrieval to the day of pregnancy test
Why it is done	The function of the corpus luteum and LH production is disrupted and therefore natural progesterone production is affected
Medication	Progesterone (sometimes with oestrogen) or hCG medication helps to maintain the endometrial lining and create a viable environment for the implantation of the embryo
How it is achieved	By exerting the same function as natural progesterone
Monitoring	None, or some clinics will check serum progesterone levels

CLINICAL TIPS

'AM I PREGNANT?'

Some women will be very anxious and look for signs that they are pregnant. They may search the Internet for symptoms of pregnancy. They may also ask the acupuncturist to comment on the possibility of the patient being pregnant.

In our experience, women who are pregnant often experience:

- Twinges/pulling sensation in the lower abdomen, particularly on movement.
- Breast tenderness and/or nipple tingling sensation.
- Extreme tiredness/sleepiness.
- Changes in appetite.

TCM pulse quality may change to slippery, but it may also remain weak and thin in patients who are constitutionally weak.

However, 'pregnancy-type symptoms' may be mimicked by stress and/or luteal support medication. Therefore it is probably best for the acupuncturist to refrain from commenting about any possible pregnancy status in order to avoid unnecessarily raising or dashing a patient's hopes. If there is nothing to be concerned about, it is probably best to reassure the patient and explain that it is better to wait until the pregnancy test result.

TCM protocol

Acupuncture provided during the luteal phase may help to improve implantation and clinical pregnancy rates. A randomized, prospective, controlled study found that acupuncture during the luteal phase in addition to the embryo transfer protocol in patients undergoing IVF/ICSI treatment significantly increased implantation, clinical, and ongoing pregnancy rates. Acupuncture points used in the luteal phase protocol were REN4, REN6, ST29, P6, SP10, and SP8. In addition, herbal seeds were placed on ear points Shenmen (55), Uterus (58), Endocrine (22), and Forehead (33), and patients were advised to press them twice daily for 2 days.[91] However, another prospective randomized trial found no additional benefit from acupuncture during the luteal phase.[83]

Acupuncture may also help to reduce the risk of miscarriages in patients undergoing IVF/ICSI. In a retrospective analysis of 238 patients undergoing IVF/ICSI, the first trimester miscarriage rate was significantly lower in the acupuncture group compared with a control group of patients who did not receive acupuncture (31.8% and 40%, respectively).[135]

During the 'two-week wait', a patient's anxiety levels can fluctuate greatly (sometimes several times a day), exacerbated by an emotional response to the thought of the possibility of IVF failure. Even in cases where all has gone seemingly well, patients may still feel anxious during this phase. The 'two-week wait' is a quieter period of time of the IVF process. Patients go from having regular scans and blood tests, egg retrieval, and embryo transfer to almost nothing while awaiting the final outcome. Therefore, emotional support is also very important.

Patients' TCM pathology may also change during this time; therefore, responding dynamically by continually reviewing acupuncture treatment principles is of paramount importance. Table 9.14 provides details of a basic luteal phase acupuncture protocol and modifications.

Pregnancy test

Orthodox medical protocol

The pregnancy test is usually done 14–16 days after egg retrieval. Pregnancy status can be checked by a home urine pregnancy test, or patients can have their blood beta-hCG levels tested at their ART clinic. Pregnancy is confirmed if beta-hCG levels are ≥ 5 IU/L.[137]

If the pregnancy test is positive, a transvaginal ultrasound scan is usually carried out between 6 and 7 weeks' gestation to assess viability of the pregnancy. If the pregnancy is viable, patients are often discharged from the ART clinic, and usual obstetric care is initiated by the patient's GP.

Some patients may not be discharged from the ART clinic until later, for example, if they need immunotherapy. In some cases a specialist referral is necessary, for example, in patients testing positive for thyroid antibodies. It is important for fertility acupuncturists to monitor and to assist patients and ensure that appropriate referrals have been made.

TCM protocol

Early pregnancy acupuncture support is discussed in Chapter 14, and miscarriage prevention is covered in depth in Chapter 12.

Table 9.14 Luteal phase ('two-week wait') acupuncture protocol (from the day of embryo transfer to pregnancy test day)

Timing and frequency	*Session 1*: during implantation window (4–8 days post egg retrieval)[124]	
	Session 2: halfway between session 1 and proposed pregnancy test date	
Main points prescription	Reinforce Yang, nourish and warm Blood, tonify the Spleen and Kidneys, calm the Shen (Spirit) to aid implantation and prevent miscarriage[136]: KID3, KID7, ST36, SP3, REN4, REN6, DU20, YINTANG moxa	
TCM acupuncture treatment modifications (also see Chapter 5)	Liver Qi Stagnation	Regulate Qi and Blood: LIV8,[17] BL18[54]
	Blood-Stasis	Eliminate Blood-Stasis, invigorate Blood: SP10,[19] SP4+P6[19]
	Dampness	Resolve Dampness: SP9,[19] REN9[28] moxa
	Cold	Warm Cold: DU4,[55] REN8[28] moxa
	Kidney Jing (Essence) Deficiency	Tonify the Kidney: BL23, BL52[54] moxa
	Blood Deficiency	Nourish Blood: LIV8,[17] REN12[28] moxa
	Qi Deficiency	Tonify and regulate Qi: HE5[23]
Orthodox medical conditions modifications	Advanced maternal age	Tonify Kidney Jing (Essence), nourish Blood, regulate the Chong and Ren Mai (Penetrating and Conception Vessels): KID13+KID12,[22] LU7+KID6,[53] SP4+P6[19] moxa (also see Chapters 10 and 12)
	History of miscarriage(s)	Tonify Kidney Jing (Essence), Qi, Yang and Blood: BL23, BL52,[54] KID2,[22] BL20[54] moxa (also see Chapter 12)
	PCOS	Raise Qi, regulate the Spleen: TITUO,[24] SP9[19] (also see Chapter 8)
	Hypothyroidism	Regulate Qi and Blood: REN12,[28] HE5[23] (also see Chapter 8)
	Hyperthyroidism	Clear Heat/Fire, nourish Blood: LIV2,[17] P7,[18] LIV8,[17] HE3[23] (also see Chapter 8)
	Endometriosis	Regulate Blood: KID5,[22] REN3,[28] SP10,[19] SP4+P6[19] (also see Chapter 8)
	OHSS	Regulate fluids, Qi, and Blood: SP9,[19] REN9[28] (also see Chapter 11)
	Immune issues	Regulate Qi and Blood: ST36,[25] SP10[19] (also see Chapter 12)
	Thrombophilia and other clotting conditions	Promote free flow of Qi and Blood: SP4+P6,[19] ST30[25] (also see Chapter 12)

Case study

Treatment of Patients During IVF

Fiona, a 34-year-old teacher, presented for acupuncture to prepare her for her third IVF/ICSI treatment cycle. Fiona and her husband Jack had been trying to conceive for over 3 years. Their Orthodox medical diagnosis was infertility due to mixed male and female factor. Fiona had mild endometriosis and Jack had a low sperm count. Fiona's ovarian reserve was good. Jack had a 10-year-old child from a previous relationship.

Previous IVF History

In their first IVF cycle, conventional IVF was used because sperm on the day of collection was good. Unfortunately, despite Fiona producing 10 mature eggs, none of them fertilized.

In the second cycle, Fiona produced 11 mature eggs and 4 were fertilized using ICSI. Only one embryo was available for transfer on day 2. Pregnancy test was negative.

Continued

Case study—cont'd

In view of Fiona's and Jack's fertility and ART history, I recommended that Jack should also have acupuncture treatment.

Jack's Manifestations

Feeling hot, especially at night, nightsweats, thirsty, back pain, scanty urination. Pulse: very weak on all positions. Tongue: slightly pale. Jack also had family history of male factor subfertility.

Fiona's Manifestations

Red face and neck, irritability, frustration, extreme tiredness, tendency to worry. Menstrual cycles were regular 28 days and bleeding lasted 6–7 days (including 1–2 days of premenstrual spotting). Dull abdominal ache persisted throughout the cycle, which was worse during menses. Her tongue was red with heat spots, and her pulse was rapid, overflowing.

TCM Diagnosis (Jack)

Kidney Yin Deficiency (primary syndrome)

TCM Diagnosis (Fiona)

- Liver Fire
- Spleen Qi Deficiency

Acupuncture Treatment (Jack)

Jack's point prescription included LU7+KID6, SP6, ST36, KID3, KID7, P6. He received a total of seven acupuncture treatments. Jack was also provided with evidence-based lifestyle advice.

Acupuncture Treatment (Fiona)

- Preparation phase: LIV2, LI11, ST44, SP3, KID3 (three sessions). Evidence-based lifestyle advice was also provided.

- Pretreatment phase: Fiona's cycle was supressed with GnRH agonist, which she began on day 21 of the cycle preceding the IVF treatment cycle. One acupuncture treatment was administered 2 days before stimulation: LU7+KID6, SP6, SP3, LIV2, ST29, ZIGONG, REN4. A heat lamp was placed over her abdomen.
- Stimulation phase prescription: LU7+KID6, SP4+P6, ST29, ZIGONG, REN4, SP6, LIV3. A total of three sessions were administered. The endometrium reached at least 8 mm (Fiona was not sure), and on the day of hCG trigger injection she had five follicles between 13 and 18 mm on the right side and one on the left.
- Egg retrieval and fertilization: 4 mature eggs were retrieved and all were fertilized using ICSI.
- Embryo transfer: one top-grade embryo was transferred on day 2 and two top-grade embryos were frozen. Paulus et al.[84] embryo transfer acupuncture protocol was done before and after the transfer.
- Luteal phase: acupuncture treatment was done on day 6 post egg retrieval (to coincide with implantation stage). Points used were: HE7, LIV2, SP3, KID7, KID9.

The pregnancy test was positive and pregnancy progressed to full term.

Summary

Treating both partners was essential in this case because their infertility was due to both male and female factor. Their previous ART history included total fertilization failure and poor fertilization rate, which in many cases is caused by suboptimal sperm. Therefore Jack was treated to optimize his fertility, and Fiona was provided with IVF support to improve her response to medication and to minimize the negative effect of endometriosis.

Case study

Treatment of a Patient of Advanced Reproductive Age During IVF

Jane was 44 when she underwent a fresh IVF cycle due to secondary infertility. She had previously undergone several other IVF cycles without success, although in some of these IVF cycles no embryo transfer took place and the embryos were frozen, as Jane preferred to 'bank' as many embryos as she could while she was still allowed to undergo stimulated IVF cycles.

Jane's ovarian reserve markers were very good given her age: FSH 7.4 IU/L, LH 1.2 IU/L and AMH 5.6 pmol/L.

Manifestations

- Feels very hot, dry mouth (especially at night)
- Stools: normal or constipation alternating with diarrhoea
- Indigestion, exacerbated by caffeine or alcohol
- Urination: frequent, every 2.5 h

Case study—cont'd

- Very mild asthma
- Headaches, occasional migraines
- Achy in upper back and shoulders
- Eyes: floaters, dry and gritty sensation
- Menstrual cycle: regular 28 days, mild premenstrual tension (irritability, sore breasts)
- Menses: last 5 days, very heavy
- Tongue: red body with small cracks
- Pulse: rapid, empty on both 3rd positions

TCM Diagnosis

- Kidney and Liver Yin Deficiency with Empty-Heat
- Liver Yang Rising

Preparation Phase

Jane received acupuncture treatment over several months while undergoing previous IVF cycles and in preparation for the current cycle. Acupuncture points used included LU7 +KID6, KID3, KID2, LIV3, LIV2, SP6, YINTANG, ST29, ZIGONG, REN4. Evidence-based lifestyle advice was also provided to Jane.

Pretreatment Phase

Jane started downregulation (Suprefact®) medication on day 21 of her menstrual cycle.

Overall Jane felt less hot, but this fluctuated. Four acupuncture sessions were administered during this phase. The same acupuncture points were used with the addition of HE7 and P6 because Jane was feeling very anxious.

Stimulation Phase

Baseline ultrasound scan on day 2 of the treatment cycle showed eight antral follicles (four on each ovary). The endometrial lining was 8 mm, but Jane was still bleeding heavily. She began stimulation medication Fostimon® 375 IU/day whilst continuing on a reduced dose of downregulation medication.

Acupuncture Treatment on Day 3

- LU7+KID6, SP6, LIV3, LIV2, ST29, ZIGONG, REN4, YINTANG, HE7, KID1.
- Semi-permanent needles were placed on KID2, SP6, ZIGONG, HE7, LIV2.
- A heat lamp was placed over the abdomen.

Ultrasound Scan on Day 6

- Left ovary: no follicles
- Right ovary: 2 × 10 mm and 3 × 4 mm follicles
- Endometrium: not developing well

- Concern: not responding to stimulation? Cycle at risk of being cancelled.

Acupuncture Treatment on Day 6

Same as on day 3

Ultrasound Scan on Day 10

- Left ovary: 5 follicles (18, 15, 14, 13, 10 mm)
- Right ovary: 6 follicles (16, 15, 12, 10, 9, 7 mm)
- Endometrium: 10 mm thick and trilaminar in appearance

Acupuncture Treatment on Day 10

Same as on day 3.

Ultrasound Scan on Day 12

- Left ovary: 6 follicles (20, 19, 17, 16, 13, 9 mm)
- Right ovary: 6 follicles (20, 18, 17, 13, 11, 11 mm)
- Endometrium: 12 mm, but of poor appearance
- Oestrogen: 7000 pmol/L
- IVF clinic placed Jane on 'OHSS watch'.
- The trigger injection to be done on the evening of day 12 and egg retrieval was scheduled for 36 h later.

My concern at this point was that the smaller follicles (<17 mm) may not contain a mature egg. Another acupuncture treatment session was scheduled on the day between ovulation trigger and egg retrieval.

Acupuncture Treatment on the Day Between Ovulation Trigger and Egg Retrieval

- LIV8, ST36, SP6, KID3, HE5, REN4, YINTANG
- Electroacupuncture on ST29 and ZIGONG
- A heat lamp over abdomen

Outcome

12 eggs retrieved, 11 were mature, 7 fertilized, and embryos were frozen until Jane was ready to go ahead with FET.

Discussion

Eleven mature eggs in a woman aged 44 is an excellent result, particularly because on day 6 of stimulation it looked likely that the treatment cycle might be cancelled due to poor response to stimulation. The success of treatment was partly due to her naturally good ovarian reserve. Frequent acupuncture treatments may have helped to rescue the cycle. Electroacupuncture on the day between ovulation trigger and egg retrieval may have helped with the process of final egg maturation, resulting in almost all follicles (including the small ones) containing a mature egg.

ADAPTING TREATMENT PRINCIPLES TO NATURAL IVF

Overview and indications

Natural or unstimulated IVF is defined by the Centres for Disease Control and Prevention as 'an ART cycle in which the woman does not receive drugs to stimulate her ovaries to produce more follicles. Instead, follicles develop naturally.'[138] In the United States, <1% of IVF cycles are natural and this type of IVF treatment is provided by only 15% of ART clinics.[138]

Natural IVF is thought to be useful for certain patient groups:

- Patients who object to hormonal stimulation on medical, religious, or psychological grounds.[2]
- Couples with extreme oligoasthenoteratospermia (low concentration, low percentage of progressively motile sperm, and low normal forms) with only 1–5 sperm available for fertilization.[2]
- Cancer patients where all types of gonadotrophins are to be avoided[139]

Natural IVF may also be considered in patients who have a history of poor response because these patients are likely to produce a low number of eggs, irrespective of the dose of the stimulation medication.[32] Natural IVF is not suitable for women with anovulatory or irregular cycles.[138]

The disadvantages of natural IVF is that the cycle cancellation rate is higher than in stimulated IVF, as only one egg is expected to be retrieved, and it may or may not fertilize. In women <35 years old, 54% of natural IVF cycles reach embryo transfer stage and have an implantation rate of 39.5%.[138]

Live birth rates are dependent on a woman's age:[138]

- <35 years of age live birth rate of 15.2%
- 35–37 years of age live birth rate of 14.9%
- 38–40 years of age live birth rate of 8.7%
- 41–42 years of age live birth rate of 2.4%
- >42 years of age live birth rate 0%

Orthodox medical protocol

Women require no pituitary suppression (or downregulation) medication. During the follicular phase of the treatment cycle no ovarian stimulation with FSH is necessary. Follicular and endometrial development is monitored by vaginal ultrasound, LH and oestradiol levels.[2]

In a modified natural cycle GnRH antagonist may be administered during the follicular phase to prevent premature ovulation. Sometimes FSH or hMG (up to 150 IU/day) may also be prescribed to compensate for a possible drop in natural FSH levels as a result of GnRH antagonist administration.[139]

Ovulation may occur spontaneously,[139] or it may be induced with hCG trigger medication.[2,139] Egg retrieval, fertilization, and embryo transfer procedures are similar to that of conventional IVF. Luteal support may or may not be administered.

TCM protocol

Treating women with acupuncture during a cycle of natural IVF is identical to the approach used in conventional IVF. The timing and frequency of acupuncture treatment administration is especially important in a natural IVF cycle because acupuncture may help to increase the blood flow and therefore reproductive hormone delivery to the ovaries and uterus.

ADAPTING TREATMENT PRINCIPLES TO MILD IVF

Overview

Mild IVF is a term used to describe a cycle of IVF treatment where a woman is prescribed a lower dose of ovarian stimulation medication. Indications for mild IVF are similar to that of natural IVF.

Orthodox medical protocol

Women require no pituitary suppression (or downregulation) medication in a mild IVF cycle. During the follicular phase of the treatment cycle, a fixed dose of FSH or hMG (up to 150 IU/day) is administered. GnRH antagonist is usually also administered during the follicular phase to prevent premature ovulation.[139]

Follicular and endometrial development is monitored by serial vaginal ultrasound scans and sometimes also by serial oestradiol blood tests.[139]

Ovulation is induced with hCG trigger medication. Egg retrieval, fertilization, and embryo transfer are similar to conventional IVF. Luteal support in the form of progesterone or hCG is administered.[139]

TCM protocol

Treating women with acupuncture during a mild IVF cycle is identical to the treatment provided in conventional IVF.

ADAPTING TREATMENT PRINCIPLES TO FROZEN EMBRYO TRANSFER

FET is a transfer of previously frozen embryos. Chapter 6 describes the indications for FET and the expected success rates. This section describes common FET protocols and how to manage patients undergoing FET.

Pretreatment (downregulation or suppression)

Orthodox medical protocol

Protocols vary significantly amongst fertility clinics. Some clinics prefer not to do any ovarian suppression. Others regulate the menstrual cycle with GnRH agonist to supress FSH and LH production. The protocol for suppression with GnRH agonist is described in detail in section 'In vitro fertilization'.

TCM protocol

Acupuncture treatment during the pretreatment cycle will depend on the protocol chosen by the fertility clinic. If the long GnRH agonist is used with the purpose of suppressing gonadotrophin secretions by the pituitary, the aim of acupuncture treatment administration will be to:

- Treat the adverse effects of medication, which for GnRH agonist tend to be quite severe because they induce low oestrogen levels; this may cause hot flashes, perspiration, headaches, mood fluctuations, insomnia, nervousness, sore breasts, and fatigue.[2]
- Support the patient emotionally.
- Continue to address any underlying TCM pathology.

With the short GnRH agonist or in cycles with no suppression, acupuncture during the pretreatment cycle aims to:

- Regulate the menstrual cycle to ensure that the ART treatment cycle can be started on schedule.
- Support the patient emotionally.
- Continue to address any underlying TCM pathology.

A 2008 Cochrane review found that pretreatment with GnRH agonist in women undergoing FET significantly increases live birth rates.[140]

Tables 9.15 and 9.16 summarize TCM acupuncture treatment during the FET pre-treatment cycle.

Follicular phase (endometrium preparation)

Orthodox medical protocol

This stage of FET focuses on adequate endometrial preparation. The main aim of the endometrial preparation phase is to synchronize the age of the embryo (after it has been thawed) with the correct stage of endometrial development.[140] Endometrial preparation can be natural or medically controlled.

Natural FET

Regular ultrasound scans are undertaken to monitor follicular and endometrial development and to help with starting LH tests at the correct time. The endometrial lining thickness should be at least 7–8 mm,[44,141–143] but ideally it should be 9–14 mm.[44] Cycles may be cancelled if the endometrium is too thin or if a woman ovulates prematurely.[144]

Table 9.15 Acupuncture protocol for FET pretreatment phase

To be used in:
- Long GnRH agonist protocol

When to provide acupuncture treatment	Up to 4 weeks before the FET cycle begins. But more commonly beginning on day 21 of the pretreatment cycle
Timing and frequency	Treat once a week until FET cycle begins
Needling method and techniques	Manual acupuncture is usually adequate. Some acupuncturists recommend not using any abdominal points to avoid thickening the endometrial lining.[15] Our experience is that abdominal points do not normally interfere with the pituitary suppression and do not usually cause the endometrium to thicken
Main points prescription	Nourish Yin, clear Heat, regulate Qi,[16] Blood, emotion, and harmonize the Liver: LIV3,[16,17] P6,[18] SP6,[16] SP10,[16,19] YINTANG
TCM acupuncture treatment modifications	Headaches · GB20,[20] LI4[16,21]
	Hot flashes · KID6, KID2, KID1,[22] HE6[23]
	Insomnia · HE7,[23] P7,[18] ANMIAN[24]
	Fatigue · ST36,[16,25] HUANMEN[24]

Table 9.16 Acupuncture protocol for FET pretreatment phase

To be used in:
- Short GnRH agonist protocol or
- Natural (unsuppressed) pretreatment cycle

When to provide acupuncture treatment	Menstrual cycle before FET cycle
Timing and frequency	Weekly sessions
Needling method and techniques	Manual acupuncture is usually adequate during the first 3 weeks
Main points prescription	*Pretreatment cycle days 1–5 (menses)*: invigorate, regulate Qi and Blood, tonify Kidney Jing (Essence): SP4 + P6,[26] LU7 + KID6,[27] REN4[28]
	Pretreatment cycle days 5–14: nourish Blood and Yin: SP4 + P6,[26] LIV8,[17] SP6,[19] HE6,[23] KID3,[22] LU7 + KID6[27]
	Pretreatment cycle days 14–16 (ovulation): tonify Jing (Essence), regulate Qi and Blood, reinforce Yang: KID1,[22] ST27,[25] REN4,[28] KID3,[22] ZIGONG[24]
	Pre-treatment cycle day 16 until FET cycle begins: SP4 + P6,[26] ZIGONG,[24] REN4,[28] ST36,[25]

From around day 9 or 10 plasma or urine LH levels are checked until the LH surge is detected. In some natural FET cycles ovulation is medically triggered by hCG injection.[140] In one study the criteria for triggering with hCG was that the leading follicle was >17 mm in diameter, serum oestradiol level >150 pg/mL, and serum progesterone level <1 ng/mL.[143]

Natural cycles are suitable for women with regular menstrual cycles and who regularly ovulate.[140] The disadvantage of a natural cycle is that ovulation may not always occur or it may be difficult to time FET.

Controlled FET

In a controlled FET cycle, the endometrium is prepared by administering exogenous oestrogen, which causes proliferation of the endometrium.[144] Administering oestrogen from day 1 of the menstrual cycle suppresses FSH levels and therefore stops a dominant follicle developing, thus preventing spontaneous ovulation. Oestrogen is usually administered in tablet form, transdermal patches, or vaginal rings or vaginal tablets.[140] One commonly used oestrogen preparation in FET is Progynova®, which can be prescribed in a tablet form or patch form. The dose used can be between 2 and 8 mg/day and is usually increased gradually until the endometrium is sufficiently thickened.[140] In cases where the lining fails to thicken, oral oestrogen may be replaced by vaginal oestrogen.[145]

Regular ultrasound scans are performed to monitor endometrial development. The scans start around day 9 or 10.[145] When the endometrium is 7–9 mm thick, progesterone supplementation is added to initiate secretory changes in the endometrium.[44,144–146] As with natural FET, an endometrial lining that is <7–8 mm thick may result in a cancellation of FET.[44,141–143] FET may also be cancelled due to premature ovulation.[144]

In women with functional ovaries, oestrogen medication may be insufficient to fully suppress the development of the dominant follicle. Therefore, the GnRH agonist may be used in addition to oestrogen to achieve suppression of ovarian function and prevent a premature LH surge and ovulation.[140,144,147] This approach has been shown to significantly increase live birth rates.[140]

Controlled cycles have the advantage of greater predictability and flexibility. Thus cancellation rates are lower, especially if GnRH agonist is used.[140]

TCM protocol

Acupuncture treatment during the follicular phase of FET may help with endometrial development. Table 9.17 summarizes the TCM acupuncture treatment during endometrial preparation in a FET cycle.

Ovulation

Orthodox medical protocol

Natural cycle

Spontaneous ovulation occurs in a natural FET cycle.

Table 9.17 FET endometrial preparation with TCM acupuncture	
Timing and frequency	Once or twice a week, ideally starting on day 1–3 of the treatment cycle
	More frequent treatments are recommended in older women, as their endometrial lining is generally thinner[46,148,149]
Needling method and technique	Electroacupuncture may be used. A heat lamp and/or moxa should be used on the abdomen
Main points prescription	Nourish Yin and regulate Blood
	LU7 + KID6,[27] SP4 + P6,[26] SP6,[19] ST29,[25] ZIGONG,[24] SP10,[19] LIV8, LIV3,[17] KID3[22]
Research-based modifications	*Protocol 1*[50]: LIV3, SP6, ST28, ZIGONG, REN6, REN4
	Protocol 2[51]: Electroacupuncture on bilateral BL23 and BL28 (100 Hz, pulses of 0.5 ms duration) plus bilateral SP6 and BL57 (2 Hz, pulses of 0.5 ms duration)

CLINICAL TIPS

INTERCOURSE DURING NATURAL FET

IVF clinics normally advise patients not to have intercourse during a natural FET cycle because doing so may result in a multiple gestation pregnancy, for example, if intercourse results in a natural conception and the transferred embryo(s) also implants.

However, some couples choose not to follow this advice and may comment to their acupuncturists about this. Acupuncturists have a responsibility to keep their patients safe and ensure a healthy pregnancy and the health of any babies that are born as a result of ART. Therefore, it is important to reinforce this advice in such cases.

Controlled cycle

No ovulation usually happens in a controlled FET cycle.

TCM protocols

No acupuncture treatment is usually necessary at this stage of FET.

Embryo transfer

Orthodox medical protocol

Depending on their stage of development and grading, embryos can be transferred on day 2, 3, or 5 (blastocyst stage) post ovulation (in a natural cycle) or post initiation of progesterone (in a controlled cycle).[145] The procedure for embryo transfer is the same as in fresh IVF.

TCM protocol

The acupuncture treatment procedure for embryo transfer in FET is identical to that in a fresh IVF cycle (see Table 9.12).

The research on acupuncture during FET is limited because most studies have looked at fresh IVF cycles. A study carried out by So *et al.* evaluated the effect of acupuncture on FET. The acupuncture protocol was as follows: acupuncture was performed 25 min after the embryo transfer on points ST36, SP6, SP10, LI4. De qi sensation was obtained during the initial insertion and again 10 min later. Needles (0.30 × 40 mm) were retained for 25 min. Streitberger placebo needles were used in the placebo acupuncture group. There was no statistically significant difference in clinical or ongoing pregnancy rates or live birth rates. However, the authors noted that both groups had a statistically significant higher ongoing pregnancy rate compared to patients who refused to join the study, potentially raising the question of whether the placebo actually was inert.[150]

Luteal support

Orthodox medical protocol

Natural FET

No luteal support is necessary in a natural uncontrolled FET.

Controlled FET

Both oestrogen and progesterone supplementation is continued until the day of the pregnancy test. If the test is positive, supplementation needs to be continued until around 8 weeks' gestation.[145]

TCM protocol

Luteal phase support with acupuncture is the same as in conventional IVF, with the emphasis on acupuncture treatment being placed on the implantation window (see Table 9.14).

ADAPTING TREATMENT PRINCIPLES TO OVULATION INDUCTION

The indications for various ovulation induction treatments are described in Chapter 8. In Chapter 6 the mode of action of various ovulation-inducing medications was explored. This section focuses on the management of patients undergoing ovulation induction treatments.

Follicular phase

Ovulation induction with Clomiphene Citrate

Clomiphene Citrate (CC) is administered as a 5-day course therapy starting on days 3, 4, or 5 of the menstrual cycle.[6] The dose administered ranges from 50 to 150 mg/day.[6] A higher dose may be needed in obese patients.[6] However, most women respond to a dosage range of between 50 mg/day (52%) and 100 mg/day (22%).[151,152] Amenorrhoeic patients will benefit from an oestrogen- or progesterone-induced withdrawal bleed to prime oestrogen receptors.[6]

Follicular development can be monitored by transvaginal ultrasound, usually with one or two scans that start on day 8 or 9 of the menstrual cycle.[6] Urinary LH surge kits can be used to detect pre-ovulatory LH surge, indicating that ovulation is likely to follow 12–24 h later.[6] Intercourse should begin around the time of LH surge and take place every day or every other day for 5 days.

Ovulation is confirmed if a collapsed follicle can be seen on transvaginal ultrasound or alternatively by checking mid-luteal phase progesterone levels.[6] A level of >9.54 nmol/L (3 ng/mL) is considered to be evidence that ovulation has occurred. Levels of $\geq$31.8 nmol/L ($\geq$10 ng/mL) are considered a sign of healthier luteal phase.[152]

The administration of CC can be repeated for up to 6 cycles.[6] If there are significant adverse effects such as headaches, abdominal pain, or visual disturbances, the CC treatment may need to be discontinued at an earlier than planned date.[6] CC has an anti-oestrogenic effect and in some women can cause thickening of cervical mucus and/or inhibit endometrial development resulting in a thin uterine lining.[6]

Ovulation induction with LHRH (GnRH) pulse pump system

For the induction of ovulation in patients with WHO grade I ovulation disorders (see Chapter 8) the LHRH (GnRH) pulse pump system is beneficial.[153] LHRH is injected intravenously via a mini pump at 90 min intervals.[153] This induces an increased production of FSH and LH and improved pituitary-ovarian feedback. The starting dose is usually 2.5 μg[34] to 5 μg[153] per pulse, and the maximum recommended dose is 20 μg.[153] The pump is usually attached on cycle day 1–3 and worn continuously until ovulation.[34]

Ovarian response is monitored by serial ultrasound scans and oestradiol levels. LH kits can be used to detect the LH surge, which normally happens around 36 h before ovulation. Intercourse should begin around the time of LH

surge and take place every day or every other day for 5 days. Ovulation is confirmed by visualization of a collapsed follicle on transvaginal ultrasound or by checking the mid-luteal phase progesterone levels.

The pregnancy rate is around 10–30% per ovulatory cycle.[34] Up to six cycles may be performed and the overall chance of pregnancy is around 75%.[153]

Ovulation induction with FSH

Ovulation induction with FSH is a second-line treatment for induction of ovulation in patients with WHO grade I ovulation disorders (see Chapter 8). It can be used if the LHRH (GnRH) pulse pump system fails to induce ovulation.

Fifty to 75 units of FSH gonadotrophins are injected subcutaneously daily. If the follicular development is poor, the dose can be increased incrementally by 37.5 units. The maximum recommended dose is 225 units/day. GnRH antagonist may be administered to stop premature LH surge.

Follicular growth is monitored by a series of ultrasound scans. Oestrogen levels are monitored after 3–4 days of stimulation.[6] Ovulation is triggered by a single hCG injection of 5000–10,000 IU intramuscularly when the follicles are 15–18 mm in size.[6] Intercourse should take place every day or every other day for 5 days, starting with the night of the hCG trigger injection.[6] This treatment protocol is 90% successful in achieving ovulation and has 50% pregnancy rate. It can be repeated for a total of 6–8 cycles.[6,153]

TCM protocol

Pretreatment cycle

Follicular recruitment normally begins when FSH rises at the end of the luteal phase of the cycle preceding the ovulation induction cycle. Administering acupuncture during the pretreatment cycle (especially during the last week) may help to improve follicular recruitment. Treatment principles are the same as in IVF pretreatment with GnRH antagonist protocol (see Table 9.4).

Follicular (stimulation) phase

Acupuncture treatment during the follicular phase of the ovulation induction cycle should ideally begin on menstrual days 1–3 because by day 3 follicular recruitment is completed.[6] Acupuncture treatment should then be repeated every 3–4 days until either the hCG trigger injection or the LH surge. Acupuncture principles and points are identical to IVF ovarian stimulation phase (Table 9.6).

Final egg maturation and ovulation trigger

As in IVF, acupuncture administered shortly after the hCG trigger or LH surge may help with the final egg(s) maturation. The acupuncture treatment protocol is the same as in IVF during this egg maturation stage (see Table 9.8).

Luteal phase

Implantation is likely to take place 6–8 days after ovulation. Therefore administering acupuncture to women on these days may help to increase the chances of implantation. Acupuncture during the luteal phase may also reduce the risk of miscarriages (as described in section 'In vitro fertilization'). The treatment principles and points utilized are identical to those outlined in Table 9.14 in section 'In vitro fertilization'.

ADAPTING TREATMENT PRINCIPLES TO IUI

Intrauterine Insemination (IUI) (sometimes referred to as artificial insemination) is a procedure that places the partner's or donor's prepared sperm into a woman's uterus via a soft catheter around the time of ovulation. Chapter 6 provided information on indications and success rates with IUI. This section describes the most common IUI medical protocols and how to treat patients undergoing IUI with acupuncture.

Pretreatment phase (suppression or downregulation)

Orthodox medical protocol

No pretreatment is usually necessary before IUI cycle.

TCM protocol

Follicular recruitment normally begins when FSH rises at the end of the luteal phase of the cycle preceding the IUI cycle. Administering acupuncture during the pretreatment cycle (especially during the last week) may help to improve follicular recruitment. Treatment principles are the same as in IVF pretreatment with GnRH antagonist protocol (see Table 9.4).

Stimulation phase

Orthodox medical protocol

IUI can be carried out during stimulated or non-stimulated (natural spontaneous) cycles. In a natural cycle, only one egg may be fertilized. In a stimulated IUI, up to three eggs may develop and be fertilized. The chances of conception are greater with a stimulated IUI because more eggs are available for fertilization, but because of this there is also an increased risk of a multiple gestation pregnancy.[154]

IUI during a stimulated cycle

In a stimulated IUI cycle, a woman usually injects herself subcutaneously with gonadotrophins, starting on day 3–5 of her menstrual cycle.[155–158] In some cases CC or other antioestrogens can be used.[155] A GnRH antagonist may also be administered to avoid a premature LH surge.[157]

On cycle days 8–13, the response to stimulation is monitored by serial blood tests to check the levels of LH and oestradiol, and the extent of follicular growth is monitored by transvaginal ultrasound.[155,156,159]

Sometimes, if a woman produces more than two follicles, IUI may be cancelled or rescue IVF may be performed.[154]

Non-stimulated (natural) IUI

In a non-stimulated IUI a woman starts monitoring her LH levels by testing her urine daily, starting usually on day 10 of her menstrual cycle. Ultrasound may also be performed to monitor follicular development and endometrial lining growth. LH surge is normally detected 36 h before ovulation.

TCM protocol

Acupuncture treatment during the follicular phase of IUI (stimulated and non-stimulated) should ideally begin on days 1–3 of the treatment cycle (or stimulation) in order to help with the recruitment of follicles. Acupuncture should then be repeated every 3–4 days until either the hCG trigger injection or the LH surge. The acupuncture principles and points are identical to the IVF ovarian stimulation phase (Table 9.6).

Ovulation trigger

Orthodox medical protocol

Stimulated IUI

Once the leading follicle is ≥16–18 mm in diameter, a woman will stop injecting gonadotrophins and inject hCG to trigger ovulation.[156,159,160] The insemination takes place 32–36 h later.[154]

Non-stimulated IUI

As soon as the LH surge is detected, then uterine insemination is normally scheduled to take place usually 24–36 h later.[158]

TCM protocol

As in IVF, acupuncture administered shortly after the hCG trigger or LH surge may help with the final egg(s) maturation. The acupuncture treatment protocol is the same as in IVF during this stage (see Table 9.8).

Insemination

Orthodox medical protocol

Freshly collected sperm or previously frozen sperm can be used in IUI. Before it can be inseminated, seminal plasma is removed to avoid prostaglandin-induced uterine contractions and to avoid pelvic infection.[154] Sperm is deposited with a small catheter in the cervix, the uterus, the peritoneum, or the fallopian tubes,[154] but the uterus is the most commonly used site of insemination.[154] Insemination can be repeated several times in the same cycle.[154]

TCM protocol

Acupuncture on the day of insemination is optional. If the practitioner feels their patient would benefit from acupuncture treatment on this day, the points can be chosen from the following:

- SP6, ST36, LIV3, LI4, KID3, ST29, SP10, HE7, P6, YINTANG. A heat lamp or moxa on the abdomen are also indicated.

This point prescription has a strong Blood and Qi moving function and can Calm the Shen (Mind).

Luteal phase

Orthodox medical protocol

As in IVF, the luteal phase will be supported with progesterone or hCG hormonal medication, the use of which usually starts after insemination. However, there is no strong evidence to support this practice.[154]

TCM protocol

Implantation is likely to take place 6–8 days after insemination. Therefore treating women on these days may help to increase the chances of implantation. Acupuncture during the luteal phase may also reduce the risk of miscarriages (as described in section 'In vitro fertilization'). The treatment principles and points are identical to those outlined in Table 9.14 in section 'In vitro fertilization'.

ADAPTING TREATMENT PRINCIPLES TO EGG DONOR IVF

Overview

Chapter 6 reviewed third-party ART treatments. This section describes how to manage patients undergoing egg donation IVF, the most common type of third-party ART treatment.

Indications for egg donation include:

- Premature ovarian failure[161]
- Ovarian ageing[162]
- Menopause[161]
- Risk of transmission of genetic disease[161,162]
- Poor-quality eggs[162]
- Inaccessible or missing ovaries[162]

Donor eggs can be successfully transferred into the uterus of post-menopausal women (even when they are in their 60s), and their pregnancy outcomes are favourable.[161] However, some people object to this use of IVF on ethical grounds (see Chapter 13).

Donors usually will only be considered if their ovarian reserve is good and if certain genetic and other diseases have been excluded. Egg donors may be financially reimbursed. The amount of reimbursement varies from country to country. All parties involved may be required to undergo implications counselling. In some countries this is compulsory.

In the authors' experience, acupuncturists may be asked to treat the donor, the recipient, or both. In some cases the male partner may also attend for acupuncture treatment.

CLINICAL TIPS

TREATING DONOR EGG RECIPIENTS

Some patients undergoing donor egg IVF may experience sadness and grief about having to give up their dream of having a genetically related baby. Some patients are very open about this. Others may grieve in privacy. Look out for signs of grief and consider using acupuncture points that may help, such as LIV14,[163] DU13,[55] KID26,[164] BL10.[165]

Pretreatment phase

Orthodox medical protocol: the recipient

Recipients may be asked to undergo a 'mock cycle' in order to have the functional adequacy of their endometrium assessed.[161] During a mock cycle, the recipient undergoes endometrial priming with oestrogen and progesterone and a mock embryo transfer. If the lining does not respond to hormonal preparation, further investigations may be necessary, for example, a hysteroscopy to exclude adhesions.[161]

Orthodox medical protocol: the donor

Pretreatment protocols for egg donors are the same as in conventional fresh IVF cycles, usually involving pituitary suppression or downregulation with a GnRH agonist or antagonist (see Table 9.2).

TCM protocol: the recipient

Acupuncture treatment can be provided to the recipient during the 'mock cycle' using the same acupuncture protocol as would be used for a real cycle (see the rest of this section).

CLINICAL TIPS

DONOR EGG IVF: MALE PARTNER

If the recipient's male partner's sperm will be used to fertilize the donated eggs, male partners may also benefit from acupuncture treatment (see Chapter 8).

TCM protocol: the donor

Acupuncture treatment of the egg donor during the pretreatment phase is the same as in fresh IVF cycles, and the acupuncture approach utilized will depend on the type of medication protocol the donor is prescribed (see Tables 9.3 and 9.4).

Follicular phase

The donor and recipient's menstrual cycles have to be synchronized so that the embryos are transferred when the recipient's endometrium is receptive.[161]

Orthodox medical protocol: the recipient

Preparation of the recipient's endometrium is very similar to that used in FET cycles, involving 2 or more weeks of oestrogen administration with the progesterone added 3–4 days before the embryo transfer.[161] As with FET, women with functional ovaries may need to take GnRH agonists or antagonists to supress premature LH surge.[161] A recipient may also need to take an oral contraceptive pill before starting her oestrogen regimen, thereby allowing synchronization of her menstrual cycle with that of the donor.

As with most types of ART, regular ultrasound scans are used to monitor the development of the endometrium. The endometrial lining should be at least 7–8 mm,[44,141–143] but ideally it should be 9–14 mm in thickness.[44] The cycle may be cancelled if the endometrium is too thin. In such circumstances the donor's eggs or the resulting embryos may be frozen.

Orthodox medical protocol: the donor

Egg donors undergo the same ovarian stimulation treatment as adopted with a fresh IVF cycle (see section 'In vitro fertilization').

TCM protocol: the recipient

The protocol for acupuncture treatment is similar to that used with FET cycles (see Table 9.17). The frequency of acupuncture treatment can be adjusted based on how the recipient responded to a 'mock cycle'. If the endometrial lining was thin (<7–8 mm), patients should be treated at least twice a week until the embryo is transferred. Otherwise treatment every 5–7 days may be sufficient.

TCM protocol: the donor

Acupuncture treatment of egg donors is similar to the acupuncture protocol provided during the ovarian stimulation phase of a fresh IVF cycle (see Table 9.6).

Ovulation trigger, egg retrieval, and embryo transfer

Orthodox medical protocol

When the donor is deemed ready for egg retrieval, with the criteria for retrieval being the same as for a fresh IVF cycle, she will inject hCG to trigger the final egg maturation. The egg retrieval procedure takes place 36 h later. The role of the donor is now fulfilled.

The eggs are fertilized using the recipient's partner's sperm or by sperm from a sperm donor. Conventional IVF or ICSI fertilization methods may be used. Depending on the number and quality of embryos, they are transferred into the recipient's uterus 2, 3, or 5 days later.

TCM protocol

Acupuncture protocols for final egg maturation, egg retrieval, and embryo transfer procedure are the same as in fresh IVF cycles.

The luteal phase

Orthodox medical protocol

The recipient continues with oestrogen and progesterone supplementation until the day of the pregnancy test. If the test is positive, oestrogen and progesterone should be continued until around 10–12 weeks' gestation.

TCM protocol

Acupuncture protocol for the recipient is identical to the luteal phase acupuncture protocol in a fresh IVF cycle (see Table 9.14).

Case study

Donor Egg IVF-acupuncture Treatment of the Recipient

Katie, aged 43, was undergoing donor egg IVF due to poor ovarian reserve. Her partner's semen analysis was excellent, and the donor was a 31-year-old relative. Katie's menstrual cycles had stopped for a year, but then restarted again a few months before IVF and were now 25–28 days long.

Manifestations

- Menses: light, no pain
- Emotions: in the run up to IVF very tearful and feeling down
- Digestion: IBS, bloated, constipation, symptoms worse before menstruation
- Tension headaches
- Tongue: slightly purple
- Pulse: wiry on the left, weak on the right

TCM Syndromes

- Liver Qi Stagnation
- Spleen Qi Deficiency
- Kidney Jing [Essence] Deficiency

Pretreatment Phase

Katie's menstrual cycle was supressed with a GnRH agonist (buserelin), 500 µg to be injected subcutaneously daily starting with day 21 of the pretreatment cycle.

Acupuncture: three acupuncture treatments were administered. Points used included LU7 + KID6, SP4 + P6, SP6, LIV3, SP3, ST29, KID3, YINTANG.

Follicular Phase

Baseline scan confirmed that the lining was thin, and Katie was prescribed oral oestrogen (Progynova®) to prime her endometrium. The dose was to be increased incrementally from 2 to 6 mg between days 1 and 10.

Two acupuncture treatments were administered on days 4 and 9 of oestrogen priming. Acupuncture points included REN4, ST29, ZIGONG, SP6, and HE7 (with a heat lamp placed over the abdomen).

On day 11 Katie attended for a monitoring ultrasound scan. Her endometrium was 9.62 mm thick and trilaminar in appearance. We decided that no further acupuncture session was necessary because the endometrium was already of good quality, and it was likely that it would increase in thickness a little more before the embryo transfer procedure.

Egg Retrieval

Egg retrieval procedure in Katie's donor went well and 13 eggs were recovered.

In addition to oestrogen, Katie started progesterone (Utrogestan vaginal capsules 2 × 200 mg twice a day) to be continued until 10 weeks' gestation (if pregnant).

Fertilization

Disappointingly, only three eggs fertilized. Embryo transfer was scheduled for 2 days later.

Embryo Transfer

The transfer went well. Two good-grade embryos were transferred. Two acupuncture sessions were administered, approximately 2 h before and 2 h after the embryo transfer. Paulus et al.[84] embryo transfer acupuncture protocol was used.

Luteal Phase

Five days after the transfer (day 7 post egg retrieval) Katie had 'cold like symptoms'. She felt breathless, tired, achy. She had some abdominal 'twinges' that felt hot. Katie was beginning to feel very anxious and was experiencing panic attacks. Her pulse was slightly rapid and very slightly slippery. Acupuncture prescription was LU7 + KID6, SP10, KID7, KID9, LIV3, LIV2, REN6, DU20, YINTANG.

Katie tested positive and the scan at 6 weeks' gestation showed two gestation sacks. Katie continued to have acupuncture treatment throughout her pregnancy. Her pregnancy was complicated by some vaginal bleeding and recurrent urinary infections, and she developed pre-eclampsia later in pregnancy. Katie's two healthy baby girls were delivered by c-section.

ADAPTING TREATMENT PRINCIPLES TO SURROGACY AND GESTATIONAL CARRIER

Overview

As outlined in Chapter 6, there are two types of surrogacy: 'traditional surrogate' and 'gestational carrier'.

Indications for a gestational carrier and/or surrogacy include:[166]

- Absent or scarred uterus/endometrium
- Hysterectomy
- Medical contraindication to pregnancy

All types of surrogacy are tightly regulated. In some cases babies must be legally adopted by the intended parents.[166] Regulations also cover areas such as financial compensation of the carrier or surrogate, informed consent, and incest.[166]

Adapting treatment to gestation carrier IVF

A pregnant woman who is not usually genetically related to the baby because the gametes or embryos are provided by the commissioning (intended) parents is known as a 'gestational carrier'.[166]

The treatment protocol for a gestational carrier IVF is very similar to egg donor IVF. The woman who is the gestation carrier is provided with the same treatment as is adopted for an egg donation recipient. The biological mother undergoes the same treatment regimen as is used with an egg donor (see section 'Adapting Treatment Principles to Egg Donor IVF'). When the baby is born, the gestation carrier 'hands over' the baby to its biological and intended parents.

Adapting treatment to traditional surrogate IVF

A 'traditional surrogate' is an arrangement where a pregnancy is carried by a woman who is also the egg donor. She can conceive as a result of IUI or IVF, using the biological father's sperm. The child is intended to be raised by its biological father and his partner. Donor sperm can be used in cases of severe male factor infertility.

The treatment protocols (Orthodox medicine and acupuncture) for the surrogate are the same as in IUI or IVF, depending on which ART method is used. There is no physiological need to treat the intended mother. Acupuncture treatment may be provided to the biological father, especially in cases of suboptimal semen parameters.

ADAPTING TREATMENT PRINCIPLES TO ZIFT/GIFT

Chapter 6 described Gamete Intra-fallopian Transfer (GIFT) and Zygote Intrafallopian Transfer (ZIFT) procedures and indications for their use. This section will explain how to adapt IVF treatment protocols for patients undergoing these procedures.

Pretreatment through to ovulation trigger phases

Orthodox medical and acupuncture procedures during the pretreatment, ovarian stimulation, final egg maturation, and ovulation trigger stages are identical to those in a fresh IVF cycle.

Egg retrieval, fertilization, and transfer

GIFT

Orthodox medical protocol

Eggs are usually retrieved laparoscopically under general anaesthesia. The retrieved unfertilized eggs are mixed with sperm and fluid and are placed during the same laparoscopic procedure into the fallopian tube to enable natural fertilization.[167] Up to three eggs can be transferred.[167]

TCM protocol

In the majority of cases acupuncturists are unlikely to be able to treat patients on the day when the gametes are replaced. However, acupuncture can be given on the day after the transfer.

In GIFT, fertilization takes place in the fallopian tubes. Therefore TCM acupuncture treatment principles that assist with ovulation and fertilization apply. The following points may be used: SP4 + P6, LIV3, KID3, P5, REN4, ST36, ST28, KID7, ZIGONG.

ZIFT

Orthodox medical protocol

The eggs are retrieved using the same procedure that is used in a conventional IVF cycle. The eggs are then fertilized in the laboratory using IVF or ICSI. On the following day, before cell division takes place, the resulting zygote(s) is transferred into the fallopian tube. The transfer is done by a laparoscopic procedure requiring general anaesthesia. Therefore, in ZIFT two surgical procedures need to be performed: one for egg collection and one for embryo transfer.[168]

TCM protocol

Since the zygote is transferred into the fallopian tube, it is essential that there is free flow of Qi and Blood to allow the resulting embryo to travel down the fallopian tube to the uterus. Some of the acupuncture points that can assist with this are KID3, HE5, ST36, LIV3, KID7. Alternatively, IVF embryo transfer protocols listed in Table 9.12 may be utilized.

Luteal support

Orthodox medical and acupuncture protocols during the luteal phase are the same as in conventional IVF.

ADAPTING TREATMENT PRINCIPLES TO IVM

Chapter 6 described IVM treatment technique and its indications. Because it is classed as an experimental procedure, acupuncturists are unlikely to see many patients undergoing this treatment. However, if a patient presents who is undergoing an IVM treatment, the following protocol may be used to assist her.

Pretreatment (downregulation or suppression)

Orthodox medical treatment

IVM protocols usually do not involve any pretreatment medication.

Acupuncture

Acupuncture treatment is the same as for IVF pretreatment with short GnRH agonist protocol (see Table 9.4).

Stimulation phase

Orthodox medical protocol

A baseline transvaginal ultrasound scan is usually carried out on days 2 or 3 of the menstrual cycle. The ovaries are observed for presence of cysts and the number of antral follicles. A blood test may be done to check that the levels of oestradiol and FSH are within an acceptable range. In one RCT investigating IVM protocols, women with oestradiol >75 pg/L (275 pmol/L) and FSH >13 mIU/mL (13 IU/L) or ovarian functional cysts ≥12 mm in diameter were excluded from the study.[169]

There are several stimulation protocols in IVM:

- FSH (usually a dose of 150 IU)[169] is administered for 3–6 days, followed by egg retrieval on days 9–10 of the treatment cycle.[170]
- A single dose of 10,000 IU of hCG is injected to prime intermediate-sized follicles 36 h prior to egg retrieval.[170]
- A combination of FSH and hCG.[170]
- No stimulation.[170]

Stimulation with both FSH and hCG results in a higher number of eggs that mature and in greater implantation rates compared with other protocols.[169] Stimulation with either FSH or hCG may benefit patients with PCOS.[170]

Regular transvaginal ultrasound scans are performed to monitor follicular growth and sometimes also to observe the extent of endometrial development. Egg retrieval is usually scheduled when the leading follicle is 10 mm in diameter. If endometrial development is also monitored, then the endometrium needs to be >5 mm thick.[170]

TCM protocol

Acupuncture treatment during the follicular phase of the IVM cycle is similar to that followed in conventional IVF (see Table 9.6). The only difference is that fewer sessions are necessary as the egg retrieval procedure is normally completed earlier in the cycle.

Egg retrieval

Orthodox medical protocol

The egg retrieval procedure is similar to that used in IVF. However, the aspiration technique, type of needle, and aspiration pressure may be different when retrieving immature eggs in IVM.[170]

TCM protocol

The acupuncture egg retrieval protocol is the same as in conventional IVF (see Table 9.10).

Egg maturation phase

Orthodox medical protocol

Retrieved eggs are placed in an IVM culture medium and periodically observed for signs of maturation. They are fertilized as soon as they become mature.

TCM protocol

In a conventional IVF cycle, there are normally only 2–5 days between the egg retrieval and embryo transfer procedures. So in the majority of cases no acupuncture treatment is necessary during this phase. In IVM, this period can last for around a week. Therefore, some patients may benefit from an extra treatment session to support their endometrial lining, to help them recover from egg retrieval procedure and to sustain them emotionally.

The following acupuncture points may be used during this stage: ST29, HE5, LIV3, KID3, ST30, REN4, ST36, YINTANG.

Fertilization

An ICSI technique may be used to fertilize IVM eggs, but ICSI is not necessary to achieve fertilization in eggs matured *in vitro*, and TCM IVF may be used instead.[170]

Embryo transfer

Orthodox medical protocol

Embryo transfer procedure is the same as in conventional IVF.

TCM protocol

Acupuncture embryo transfer protocols are the same as in conventional IVF (see Table 9.12).

Luteal phase (the 'two-week wait')

Orthodox medical protocol

Endometrial support may include oral oestradiol supplementation (for example, 6 mg/day starting on the day of egg retrieval), and luteal support may include progesterone supplementation (for example, intravaginal progesterone 600 mg/day starting on the day after egg retrieval).[169]

TCM protocol

Acupuncture luteal support is the same as in conventional IVF (see Table 9.14).

SUMMARY

In most ART treatment modalities, a woman's hormones are pharmaceutically manipulated in order to suppress the natural menstrual cycle and to artificially control it. Acupuncture treatment is similar in most types of ART, aiming to enhance patient's response to medication, treat any adverse effects, and support the patient emotionally.

This chapter provides several acupuncture protocols. However, acupuncture treatment is most likely to be beneficial if it is individualized based on the personal circumstances of each member of the couple.

REFERENCES

1. Assisted Reproductive Technology (ART) – glossary. Available from: http://www.eshre.eu/ESHRE/English/Guidelines-Legal/ART-glossary/page.aspx/1062 (accessed 26 January 2013).

2. Blok L, Kremer J. In vitro fertilisation and intracytoplasmic sperm injection. In: de Haan N, Spelt M, Gobel R, editors. Reproductive medicine: a textbook for paramedics. Amsterdam: Elsevier Gezondheidszorg; 2010. p. 105–26 [chapter 8].

3. Reh A, Krey L, Noyes N. Are gonadotropin-releasing hormone agonists losing popularity? Current trends at a large fertility center. Fertil Steril 2010;93:101–8.

4. Muasher SJ, Abdallah RT, Hubayter ZR. Optimal stimulation protocols for in vitro fertilization. Fertil Steril 2006;86:267–73.

5. Sunkara SK, Coomarasamy A, Khalaf Y, et al. A three-arm randomised controlled trial comparing gonadotrophin releasing hormone (GnRH) agonist long regimen versus GnRH agonist short regimen versus GnRH antagonist regimen in women with a history of poor ovarian response undergoing in vitro fertilisation (IVF) treatment: poor responders intervention trial (PRINT). Reprod Health 2007;4:12.

6. MD024 female infertility pharmacotherapy – stimulation protocols. ASRM elearning course notes; 2010.

7. Al-Inany HG, Youssef MA, Aboulghar M, et al. Gonadotrophin-releasing hormone antagonists for assisted reproductive technology. Cochrane Database Syst Rev 2011;(5): CD001750.

8. Pandian Z, McTavish AR, Aucott L, et al. Interventions for 'poor responders' to controlled ovarian hyper stimulation (COH) in in-vitro fertilisation (IVF). Cochrane Database Syst Rev 2010; (1):CD004379.

9. Bosch E. Can we skip weekends in GnRH antagonist cycles without compromising the final outcome? Fertil Steril 2012;97:1299–300.

10. Griesinger G, Kolibianakis EM, Venetis C, et al. Oral contraceptive pretreatment significantly reduces ongoing pregnancy likelihood in gonadotropin-releasing hormone antagonist cycles: an updated meta-analysis. Fertil Steril 2010;94:2382–4.

11. Zeleznik AJ. The physiology of follicle selection. Reprod Biol Endocrinol 2004;2:31.

12. Anderson BJ, Haimovici F, Ginsburg ES, et al. In vitro fertilization and acupuncture: clinical efficacy and mechanistic basis. Altern Ther Health Med 2007;13:38–48.

13. Anderson B, Rosenthal L. Acupuncture and in vitro fertilization: critique of the evidence and application to clinical practice. Complement Ther Clin Pract 2013;19:1–5.

14. Cheong YC, Hung Yu Ng E, Ledger WL. Acupuncture and assisted conception. Cochrane Database Syst Rev 2008;(4):CD006920.

15. Mao Q. Acupuncture protocol in the process of in vitro fertilization (IVF) – an integrated approach. J Assoc Tradit Chin Med Acupunct 2012;19:35–8.

16. Rosenthal L, Anderson B. Acupuncture and in vitro fertilisation: recent research and clinical guidelines. J Chin Med 2007;84:28–35.

17. Deadman P, Al-Khafaji M, Baker K. The Liver channel. In: A manual of acupuncture. England: Journal of Chinese Medicine Publications; 1998. p. 467–92.

18. Deadman P, Al-Khafaji M, Baker K. The Pericardium channel. In: A manual of acupuncture. England: Journal of Chinese Medicine Publications; 1998. p. 365–84.

19. Deadman P, Al-Khafaji M, Baker K. The Spleen channel. In: A manual of acupuncture. England: Journal of Chinese Medicine Publications; 1998. p. 175–206.

20. Deadman P, Al-Khafaji M, Baker K. The Gallbladder channel. In: A manual of acupuncture. England: Journal of Chinese Medicine Publications; 1998. p. 415–66.

21. Deadman P, Al-Khafaji M, Baker K. The Large Intestine channel. In: A manual of acupuncture. England: Journal of Chinese Medicine Publications; 1998. p. 93–122.

22. Deadman P, Al-Khafaji M, Baker K. The Kidney channel. In: A manual of acupuncture. England: Journal of Chinese Medicine Publications; 1998. p. 329–64.

23. Deadman P, Al-Khafaji M, Baker K. The Heart channel. In: A manual of acupuncture. England: Journal of Chinese Medicine Publications; 1998. p. 207–24.

24. Deadman P, Al-Khafaji M, Baker K. The Extraordinary points. In: A manual of acupuncture. England: Journal of Chinese Medicine Publications; 1998. p. 563–86.

25. Deadman P, Al-Khafaji M, Baker K. The Stomach channel. In: A manual of acupuncture. England: Journal of Chinese Medicine Publications; 1998. p. 123–74.

26. Maciocia G. Women's physiology. In: Obstetrics and gynecology in Chinese medicine. New York: Churchill Livingstone; 1998. p. 7–29 [chapter 2].

27. Maciocia G. Women's pathology. In: Obstetrics and gynecology in Chinese medicine. New York: Churchill Livingstone; 1998. p. 31–49 [chapter 3].

28. Deadman P, Al-Khafaji M, Baker K. The conception vessel. In: A manual of acupuncture. England: Journal of Chinese Medicine Publications; 1998. p. 493–526.

29. Smith CA, Grant S, Lyttleton J, et al. Development of an acupuncture treatment protocol by consensus for women undergoing Assisted Reproductive Technology (ART) treatment. BMC Complement Altern Med 2012;12:88.

30. Loutradis D, Drakakis P, Vomvolaki E, et al. Different ovarian stimulation protocols for women with diminished ovarian reserve. J Assist Reprod Genet 2007;24:597–611.

31. Kwan I, Bhattacharya S, McNeil A, et al. Monitoring of stimulated cycles in assisted reproduction (IVF and ICSI). Cochrane Database Syst Rev 2008;(2):CD005289.

32. Keltz M, Sauerbrun-Cutler M-T, Breborowicz A. Managing poor responders in IVF. Expert Review of Obstretics and Gynecology 2013;8:121–34.

33. Weissman A, Howles C. Treatment strategies in assisted reproduction for the poor responder patient. In: Gardner DK, Shoham Z, editors. Textbook of assisted reproductive techniques. Revised ed. Clinical perspectives, 4, illustrated, vol. 2.

Essex: Informa Healthcare; 2012. p. 162–207 [chapter 46].

34. MD023 female infertility pharmacotherapy. ELearning course notes; 2012.

35. van Wely M, Kwan I, Burt AL, et al. Recombinant versus urinary gonadotrophin for ovarian stimulation in assisted reproductive technology cycles. Cochrane Database Syst Rev 2011;(2):CD005354.

36. Baerwald AR, Walker RA, Pierson RA. Growth rates of ovarian follicles during natural menstrual cycles, oral contraception cycles, and ovarian stimulation cycles. Fertil Steril 2009;91:440–9.

37. Yoldemir T, Erenus M, Durmusoglu F. Follicular dominance on the fifth day of controlled ovarian stimulation reduces implantation in long down-regulated ICSI cycles. Eur J Obstet Gynecol Reprod Biol 2011;156:186–9.

38. Orvieto R, Zohav E, Scharf S, et al. The influence of estradiol/follicle and estradiol/oocyte ratios on the outcome of controlled ovarian stimulation for in vitro fertilization. Gynecol Endocrinol 2007;23:72–5.

39. Practice Committee of American Society for Reproductive Medicine. Ovarian hyperstimulation syndrome. Fertil Steril 2008;90:S188–S193.

40. Simon A, Laufer N. Repeated implantation failure: clinical approach. Fertil Steril 2012;97:1039–43.

41. Richter KS, Bugge KR, Bromer JG, et al. Relationship between endometrial thickness and embryo implantation, based on 1,294 cycles of in vitro fertilization with transfer of two blastocyst-stage embryos. Fertil Steril 2007;87:53–9.

42. Al-Ghamdi A, Coskun S, Al-Hassan S, et al. The correlation between endometrial thickness and outcome of in vitro fertilization and embryo transfer (IVF-ET) outcome. Reprod Biol Endocrinol 2008;6:37.

43. Kovacs P, Matyas S, Boda K, et al. The effect of endometrial thickness on IVF/ICSI outcome. Hum Reprod 2003;18:2337–41.

44. El-Toukhy T, Coomarasamy A, Khairy M, et al. The relationship between endometrial thickness and outcome of medicated frozen

embryo replacement cycles. Fertil Steril 2008;89:832–9.

45. Dietterich C, Check JH, Choe JK, et al. Increased endometrial thickness on the day of human chorionic gonadotropin injection does not adversely affect pregnancy or implantation rates following in vitro fertilization-embryo transfer. Fertil Steril 2002;77:781–6.

46. Yoeli R, Ashkenazi J, Orvieto R, et al. Significance of increased endometrial thickness in assisted reproduction technology treatments. J Assist Reprod Genet 2004;21:285–9.

47. Zheng CH, Huang GY, Zhang MM, et al. Effects of acupuncture on pregnancy rates in women undergoing in vitro fertilization: a systematic review and meta-analysis. Fertil Steril 2012;97:599–611.

48. Isoyama Manca di Villahermosa D, Dos Santos LG, Nogueira MB, et al. Influence of acupuncture on the outcomes of in vitro fertilisation when embryo implantation has failed: a prospective randomised controlled clinical trial. Acupunct Med 2013;31:157–61.

49. Yu W, Horn B, Acacio B, et al. A pilot study evaluating the combination of acupuncture with sildenafil on endometrial thickness. Fertil Steril 2007;87:23.

50. Ho M, Huang LC, Chang YY, et al. Electroacupuncture reduces uterine artery blood flow impedance in infertile women. Taiwan J Obstet Gynecol 2009;48:148–51.

51. Stener-Victorin E, Waldenström U, Andersson SA, et al. Reduction of blood flow impedance in the uterine arteries of infertile women with electro-acupuncture. Hum Reprod 1996;11:1314–7.

52. Deadman P, Al-Khafaji M, Baker K. The Sanjiao channel. In: A manual of acupuncture. England: Journal of Chinese Medicine Publications; 1998. p. 385–414.

53. Deadman P, Al-Khafaji M, Baker K. The Lung channel. In: A manual of acupuncture. England: Journal of Chinese Medicine Publications; 1998. p. 71–92.

54. Deadman P, Al-Khafaji M, Baker K. The Bladder channel. In: A manual of acupuncture. England: Journal of

Chinese Medicine Publications; 1998. p. 249–328.

55. Deadman P, Al-Khafaji M, Baker K. The Governing Vessel. In: A manual of acupuncture. England: Journal of Chinese Medicine Publications; 1998. p. 527–62.

56. Practice Committee of American Society for Reproductive Medicine, Birmingham, Alabama. Gonadotropin preparations: past, present, and future perspectives. Fertil Steril 2008;90:S13–S20.

57. Griesinger G, Diedrich K, Devroey P, et al. GnRH agonist for triggering final oocyte maturation in the GnRH antagonist ovarian hyperstimulation protocol: a systematic review and meta-analysis. Hum Reprod Update 2006;12:159–68.

58. Humaidan P, Papanikolaou EG, Tarlatzis BC. GnRHa to trigger final oocyte maturation: a time to reconsider. Hum Reprod 2009;24:2389–94.

59. Humaidan P, Quartarolo J, Papanikolaou EG. Preventing ovarian hyperstimulation syndrome: guidance for the clinician. Fertil Steril 2010;94:389–400.

60. Youssef MA, Van der Veen F, Al-Inany HG, et al. Gonadotropin-releasing hormone agonist versus HCG for oocyte triggering in antagonist assisted reproductive technology cycles. Cochrane Database Syst Rev 2011; (1):CD008046.

61. McClure N, Macpherson AM, Healy DL, et al. An immunohistochemical study of the vascularization of the human graafian follicle. Hum Reprod 1994;9:1401–5.

62. Kim KH, Oh DS, Jeong JH, et al. Follicular blood flow is a better predictor of the outcome of in vitro fertilization-embryo transfer than follicular fluid vascular endothelial growth factor and nitric oxide concentrations. Fertil Steril 2004;82:586–92.

63. Bhal PS, Pugh ND, Gregory L, et al. Perifollicular vascularity as a potential variable affecting outcome in stimulated intrauterine insemination treatment cycles: a study using transvaginal power doppler. Hum Reprod 2001;16:1682–9.

64. Stener-Victorin E, Kobayashi R, Kurosawa M. Ovarian blood flow responses to electro-acupuncture stimulation at different frequencies and intensities in anaesthetized rats. Auton Neurosci 2003;108:50–6.

65. Yu YP, Ma LX, Ma YX, et al. Immediate effect of acupuncture at Sanyinjiao (SP6) and Xuanzhong (GB39) on uterine arterial blood flow in primary dysmenorrhea. J Altern Complement Med 2010;16:1073–8.

66. Vergouw C. Egg cells. In: de Haan N, Spelt M, Gobel R, editors. Reproductive medicine: a textbook for paramedics. Amsterdam: Elsevier Gezondheids-zorg; 2010. p. 73–8 [chapter 4].

67. Humaidan P, Stener-Victorin E. Pain relief during oocyte retrieval with a new short duration electro-acupuncture technique – an alternative to conventional analgesic methods. Hum Reprod 2004;19:1367–72.

68. Sator-Katzenschlager SM, Wölfler MM, Kozek-Langenecker SA, et al. Auricular electro-acupuncture as an additional perioperative analgesic method during oocyte aspiration in IVF treatment. Hum Reprod 2006;21:2114–20.

69. Humaidan P, Brock K, Bungum L, et al. Pain relief during oocyte retrieval – exploring the role of different frequencies of electro-acupuncture. Reprod Biomed Online 2006;13:120–5.

70. Stener-Victorin E, Waldenström U, Wikland M, et al. Electro-acupuncture as a peroperative analgesic method and its effects on implantation rate and neuropeptide Y concentrations in follicular fluid. Hum Reprod 2003;18:1454–60.

71. Humaidan PS, Bungum L, Andersen KB. Electro-acupuncture for ovum pick-up – a good alternative to conventional anesthetics. Fertil Steril 2003;80:95.

72. Papale L, Fiorentino A, Montag M, et al. The zygote. Hum Reprod 2012;27(Suppl. 1):i22–i49.

73. Mahutte NG, Arici A. Failed fertilization: is it predictable? Curr Opin Obstet Gynecol 2003;15:211–8.

74. Schats R. Ovarian hyperstimulation syndrome. In: de Haan N, Spelt M, Gobel R, editors. Reproductive medicine: a textbook for paramedics. Amsterdam: Elsevier Gezondheids-zorg; 2010. p. 127–34 [chapter 9].

75. Meseguer M, Rubio I, Cruz M, et al. Embryo incubation and selection in a time-lapse monitoring system improves pregnancy outcome compared with a standard incubator: a retrospective cohort study. Fertil Steril 2012;98:1481-9.e10.

76. Gunby J, Daya S, Olive D, et al. Day three versus day two embryo transfer following in vitro fertilization or intracytoplasmic sperm injection. Cochrane Database Syst Rev 2004; (2):CD004378.

77. Abou-Setta AM, Mansour RT, Al-Inany HG, et al. Among women undergoing embryo transfer, is the probability of pregnancy and live birth improved with ultrasound guidance over clinical touch alone? A systemic review and meta-analysis of prospective randomized trials. Fertil Steril 2007;88:333–41.

78. Kojima K, Nomiyama M, Kumamoto T, et al. Transvaginal ultrasound-guided embryo transfer improves pregnancy and implantation rates after IVF. Hum Reprod 2001;16:2578–82.

79. Spitzer D, Haidbauer R, Corn C, et al. Effects of embryo transfer quality on pregnancy and live birth delivery rates. J Assist Reprod Genet 2012;29:131–5.

80. Spandorfer SD, Goldstein J, Navarro J, et al. Difficult embryo transfer has a negative impact on the outcome of in vitro fertilization. Fertil Steril 2003;79:654–5.

81. Tomás C, Tikkinen K, Tuomivaara L, et al. The degree of difficulty of embryo transfer is an independent factor for predicting pregnancy. Hum Reprod 2002;17:2632–5.

82. Woolcott R, Stanger J. Potentially important variables identified by transvaginal ultrasound-guided embryo transfer. Hum Reprod 1997;12:963–6.

83. Westergaard LG, Mao Q, Krogslund M, et al. Acupuncture on the day of embryo transfer significantly improves the reproductive outcome in infertile women: a prospective, randomized trial. Fertil Steril 2006;85:1341–6.

84. Paulus WE, Zhang M, Strehler E, et al. Influence of acupuncture on the pregnancy rate in patients who undergo assisted reproduction therapy. Fertil Steril 2002;77:721–4.

85. Johnson D. Acupuncture prior to and at embryo transfer in an assisted conception unit – a case series. Acupunct Med 2006;24:23–8.

86. Omodei U, Piccioni G, Tombesi S, et al. Effect of acupuncture on rates of pregnancy among women undergoing in vitro fertilization. Fertil Steril 2010;94:S170.

87. Andersen D, Løssl K, Nyboe Andersen A, et al. Acupuncture on the day of embryo transfer: a randomized controlled trial of 635 patients. Reprod Biomed Online 2010;21:366–72.

88. So EW, Ng EH, Wong YY, et al. A randomized double blind comparison of real and placebo acupuncture in IVF treatment. Hum Reprod 2009;24:341–8.

89. Domar AD, Meshay I, Kelliher J, et al. The impact of acupuncture on in vitro fertilization outcome. Fertil Steril 2009;91:723–6.

90. Smith C, Coyle M, Norman RJ. Influence of acupuncture stimulation on pregnancy rates for women undergoing embryo transfer. Fertil Steril 2006;85:1352–8.

91. Dieterle S, Ying G, Hatzmann W, et al. Effect of acupuncture on the outcome of in vitro fertilization and intracytoplasmic sperm injection: a randomized, prospective, controlled clinical study. Fertil Steril 2006;85:1347–51.

92. Manheimer E, Zhang G, Udoff L, et al. Effects of acupuncture on rates of pregnancy and live birth among women undergoing in vitro fertilisation: systematic review and meta-analysis. BMJ 2008;336:545–9.

93. El-Toukhy T, Sunkara SK, Khairy M, et al. A systematic review and meta-analysis of acupuncture in in vitro fertilisation. BJOG 2008;115:1203–13.

94. Rubio C, Giménez C, Fernández E, et al. Acupuncture and in vitro fertilization: updated meta-analysis. Hum Reprod 2009;24:2045–7.

95. Qu F, Zhou J, Ren RX. Effects of acupuncture on the outcomes of in vitro fertilization: a systematic review and meta-analysis. J Altern Complement Med 2012;18:429–39.

96. Manheimer E, van der Windt D, Cheng K, et al. The effects of acupuncture on rates of clinical pregnancy among women undergoing in vitro fertilization: a systematic review and meta-analysis. Hum Reprod Update 2013;19:696–713.

97. Cheong YC, Dix S, Hung Yu Ng E, et al. Acupuncture and assisted reproductive technology. Cochrane Database Syst Rev 2013;(7): CD006920.

98. Stener Victorin E. Acupuncture in in vitro fertilization: why do reviews produce contradictory results? Focus Altern Complement Ther 2009;14:8–11.

99. Meldrum DR, Fisher AR, Butts SF, et al. Acupuncture-help, harm, or placebo? Fertil Steril 2013;99:1821–4.

100. Qu F, Zhou J, Bovey M, et al. Does acupuncture improve the outcome of in vitro fertilization? Guidance for future trials. Eur J Integr Med 2012;4:e234–e244.

101. El-Toukhy T, Khalaf Y. A new study of acupuncture in IVF: pointing in the right direction. Reprod Biomed Online 2010;21:278–9.

102. Zhu D, Gao Y, Chang J, et al. Placebo acupuncture devices: considerations for acupuncture research. Evid Based Complement Alternat Med 2013;2013:628907.

103. Zheng CH, Zhang MM, Huang GY, et al. The role of acupuncture in assisted reproductive technology. Evid Based Complement Alternat Med 2012;2012:543924.

104. Streitberger K, Kleinhenz J. Introducing a placebo needle into acupuncture research. Lancet 1998;352:364–5.

105. White P, Lewith G, Hopwood V, et al. The placebo needle, is it a valid and convincing placebo for use in acupuncture trials? A randomised, single-blind, cross-over pilot trial. Pain 2003;106:401–9.

106. MacPherson H, Altman DG, Hammerschlag R, et al. Revised standards for reporting interventions in clinical trials of acupuncture (STRICTA): extending the CONSORT statement. Acupunct Med 2010;28:83–93.

107. El-Toukhy T, Khalaf Y. The impact of acupuncture on assisted reproductive technology outcome. Curr Opin Obstet Gynecol 2009;21:240–6.

108. Wang W, Check JH, Liss JR, et al. A matched controlled study to evaluate the efficacy of acupuncture for improving pregnancy rates following in vitro fertilization-embryo transfer. Clin Exp Obstet Gynecol 2007;34:137–8.

109. Wang YA, Healy D, Black D, et al. Age-specific success rate for women undertaking their first assisted reproduction technology treatment using their own oocytes in Australia, 2002-2005. Hum Reprod 2008;23:1633–8.

110. Thum MY, Abdalla HI, Taylor D. Relationship between women's age and basal follicle-stimulating hormone levels with aneuploidy risk in in vitro fertilization treatment. Fertil Steril 2008;90:315–21.

111. Farhi J, Ben-Haroush A, Dresler H, et al. Male factor infertility, low fertilisation rate following ICSI and low number of high-quality embryos are associated with high order recurrent implantation failure in young IVF patients. Acta Obstet Gynecol Scand 2008;87:76–80.

112. Zini A. Are sperm chromatin and DNA defects relevant in the clinic? Syst Biol Reprod Med 2011;57:78–85.

113. Evenson D, Wixon R. Meta-analysis of sperm DNA fragmentation using the sperm chromatin structure assay. Reprod Biomed Online 2006;12:466–72.

114. Terriou P, Sapin C, Giorgetti C, et al. Embryo score is a better predictor of pregnancy than the number of transferred embryos or female age. Fertil Steril 2001;75:525–31.

115. Gougeon A. Regulation of ovarian follicular development in primates: facts and hypotheses. Endocr Rev 1996;17:121–55.

116. Balakier H, Stronell RD. Color doppler assessment of folliculogenesis in in vitro fertilization patients. Fertil Steril 1994;62:1211–6.

117. Nargund G, Bourne T, Doyle P, et al. Associations between ultrasound

indices of follicular blood flow, oocyte recovery and preimplantation embryo quality. Hum Reprod 1996;11:109–13.

118. Borini A, Maccolini A, Tallarini A, et al. Perifollicular vascularity and its relationship with oocyte maturity and IVF outcome. Ann N Y Acad Sci 2001;943:64–7.

119. Coulam CB, Goodman C, Rinehart JS. Colour doppler indices of follicular blood flow as predictors of pregnancy after in-vitro fertilization and embryo transfer. Hum Reprod 1999;14:1979–82.

120. Ozturk O, Bhattacharya S, Saridogan E, et al. Role of utero-ovarian vascular impedance: predictor of ongoing pregnancy in an IVF – embryo transfer programme. Reprod Biomed Online 2004;9:299–305.

121. Bassil S, Wyns C, Toussaint-Demylle D, et al. The relationship between ovarian vascularity and the duration of stimulation in in-vitro fertilization. Hum Reprod 1997;12:1240–5.

122. Macklon NS, Stouffer RL, Giudice LC, et al. The science behind 25 years of ovarian stimulation for in vitro fertilization. Endocr Rev 2006;27:170–207.

123. Stener-Victorin E, Waldenström U, Nilsson L, et al. A prospective randomized study of electro-acupuncture versus alfentanil as anaesthesia during oocyte aspiration in in-vitro fertilization. Hum Reprod 1999;14:2480–4.

124. Nikas G, Makrigiannakis A, Hovatta O, et al. Surface morphology of the human endometrium. Basic and clinical aspects. Ann N Y Acad Sci 2000;900:316–24.

125. Chien LW, Lee WS, Au HK, et al. Assessment of changes in utero-ovarian arterial impedance during the peri-implantation period by doppler sonography in women undergoing assisted reproduction. Ultrasound Obstet Gynecol 2004;23:496–500.

126. Ivanovski M, Damcevski N, Radevska B, et al. Assessment of uterine artery and arcuate artery blood flow by transvaginal color doppler ultrasound on the day of

human chorionic gonadotropin administration as predictors of pregnancy in an in vitro fertilization program. Akush Ginekol (Sofiia) 2012;51:55–60.

127. Craig LB, Criniti AR, Hansen KR, et al. Acupuncture lowers pregnancy rates when performed before and after embryo transfer. Fertil Steril 2007;92:1870–9.

128. ESHRE ART fact sheet. Available from: http://www.eshre.eu/ESHRE/English/Guidelines-Legal/ART-fact-sheet/page.aspx/1061 (accessed 13 December 2012).

129. Robinson L, Gallos ID, Conner SJ, et al. The effect of sperm DNA fragmentation on miscarriage rates: a systematic review and meta-analysis. Hum Reprod 2012;27:2908–17.

130. Zini A, Boman JM, Belzile E, et al. Sperm DNA damage is associated with an increased risk of pregnancy loss after IVF and ICSI: systematic review and meta-analysis. Hum Reprod 2008;23:2663–8.

131. Pritts EA, Atwood AK. Luteal phase support in infertility treatment: a meta-analysis of the randomized trials. Hum Reprod 2002;17:2287–99.

132. Zarutskie PW, Phillips JA. A meta-analysis of the route of administration of luteal phase support in assisted reproductive technology: vaginal versus intramuscular progesterone. Fertil Steril 2009;92:163–9.

133. Var T, Tonguc EA, Doğanay M, et al. A comparison of the effects of three different luteal phase support protocols on in vitro fertilization outcomes: a randomized clinical trial. Fertil Steril 2011;95:985–9.

134. van der Linden M, Buckingham K, Farquhar C, et al. Luteal phase support for assisted reproduction cycles. Cochrane Database Syst Rev 2011;(10):CD009154.

135. Khorram NM. Adjuvant acupuncture reduces first trimester pregnancy loss after IVF. Open J Obstet Gynecol 2012;02:283–6.

136. Ke SX. Treating infertility in Traditional Chinese medicine. Eur J Orient Med 2008;6:10–1.

137. Lawler CC, Budrys NM, Rodgers AK, et al. Serum beta human chorionic gonadotropin levels can inform

outcome counseling after in vitro fertilization. Fertil Steril 2011;96:505–7.

138. Gordon JD, Dimattina M, Reh A, et al. Utilization and success rates of unstimulated in vitro fertilization in the United States: an analysis of the Society for Assisted Reproductive Technology database. Fertil Steril 2013;100:392–5.

139. Nargund G, Fauser BC, Macklon NS, et al. The ISMAAR proposal on terminology for ovarian stimulation for IVF. Hum Reprod 2007;22:2801–4.

140. Ghobara T, Vandekerckhove P. Cycle regimens for frozen-thawed embryo transfer. Cochrane Database Syst Rev 2008;(1):CD003414.

141. Al-Shawaf T, Yang D, Al-Magid Y, et al. Infertility: ultrasonic monitoring during replacement of frozen/thawed embryos in natural and hormone replacement cycles. Hum Reprod 1993;8:2068–74.

142. Ashrafi M, Jahangiri N, Hassani F, et al. The factors affecting the outcome of frozen-thawed embryo transfer cycle. Taiwan J Obstet Gynecol 2011;50:159–64.

143. Weissman A, Levin D, Ravhon A, et al. What is the preferred method for timing natural cycle frozen-thawed embryo transfer? Reprod Biomed Online 2009;19:66–71.

144. Groenewoud ER, Cantineau AE, Kollen BJ, et al. What is the optimal means of preparing the endometrium in frozen-thawed embryo transfer cycles? A systematic review and meta-analysis. Hum Reprod Update 2013;19:458–70.

145. Wright KP, Guibert J, Weitzen S, et al. Artificial versus stimulated cycles for endometrial preparation prior to frozen-thawed embryo transfer. Reprod Biomed Online 2006;13:321–5.

146. Nawroth F, Ludwig M. What is the 'ideal' duration of progesterone supplementation before the transfer of cryopreserved-thawed embryos in estrogen/progesterone replacement protocols? Hum Reprod 2005;20:1127–34.

147. Glujovsky D, Pesce R, Fiszbajn G, et al. Endometrial preparation for women undergoing embryo transfer with frozen embryos or

embryos derived from donor oocytes. Cochrane Database Syst Rev 2010;(1):CD006359.

148. Amir W, Micha B, Ariel H, et al. Predicting factors for endometrial thickness during treatment with assisted reproductive technology. Fertil Steril 2007;87:799–804.

149. Zhang X, Chen CH, Confino E, et al. Increased endometrial thickness is associated with improved treatment outcome for selected patients undergoing in vitro fertilization-embryo transfer. Fertil Steril 2005;83:336–40.

150. So EW, Ng EH, Wong YY, et al. Acupuncture for frozen-thawed embryo transfer cycles: a double-blind randomized controlled trial. Reprod Biomed Online 2010;20:814–21.

151. Gysler M, March CM, Mishell DR, et al. A decade's experience with an individualized clomiphene treatment regimen including its effect on the postcoital test. Fertil Steril 1982;37:161–7.

152. Practice Committee of the American Society for Reproductive Medicine. Use of clomiphene citrate in women. Fertil Steril 2006;86:S187–S193.

153. Broekmans F. The initial fertility assessment: a medical check-up of the couple experiencing difficulties conceiving. In: de Haan N, Spelt M, Gobel R, editors. Reproductive medicine: a textbook for paramedics. Amsterdam: Elsevier Gezondheidszorg; 2010. p. 21–39 [chapter 1].

154. ESHRE Capri Workshop Group. Intrauterine insemination. Hum Reprod Update 2009;15:265–77.

155. Kosterman M. Intrauterine insemination. In: de Haan N, Spelt M, Gobel R, editors. Reproductive medicine: a textbook for paramedics. Amsterdam: Elsevier Gezondheidszorg; 2010. p. 101–4 [chapter 7].

156. Tonguc E, Var T, Onalan G, et al. Comparison of the effectiveness of single versus double intrauterine insemination with three different timing regimens. Fertil Steril 2010;94:1267–70.

157. Matorras R, Ramón O, Expósito A, et al. Gn-RH antagonists in intrauterine insemination: the weekend-free protocol. J Assist Reprod Genet 2006;23:51–4.

158. Yulian YZ. Impact of semen characteristics on the success of intrauterine insemination. J Assist Reprod Genet 2004;21:143–8.

159. Zadehmodarres S, Oladi B, Saeedi S, et al. Intrauterine insemination with husband semen: an evaluation of pregnancy rate and factors affecting outcome. J Assist Reprod Genet 2009;26:7–11.

160. Lucchini C, Volpe E, Tocci A. Comparison of intrafollicular sperm injection and intrauterine insemination in the treatment of subfertility. J Assist Reprod Genet 2012;29:1103–9.

161. Klein J, Sauer MV. Oocyte donation. Best Pract Res Clin Obstet Gynaecol 2002;16:277–91.

162. Kortman M. Egg cell donation. In: de Haan N, Spelt M, Gobel R, editors. Reproductive medicine: a textbook for paramedics. Amsterdam: Elsevier Gezondheidszorg; 2010. p. 135–44 [chapter 10].

163. Jarrett LS. The Liver. In: The clinical practice of Chinese medicine. Stockbridge, Mass: Spirit Path Press; 2003. p. 549–70 [chapter 31].

164. Jarrett LS. Kidney. In: The clinical practice of Chinese medicine. Stockbridge, Mass: Spirit Path Press; 2003. p. 427–59 [chapter 27].

165. Lu HC. Section three: Spiritual pivot [Ling Shu]. Verbal questions. In: A complete translation of the Yellow Emperor's classics of internal medicine and the difficult classic (Nei-Jing and Nan-Jing). Vancouver: International College of Traditional Chinese Medicine; 2004. p. 481–7 [chapter 28].

166. Shenfield F, Pennings G, Cohen J, et al. ESHRE task force on ethics and law 10: surrogacy. Hum Reprod 2005;20:2705–7.

167. Rowell P, Braude P. Assisted conception. I – General principles. BMJ 2003;327:799–801.

168. Friel KS, Penzias AS. Intratubal gamete transfer. In: Collins RL, Seifer DB, editors. Office-based infertility practice. London: Springer; 2012. p. 184–94 [chapter 18].

169. Fadini R, Dal Canto MB, Mignini Renzini M, et al. Effect of different gonadotrophin priming on IVM of oocytes from women with normal ovaries: a prospective randomized study. Reprod Biomed Online 2009;19:343–51.

170. The Practice Committees of the American Society for Reproductive Medicine and the Society for Assisted Reproductive Technology. In vitro maturation: a committee opinion. Fertil Steril 2013;99:663–6.

Chapter | 10 |

Clinical issues during ART

It is often assumed that the only hurdle to overcome during Assisted Reproductive Technology (ART) treatment is whether the treatment results in a pregnancy. However, in reality, various problems can arise before a pregnancy test day, as the following examples illustrate.

During the downregulation phase when medication is used to block the release of Follicle Stimulating Hormone (FSH) and Luteinizing Hormone (LH) in order to suppress follicular growth, women may not respond as expected physiologically, and they may fail to downregulate. This problem is relatively easily overcome, and most clinics will extend the period for downregulation until the woman has appropriately downregulated. Issues may develop during the stimulation phase. For example, the follicles may not grow sufficiently well, there may be too few follicles, or the endometrium may not develop adequately. Sometimes, at the egg retrieval stage, not all follicles will contain an egg, and not all of the eggs that are retrieved will be mature; in some cases, no eggs will be retrieved. On some rare occasions, men may fail to produce a semen sample on the day of egg retrieval or may produce a very poor sample.

The *In Vitro* Fertilization (IVF) fertilization rate (that is, the percentage of eggs expected to be fertilized in the laboratory) is about 60–70%.[1] However, some couples will consistently have lower than average fertilization rates. In exceptional cases, none of the eggs will be fertilized. This can occasionally happen even in couples who have a good number of retrieved eggs.

The next stage at which problems can arise is during embryo development. Embryos develop for up to 6 days following egg retrieval. Not all embryos are expected to continue developing. But, in some cases, the embryo demise rate is higher than the expected frequency. Occasionally, no embryos survive to the embryo transfer stage. This is one of the most devastating psycho-emotional blows for couples because they feel cheated of their chance of succeeding with IVF.

The next potential stumbling block is the embryo transfer procedure. Most procedures are carried out without any complications. However, in a few cases, things go wrong.

The next few sections will discuss in more detail what problems may arise during each stage of the IVF cycle and what solutions are available to manage the resulting issues. Figure 10.1 summarizes the clinical complications that can arise at different stages of a typical IVF cycle.

POOR FOLLICULAR DEVELOPMENT

Poor ovarian response is a situation where too few follicles develop during the ovarian stimulation phase.

As discussed in Chapter 9, follicular growth during the stimulation phase is monitored by regular transvaginal ultrasound scans, which usually start on day 5–7 of the ovarian stimulation phase and are repeated every 1–3 days. Average follicular size is determined after two-plane measurements of individual follicles. Sizes are plotted on a chart.

A review by Baerwald *et al.* established that, during ovarian stimulation cycles, ovulatory follicles' mean growth rate is 1.64 ± 0.02 mm/day.[2] Interestingly, anovulatory follicles grow at a slightly faster rate of 1.85 ± 0.04 mm/day[2] as compared to a natural cycle (1.48 ± 0.10 mm for ovulatory and 1.41 ± 0.06 mm for anovulatory follicles).[2] Basically, this means that it is undesirable for follicles to develop too quickly or too slowly.

In some individuals, only one or two follicles will develop. In these cases, the treatment cycle may be cancelled (except in natural or mild IVF, where the aim is to only retrieve one or two eggs).

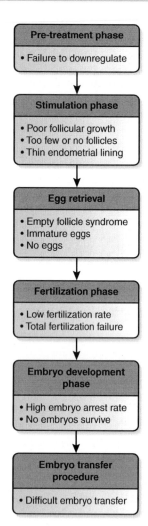

Figure 10.1 Steps in the typical IVF cycle, and clinical complications that may arise during these steps.

According to the European Society of Human Reproduction and Embryology consensus, patients are at risk of poor response to stimulation if they meet at least two of the following three criteria:[3]

- Advanced maternal age (more than 40 years old) or any other risk factor for poor ovarian response (for example, genetic or acquired conditions linked to reduced ovarian reserve)
- A previous poor ovarian response (cancelled cycle or collection of three or fewer eggs with a conventional stimulation protocol)
- An abnormal ovarian reserve test (for example, an Antral Follicle Count of fewer than five to seven follicles or Anti-Müllerian Hormone <0.5–1.1 ng/mL or <3.6–7.9 pmol/L)

Orthodox medical therapeutic options in the affected cycle

Longer gonadotrophin stimulation

Longer stimulation may be required if follicles develop too slowly. However, some studies show that prolonged stimulation (≥ 13 days)[4] is associated with a reduced probability of pregnancy[5] and a significant reduction in live birth rates.[4] However, not all studies agree with this finding. For example, in another study, no significant differences were observed in fertilization rates or clinical and ongoing pregnancy rates in patients who were stimulated for fewer than 9, 10–11, and more than 12 days.[6]

Increasing the dose of stimulation medication

Increasing the dose of ovarian stimulation medication after the first monitoring scan ('step up' approach) is ineffective because the follicular recruitment will have happened by that stage.[7]

Conversion to Intrauterine Insemination

In patients with only one or two follicles, the treatment cycle can be converted to Intrauterine Insemination. This is only suitable in patients in which the male partner has good semen parameters and the female partner has no evidence of blocked fallopian tubes.

Orthodox medical preventative options

Androgen pretreatment (DHEA or testosterone)

Women with a reduced ovarian reserve have low testosterone levels. In women with reduced ovarian reserve, androgen supplementation seems to improve ovarian response to stimulation.[8–12]

Dehydroepiandrosterone (DHEA) supplementation has been shown to improve ovarian response to stimulation.[13–15] It is usually necessary to take DHEA for 3–4 months prior to IVF. DHEA is not suitable for all patients. Therefore, potential female candidates for DHEA supplementation should be advised to discuss its use in their individual case with their ART consultant prior to taking it.

Pretreatment with testosterone for 2 weeks before stimulation may also help to improve ovarian response.[7,16,17]

Treatment protocol

It has been claimed that certain stimulation protocols are therapeutically more effective in patients at risk of poor response. Gonadotrophin-Releasing Hormone (GnRH) flare and antagonist protocols are therapeutically indicated in poor responders compared to luteal pretreatment with GnRH agonist or oral contraceptive pills.[18]

Higher stimulation dose

The standard dose of stimulation is between 150 and 300 IU of Follicle Stimulating Hormone (FSH) per day.[18] In patients at risk of poor response, the starting dose of FSH may need to be between 300 and 450 IU/day.[18] However, doses higher than this are ineffective.[7,18] A higher starting dose of medication is necessary in order to maximize the amount of follicular recruitment, which happens during the late luteal and early follicular phases.[18]

Minimal stimulation dose or natural IVF

A criticism of increasing the dose of stimulation medication is that ovarian response is largely determined by the number of antral follicles.[7] If there are not many follicles to start with, a higher dose of medication will not make any difference. Therefore, minimal stimulation or natural IVF should be considered in patients who have a history of poor response because these patients are likely to produce a low number of eggs, irrespective of the dose of the stimulation medication.[18]

Weight loss

Overweight women undergoing ART require more gonadotropin stimulation, and they have poorer response rates and produce fewer eggs.[19] Therefore, women who are overweight or obese should be encouraged to lose weight (see Chapter 7).

Acupuncture: Rescue treatment

Follicles develop too quickly

If follicles develop too quickly, Full or Empty Heat is usually implicated. Empty Heat may arise as a result of underlying Kidney Yin Deficiency and/or Liver Yin and/or Blood Deficiency. Full Heat is usually from Liver Qi Stagnation. In the authors' experience, the following points are helpful:

* Clear Heat, Regulate the Chong and Ren Mai (Penetrating and Conception Vessels), Nourish Blood: KID2, LIV2, LIV3, REN3, P7, KID8, LI11, ST36

Follicles develop too slowly

When follicles grow too slowly, this problem may be due to different combinations of underlying deficiencies of Qi, Blood, Yin, and/or Jing (Essence). In the authors' experience, the following points and treatments may be helpful:

* Tonify Qi and facilitate Blood flow to the Uterus: ginger with moxa cones on the ovary area[20] or heat on the lower abdominal area (for example, a moxa box or a heat lamp)
* LU7 + KID6, SP4 + P6, REN8, REN12, REN14, REN15, KID13, ST27, and ZIGONG
* Acupuncture treatment frequency may need to be increased to every 2–3 days

Combination of very large and small follicles

In addition to the syndromes listed above, Liver Qi Stagnation may be involved. Additional points include LIV3, LIV2, LI4, ST29, KID13, and SP10.

Acupuncture: Preventative treatment

Other long-term approaches to managing patients with a history of poor response to stimulation are described in Chapter 9 in the sections on ovarian stimulation.

IMMATURE OR NO EGGS

Overview

The previous section discussed poor follicular development, where a woman does not respond well to stimulation medication and there is inadequate development of only a few follicles. This section will discuss a situation where the follicles develop normally but yield few or no eggs (referred to as Empty Follicle Syndrome or EFS) or yield immature eggs. This event is usually unexpected and can potentially lead to the cancellation of a treatment cycle. EFS results in significant psycho-emotional effects and financial implications for a couple.

As discussed in Chapter 9, the Human Chorionic Gonadotrophin (hCG) trigger medication is usually injected 36 h before the retrieval of the eggs. It initiates the final egg maturation process. It is normal for a small number of follicles to not have an egg within them or to produce an immature egg. However, the majority of follicles should produce a mature egg. Research shows that the chances of a live birth are greater if 6[21] to at least 13[22] mature eggs are retrieved.

Empty follicle syndrome

EFS can be 'genuine' or 'false'. In genuine EFS, hCH level on the day of egg retrieval is >40 IU/L, whereas, in false EFS, hCH level is <40 IU/L, either because the patient did not administer the trigger hCG correctly, because the patient administered a faulty batch of hCG, or because of issues with the bioavailability of hCG.[23] False EFS is more common compared to genuine EFS (0.072% and 0.016%, respectively).[24] Borderline EFS is where some eggs are retrieved but not from all follicles. In the authors' experience, this situation is more common in patients who, having experienced EFS, then decide to seek acupuncture to prevent EFS in subsequent IVF treatment cycles.

Some studies show that the occurrence of genuine EFS is a prognostic indicator of a poor IVF outcome in subsequent IVF cycles[25,26] and is associated with reduced ovarian reserve.[27]

Follicular flushing

Sometimes the follicle is classed as empty, but, in reality, the egg is 'stuck' inside the follicle, giving the impression that the follicle is empty. This is referred to as egg (oocyte) retention. A 2012 systematic review claims that potentially about 50% of eggs may be retained inside the follicles after standard follicular aspiration, especially in patients with poor response to ovarian stimulation.[28]

The technique of follicular flushing is believed to help minimize the risk of retained eggs. In a standard egg retrieval procedure, a single lumen needle is used for follicular aspiration. With follicular flushing, a double-lumen needle is used to retrieve eggs. With this technique, as the follicular fluid is extracted with one channel in the needle, saline fluid is instilled into the follicle via another channel. This is thought to help flush out the egg, which might not be picked up with standard aspiration.

Currently, the research evidence is equivocal for the use of this technique. For example, a systematic review and meta-analysis of five trials and 428 patients evaluated if follicular flushing can improve the outcomes of ART. The review authors concluded that while there is no evidence that routine use of follicular flushing is beneficial, the technique may be of benefit in patients with a history of poor response to ovarian stimulation and in natural or mild IVF cycles, where even a marginal improvement in the oocyte retrieval rate could make a difference to the ART outcome.[28]

However, another systematic review and meta-analysis of six randomized trials and 518 patients found that follicular flushing did not improve ART rates in normal responding patients or in poor responders.[29]

Higher dose or different 'trigger' medication

Genuine EFS can be managed in subsequent cycles by using a different trigger medication instead of urinary hCG, for example, recombinant hCG, recombinant Luteinizing Hormone, or GnRH agonist in an antagonist cycle.[30] Adding FSH at the time of hCG trigger increases the likelihood of egg recovery.[31,32]

The other option is to increase the dose of hCG trigger, usually from 5000 to 10,000 IU.

Timing of hCG trigger

Follicles as small as 10 mm in diameter can contain a mature egg capable of being fertilized.[33] ART clinics have different policies on when patients are ready for the trigger injection. For example, some clinics will do the trigger when three or more follicles are ≥ 16 mm, others when the follicles are ≥ 18 mm in diameter. In some clinics, the decision is dictated by practical logistical aspects, for example, triggering a day sooner or a day later in order to avoid a weekend egg retrieval.

The research evidence on this is very mixed. Some studies show that the size of the follicles on the day of egg retrieval makes no difference to the number of eggs retrieved while other studies show that delaying the time of egg retrieval results in more eggs. The following studies illustrate the difficulty that presently exists in making any convincing evidence-based recommendations about when hCG should be administered, the quality of eggs retrieved, and subsequent live birth rates.

- A study of 423 patients undergoing IVF found that triggering when three or more follicles were ≥ 17 mm in diameter compared to triggering 2 days later resulted in no difference in egg quality although there was a significantly higher ongoing pregnancy rate in the group who triggered early.[34]

- Another study analysed 1577 IVF cycles and found no significant differences in the number of mature eggs retrieved, the number of embryos, and the live birth rates from four different follicular size groups (two or more lead follicles <18 mm, 18–18.9 mm, 19–19.9 mm, and ≥ 20 mm). However, there was a nonsignificant decline in live birth rates as lead follicle sizes increased.[35]

- In one study, 125 women undergoing IVF/ICSI (Intracytoplasmic Sperm Injection) were randomized into three groups: (A) trigger administered when three or more follicles were ≥ 17 mm in diameter, (B) 1 day later, (C) 2 days later. There were no statistically significant differences among the three groups in the number of eggs retrieved. However, pregnancies and live birth rates were nonsignificantly higher in groups B and C (A = 30.8%, B = 54.1%, C = 38.7%; A = 17.9%, B = 27.0%, C = 25.8%, respectively). The authors therefore suggested that egg retrieval can be scheduled to suit the clinic, for example, to avoid weekend procedures.[36]

- In another study of 120 women undergoing IVF or ICSI, significantly more mature eggs were retrieved from the early hCG administration group (three or more follicles ≥ 16 mm in diameter) compared to the late (1 day later) hCG administration group. However, no significant differences were found in pregnancy rates or ongoing pregnancy rates.[37]

- A large study of 1642 IVF antagonist cycles analysed if delaying egg retrieval by 1 day or bringing it forward by 1 day from the ideal day negatively affects the outcome. While more eggs were retrieved in the group where the egg retrieval was delayed by 1 day, no significant difference in live birth rates was detected.[38]

- Another study, which analysed 235 cycles and 2934 retrieved eggs, found that the odds of retrieving a mature egg from follicles 16–18 mm in diameter compared to >18 mm were 37% lower and declined progressively with each smaller size.[33]
- In a large retrospective analysis of 1109 IVF cycles and 606 patients, egg retrieval rate was highest (at 83.5%) from follicles 16–18 mm in diameter on the day of egg retrieval and lowest from follicles ≤12 mm or >24 mm in diameter.[39]

Although per cycle pregnancy rates seem to be similar in different follicle groups, there is a weak trend of evidence that cumulative pregnancy rates may be higher when hCG is delayed by a day or two because slightly more eggs are retrieved.[40]

>36 h between the trigger injection and egg retrieval

The time interval between the trigger injection and egg retrieval has historically been set at around 36 h. However, this has not been extensively studied. One study found that trigger injection can be done any time between 34 and 38 h before egg retrieval without any detrimental effects.[41] Another study also found no difference in egg yield in <36.5 and ≥36.5 h intervals although a longer time interval resulted in better implantation, clinical pregnancy rates, and live birth rates in women more than 40 years of age.[42] A longer time interval between trigger injection and egg retrieval may be useful in patients with a previous history of a large number of immature eggs.

Rescue hCG

In patients with false EFS (where hCG is <40 IU/L), hCG can be readministered, and egg retrieval can be rescheduled 36 h later.[43]

Donor eggs

In cases of recurrent genuine EFS, egg donation may be the only option available to these patients.

Immature eggs

A rate of ≤25% of immature eggs is not associated with adverse ART outcomes.[44] If the eggs are immature, they can be left to mature in the laboratory in a procedure called *In Vitro* Maturation or IVM (discussed in more detail in Chapter 6). IVM may be a feasible option for patients who have a history of genuine EFS or in cases where the retrieved eggs are not mature.[45]

The role of the acupuncturist

As already discussed in Chapter 2, acupuncture may improve the quality of the follicles and eggs within them by improving the blood flow to the ovary.[46]

Regular and frequent treatment during the stimulation phase may help with follicular development. In one study of acupuncture in mice undergoing ovarian stimulation, it was found that acupuncture on SP6 three times during the stimulation period resulted in an almost twofold increase in the number of mature eggs in the acupuncture group compared with the control group, where some of the eggs were retained in unruptured follicles. SP6 was chosen because of its connection with Kidneys, Liver, and Spleen Zangfu organs and their function of regulating Qi and Blood. The authors hypothesized that acupuncture enhances follicular recruitment, inhibits follicular atresia, and enhances action of hCG in promoting ovulation.[47]

In our experience, if on the day of the trigger injection there are several smaller to medium-size follicles (10–15 mm in diameter), acupuncture treatment on the day before egg retrieval aids hCG's function of final follicular maturation and seems to increase the number of mature eggs retrieved from these follicles. The following acupuncture point prescription works particularly well: SP4 + P6, SP6, ST36, SP10, LIV8, KID3 plus abdominal points ST29, ZIGONG, and REN4. Moxa or a heat lamp on abdominal points is indicated. Acupuncture treatment on this day has also been recommended by other authors.[48]

In the authors' experience, the following Traditional Chinese Medicine (TCM) syndromes can cause a low number of eggs and/or immature eggs:

- Pre/Post-Natal Jing (Essence) Deficiency
- Yin and/or Yang Deficiency
- Blood Deficiency
- Qi Deficiency
- Qi Stagnation
- Phlegm-Damp
- Blood-Stasis

Acupuncture treatment of these syndromes is discussed in Chapter 5.

SUBOPTIMAL ENDOMETRIAL LINING

Overview

In order for the embryo to implant, the endometrial lining needs to be of appropriate thickness and receptive to the embryo. The lining also needs to be trilaminar (triple layer) in appearance. Chapter 2 described in detail how the endometrial lining develops.

The endometrial lining during the late follicular phase needs to be at least 6–8 mm thick,[49] and it can be up to 16–17 mm thick or, in a few cases, even thicker.[50,51]

Implantation and clinical and ongoing pregnancy rates are significantly increased if the endometrial lining is thicker than 9–10 mm.[50,52,53] Clinical pregnancies and live birth rates increase linearly with increasing thickness of the endometrium, even after adjusting for age and embryo quality.[50,51] There does not appear to be an upper limit to the endometrial thickness, with a lining >14 mm thick not associated with adverse outcomes.[54,55]

Some studies, however, have not found any correlation between the thickness of the endometrial lining and pregnancy rates.[56,57]

All fertility clinics have different cutoff points for what they consider to be adequate endometrial thickness. It is not uncommon for clinics to recommend freezing all embryos if the lining is <6–7 mm thick.

Causes and therapeutic options

Age may affect the endometrial lining, with older women having thinner linings.[55,58,59] This may be because endometrial development depends on good oestrogen levels.[59]

A repeatedly thin endometrium (<7 mm) might be caused by previous surgical curettage, even if, subsequently, no signs of adhesions are found.[60] Therefore, in cases of repeatedly thin endometrium, advanced uterine investigations should be undertaken. In cases where adhesions are found, they should be surgically removed.

Therapeutic options include:

- Stimulation with a high dose of oestrogens or vaginal oestrogen pills[49]
- Medication that may increase the blood flow to the endometrium.[49] For example, aspirin[61] and/or low-molecular weight heparin, a high dose (400–500 IU/day) of vitamin E from day 3 to hCG trigger,[62] pentoxifylline,[63] sildenafil (vaginal Viagra)[64]
- Investigative and therapeutic uterine evaluation
- Surrogacy if other treatments fail[49]

Lifestyle advice

TCM advocates applying heat to the surface of the abdomen (for example, a hot wheat pack), which may help to move stagnant Blood in the Uterus. Moderate exercise or physical activity may also help with blood circulation.

Role of the acupuncturist

As with all other aspects of treating patients undergoing ART, one of the roles as acupuncturists is to provide information to patients. In the cases of thin endometrial lining, informing patients of other treatment options may help to optimize their Orthodox medical care.

Acupuncture treatment has been shown to improve endometrial lining. Two types of outcome measures have been used in research. One is to see if there are any changes

to the Pulsatile Index (PI) of the uterine arteries (that is, the resistance of the blood flow to the uterus). In one study, electro-acupuncture significantly reduced PI. Acupuncture was administered four times, twice a week from day 2 of ovarian stimulation until the day before egg retrieval. Acupuncture points needled bilaterally were: LIV3, SP6, ST28, ZIGONG, REN6, and REN4.[65]

In another study, eight sessions of electro-acupuncture were administered twice a week for 4 weeks. PI was significantly reduced after the eighth session and 10–14 days later. Acupuncture points used were bilateral BL23 and BL28 (100 Hz, pulses of 0.5 ms duration) plus bilateral SP6 and BL57 (2 Hz, pulses of 0.5 ms duration).[66]

Other studies have investigated if acupuncture treatment increases endometrial thickness. In a pilot study combining acupuncture and sildenafil (vaginal Viagra) in four patients who previously failed to achieve a uterine lining of ≥ 8 mm, five sessions of acupuncture treatment during the IVF cycle resulted in all four patients developing a lining of >9 mm (even in those who had received Viagra in previous IVF cycles without success).[67]

In another pilot study evaluating 14 women in the acupuncture group and 14 women in a control group, no changes to the endometrium were detected between the two groups. However, in this study, only one acupuncture treatment was performed during the stimulation phase (day 9), followed by acupuncture treatment before and after the embryo transfer.[68] We would argue that one acupuncture treatment session during the stimulation phase is not enough to achieve the desired therapeutic effect.

A recently published randomized controlled trial showed that patients who received acupuncture treatment during the stimulation phase of an IVF cycle had significantly thicker endometrial linings compared to the control and sham groups (10.3 mm vs. 8.7 mm vs. 8.5 mm, respectively). Acupuncture treatment was done on days 1 and 7 of ovarian stimulation, on the day before the egg retrieval, and on the day after the embryo transfer. The acupuncture point prescription was as follows: unilateral moxibustion was administered for 5 min on BL18, BL22, BL23, BL52, REN3, REN4, REN5, REN7, DU4, followed by unilateral acupuncture on P6, KID3, KID6, KID7, KID10, LIV3, SP4, SP6, SP10, ST40, LU7, and bilateral ZIGONG. De qi was obtained, and needles were retained for 20 min.[69]

Case study

Thin Endometrium

Sue, a 39-year-old administrator, presented to the clinic for acupuncture treatment to help improve her endometrial thickness in preparation for a frozen embryo transfer (FET). The embryos were frozen because of a thin endometrium (4 mm) following a fresh IVF cycle.

Case study—cont'd

Her primary TCM diagnosis was Blood Deficiency with some evidence of Cold in the Uterus. Sue received several months of regular acupuncture treatment. Acupuncture points included SP4+P6, SP6, SP10, ST36, LIV8, and HE5.

When FET was attempted, the lining was thicker (6 mm), but the ART consultant decided that it was still insufficiently thick for the transfer to proceed. Sue was prescribed a high dose of vitamin E and pentoxifylline. However, the treatment did not improve the lining thickness. Sue's consultant offered no further options.

I then informed Sue about research on sildenafil (vaginal Viagra) and thin endometrium. Sue was very interested in trying this treatment, but her consultant refused to support her. She was forced to move to a different clinic. Her new consultant prescribed sildenafil, and, together with more acupuncture treatment, Sue's lining reached 7 mm. The transfer went ahead, and she conceived, but, unfortunately, the pregnancy failed in the very early stages. Subsequent fresh IVF resulted in conception, and Sue gave birth to a healthy baby girl.

This case demonstrates how the integrated use of Orthodox medicine and acupuncture can help patients conceive where it is quite possible that the use of either medical system on its own may not have a successful outcome. It also shows how our role as advisers can help in some cases.

NO SPERM

In many cases, men are able to produce a semen sample on the day of egg retrieval without any problems. However, in rare cases, they may produce a poor sample or fail to produce a sample at all. This inability to produce a sperm sample on demand is often caused by the stress of the situation (i.e., having to masturbate in a small room in a fertility clinic).

If the produced sperm sample is poor, ICSI may be used instead of IVF (Chapter 6 discusses ICSI in more detail).

If a male partner fails to produce a semen sample on the day of egg retrieval and a previously frozen sample is not available, specialist sperm retrieval methods, such as Percutaneous Epididymal Sperm Aspiration or Testicular Sperm Extraction may be used (described in more detail in Chapter 6).

In patients with a history of poor semen samples or no sample at all on the day of egg retrieval, freezing sperm in advance is a good policy in case of any future issues.

One study showed that the longer men take to produce a sample, the more likely they are to produce a better sample.[70] Average time to produce a sample was 15.5 min (range of 3–55 min).[70] However, these findings have not been replicated in another study.[71] Men who find it

stressful to produce a sample need to be reassured that they can take their time to do so and that it might be possibly advantageous to take more time.

In extreme cases, when men find it very stressful to produce a sample on the clinic premises, they can rent a room in a nearby hotel and produce a sample in the privacy of their room. The sperm sample needs to be delivered to the clinic within 1 h. Delay in doing so may compromise the integrity of the sperm.[72]

In some cases, men may find it difficult to ejaculate into a plastic container, and the fertility clinic may provide a special condom, which can be helpful.[72]

In cases where no sperm is available even after surgical extraction, third-party sperm donation may be the only option.

Case study

Poor Semen Sample on the Day of Egg Retrieval

Ben produced a very poor semen sample on the day of egg retrieval. This was completely unexpected because his previous samples had always been good. Ben's partner's eggs had to be donated to another couple, something that they both found extremely difficult to deal with.

The most likely reason for such a poor sample is that Ben found it extremely stressful to produce a sample in a clinical environment. It was decided that several samples of semen would be frozen in advance of any future IVF treatment, just in case such a situation should arise again. In the next round of treatment, Ben also rented a room in a hotel near his IVF clinic and produced a much better sample.

The role of the acupuncturist

As acupuncturists, there is nothing we can do on the day when men fail to produce a (good) sample. However, acupuncture treatment may help to reduce the risk of this happening in the future. Male partners should be advised to consider having a course of acupuncture to improve sperm parameters in preparation for any future IVF treatment (see the section 'Male Factor Subfertility' in Chapter 8). Lifestyle factors should be assessed, and, if necessary, appropriate advice should be provided (see Chapter 7).

FERTILIZATION FAILURE

Fertilization failure incidence and implications

The presence of two centrally positioned pronuclei with clearly defined membranes and two polar bodies 17 h (in IVF) and 18 h (in ICSI) after insemination confirms fertilization.[73] If the pronuclei cannot be seen, it could mean that either the eggs failed to fertilize or the fertilization is delayed.

About 60–70% of retrieved eggs normally are fertilized, and the rates are similar in IVF and ICSI.[1] Fertilization rates strongly predict the outcome of the ART cycle.[74] Total Fertilization Failure (TFF) is when none of the available eggs fertilize. TFF happens in 5–16% of IVF cycles.[75–78] In cases where TFF occurs, there is a 29% chance of it recurring.[78]

There is an inverse relationship between eggs retrieved and TFF. TFF becomes much less likely the more eggs are retrieved. When TFF does happen, it is unlikely to be caused by a random event. A recent review found that most cases of failed fertilization can be broadly attributed to the following causes:[1]

- Insufficient number or poor-quality eggs
- Low number or poor-quality sperm
- Defective culture medium

Fertilization failure in IVF

Sperm factor is implicated in the majority of cases of failed fertilization with IVF. Interestingly, 52% of couples with TFF have normal pre-IVF semen parameters.[79] However, sperm parameters on the day of insemination appear to be strongly correlated with fertilization rates.[1] The main issue lies with failure by sperm to penetrate the zona pellucida (outer shell of the egg).[1] Tests are available to assess sperm–zona pellucida binding. However, in most cases where there is a history of failed fertilization, the ICSI technique should be used in any future treatment cycles. In ICSI, one sperm is injected inside the egg, thereby bypassing the need for sperm to penetrate the zona pellucida (see Chapter 6 for more details on ICSI). ICSI outcomes are independent of semen quality and quantity.[1]

The egg is less frequently implicated in TFF in IVF. Cases that do happen are usually because there are too few eggs or the eggs are abnormal, usually related to advanced maternal age.[1] In cases where fewer than three eggs are retrieved, TFF is common.[80] Animal studies show that omega-3 supplementation may improve egg quality.[81]

Fertilization failure in ICSI

Up to 50% of cases of failed fertilization following ICSI are attributed to DNA damage of the spermatozoon and the egg (in equal proportion), and about 40% of cases are caused by failure of egg activation. TFF in ICSI cycles can also be caused by a low number of retrieved eggs.[1]

Antioxidant supplementation[82] and shorter abstinence time before ejaculation[83] have been reported to improve sperm DNA.

If after ICSI, there has been a failure of fertilization, then assisted egg activation (usually chemical or electrical) can be used to try and achieve fertilization.[84,85]

Some clinics offer ICSI to all couples, including those with nonmale factor subfertility. However, the routine use of ICSI in couples with nonmale factor subfertility is questionable. For example, one study assessed the routine use of ICSI in nonmale factor cases. The fertilization failure rate was significantly higher in the IVF group than in the ICSI group (5% and 2%, respectively), and implantation rates were significantly higher in the IVF group than in the ICSI group (30% vs. 22%). Clinical pregnancy rates, however, were not significantly different.[75]

The skill of the embryologist can also influence ICSI success rates.[74]

Other causes of fertilization failure

Women with hypothyroidism have a lower fertilization rate than euthyroid women.[86–89] A meta-analysis found that treatment with Levothyroxine (LT4) improves the fertilization rates in these women.[86]

A lower fertilization rate may also be related to the size of the follicles. A study of 412 IVF/ICSI cycles and 340 women that compared different-sized follicles' fertilization competence found that medium-sized follicles (16–23 mm on the day of aspiration) produced significantly better fertilization rates compared to small (<16 mm) and large (>23 mm) follicles.[90] Another study that analysed 235 cycles and 2934 retrieved eggs found that eggs retrieved from follicles 16–18 mm in diameter were 28% less likely to result in fertilization compared to eggs from follicles >18 mm.[33] So, in cases with fertilization issues, it is important to ensure that egg retrieval is carefully timed.

Table 10.1 summarizes common causes of fertilization failure and therapeutic options.

The role of the acupuncturist

When patients suffer failed fertilization, they are devastated. As acupuncturists, we can support them by providing them with information (especially if the provision of information is time critical) and by helping them to deal with the emotional fallout.

In cases where the preparatory phase of acupuncture treatment was not long enough or where TCM pathology was not adequately addressed in both partners, it may be appropriate to suggest a longer course of preparatory acupuncture before undergoing further IVF treatment. An assessment and treatment with acupuncture of male partners is essential in most cases with fertilization issues.

In the authors' experience, the following syndromes may cause fertilization issues:

- Kidney Jing (Essence) Deficiency
- Qi Deficiency
- Blood Deficiency[91]
- Yin and/or Yang Deficiency
- Shen (Spirit) affected

Table 10.1 Summary of fertilization methods, causes of failure, and treatment options available

Fertilization method	Causes of failure	Immediate treatment options	Future treatment options
IVF (failure rate 10–20%)	Low quantity or quality of sperm (mostly related to ability of sperm to bind to zona pellucida)	Re-insemination on day 1 (IVF or ICSI), but this is of debatable benefit	ICSI
	Low quantity or quality of eggs		ICSI (of debatable benefit) or donor eggs
	Defective culture medium	–	If trust in the clinic is lost, change of clinic may be necessary
	Cause not identified	Re-insemination on day 1 (IVF or ICSI), but this is of debatable benefit	Test insemination: • Patient's eggs with donor sperm and/or • Donor eggs with patient's sperm
ICSI (failure rate 1–5%)	Sperm and/or egg DNA damage (50%)	–	Sperm: shorter abstinence times and/or antioxidant supplementation or donor sperm Eggs: possibly omega-3 supplementation or donor eggs
	Lack of egg activation (40%)	Assisted egg activation (on day 1): • Chemical • Electrical	Assisted egg activation (at the time of ICSI): • Chemical • Electrical
	Too few eggs	–	Change of ART protocol or donor eggs
	Clinician skills	–	Change of clinician or clinic
	Cause not identified	Re-insemination on day 1 (debatable benefit)	Test insemination: • Patient's eggs with donor sperm and/or • Donor eggs with patient's sperm

- Cold
- Fire
- Phlegm and/or Dampness

Acupuncture treatment of these syndromes is discussed in Chapter 5.

POOR EMBRYO GROWTH OR GROWTH ARREST

The section 'Embryo Grading' in Chapter 6 provides detailed information about normal embryonic development. This section will briefly review the causes of poor embryo development and, where available, will provide details of therapeutic options.

It is normal for some of the embryos to arrest during the culturing period (day of egg retrieval up to 5 days later). However, in some cases, the embryo demise rate is greater than expected, and, in a few cases, all embryos arrest before the transfer. For patients, waiting for the day of transfer is very stressful because they have no control over what happens to their embryos. Patients usually have regular updates from an embryologist on how their embryos are developing. If the embryos are not developing well, patients may be asked to come in for a transfer at short notice.

Causes of poor embryo development

Maternal influences

The majority of embryos fail to develop because of faulty DNA. Embryo development depends on the quality of the egg, particularly embryo fragmentation and cell division.[92] Maternal age is believed to influence embryo quality. In their review, Fujimoto et al. found insufficient evidence to support this belief.[93] Egg quality, however, does influence the quality of the embryo.[93]

The size of follicles on the day of egg collection may also affect embryo development. A study that analysed 235 cycles and 2934 retrieved eggs found that embryos resulting from eggs retrieved from smaller follicles (≤ 18 mm in diameter) had a significantly higher degree of fragmentation.[33] In a large retrospective analysis of 1109 IVF cycles and 606 patients, embryos resulting from follicles 21.6–24 mm in diameter on the day of egg retrieval had the highest cleavage rate at 92%.[39]

This finding was contradicted by another smaller study, in which 819 eggs were assessed according to the size of follicles from which they were retrieved. It was found that all sizes of follicles (small, medium, and large) were capable of producing a good-quality cleavage-stage embryo with no significant difference among them.[94]

Maternal prenatal high-level omega-3 supplementation improves embryo morphology.[95]

Paternal influences

Embryo development, especially embryo cell division, also depends on the quality of the sperm.[92] Paternal genes are switched on at the four-cell stage, and, therefore, sperm DNA may be implicated if embryos stop developing at this time or soon afterward.[96] A meta-analysis found very little consistent evidence that sperm DNA damage influences embryo quality although the authors acknowledge that sperm DNA damage may be a more significant factor in ICSI cycles.[97]

Other factors

The quality of culture medium used in the laboratory, the skill of the embryologist, and the environment in the laboratory are other factors that influence embryo development.

INTERESTING FACTS

EFFECT OF SEASONS ON EMBRYO QUALITY

In a retrospective study, 1072 consecutive IVF cycles were categorized according to the seasons, based on the day on which women started their medication. There was a significant difference in embryo quality (expressed as percentage) depending on the season, with the best quality embryos developing in spring:[98]

- ◆ Winter (December–February): 38.2%
- ◆ Spring (March–May): 54.2%
- ◆ Summer (June–August): 48.2%

INTERESTING FACTS—cont'd

- ◆ Autumn (September–November): 33.6%

Acupuncture may be used to help strengthen patients' constitutions during various seasons, and, therefore, it may positively influence embryo quality:

- ◆ Winter: BL66+KID10[99]
- ◆ Spring: GB44+LIV1[99]
- ◆ Summer: SI2+HE8[99]
- ◆ Autumn: LI1+LU8[99]

Role of the acupuncturist

Acupuncture has a major role during the preparation phase. By optimizing our patients' care, we can influence the quality of eggs and sperm and, therefore, reduce the chances of poor embryo development. Chapters 7 and 8 explain in detail how to prepare patients for ART treatment.

We have no influence over the development of embryos in the laboratory. However, if patients find the waiting time very stressful, acupuncture treatment may be used to help reduce their stress levels.[100,101]

DIFFICULT EMBRYO TRANSFER

What can go wrong and the consequences

Chapter 9 provides detailed information about what happens during the embryo transfer procedure. Most embryo transfers go smoothly and take only few minutes. However, in some cases, there may be complications, referred to as *difficult transfers*. The most common embryo transfer complications are:

- • Painful transfer
- • Technically difficult transfer for the clinician (difficulty inserting the speculum and/or catheter)
- • Issues with embryo(s) discharge from the catheter into the uterus

Difficult transfers are associated with lower success rates[102–104] possibly because they stimulate uterine contractions[105,106] or because the embryos get damaged in the process of transfer. Successful cycles have shorter times between the embryo being loaded into a catheter and its discharge into the uterus, compared to unsuccessful cycles. Intervals of >120 s are associated with poor prognosis.[107] However, too fast an ejection of the embryos can also damage them.[108]

Therapeutic options

Several options are available to patients with a history of difficult or painful embryo transfer:

- Sedation or general anaesthesia may be offered for future embryo transfers.
- Holding the cervix by volsellum should be avoided except in few rare cases.[106]
- A dummy (trial) embryo transfer may be performed to assess the uterine cavity.[105]
- Cervical mucus should be removed with saline liquid because mucus may block the tip of the catheter, thus blocking the embryos' passage or causing them to stick to the mucus and therefore be extracted with the catheter when it is removed from the uterus.[106]
- Different catheters may be used.[105]
- Ultrasound-guided transfer may be used, if it was not used previously.[109]
- Transfer may be performed by a more experienced clinician.[110]
- Cervical dilation prior to gonadotrophin stimulation may help to 'stretch' the cervix.[111,112]
- In extremely severe cases, alternative methods of transfer can be used. For example, transmyometrial[105] or Zygote Intrafallopian Transfer.[113]
- Following the transfer, if embryos are found inside the catheter, they need to be retransferred immediately. This way the pregnancy is not compromised.[114]

The role of the acupuncturist

Acupuncture practitioners cannot directly influence what happens during the embryo transfer. However, there are several things they can do to help the patient who has a history of difficult embryo transfers.

We can inform patients about various therapeutic options available to them to reduce the risk of future difficult transfers.

Transfer can be more difficult if patients are tense as it is harder for a clinician to insert the speculum. Using semipermanent needles or magnetic or herbal seeds on acupuncture ear point Shenmen and instructing the patient to stimulate the point during embryo transfer may help, both as a distraction and as means of helping her to relax.

Patients who have previously experienced difficult transfers prior to starting acupuncture treatment often comment how much easier their transfer was after acupuncture. Most acupuncture embryo transfer protocols outlined in Chapter 9 include strong calming points, and these will help the patient to feel more relaxed for the transfer.

SP6 is known for its effect on the cervix. Applying a semipermanent needle to SP6 before the transfer and removing it after the transfer can help to soften the cervix. Alternatively, the ear cervix point may also be used. The point LI4 can be used for managing the pain of those patients who have previously experienced painful embryo transfer.

Immediately after a difficult transfer, it is important to use the points that decrease uterine contractions. Animal studies show that LI4[115] and SP6[116] can reduce uterine motility. Interestingly, both these points are commonly used in postembryo transfer acupuncture protocols although a study on human participants using LI4 and SP6 in combination with other points did not find any reduction in uterine contractions.[117] This may be because of a combination of points otherwise used in this study or, alternatively, because LI4 and SP6 are not effective at reducing uterine contractions in humans.

SUMMARY

Fertility acupuncturists must be aware of and anticipate what could go wrong during the ART process and take adequate steps to reduce the identified risk factors and to adequately support their patients.

When patients present for acupuncture to help them conceive a baby, it is important to ask them about their previous ART history and whether any clinical issues arose. Then we can advise patients about the available Orthodox medical and TCM interventions that can be used to minimize or prevent the same issue(s) arising again.

REFERENCES

1. Mahutte NG, Arici A. Failed fertilization: is it predictable? Curr Opin Obstet Gynecol 2003;15:211–8.
2. Baerwald AR, Walker RA, Pierson RA. Growth rates of ovarian follicles during natural menstrual cycles, oral contraception cycles, and ovarian stimulation cycles. Fertil Steril 2009;91:440–9.
3. Ferraretti AP, La Marca A, Fauser BC, et al. ESHRE consensus on the definition of 'poor response' to ovarian stimulation for in vitro fertilization: the Bologna criteria. Hum Reprod 2011;26:1616–24.
4. Chuang M, Zapantis A, Taylor M, et al. Prolonged gonadotropin stimulation is associated with decreased ART success. J Assist Reprod Genet 2010;27:711–7.
5. Kolibianakis EM, Papanikolaou EG, Camus M, et al. Menstruation-free interval and ongoing pregnancy in IVF using GnRH antagonists. Hum Reprod 2006;21:1012–7.
6. Martin JR, Mahutte NG, Arici A, et al. Impact of duration and dose of gonadotrophins on IVF outcomes. Reprod Biomed Online 2006;13:645–50.
7. Weissman A, Howles C. Treatment strategies in assisted reproduction for the poor responder patient. In: Gardner DK, Shoham Z, editors. Textbook of assisted reproductive

techniques. 4. Clinical perspectives. Volume 2. Essex: Informa Healthcare; 2012. p. 162–207. [chapter 46].

8. Qin Y, Zhao Z, Sun M, et al. Association of basal serum testosterone levels with ovarian response and in vitro fertilization outcome. Reprod Biol Endocrinol 2011;9:9.

9. Gleicher N, Kim A, Weghofer A, et al. Hypoandrogenism in association with diminished functional ovarian reserve. Hum Reprod 2013;1–8.

10. Meldrum DR, Chang RJ, Giudice LC, et al. Role of decreased androgens in the ovarian response to stimulation in older women. Fertil Steril 2013;99:5–11.

11. Gleicher N, Kim A, Weghofer A, et al. Starting and resulting testosterone levels after androgen supplementation determine at all ages in vitro fertilization (IVF) pregnancy rates in women with diminished ovarian reserve (DOR). J Assist Reprod Genet 2013;30:49–62.

12. Drillich A, Davis SR. Androgen therapy in women: what we think we know. Exp Gerontol 2007;42:457–62.

13. Hyman JH, Margalioth EJ, Rabinowitz R, et al. DHEA supplementation may improve IVF outcome in poor responders: a proposed mechanism. Eur J Obstet Gynecol Reprod Biol 2013;168 (1):49–53. Available from: http://dx.doi.org/10.1016/j.ejogrb.2012.12.017.

14. Wiser A, Gonen O, Ghetler Y, et al. Addition of dehydroepiandrosterone (DHEA) for poor-responder patients before and during IVF treatment improves the pregnancy rate: a randomized prospective study. Hum Reprod 2010;25:2496–500.

15. Gleicher N, Barad DH. Dehydroepiandrosterone (DHEA) supplementation in diminished ovarian reserve (DOR). Reprod Biol Endocrinol 2011;9:67.

16. Kim CH, Howles CM, Lee HA. The effect of transdermal testosterone gel pretreatment on controlled ovarian stimulation and IVF outcome in low responders. Fertil Steril 2011;95:679–83.

17. Bosdou JK, Venetis CA, Kolibianakis EM, et al. The use of androgens or androgen-modulating agents in poor responders undergoing in vitro fertilization: a systematic review and meta-analysis. Hum Reprod Update 2012;18:127–45.

18. Keltz M, Sauerbrun-Cutler M-T, Breborowicz A. Managing poor responders in IVF. Expert Rev Obstet Gynecol 2013;8:121–34.

19. Practice Committee of American Society for Reproductive Medicine. Obesity and reproduction: an educational bulletin. Fertil Steril 2008;90:S21–9.

20. Auteroche B, Kivity O. Moxibustion and other techniques. In: Acupuncture and moxibustion: a guide to clinical practice. Edinburgh: Churchill Livingstone; 1992. p. 75–92, Section 2 [chapter 1].

21. McAvey B, Zapantis A, Jindal SK, et al. How many eggs are needed to produce an assisted reproductive technology baby: is more always better? Fertil Steril 2011;96:332–5.

22. Van der Gaast MH, Eijkemans MJC, Van der Net JB, et al. Optimum number of oocytes for a successful first IVF treatment cycle. Reprod Biomed Online 2006;13:476–80.

23. Kim JH, Jee BC. Empty follicle syndrome. Clin Exp Reprod Med 2012;39:132–7.

24. Mesen TB, Yu B, Richter KS, et al. The prevalence of genuine empty follicle syndrome. Fertil Steril 2011;96:1375–7.

25. Coskun S, Madan S, Bukhari I, et al. Poor prognosis in cycles following "genuine" empty follicle syndrome. Eur J Obstet Gynecol Reprod Biol 2010;150:157–9.

26. Lorusso F, Depalo R, Tsadilas S, et al. Is the occurrence of the empty follicle syndrome a predictor that a subsequent stimulated cycle will be an unfavourable one? Reprod Biomed Online 2005;10:571–4.

27. Zreik TG, Garcia-Velasco JA, Vergara TM, et al. Empty follicle syndrome: evidence for recurrence. Hum Reprod 2000;15:999–1002.

28. Roque M, Sampaio M, Geber S. Follicular flushing during oocyte retrieval: a systematic review and meta-analysis. J Assist Reprod Genet 2012;29:1249–54.

29. Levy G, Hill MJ, Ramirez CI, et al. The use of follicle flushing during oocyte retrieval in assisted reproductive technologies: a systematic review and meta-analysis. Hum Reprod 2012;27:2373–9.

30. Smisha M, Sankar K, Thomas B, et al. Recurrent genuine empty follicle syndrome. J Hum Reprod Sci 2011;4:147–9.

31. Lamb JD, Shen S, McCulloch C, et al. Follicle-stimulating hormone administered at the time of human chorionic gonadotropin trigger improves oocyte developmental competence in in vitro fertilization cycles: a randomized, double-blind, placebo-controlled trial. Fertil Steril 2011;95(5):1655–60.

32. Kol S, Humaidan P. LH (as HCG) and FSH surges for final oocyte maturation: sometimes it takes two to tango? Reprod Biomed Online 2010;21:590–2.

33. Rosen MP, Shen S, Dobson AT, et al. A quantitative assessment of follicle size on oocyte developmental competence. Fertil Steril 2008;90:684–90.

34. Kolibianakis EM, Albano C, Camus M, et al. Prolongation of the follicular phase in in vitro fertilization results in a lower ongoing pregnancy rate in cycles stimulated with recombinant follicle-stimulating hormone and gonadotropin-releasing hormone antagonists. Fertil Steril 2004;82:102–7.

35. Knopman J, Frifo J, Novetsky A, et al. Is bigger better: the association between follicle size and live birth rate following IVF? Open J Obstet Gynecol 2012;02:361–6.

36. Morley L, Tang T, Yasmin E, et al. Timing of human chorionic gonadotrophin (hCG) hormone administration in IVF protocols using GnRH antagonists: a randomized controlled trial. Hum Fertil (Camb) 2012;15:134–9.

37. Kyrou D, Kolibianakis EM, Fatemi HM, et al. Is earlier administration of human chorionic gonadotropin (hCG) associated with the probability of pregnancy in cycles stimulated with recombinant follicle-stimulating hormone and gonadotropin-releasing hormone (GnRH) antagonists? A prospective

randomized trial. Fertil Steril 2011;96:1112–5.

38. Tremellen KP, Lane M. Avoidance of weekend oocyte retrievals during GnRH antagonist treatment by simple advancement or delay of hCG administration does not adversely affect IVF live birth outcomes. Hum Reprod 2010;25:1219–24.

39. Wittmaack FM, Kreger DO, Blasco L, et al. Effect of follicular size on oocyte retrieval, fertilization, cleavage, and embryo quality in in vitro fertilization cycles: a 6-year data collection. Fertil Steril 1994;62:1205–10.

40. Zhang P. Late hCG administration yields more good quality embryos and favors the overall IVF outcome. Open J Obstet Gynecol 2012;02:331–6.

41. Bjercke S, Tanbo T, Dale PO, et al. Comparison between two hCG-to-oocyte aspiration intervals on the outcome of in vitro fertilization. J Assist Reprod Genet 2000;17:319–22.

42. Reichman DE, Missmer SA, Berry KF, et al. Effect of time between human chorionic gonadotropin injection and egg retrieval is age dependent. Fertil Steril 2011;95:1990–5.

43. Doyle JO, Attaman JA, Styer AK, et al. Rescue human chorionic gonadotropin for false empty follicle syndrome: optimism for successful pregnancy outcome. Fertil Steril 2012;98:450–2.

44. Bar-Ami S, Zlotkin E, Brandes JM, et al. Failure of meiotic competence in human oocytes. Biol Reprod 1994;50:1100–7.

45. Hourvitz A, Maman E, Brengauz M, et al. In vitro maturation for patients with repeated in vitro fertilization failure due to "oocyte maturation abnormalities". Fertil Steril 2010;94:496–501.

46. Anderson BJ, Haimovici F, Ginsburg ES, et al. In vitro fertilization and acupuncture: clinical efficacy and mechanistic basis. Altern Ther Health Med 2007;13:38–48.

47. Jin C, Tohya K, Kuribayashi K, et al. Increased oocyte production after acupuncture treatment during superovulation process in mice. J Reprod Contracept 2009;20:35–44.

48. Anderson B, Rosenthal L. Acupuncture and in vitro fertilization: critique of the evidence and application to clinical practice. Complement Ther Clin Pract 2013;19:1–5.

49. Simon A, Laufer N. Repeated implantation failure: clinical approach. Fertil Steril 2012;97:1039–43.

50. Richter KS, Bugge KR, Bromer JG, et al. Relationship between endometrial thickness and embryo implantation, based on 1,294 cycles of in vitro fertilization with transfer of two blastocyst-stage embryos. Fertil Steril 2007;87:53–9.

51. Al-Ghamdi A, Coskun S, Al-Hassan S, et al. The correlation between endometrial thickness and outcome of in vitro fertilization and embryo transfer (IVF-ET) outcome. Reprod Biol Endocrinol 2008;6:37.

52. Kovacs P, Matyas S, Boda K, et al. The effect of endometrial thickness on IVF/ICSI outcome. Hum Reprod 2003;18:2337–41.

53. El-Toukhy T, Coomarasamy A, Khairy M, et al. The relationship between endometrial thickness and outcome of medicated frozen embryo replacement cycles. Fertil Steril 2008;89:832–9.

54. Dietterich C, Check JH, Choe JK, et al. Increased endometrial thickness on the day of human chorionic gonadotropin injection does not adversely affect pregnancy or implantation rates following in vitro fertilization-embryo transfer. Fertil Steril 2002;77:781–6.

55. Yoeli R, Ashkenazi J, Orvieto R, et al. Significance of increased endometrial thickness in assisted reproduction technology treatments. J Assist Reprod Genet 2004;21:285–9.

56. Rashidi BH, Sadeghi M, Jafarabadi M, et al. Relationships between pregnancy rates following in vitro fertilization or intracytoplasmic sperm injection and endometrial thickness and pattern. Eur J Obstet Gynecol Reprod Biol 2005;120:179–84.

57. Bassil S. Changes in endometrial thickness, width, length and pattern in predicting pregnancy outcome during ovarian stimulation in in vitro fertilization. Ultrasound Obstet Gynecol 2001;18:258–63.

58. Amir W, Micha B, Ariel H, et al. Predicting factors for endometrial thickness during treatment with assisted reproductive technology. Fertil Steril 2007;87:799–804.

59. Zhang X, Chen CH, Confino E, et al. Increased endometrial thickness is associated with improved treatment outcome for selected patients undergoing in vitro fertilization-embryo transfer. Fertil Steril 2005;83:336–40.

60. Shufaro Y, Simon A, Laufer N, et al. Thin unresponsive endometrium – a possible complication of surgical curettage compromising ART outcome. J Assist Reprod Genet 2008;25:421–5.

61. Hsieh YY, Tsai HD, Chang CC, et al. Low-dose aspirin for infertile women with thin endometrium receiving intrauterine insemination: a prospective, randomized study. J Assist Reprod Genet 2000;17:174–7.

62. Cicek N, Eryilmaz OG, Sarikaya E, et al. Vitamin E effect on controlled ovarian stimulation of unexplained infertile women. J Assist Reprod Genet 2012;29:325–8.

63. Acharya S, Yasmin E, Balen AH. The use of a combination of pentoxifylline and tocopherol in women with a thin endometrium undergoing assisted conception therapies – a report of 20 cases. Hum Fertil (Camb) 2009;12:198–203.

64. Sher G, Fisch JD. Effect of vaginal sildenafil on the outcome of in vitro fertilization (IVF) after multiple IVF failures attributed to poor endometrial development. Fertil Steril 2002;78:1073–6.

65. Ho M, Huang LC, Chang YY, et al. Electroacupuncture reduces uterine artery blood flow impedance in infertile women. Taiwan J Obstet Gynecol 2009;48:148–51.

66. Stener-Victorin E, Waldenström U, Andersson SA, et al. Reduction of blood flow impedance in the uterine arteries of infertile women with electro-acupuncture. Hum Reprod 1996;11:1314–7.

67. Yu W, Horn B, Acacio B, et al. A pilot study evaluating the combination of

acupuncture with sildenafil on endometrial thickness. Fertil Steril 2007;87:23.

68. Smith CA, Coyle ME, Norman RJ. Does acupuncture improve the endometrium for women undergoing an embryo transfer: a pilot randomised controlled trial. Aust. J Acupuncture Chinese Med 2009;4:7–13.

69. Isoyama Manca di Villahermosa D, Dos Santos LG, Nogueira MB, et al. Influence of acupuncture on the outcomes of in vitro fertilisation when embryo implantation has failed: a prospective randomised controlled clinical trial. Acupunct Med 2013;31:157–61.

70. Pound N, Javed MH, Ruberto C, et al. Duration of sexual arousal predicts semen parameters for masturbatory ejaculates. Physiol Behav 2002;76:685–9.

71. Elzanaty S. Time-to-ejaculation and the quality of semen produced by masturbation at a clinic. Urology 2008;71:883–8.

72. WHO. Standard procedures. In: Cooper TG, editor-in-chief. WHO laboratory manual for the examination and processing of human semen. 5th ed. Geneva: World Health Organization; 2010. p. 7–114. [chapter 2].

73. Papale L, Fiorentino A, Montag M, et al. The zygote. Hum Reprod 2012;27(Suppl. 1):i22–49.

74. Rosen MP, Shen S, Rinaudo PF, et al. Fertilization rate is an independent predictor of implantation rate. Fertil Steril 2010;94:1328–33.

75. Bhattacharya S, Hamilton MP, Shaaban M, et al. Conventional in-vitro fertilisation versus intracytoplasmic sperm injection for the treatment of non-male-factor infertility: a randomised controlled trial. Lancet 2001;357:2075–9.

76. Repping S, van Weert JM, Mol BW, et al. Use of the total motile sperm count to predict total fertilization failure in in vitro fertilization. Fertil Steril 2002;78:22–8.

77. Ruiz A, Remohí J, Minguez Y, et al. The role of in vitro fertilization and intracytoplasmic sperm injection in couples with unexplained infertility after failed intrauterine insemination. Fertil Steril 1997;68:171–3.

78. Barlow PP, Englert YY, Puissant FF, et al. Fertilization failure in IVF: why and what next? Hum Reprod 1990;5:451–6.

79. Liu DY, Baker HW. Defective sperm-zona pellucida interaction: a major cause of failure of fertilization in clinical in-vitro fertilization. Hum Reprod 2000;15:702–8.

80. Luna M, Bigelow C, Duke M, et al. Should ICSI be recommended routinely in patients with four or fewer oocytes retrieved?, J Assist Reprod Genet 2011;28:911–5. Available from: http://dx.doi.org/10.1007/s10815-011-9614-9.

81. Nehra D, Le HD, Fallon EM, et al. Prolonging the female reproductive lifespan and improving egg quality with dietary omega-3 fatty acids. Aging Cell 2012;11:1046–54.

82. Comhaire FH, Mahmoud A. The role of food supplements in the treatment of the infertile man. Reprod Biomed Online 2003;7:385–91.

83. Gosálvez J, González-Martínez M, López-Fernández C, et al. Shorter abstinence decreases sperm deoxyribonucleic acid fragmentation in ejaculate. Fertil Steril 2011;96:1083–6.

84. Nasr-Esfahani MH, Razavi S, Javdan Z, et al. Artificial oocyte activation in severe teratozoospermia undergoing intracytoplasmic sperm injection. Fertil Steril 2008;90:2231–7.

85. Heindryckx B, Van der Elst J, De Sutter P, et al. Treatment option for sperm- or oocyte-related fertilization failure: assisted oocyte activation following diagnostic heterologous ICSI. Hum Reprod 2005;20:2237–41.

86. Velkeniers B, Van Meerhaeghe A, Poppe K, et al. Levothyroxine treatment and pregnancy outcome in women with subclinical hypothyroidism undergoing assisted reproduction technologies: systematic review and meta-analysis of RCTs. Hum Reprod Update 2013;19:251–8.

87. Kilic S, Tasdemir N, Yilmaz N, et al. The effect of anti-thyroid antibodies on endometrial volume, embryo grade and IVF outcome. Gynecol Endocrinol 2008;24:649–55.

88. Scoccia B, Demir H, Kang Y, et al. In vitro fertilization pregnancy rates in levothyroxine-treated women with hypothyroidism compared to women without thyroid dysfunction disorders. Thyroid 2012;22:631–6.

89. Cramer DW, Sluss PM, Powers RD, et al. Serum prolactin and TSH in an in vitro fertilization population: is there a link between fertilization and thyroid function? J Assist Reprod Genet 2003;20:210–5.

90. Ectors FJ, Vanderzwalmen P, Van Hoeck J, et al. Relationship of human follicular diameter with oocyte fertilization and development after in-vitro fertilization or intracytoplasmic sperm injection. Hum Reprod 1997;12:2002–5.

91. Liang L. The pathology of infertility. In: Acupuncture & IVF. Boulder, CO: Blue Poppy Press; 2003. p. 9–16. [chapter 2].

92. Salumets A, Suikkari AM, Möls T, et al. Influence of oocytes and spermatozoa on early embryonic development. Fertil Steril 2002;78:1082–7.

93. Fujimoto VY, Browne RW, Bloom MS, et al. Pathogenesis, developmental consequences, and clinical correlations of human embryo fragmentation. Fertil Steril 2011;95:1197–204.

94. Lee TF, Lee RK, Hwu YM, et al. Relationship of follicular size to the development of intracytoplasmic sperm injection-derived human embryos. Taiwan J Obstet Gynecol 2010;49:302–5.

95. Hammiche F, Vujkovic M, Wijburg W, et al. Increased preconception omega-3 polyunsaturated fatty acid intake improves embryo morphology. Fertil Steril 2011;95:1820–3.

96. Henkel R, Hajimohammad M, Stalf T, et al. Influence of deoxyribonucleic acid damage on fertilization and pregnancy. Fertil Steril 2004;81:965–72.

97. Zini A, Jamal W, Cowan L, et al. Is sperm DNA damage associated with IVF embryo quality? A systematic review. J Assist Reprod Genet 2011;28:391–7.

98. Rojansky N, Benshushan A, Meirsdorf S, et al. Seasonal variability in fertilization and embryo quality rates in women undergoing IVF. Fertil Steril 2000;74:476–81.

99. Hicks A, Hicks J, Mole P. The use of acupuncture points. In: Five element constitutional acupuncture. Edinburgh: Churchill Livingstone; 2005. p. 261–78. [chapter 36].

100. So EW, Ng EH, Wong YY, et al. A randomized double blind comparison of real and placebo acupuncture in IVF treatment. Hum Reprod 2009;24:341–8.

101. Magarelli PC, Cridennda DK, Cohen M. Changes in serum cortisol and prolactin associated with acupuncture during controlled ovarian hyperstimulation in women undergoing in vitro fertilization-embryo transfer treatment. Fertil Steril 2009;92:1870–9.

102. Tomás C, Tikkinen K, Tuomivaara L, et al. The degree of difficulty of embryo transfer is an independent factor for predicting pregnancy. Hum Reprod 2002;17:2632–5.

103. Spitzer D, Haidbauer R, Corn C, et al. Effects of embryo transfer quality on pregnancy and live birth delivery rates. J Assist Reprod Genet 2012;29:131–5.

104. Spandorfer SD, Goldstein J, Navarro J, et al. Difficult embryo transfer has a negative impact on the outcome of in vitro fertilization. Fertil Steril 2003;79:654–5.

105. Mains L, Van Voorhis BJ. Optimizing the technique of embryo transfer. Fertil Steril 2010;94:785–90.

106. Mansour RT, Aboulghar MA. Optimizing the embryo transfer technique. Hum Reprod 2002;17:1149–53.

107. Matorras R, Mendoza R, Expósito A, et al. Influence of the time interval between embryo catheter loading and discharging on the success of IVF. Hum Reprod 2004;19:2027–30.

108. Grygoruk C, Sieczynski P, Modlinski JA, et al. Influence of embryo transfer on blastocyst viability. Fertil Steril 2011;95:1458–61.

109. Abou-Setta AM, Mansour RT, Al-Inany HG, et al. Among women undergoing embryo transfer, is the probability of pregnancy and live birth improved with ultrasound guidance over clinical touch alone? A systemic review and meta-analysis of prospective randomized trials. Fertil Steril 2007;88:333–41.

110. De Placido G, Wilding M, Stina I, et al. The effect of ease of transfer and type of catheter used on pregnancy and implantation rates in an IVF program. J Assist Reprod Genet 2002;19:14–8.

111. Abusheikha N, Lass A, Akagbosu F, et al. How useful is cervical dilatation in patients with cervical stenosis who are participating in an in vitro fertilization-embryo transfer program? The Bourn Hall experience. Fertil Steril 1999;72:610–2.

112. Noyes N, Licciardi F, Grifo J, et al. In vitro fertilization outcome relative to embryo transfer difficulty: a novel approach to the forbidding cervix. Fertil Steril 1999;72:261–5.

113. Das M, Holzer HE. Recurrent implantation failure: gamete and embryo factors. Fertil Steril 2012;97:1021–7.

114. Nabi A, Awonuga A, Birch H, et al. Multiple attempts at embryo transfer: does this affect in-vitro fertilization treatment outcome? Hum Reprod 1997;12:1188–90.

115. Kim J-S, Shin KH, Na CS. Effect of acupuncture treatment on uterine motility and cyclooxygenase-2 expression in pregnant rats. Gynecol Obstet Invest 2000;50:225–30.

116. Kim JS, Na CS, Hwang WJ, et al. Immunohistochemical localization of cyclooxygenase-2 in pregnant rat uterus by Sp-6 acupuncture. Am J Chin Med 2003;31:481–8.

117. Paulus WE, Zhang M, Strehler E, et al. Motility of the endometrium after acupuncture treatment. Fertil Steril 2003;80:131.

Chapter 11

ART complications

Assisted Reproductive Technology (ART) treatment is generally safe, but it is not without risks. Some patients may suffer medication-related side effects. One common side effect is when women over-respond to ovarian stimulation drugs, which may lead to a condition called Ovarian Hyper-Stimulation Syndrome (OHSS). When a woman has severe OHSS, it can lead to cancellation of her embryo transfer procedure and cryopreservation of all her embryos, hospitalization, or termination of her pregnancy, blood clotting, kidney damage, ovarian torsion, and, in a very few cases, death. However, because of better patient management practices, severe OHSS is now very rare.

Multiple-gestation pregnancy (pregnancy with more than one foetus) is still a very common complication following ART treatment. Multiple-gestation pregnancies put mothers' and babies' health and lives at risk. In terms of ART's long-term effects on women, currently there is no evidence that ART has any effect on genital or breast cancer rates.[1–3]

OVARIAN HYPER-STIMULATION SYNDROME

Introduction

OHSS is a complication of *In Vitro* Fertilization (IVF) treatment where, along with ovarian enlargement, the ovaries produce too many (hypertrophic) follicles, with the result that fluid may leak and accumulate in the abdominal cavity and chest. OHSS is not very well understood, but it is believed to be a result of women producing too many intermediate-size follicles (10–14 mm in diameter on the day of Human Chorionic Gonadotrophin (hCG) trigger injection).[4] Following egg retrieval, multiple corpora lutea

form. This is accompanied by neovascularization in the ovaries (angiogenesis).[4] Newly formed and existing blood vessels leak fluid into the abdominal cavity and sometimes the pleural cavities and the pericardium, which may lead to hypovolaemia (low circulating blood volume)[4] and can even cause thrombosis, organ failure, and, in very rare cases, death.

Orthodox medical management of OHSS

OHSS usually presents soon after egg retrieval in an ART cycle or after ovulation in superovulation cycles, but it can present later.[5] OHSS can be classified according to when it presents:[6]

- Early OHSS ($\leq$9 days after oocyte retrieval) or
- Late OHSS ($\geq$9 days after oocyte retrieval)

Early onset OHSS tends to be mild and often self-limiting whereas late onset OHSS is usually more severe and almost always associated with conception because hCG is necessary for OHSS to develop. Mild OHSS affects up to 30% of women and is usually managed by over-the-counter painkillers and outpatient checkups.[7] Severe OHSS affects up to 2% of women and can be fatal if not appropriately managed.[7]

Any woman undergoing ART can develop OHSS, but the disease is associated with the following risk factors:

- Patients less than 35 years old[8]
- Previous OHSS history[8–10]
- Low body weight[5,9,11]
- Oligomenorrhoea or amenorrhoea[8]
- High Luteinizing to Follicle Stimulating Hormone ratio[8]

- High serum oestradiol (E2) levels (>2500 pg/mL or 9000 pmol/L)[5]
- More than 11 follicles of 10 mm diameter on the day of hCG administration[12]
- Polycystic Ovaries/Polycystic Ovary Syndrome (PCOS)[5,8,9]
- More common and severe when conception occurs[6] or in multiple-gestation conceptions[6]
- Egg donors are more at risk[8]

OHSS is very strongly associated with the hCG hormone, which is produced by the embryo after it is implanted and rises rapidly. hCG adversely affects OHSS in a number of ways:

- hCG supplementation during the luteal phase makes OHSS worse.[9]
- Pregnancy and, therefore, rising levels of hCG make OHSS much worse. Multiple-gestation pregnancy produces even higher levels of hCG, which is associated with more severe OHSS.
- Using the lowest possible effective dose of hCG in IVF cycles to trigger final oocyte maturation before egg

retrieval is recommended because a high dose of hCG is a known risk factor for developing OHSS.[9]

The Orthodox medical management of OHSS is based on identifying women at risk of OHSS and taking preventative measures, such as:

- Lower dose Gonadotrophin-Releasing Hormone (GnRH) in high-risk women[6] (75–150 IU/day)[8]
- GnRH antagonist instead of agonist protocol[6,8,9]
- Co-treating women who have PCOS with metformin[6,8]
- Coasting (withholding the hCG trigger for a few days until oestradiol drops to <2500–4000 pg/mL)[6,8,13]
- Cancelling embryo transfer and cryopreserving all embryos[6]
- Using dopamine agonists[6,13,14]
- Avoiding hCG as luteal support[6,13]
- *In Vitro* Maturation[13]

Once a woman develops OHSS, treatment depends on the severity of the symptoms. Table 11.1 provides staging and common signs and symptoms of OHSS, and Figure 11.1 provides an algorithm for managing OHSS patients.

Table 11.1 OHSS classifications and common signs and symptoms[4,5,15]			
	Mild	**Progressive**	**Life threatening**
Abdominal pain	Mild, transient, improves with medication	Severe, does not improve with medication	
Abdominal distension, ascites (caused by build up of fluid in the abdominal cavity)	Mild, only visible on ultrasound	Yes, visible and palpable on physical examination	
Thirst	Sometimes	Yes	
Weight gain (caused by fluid build up)	<1 kg (2 lb)/day	≥1 kg (2 lb)/day	
Nausea	Mild	Yes, more pronounced	
Vomiting	Sometimes	Yes	Severe, prevents ingestion of food or fluids
Urination	Normal	Reduced	Severely reduced or completely stopped
Stools	May be diarrhoea		
Orthostatic hypotension (posture-related dizziness)	–	Yes	
Tachycardia (rapid heart rate: >100 beats per minute)	–	Yes	
Tachypnoea (rapid breathing >20 breaths per minute), shortness of breath	–	Yes	
Enlarged ovaries on ultrasound	5–12 cm	>12 cm	
Signs of thrombosis or embolism (e.g., redness and swelling in the leg caused by blood clot)	–	–	Possible
Laboratory findings	Normal	Abnormal	Severely abnormal

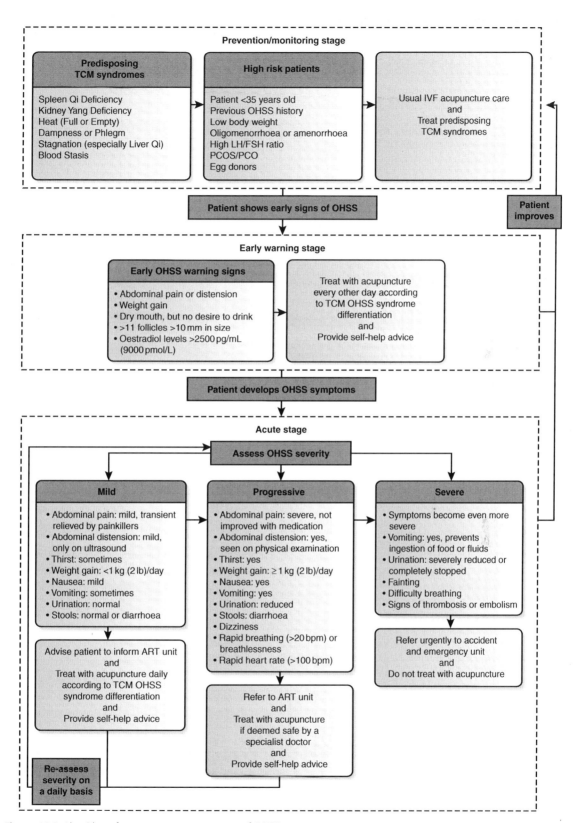

Figure 11.1 Algorithm of acupuncture management of OHSS.

Mild OHSS is characterized by mild abdominal discomfort, which improves with over-the-counter painkillers such as paracetamol.[5] Women with mild OHSS should be monitored on an outpatient basis for signs of OHSS deterioration. Increased abdominal distension and pain, rapid weight gain (≥ 1 kg (2 lb) a day), reduced urine output, and respiratory system symptoms such as shortness of breath or rapid breathing[5] are common indications. An increase in symptom severity requires hospitalization and further investigations, such as ultrasonography, X-ray scans, and laboratory tests. Treatment is supportive, including fluid and electrolyte management.

If the condition is allowed to progress still further, most major organs will be affected, and blood clots may form. These patients require very intensive medical management.

Acupuncture management of OHSS

TCM view of OHSS

OHSS is a modern condition that almost always results from ART treatment (apart from a few reported cases of spontaneous OHSS).

OHSS commonly arises in patients with underlying pathology, including:

- Spleen Qi Deficiency
- Kidney Yang Deficiency
- Heat (Full or Empty)
- Dampness or Phlegm
- Stagnation (especially Liver Qi)
- Blood Stasis

Many fertility patients have underlying Liver Qi Stagnation and also possibly Blood Stasis. Stagnation of Liver Qi can be caused by side effects of medication, the emotional impact of subfertility and IVF, or pre-existing Liver Blood Deficiency. Stagnation of Qi is marked by mood changes, tearfulness, or irritability during downregulation.

The accumulation of fluid, which features in OHSS, exacerbates Qi Stagnation. Severe obstruction of Qi will generate Heat. Pathological Heat can also cause Blood Stasis or make pre-existing Blood Stasis worse. Ovarian stimulation drugs commonly create Heat, Qi Deficiency, and/or Stagnation.

Interestingly, PCOS patients have a high risk of developing OHSS, and, in TCM, they are often diagnosed with underlying Damp-Phlegm and/or Blood Stasis. This also suggests that Dampness, Phlegm, and/or Blood Stasis play a big role in the pathophysiology of OHSS.

Once OHSS develops, it can be in a complex combination of any of the patterns below:

- Heat (thirst, scanty urine, constipation, dryness, and, in some cases, fever)
- Stagnation of Qi and/or Blood (distension, nausea, pain, blood clots)

- Phlegm/Damp (weight gain caused by sudden accumulation of fluids)

Acupuncture points that may be used include:

- REN9, SP9, ST40:[16] to drain Damp and resolve Phlegm
- REN12, LIV3:[16] to regulate Qi
- KID2, LIV2:[16] to clear Heat and Fire
- KID14:[17] to dispel the 'four fullnesses' (Qi, water, food, and Blood Stagnation)
- SP10:[18] to move Blood Stasis
- SP6:[18] to resolve Dampness, regulate Qi, and move Blood Stasis (contraindicated in confirmed pregnancy; use SP10 instead)

OHSS patient management

Principles of management and treatment of OHSS include:

- Identifying patients at risk of OHSS (from both an Orthodox and a TCM perspective)
- Prophylactic acupuncture treatment of patients identified at risk of developing OHSS
- If OHSS develops, minimizing OHSS symptomatology and progression

Prevention is definitely better than cure when it comes to managing patients at risk of developing OHSS. Extreme caution and vigilance is required by less experienced acupuncturists when managing OHSS in order to minimize its progression.

When treating patients at high risk of developing OHSS during the stimulation phase of the IVF treatment, the acupuncturist should place less emphasis on enhancing ovarian response and more on supporting the Spleen and Kidney functions of transforming and transporting Body Fluids and on clearing Damp and Heat and moving Qi and Blood.

Although OHSS is more common in high-risk patients, every patient should be monitored for signs of OHSS. If the early warning signs become apparent, the patient should be treated every other day in order to prevent OHSS from developing. Practitioners need to look for early warning signs of OHSS, such as:

- Any abdominal pain
- Any abdominal distension
- Weight gain
- Nausea
- Dry mouth with little desire to drink[16]
- More than 11 follicles of ≥ 10 mm diameter on the day of hCG administration[12]
- Serum oestradiol levels >2500 pg/mL (>9000 pmol/L)

Patients at risk of OHSS or patients who show early warning signs should be provided with self-help advice, as outlined in Box 11.1.

If OHSS develops, the severity should be assessed. If OHSS is mild, acupuncture may help to reduce the symptoms and the risk of progression and, hence, optimize ART

Box 11.1 **OHSS patient self-help advice**

OHSS patient self-help advice

- Contact your ART unit, and inform them of your symptoms.
- Take over-the-counter medication, such as paracetamol, to help with pain. Avoid ibuprofen.
- Drink until thirst is quenched,[15] but drink a minimum of 1 L of fluids a day.[5]
- Ideal fluids to drink are any commercially available electrolyte-supplemented drinks.[5]
- Avoid intercourse.[5]
- Avoid heavy lifting.[5]

- Maintain light activity and avoid strict bed rest.[5]
- Check weight daily and log it. Immediately report a weight increase of $\geq$ 1 kg (2 lb) per day to your doctor.[5]
- Record frequency and volume of urination.[5] Report reduction in urination to your doctor.
- Other symptoms that you need to report immediately to your doctor are dizziness, severe nausea and vomiting where you cannot keep food or fluids down, severe pain that does not improve with painkillers, shortness of breath, fainting, and burning and swelling anywhere in the body.

outcome. It is very important to appreciate that the severity of OHSS can change very quickly; therefore, it is essential that patients are monitored and reassessed on a daily basis. Patients should be advised to contact their ART unit and inform the unit (and preferably a senior clinician) of their symptoms. Acupuncture treatment frequency will depend on the number and severity of symptoms. Ideally, acupuncture treatment needs to take place every other day or even daily[16] in order to stop OHSS progression.

If symptoms progress to severe OHSS, patients must be advised to seek urgent medical help. They should be referred as an emergency case to an accident and emergency department or a gynaecological ward, depending on the local hospital policy on managing OHSS. Some hospitals lack the necessary expertise to manage OHSS. This may mean that patients might even be turned away from some medical units. So it is essential that IVF acupuncturists follow up with their patients who have OHSS to ensure that they receive appropriate medical care. It may be useful for fertility acupuncturists to know which local medical facilities are able to manage OHSS.

Figure 11.1 summarizes how to manage patients with OHSS.

 Case study

OHSS

Emily, a 29-year-old manager, has a history of 3 years of subfertility caused by endometriosis.

She underwent IVF and produced 13 eggs, all fertilized by IVF. One embryo was transferred at the blastocyst stage, and six blastocysts were frozen. After egg retrieval, she 'felt a bit tender'. On the day of embryo transfer, she had a 'sore tummy' and some bloating. I advised her during her acupuncture session to inform the ART clinic of her symptoms and, if symptoms got worse, to go to her local

Continued

 Case study—cont'd

hospital accident and emergency department. Emily informed her ART clinic, but they were not concerned.

In the days following transfer, Emily's symptoms gradually became worse. She felt hot, had tummy cramps, had retching, and was breathless, randomly gasping for air.

Three days after the transfer, Emily went to the A&E. By this time, she was sweating and shivering. After waiting for 5 h to be assessed, she was advised by a nurse that she '[could] not get OHSS after embryo transfer' and was sent home.

When she arrived home, she telephoned her ART clinic. However, because the consultant was away, she was left without any help. The next day, her IVF consultant telephoned and asked her to come straight to the emergency gynaecology department. She was scanned, and her ovaries were described as 'very enlarged'. A drip was administered, along with painkillers and anti-sickness medication. Her blood was monitored daily, her blood pressure and heart rate were monitored every 4 h, and she had continuous monitoring of urine output. Her waist increased dramatically in size, she 'ballooned' (her skin was tight and fluid was also on her back, which felt 'squishy on touch').

On discharge, her blood test results showed that she was pregnant. She felt tired, had no energy, and was drinking a lot of water. One week later, she had an acupuncture treatment, which helped with her recovery. Her primary syndrome at this stage was Kidney and Spleen Yang Deficiency, and acupuncture points KID7 and ST36 were used. She was well after a week. However, her abdomen felt uncomfortable for almost 3 months of her pregnancy.

The importance of follow-up is evident in this case. Emily was turned away twice (by her ART clinic and by her local A&E unit), even though her OHSS was progressing rapidly. The ART clinic's policy has since changed to ensure that OHSS patients are dealt with by the emergency gynaecology department. Emily has a healthy baby girl.

MULTIPLE GESTATION

Introduction

Multiple gestation is a term used to describe a pregnancy with more than one foetus. It includes twins, triplets, quadruplets, or more. The most common type of multiple-gestation pregnancy is a twin pregnancy. There are two main types of twinning:

- Dizygotic (nonidentical or fraternal) twinning occurs when two eggs are released in the same menstrual cycle, and each is fertilized by different sperm.
- Monozygotic (identical) twinning occurs when one egg is fertilized by one sperm, which later divides into separate embryos. If these embryos share the same placenta (around 60–70% of pregnancies), they are called monochorionic twins.

Risk factors for dizygotic (nonidentical) twins include:[19]

- Increased maternal age
- Greater parity (the number of times a woman has given birth to a foetus ≥24 weeks gestation, regardless if the child was born alive or stillborn)
- Maternal family history of twins (but not paternal)
- Ethnic predisposition (for example, the incidence of dizygotic twins is 1.3 per 1000 live births in Japan, 8 per 1000 in Europe, and 50 per 1000 in Nigeria)
- ART such as ovarian induction or superovulation induction (because of multiple follicular development)
- ART such as IVF (because of two or more embryos being transferred)

Interestingly, the incidence of monozygotic (identical) twins is not influenced by ethnicity and is relatively constant at 4 per 1000 live births. The biggest risk factor for monozygotic (identical) twins is ART treatment:[19]

- Two- to threefold increase with conventional IVF cycles
- Risks increase further if Intracytoplasmic Sperm Injection (ICSI) is used
- Blastocyst culture
- Possible increased risk with assisted hatching technique
- Risks increase further with blastocyst culture and ICSI

Risks associated with multiple pregnancy following ART

In the last three decades, the incidence of multiple pregnancies in the UK has gone up considerably, from 1 in every 100 births in 1978 to 1 in every 67 births in 2004.[20] Many other countries have seen similar increases. This is largely attributed to improved success rates of ART treatments.[20]

However, babies conceived as part of multiple-gestation pregnancy following ART are at a greater risk of morbidity[19,21] and mortality.[19] The risks include:

- Perinatal death (risk of death around the time of birth is three to six times greater for twins and nine times greater for triplets)[20]
- Low and very low birth weight. On average, singleton babies are born at 39.1 weeks gestation compared to 35.3 weeks for twins and 32.2 weeks for triplets. Birth weight in singleton babies averages at 3.4 kg compared to 2.4 kg in twins and 1.7 kg in triplets.[19]
- Preterm birth and its consequences, such as cerebral palsy, retinopathy, and bronchopulmonarydysplasia[19]
- Restricted foetal growth and its consequences[19]
- Behavioural problems[19]
- Lower IQ levels in children who were born prematurely[19]

Multiple gestations also increase the risk of maternal morbidity. Maternal complications include:

- Induced hypertension (in 20% of twin pregnancies compared to only 1–5% of singleton pregnancies)[20]
- Pre-eclampsia[19] (in up to 30% of twin pregnancies compared to 2–10% of singleton pregnancies)[20]
- Gestational diabetes[19] (in 12% in twin pregnancies compared to only 4% of singleton pregnancies)
- Pre-term labour[19]
- Premature delivery[19]
- Placenta previa, vasa previa, and abruption placentae[19]
- C-section delivery is more likely in multiple pregnancies than in singleton pregnancies[20]
- Postpartum haemorrhage[19,20]
- Maternal death during pregnancy or birth (twice as high in twin pregnancy compared to singleton pregnancy, 2 in 25,000 vs. 1 in 25,000, respectively)[20]
- Depression and anxiety as a result of physical, emotional, and financial pressures[19,20]

How to minimize the risks of ART while maximizing the chances of pregnancy

The main objective of ART is to 'maximize the probability of pregnancy while minimizing the risk of a multiple gestation – one healthy child at a time'.[19] However, there is evidence that patients prefer to have more than one embryo transferred in order to increase their chances of conception. Many also hope to conceive with more than one baby and, therefore, have a 'ready-made family'. The motivation for this is primarily financial, physical, and emotional because having more than one baby means patients are unlikely to need any more ART treatments.

Currently, the only direct method of reducing the chance of a multiple-gestation pregnancy following ART is elective single embryo transfer (eSET). There is a growing body of evidence that suggests that, in correctly identified patients, total pregnancy rates from eSET compared to double embryo transfer are similar.[22] However, eSET is still not favoured by many patients or by some fertility specialists.

Conception rates following eSET, and, therefore, its acceptance by patients and physicians, can be improved by developing better methods of identifying embryos with the highest implantation potential and by more accurately identifying which patients would be the best candidates for eSET. Many countries have issued guidelines and, in some cases, introduced legal limits on how many embryos should be transferred (see Table 11.2).

Other ways of reducing the chance of a multiple-gestation pregnancy include individualizing ART stimulation protocols

and reducing doses of gonadotrophins used for ovarian stimulation.

In some countries, (multiple) foetal reduction is practised. This method reduces the risks associated with multiple pregnancies by aborting one or more foetuses.

Implications for fertility acupuncturists

Although the main responsibility of a fertility acupuncturist is to advise patients that the number of embryos to be

Table 11.2 Elective single embryo transfer (eSET) policies[19,23]

Country	Policy	Effect of policies
Sweden	Mandatory eSET (except in patients with very low risk of twin gestation). About 70% of transfers are eSET	Twin rates: about 5%. Pregnancy rates: maintained
Finland	No state regulation, but eSET is used in about 60% of transfers	Triplet rates: 'almost completely avoided'. Twin rates: still decreasing. Pregnancy rates: maintained
Germany, Austria, and Switzerland	In Germany, a maximum of three eggs can be cultured, no 2- to 3-day embryos can be frozen, and no embryo selection is allowed. Therefore, all embryos tend to be transferred Austria and Switzerland have similar policies although restrictions are not mandatory	Triplet rates: very high. Twin rates: very high
France, Greece, Portugal, and Spain	No formal policy. This situation is under review	n/a
Netherlands, Norway, Denmark	No state regulation. eSET is widely used	Pregnancy rates: good
Hungary	Maximum of three (or, in special cases, a maximum four) embryos can be transferred	Twin rates: about 30%
Italy	Legislation states that a maximum of three eggs can be fertilized, and all resulting embryos must be transferred	Triplet rates: rising
United Kingdom	Formal limit of number of embryos that can be transferred introduced by The Human Fertilization and Embryology Authority (HFEA) in 2004: A maximum of two embryos can be transferred in women less than 40 years of age and a maximum of three embryos in women 40 or more years old In 2009, HFEA set a maximum multiple birth target of 24%, and this target has been progressively lowered in subsequent years	Triplet rates: reduced. Twin rates: still rising
Belgium	More flexible 'prognosis-dependent guidelines' for patients and physicians. Factors such as patient age, embryo quality, and previous ART history should be considered However, patients less than 36 years old must have eSET in their first IVF cycle eSET rates are around 48%[22]	Triplet rates: 'almost completely avoided'. Twin rates: dropped to 7%. Pregnancy rates: no significant decrease

Continued

Table 11.2 Elective single embryo transfer (eSET) policies—cont'd

Country	Policy	Effect of policies
Australia	Guidelines state that a maximum of two embryos can be transferred in women less than 40 years of age. It is recommended that, in women less than 35 years of age, only one embryo is transferred on their first IVF cycle. eSET accounted for 57% of embryo transfers in 2006	Multiple-gestation pregnancy rate has been reduced to 14%. Pregnancy rates: maintained
Canada	Following continued rise in multiple-gestation pregnancies, a Canadian framework was established in 2009, which set the following targets: • Decrease the twin rate per clinic to 25% by 2012 and 15% by 2015 • Increase the proportion of elective single embryo transfer to at least 50% of good prognosis patients by 2012 • Eliminate higher order multiple births caused by assisted human reproduction by 2015[24] Clinical practice guidelines were published in 2010. Recommendations include:[25] • In women less than 35 years old with good prognosis (first or second IVF attempt with at least two good quality embryos), eSET should be performed, and eSET should be performed in any subsequent frozen–thawed transfers • In women 36–37 years old with good prognosis (especially if blastocysts are available), eSET should be considered In 2010, 12.1% of transfers were eSET[26]	In 2010, multiple pregnancy rates dropped to 24.2% (largely because of excellent rates of uptake of eSET in Quebec)[26]
United States	Voluntary guidelines were issued in 2009 in the hope of reducing the rates of multiple pregnancies, but adoption of eSET has been very slow. Recommendations include:[27] • In women less than 35 years old with good prognosis (first IVF cycle, good-quality embryos, excess embryos suitable for cryopreservation), eSET should be considered, and a maximum of two embryos should be transferred • In women 38–40 years old with good prognosis, a maximum of three cleavage-stage or two blastocyst-stage embryos should be transferred • In women 38–40 years old with poor prognosis, a maximum of four cleavage-stage or three blastocyst-stage embryos should be transferred • In women 41–42 years old, a maximum of five cleavage-stage or three blastocyst-stage embryos should be transferred Other recommendations have been made for older women and women with exceptional circumstances. However, the final decision rests with patients and their physicians.	In 2009, about 10% of transfers in patients less than 35 years of age were eSET. Triplet rates: reduced. Twin rates: continue to rise[22]

transferred rests with their fertility specialist, in clinical reality, many patients turn to us for advice because they trust our opinion. As fertility acupuncturists, we are in a position to influence what choices our patients make. It is therefore our responsibility to ensure that we provide our patients with accurate information about the risks and benefits of multiple embryo transfer to help our patients make an informed decision. It is important to note that, although fertility patients present for acupuncture at all stages of their ART treatment, many come after one or more failed ART cycles. For the majority of these patients, eSET is not the best option.

Our secondary role is to look after our patients once they are pregnant and help to minimize the risks associated with multiple-gestation pregnancies, both prenatally and postnatally. That usually means treating patients on a regular basis throughout pregnancy and ideally postdelivery. The aim of treatment is to continue addressing any imbalances identified before conception and to monitor patients for any new emerging patterns. For more information about how to manage patients during early pregnancy following ART treatment, see Chapter 14.

SUMMARY

The primary objective of ART treatment is to help a couple conceive. However, the treatment should be as safe as possible for the mother and any resulting babies. Acupuncture practitioners need to be aware of the major risks of ART and manage patients as safely as possible.

REFERENCES

1. Land JA, Evers JLH. Risks and complications in assisted reproduction techniques: report of an ESHRE consensus meeting. Hum Reprod 2003;18:455–7.

2. Brinton LA, Trabert B, Shalev V, et al. In vitro fertilization and risk of breast and gynecologic cancers: a retrospective cohort study within the Israeli Maccabi healthcare services. Fertil Steril 2013;99:1189–96.

3. Källén B, Finnström O, Lindam A, et al. Malignancies among women who gave birth after in vitro fertilization. Hum Reprod 2011;26:253–8.

4. Schats R. The application of ultrasound in fertility investigations and treatment. In: de Haan N, Spelt M, Gobel R, editors. Reproductive medicine: a textbook for paramedics. Amsterdam: Elsevier Gezondheidszorg; 2010. p. 41–56 [chapter 2].

5. Practice Committee of American Society for Reproductive Medicine. Ovarian hyperstimulation syndrome. Fertil Steril 2008;90:S188–93.

6. Mathur R. OHSS – an overview, In: Presentation to the scientific and clinical advisory committee of the HFEA, Proceedings of the HFEA, Cambridge, UK; 2011.

7. ASRM. Assisted reproductive technologies. A guide for patients. Report of the ASRM. Birmingham, Alabama; 2008.

8. Radunovic N. OHSS – old dilemma new insights, In: Proceedings of the ESHRE campus symposium. Reproductive Medicine Across Europe, Belgrade, Serbia; 2012.

9. Kasum M, Oresković S. New insights in prediction of ovarian hyperstimulation syndrome. Acta Clin Croat 2011;50:281–8.

10. Humaidan P, Quartarolo J, Papanikolaou EG. Preventing ovarian hyperstimulation syndrome: guidance for the clinician. Fertil Steril 2010;94:389–400.

11. Alper MM, Smith LP, Sills ES. Ovarian hyperstimulation syndrome: current views on pathophysiology, risk factors, prevention, and management. J Exp Clin Assist Reprod 2009;6:3.

12. Lee TH, Liu CH, Huang CC, et al. Serum anti-Müllerian hormone and estradiol levels as predictors of ovarian hyperstimulation syndrome in assisted reproduction technology cycles. Hum Reprod 2008;23:160–7.

13. Nastri CO, Ferriani RA, Rocha IA, et al. Ovarian hyperstimulation syndrome: pathophysiology and prevention. J Assist Reprod Genet 2010;27:121–8.

14. Youssef MA, van Wely M, Hassan MA, et al. Can dopamine agonists reduce the incidence and severity of OHSS in IVF/ICSI treatment cycles? A systematic review and meta-analysis. Hum Reprod Update 2010;16:459–66.

15. Royal College of Obstetricians and Gynaecologists. The management of ovarian hyperstimulation syndrome. Green-top guidelines no.5. Report of the Royal College of Obstetricians and Gynaecologists; 2006.

16. Carman N. The treatment of ovarian hyperstimulation syndrome (OHSS) with acupuncture in women undergoing assisted reproductive techniques (ART). J Chin Med 2007;85:16–25.

17. Deadman P, Al-Khafaji M, Baker K. The Kidney channel. In: A manual of acupuncture. England: Journal of Chinese Medicine Publications; 1998. p. 329–64.

18. Deadman P, Al-Khafaji M, Baker K. The Spleen channel. In: A manual of acupuncture. England: Journal of Chinese Medicine Publications; 1998. p. 175–206.

19. ASRM. Practice committee opinion: multiple pregnancy associated with infertility therapy. American Society for Reproductive Medicine. Continuing medical education for physicians. Online course. Syllabus COM003; 2012.

20. Research and evidence – facts and figures. Available from: http://www.oneatatime.org.uk/126. htm [accessed 23 September 2012].

21. Barnhart KT. Epidemiology of male and female reproductive disorders and impact on fertility regulation and population growth. Fertil Steril 2011;95:2200–3.

22. Practice Committee of the American Society for Reproductive Medicine. Elective single-embryo transfer. Fertil Steril 2012;97:835–42.

23. Research and evidence – what other countires are doing – Europe. Available from: http://www.oneatatime.org.uk/372.htm [accessed 23 September 2012].

24. Annual report – 2010–2011. Available from: http://www.ahrc-pac.gc.ca/v2/pubs/ar-ra-2010–2011-eng.php [accessed 28 September 2012].

25. Min JK, Hughes E, Young D, et al. Elective single embryo transfer following in vitro fertilization. J Obstet Gynaecol Can 2010;32:363–77.

26. Canadian Fertility and Andrology Society. Reduction of multiple pregnancy risk associated with IVF/ICSI IVF. Medical directors of Canada position statement 2012. Report of the Canadian Fertility and Andrology Society; 2012.

27. Practice Committee of the Society for Assisted Reproductive Technology. Guidelines on number of embryos transferred. Fertil Steril 2009;92:1518–9.

Chapter 12

Managing the patient with a complex medical history

REPEATED IMPLANTATION FAILURE

Overview

Definition

The European Society of Human Reproduction and Embryology (ESHRE) defines implantation failure as 'The absence of a gestational sac on ultrasound at ≥ 5 weeks post-embryo transfer' and the term *Repeated Implantation Failure* (RIF) applies after '... >3 embryo transfers of high quality embryos or the transfer of ≥ 10 embryos in multiple transfers'.[1]

Other definitions of RIF range from 2 to 4 failed embryo transfers and/or 8 to 10 transferred embryos.[2] This may mean that, in some Assisted Reproductive Technology (ART) facilities, some patients may experience twice as many embryo failures compared to patients of other facilities, which may have higher indexes of suspicion of RIF. Unfortunately, the variations in the definition mean that some patients who are subsequently diagnosed with RIF experience a significant delay before being referred for RIF investigations.

Implantation failure versus preclinical pregnancy failure

The rate of pregnancy loss prior to implantation is approximately 30% in natural cycles.[3] A further 30% of pregnancies are lost between implantation and the missed period.[3]

In IVF cycles, 49% of embryos fail to implant.[4] Of the remaining 51% that do implant, 34% of pregnancies are lost between implantation and a positive pregnancy test, 4% are lost shortly after a positive pregnancy test, and 15% of pregnancies are lost after that.[4] It is therefore important to differentiate between implantation failure and a very early pregnancy loss, which may have different aetiologies and therapeutic solutions (Figure 12.1).

Early pregnancy testing may help to differentiate between RIF and early pregnancy loss.[2] Some clinics advise their patients to do an early pregnancy test (10–14 days after the Human Chorionic Gonadotrophin (hCG) trigger injection). Urine-based tests may not be sufficiently sensitive to register low levels of hCG. Therefore, ideally, a serum hCG blood test should be performed. If hCG is detected but then fails to rise exponentially or declines, this suggests a very early pregnancy failure. If the implantation of the embryo is delayed, the rate of hCG rise is reduced, and detection occurs later in the cycle, this can indicate abnormal embryonic development occurring after implantation.[5]

When advising patients to test early, it is important to warn them about a possible false negative result. Patients who do test early also need to be prepared for the possibility that a very early positive test to become negative a few days later because of failure of the pregnancy. Testing earlier than 10 days may result in a false positive test because hCG from the trigger hCG injection may still be in the body.

Causes of RIF

Causes of RIF are classified into uterine (or maternal) factors, paternal factors (mainly sperm issues), embryo factors, and other factors, for example, an incorrect treatment protocol (Figure 12.2). This section outlines the most common causes of RIF and the therapeutic management options.

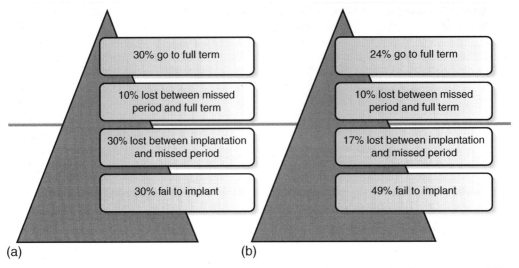

Figure 12.1 Estimates of pregnancies lost at different stages from ovulation to full term; (a) natural conceptions and (b) IVF conceptions.[3,4]

Uterine and maternal factors

As described in Chapter 3, the blastocyst is only able to implant when the endometrial surface is receptive to the embryo. This phase is referred to as an 'implantation window', and it lasts for approximately 48 h, but the exact cycle days vary in different women and in natural and stimulated cycles.[6] Approximately two-thirds of RIFs are attributed to defective endometrial receptivity and one-third to the embryo itself.[7] Endometrial receptivity can be compromised by a number of factors.

Anatomical abnormalities and hysteroscopy

Congenital uterine abnormalities are found in 5.5% of the normal female population, 8% of infertile women, 13.3% of women with a history of miscarriages, and 24.5% of women with a combined history of infertility and miscarriages.[8] Commonly, as part of the initial infertility investigations, the uterus is assessed by transvaginal ultrasound or hysterosalpingography (HSG). However, uterine abnormalities might be missed during the initial infertility investigations.[9,10]

In their review, Makrakis and Pantos found that the incidence of abnormal hysteroscopic findings in women with a history of RIFs is between 25% and 50%.[11] Common intrauterine findings in RIF are endometrial polyps, endometrial and endocervical adhesions, endometritis, uterine septa, and submucous myomas/fibroids.[10]

Hysteroscopy is a direct and definitive method of assessing intrauterine pathology (see Chapter 4 for more details). When compared with transvaginal ultrasonography (which is the usual first-line non-invasive uterine cavity assessment), hysteroscopy has been shown to detect 19%[12] to 22.2%[10] more abnormal findings, which were missed by

an ultrasound scan.[12] There is a growing body of evidence that hysteroscopy significantly increases the clinical pregnancy rate in a subsequent IVF cycle.[11,13] This seems to be the case even if no pathology was detected or treated, suggesting that the procedure itself has therapeutic value.[10,11]

Endometrial injury (biopsy or 'scratch')

Endometrial injury (biopsy or 'scratch') in the cycle before an ovarian stimulation cycle appears to improve clinical pregnancy rates in patients with unexplained RIF. A meta-analysis of seven studies and 2062 participants showed that patients who had an endometrial biopsy had a 38.1% clinical pregnancy rate compared to 36.8% in patients who only had hysteroscopy and 18.4% in patients who had no hysteroscopy or biopsy.[14] There was not enough evidence to make recommendations as to exactly when in the preceding cycle the biopsy should be done, nor if one or more injuries are necessary.[14] The endometrial injury initiates changes to the endometrium, the immune system, and gene expression, all of which help with endometrial receptivity.[14]

Interval (sequential) embryo transfer

Interval (sequential) embryo transfer is where two embryos are transferred at least 24 h apart (for example, one on day 2 and one on day 5 after egg retrieval). Several studies have shown that interval embryo transfer increases implantation rates.[15–18] The endometrial receptivity and maturation varies on different days of the luteal phase and is not an exact science. By transferring embryos on two different days, it is hypothesized that the chance of transferring the embryos when the endometrium is at its peak level of receptivity is increased.[18,19]

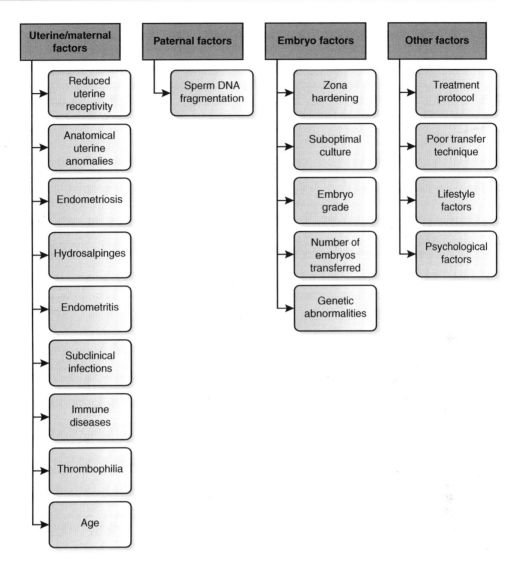

Figure 12.2 Overview of causes of RIF.

Frozen Embryo Transfer

A recent systematic review and meta-analysis of three trials and 633 IVF cycles found that Frozen Embryo Transfer (FET) results in significantly higher clinical and ongoing pregnancy rates compared with fresh IVF cycles.[20] There are two reasons why FET might work better than fresh embryo transfer. First, high levels of oestrogen resulting from ovarian stimulation may negatively affect uterine receptivity.[20–22] Second, embryos that survive cryopreservation may be stronger and, therefore, allow a form of natural selection to take place.[21]

'Embryo glue'

A 2010 Cochrane review of 16 studies with a total of 3698 participants analysed the effects of different adherence compounds in the embryo transfer media. The authors concluded that there was no evidence that fibrin sealant improved pregnancy rates or live birth rates. However, the hyaluronic acid adherence compound significantly increased clinical pregnancy rates by 8%. The rate of multiple pregnancies was also higher with hyaluronic acid. Live birth rates were not affected, and the authors attributed this lack of effect to the fact that only 4 of the 16 studies reported live birth rates.[23]

Endometriosis

A meta-analysis of 22 studies found that the pregnancy rate of women undergoing IVF because of endometriosis-related subfertility was almost half that of women with other pathologies.[24] Endometriosis is thought to affect endometrial receptivity as well as the development of the egg and the embryo.[24] Chapter 8 discusses endometriosis in greater detail.

Hydrosalpinges

Hydrosalpinx is defined as a 'collection of watery fluid in the uterine tube, occurring as the end-stage of pyosalpinx'.[25] It is strongly associated with reduced implantation.[25] The fluid within the tube is believed to be toxic to the embryo. An alternative explanation is that the fluid mechanically washes out the embryo.[25] Laparoscopic salpingectomy (removal of the affected fallopian tube(s)) prior to IVF has been shown to be beneficial.[25]

Endometrial thickness

A retrospective analysis of 2464 IVF cycles found that there was a linear relationship between endometrial thickness on the day of hCG administration and pregnancy rates, with a 29.4% pregnancy rate in women who had linings of ≤ 6 mm and 44.4% in women who had linings of ≥ 17 mm.[26] Another retrospective analysis of 768 medicated FET cycles found that implantation, clinical pregnancy, ongoing pregnancy, and live birth rates were all significantly higher in women with endometrial thickness measuring between 9 and 14 mm on the start day of progesterone supplementation.[27] Chapter 10 discusses endometrial lining thickness in greater detail.

Infections

Infections introduced inside the uterus during the embryo transfer procedure have been implicated in RIF.[28,29] The use of antibiotics before embryo transfer has not been shown to increase pregnancy rates.[28,30] Cleaning the cervix and vagina with saline liquid may help to reduce the possibility of bacterial contamination.[28]

Controversially, menstrual blood can be tested for the presence of 'hidden' intrauterine infections such as chlamydia, which a standard vaginal swab is believed to miss. A course of very strong antibiotics is prescribed for patients who test positive for infection(s).

Immune disease

Several different immune conditions may be associated with RIF.[31–38] However, the evidence is mixed and, for some conditions, controversial.

Thrombophilia

Thrombophilia is a group of different disorders that cause blood to clot abnormally.[39] Thrombophilia is linked to recurrent pregnancy loss and other pregnancy complications, such as foetal growth restriction, stillbirth, and severe preeclampsia.[39] Some studies have shown that thrombophilia is associated with RIF,[40–43] yet other studies failed to find such a link.[44,45] A 2006 literature review by the American Society for Reproductive Medicine (ASRM) concluded that antiphospholipid antibodies (acquired thrombophilia) do not negatively affect IVF success rates.[46]

Low molecular-weight heparin is the first-line treatment for thrombophilia disorders. Several studies have investigated whether heparin improves pregnancy rates in patients with a history of RIF. Some studies have shown improved success rates,[47–49] and others failed to demonstrate an improvement.[50,51]

One of the criticisms of many studies examining the link between thrombophilia and RIF is that women without clear thrombophilia are often included in the analysis. Better-quality studies are needed where only women with confirmed thrombophilia disease are included in the research methodology.

Maternal age

As women age, the rate of aneuploidy of embryos increases significantly.[52] Maternal age is an independent factor in the success rates of ART treatment when patients use their own (autologous) eggs.[53] A large retrospective analysis of 36,412 ART cycles found that for women aged 30 or older, each additional year was associated with an 11% reduction in pregnancy rates and a 13% reduction in live birth rates.[53]

In a retrospective analysis of 1263 women aged 40 or older undergoing 2705 ART cycles, cumulative birth rates varied from 28.4% if starting treatment at the age of 40 to 0% by age 46.[54] The effect is even more pronounced in women aged 43 or older, with live birth rates of 1.1% in women aged 43 or older[55] and in women aged 45 or older only 0.5%[56] to 0.7%.[57]

However, what may give some hope to older prospective mothers is that other factors such as menstrual cycle length may be even more important than maternal age. A prospective study of 6271 IVF/Intracytoplasmic Sperm Injection (ICSI) treatment cycles showed a direct significant relationship between mean cycle length and implantation, the response to ovarian stimulation, and pregnancy and live birth rates even after adjusting for women's age, with live birth rates almost double in women who had cycle lengths of >34 days compared with women who had cycle lengths of <26 days.[58]

The grade of an embryo rather than a woman's age is a better predictor of pregnancy rates following IVF according to the results of a prospective study of 10,000 embryo transfers.[59]

Mild IVF (see Chapter 9), androgen/dehydroepiandrosterone supplementation, preimplantation genetic screening (PGS), and egg donation are possible strategies for dealing with advanced maternal age and IVF.[60] Embryo banking is another viable strategy.[61]

Male factor

Male factor is associated with high order (≥ 6) RIFs.[62] High levels of sperm DNA fragmentation is linked to reduced pregnancy rates following IVF[63,64] and IVF/ICSI.[65,66] DNA fragmentation may be due to advanced paternal age or other environmental factors, increased levels of reactive oxygen species (ROS), toxins, varicoceles, and exogenous heat.[67] Some authors recommend that couples who have RIF have the man's sperm cells tested for DNA fragmentation.[68] However, due to the low predictive ability of DNA fragmentation testing to identify subsequent pregnancies, the ASRM does not recommend routine use of the procedure.[69]

The use of the Intracytoplasmic Morphologically Selected Sperm Injection (IMSI) may help to overcome high DNA fragmentation problems (see Chapter 6 for details about ICSI and IMSI).[68] For example, in one very recent cohort study, it was found that using IMSI in patients who failed to conceive following ICSI increased their chances of pregnancy and live birth rate almost threefold.[70]

Chapter 7 provides information on the possible use of antioxidant supplements in cases where there is DNA damage caused by ROSs. In severe cases of male factor genetic abnormalities, donor sperm may be required.

Embryo factors

Zona hardening and assisted hatching

Assisted hatching may be helpful in patients with RIF (see Chapter 6 for more details on assisted hatching).

Inadequate culture conditions

The quality of culture media used by the fertility clinic may affect embryo development and therefore subsequent implantation rates.[71,72] There are many different culture media available, containing between 11 and more than 30 different components.[72] A recent meta-analysis of 22 RCTs that evaluated 31 different formulations could not make any recommendations as to which media produce better results.[73] This was in part due to nearly all trials comparing different culture media and also studies reported different outcome measures (some reported live birth rates and some clinical pregnancy rates).[73] The authors of the review concluded that more better-quality studies are needed and new and better culture media need to be developed.[73]

Blastocysts versus day 2 versus day 3 transfer

A Cochrane review of 23 RCTs concluded that blastocyst (day 5/6) transfer is associated with increased live birth rates when compared to cleavage (day 2/3) stage embryo transfer.[74] Another Cochrane review assessed day 2 and day 3 transfers and found no difference in live birth rates between them.[75] However, day 2 transfer may produce better results in poor responders.[76,77]

Zygote Intra Fallopian Transfer

It has been suggested that Zygote Intra Fallopian Transfer (ZIFT) may be an effective alternative to standard IVF in patients with RIF,[78] the presumption being that the embryo would develop better in a natural environment and that ZIFT helps to overcome issues of difficult embryo transfers.[71] However, a meta-analysis of 6 RCTs and 548 cycles found no difference in implantation rates or pregnancy rates between ZIFT and IVF.[79]

Number of embryos transferred

In the United Kingdom over the past three decades, the incidence of multiple pregnancies has increased considerably. In 1978 they accounted for one in every 100 births, while by 2004 one in every 67 births was a multiple pregnancy.[80] Many other countries have seen similar increases. However, there is a greater risk of morbidity[81,82] and mortality[82] in multiple-gestation pregnancy babies conceived following ART. Multiple-gestation pregnancies also increase the risk of maternal morbidity. To reduce the rates of multiple-gestation pregnancies following ART, many countries have issued guidelines and some countries have introduced legal limits on how many embryos should be transferred (see Chapter 11).

However, research shows that elective single embryo transfer (eSET) has a lower rate of live birth. A meta-analysis by Baruffi *et al.* concluded that fresh double embryo transfer (DET) resulted in 1.64–2.60 times greater ongoing pregnancy rates and 1.44–2.42 times greater live birth rates compared to eSET.[83] A Cochrane review the same year concluded that eSET is associated with lower live birth rates when compared with DET.[84] Analysis of 124,148 IVF cycles showed that the live birth rate in women aged ≥ 40 was significantly lower with eSET compared to DET.[85] However, live birth rates did not increase with three embryos, but was associated with an increased risk of perinatal morbidity.[85]

Therefore, in couples with RIF a DET may maximize the chances of a live birth, while also balancing the risks associated with a multiple-gestation pregnancy.

Genetic causes: Parental

Chromosomal abnormalities are found in 1.14%[86] to 1.3%[87] of subfertile female partners and 1.5% of male partners.[87] This is a higher incidence than in the general population.[86,87] When comparing the incidence of chromosomal abnormalities in patients with RIF (transfer of ≥ 10 embryos) and ≥ 3 consecutive first-trimester miscarriages, the rates of chromosomal abnormalities were 2.5% in RIF and 4.7% in miscarriage patients.[88] In patients with ≥ 16 RIFs and ≥ 15 embryo transfers, the rate of parental chromosomal abnormalities is even higher at 15.4%.[89] Therefore, it is recommend that karyotyping should be undertaken in RIF patients.[88,89]

If a partner is found to have a structural genetic abnormality, he or she may be offered preimplantation genetic testing (PGT), amniocentesis, or chorionic villus sampling to detect genetic abnormalities in offspring. Available interventions include preimplantation genetic diagnosis (PGD) or the use of donor gametes.[67] Comparative genomic hybridization (CGH), however, should not be offered to patients with RIF, because it cannot detect balanced translocations.[68]

Genetic abnormalities: Embryo

Some couples experience RIF, even after the transfer of seemingly good-quality embryos. Conceivably, these embryos may be genetically abnormal. PGS is a procedure where one or more nuclei from eggs or embryo cells (blastomeres or trophoectoderm) are removed for genetic testing.[90]

There are two main types of genetic screening of embryos: PGD and PGS. PGD is recommended for patients at high risk of transmitting a genetic or chromosomal abnormality to their offspring.[90,91] PGS is reserved for couples who are known or presumed to have normal chromosomes, but their embryos are still screened for aneuploidy.[90] The ESHRE recommends PGS for IVF patients with a history of RIF, miscarriages (but normal parental karyotyping), and in women of advanced maternal age.[1] However, the ASRM currently does not recommend PGS in patients with RIF due to the contradictory evidence base for its ability to help improve pregnancy rates.[90]

Another method of genetic screening is Fluorescence In Situ Hybridization (FISH). FISH is used to check for missing or excessive chromosomal material in eggs (if the female partner is a carrier) or in the embryo (if both partners are carriers) in patients known to have genetic abnormalities.[90] FISH can also be used for embryo sexing for x-linked diseases or social reasons such as gender selection.[92] However, the application of FISH is limited by the number of chromosomes it can examine[93] and is not recommended.[71,90]

The CGH genetic screening method may overcome some of the limitations of PGS and FISH.[71] CGH cannot detect all types of abnormalities.[93] It is a time-consuming procedure with the embryos needing to be cryopreserved.

Newer methods of genetic embryo screening are emerging.[93] However, it will be some time before evidence is available about their effectiveness.

Non-invasive embryo assessment (morphokinetic analysis)

Normally, embryos are assessed by an embryologist at distinct points in time, usually chosen for the convenience of the clinical facility, rather than for biologically relevant reasons.[94] Identification of better-quality embryos is now possible with new non-invasive technologies. For example, time-lapse microscopy (TLM) has been developed, where through an embryoscope an embryo's development is monitored by capturing frequent images (every 20 min, 5 min, or even at 10 s intervals).[94] From these images, the embryo's appearance (morphology) and its cellular development (kinetics) are analysed either by an embryologist or by computer software (e.g., Early Embryo Viability Assessment or EEVA™), with the procedure known as morphokinetic analysis.[95,96]

A recent study by Campbell et al. showed that TLM analysis can be used to predict embryo aneuploidy.[97] If the first cellular division happens before 26 ± 1 h in ICSI and 28 ± 1 h in IVF, this is associated with better numbers and quality of blastocysts and higher pregnancy rates.[98] This information could be potentially missed with traditional embryo monitoring methods, whereas with TLM monitoring this would be accurately recorded, and embryos that reach the relevant developmental milestones at the right time would be transferred.

Other causes

Treatment protocol

Tailoring the stimulation protocol has been suggested to help improve implantation rates.[71,78,99] For example, the use of a Gonadotrophin Releasing Hormone (GnRH) agonist has been proposed to be preferable in poor responders[100] and in RIF.[101] However, there is little evidence to suggest that any particular protocol is the best. For example, a 2011 Cochrane review compared the use of GnRH antagonist protocol against the GnRH agonist protocol. No statistically significant difference in live birth rate was found. However, there was a significant reduction in the incidence of Ovarian Hyperstimulation Syndrome (OHSS) with GnRH antagonist protocol. Thus the GnRH antagonist protocol is probably more suitable for women at risk of OHSS.[102] There may be a case, however, for trying a different protocol in patients with RIF or with a history of poor ovarian response, in case a new protocol produces a different outcome in their individual cases.

The dose of ovarian stimulation medication should also be individualized on the basis of patient's ovarian reserve markers (Follicle Stimulating Hormone and Anti-Müllerian Hormone levels and antral follicle count scan results) and the patient's previous history of response to stimulation medication.

While synthetic progesterone is superior to micronized progesterone, there is no evidence that any particular way of administering progesterone supplementation is superior.[103]

Poor embryo transfer techniques

There are lower success rates with difficult embryo trans-fers,[104–106] possibly because difficult transfers induce uterine contractions[28,107] or because of iatrogenesis to the embryo during the transfer procedure. Chapter 10 provides more details about difficult embryo transfers.

Lifestyle factors

Poor lifestyle factors (for example smoking, obesity, a nutritionally poor diet, exposure to environmental toxins) may also increase the risk of RIF. See Chapter 7 for greater discussion of these.

Psychological

A recent meta-analysis of 31 studies found that there was small but significant association between stress, distress, and pregnancy rates following ART treatment.[108] Reducing the stress response and improving the ability to cope with anxiety and depression may enhance conception in some patients with RIF.[109] Chapter 7 discusses stress in greater detail.

Clinical perspective

Opinions vary about if and when to do additional tests in patients with RIF. One study found that 32% of ART clinics would not undertake any additional investigations,[110] and those that do may not offer all of the available tests. It is therefore logical to assume that some patients managed by such clinics keep having treatment cycles and keep failing to conceive. Other patients may give up, not realizing that there may be other options available to them. The timing of when tests are undertaken also varies. Some clinics carry out additional tests as part of the initial investigations, some after one failed IVF, and others after three or more failed cycles.

Deciding when additional investigations should be undertaken may need careful consideration, for example, the age and/or ovarian reserve of the female partner. So if a female partner has a reduced ovarian reserve, waiting for three or four failed IVF cycles (which are likely to take around a year) will only serve to exacerbate the problem of reduced ovarian reserve. The cost of treatment also needs to be factored into the decision-making equation. Patients may not be able to afford the cost of three or four cycles of IVF. The degree of psychological distress of the couple cannot be ignored.

CLINICAL TIPS

RIF INVESTIGATION REFERRAL

Not all ART units are willing to investigate RIF or have the means and treatments available to do so. Find out which ART units have expertise in RIF and refer patients to those clinics.

RIF from a TCM point of view

Introduction

RIF following ART is a very recent concept in Traditional Chinese Medicine (TCM) with very few good-quality publications available. Therefore, some of the material in this section will be based on our experience of this topic. Hopefully, encouraging discussion in the acupuncture profession will lead to good-quality studies being undertaken.

Acupuncture may potentially play an important role in RIF, as demonstrated in a recent study. A prospective RCT of acupuncture in RIF patients (≥ 2 failed cycles) showed that the clinical pregnancy rate in the acupuncture group ($n = 28$) was significantly higher than in the control ($n = 28$) and sham ($n = 28$) groups (35.7% vs. 7.1% vs. 10.7%, respectively).[111]

Common syndromes causing RIF

TCM syndromes associated with RIF include:

- Kidney Yin Deficiency[112,113]
- Kidney Yang Deficiency[112,113]
- Liver and Spleen Blood Deficiency[113]
- Liver Qi Stagnation[112,113]
- Blood Stasis[112,113]
- Phlegm-Damp[112,113]

In the authors' experience, RIF may also be due to:

- Spleen Qi Deficiency
- Kidney Jing (Essence) Deficiency
- Cold-Uterus
- Empty or Full Heat/Fire

TCM pathophysiology of RIF

Kidney pathology

Deficiencies in Kidney Jing (Essence), Yin, or Yang can adversely affect the quality of an embryo. This may stop the embryo from developing in the laboratory or soon after the transfer. If the embryo continues to develop, maternal Kidney pathologies can affect the circulation of Jing (Essence), Qi, Blood, and essential Yin and Yang energies required for the baby to continue to develop. Kidney deficiencies can also weaken the energy of the Extraordinary Vessels, in particular the Chong and Ren Mai (Penetrating and Conception Vessels), which in turn can reduce the amount and flow of nourishment getting to the Uterus and the embryo, thus preventing embryonic growth.

Kidney Yang Deficiency is also associated with the decline of Ming Men (Life Fire). When Ming Men fails to warm the Zangfu organs, it can impair the Extraordinary Vessels.[112] The embryo's vitality as well as the role of the

Uterus in facilitating conception is also impaired. Kidney (and Spleen) Yang Deficiency can also adversely affect the luteal phase, thus impairing implantation.[113]

As already discussed, a considerable proportion of RIFs can be attributed to the quality of embryos (pre-conceptual factors) and the interaction between the embryo and its mother. The transfer of embryos that are weak in Kidney Jing (Essence) (for example, due to parental weakness of Jing (Essence) being passed onto the embryos) fails to resolve such deficiency and may therefore result in a failure. Furthermore, in these cases, maternal Jing (Essence) is likely to be weak, so the embryo(s) are thus transferred into an environment unfavourable for conception and growth.

Congenital anatomical uterine anomalies, which are common in patients with RIF, may well indicate congenital Kidney pathology. However, it is unlikely that we can correct these with acupuncture. Table 12.1 lists signs and symptoms and treatment of Kidney pathology.

Liver pathology

The Chong and Ren Mai (Penetrating and Conception Vessels) supply and coordinate Qi, Blood, and Jing (Essence) to the Uterus to support the embryo's gestation.[116] Liver Blood Deficiency and Qi Stagnation can alter the amount, flow, and quality of Qi and Blood circulation in the Extraordinary Vessels.[116] When the Uterus lacks the optimal level of nourishment, ultimately so may the embryo. Stagnation blocks Qi and Blood in the Uterus and prevents implantation.

The embryo needs to attach to the endometrium and establish a stable connection to receive nutrition. Blood Deficiency and Stagnation make this difficult. Successful attachment also depends on changes in the endometrium. The endometrium can fail due to disordered functioning of Qi and Blood in the Uterus. Blood Deficiency may reduce the thickness of the endometrial lining, thus adversely affecting implantation.[113,117] Liver Qi Stagnation,[113] particularly when the woman is more acutely distressed at the time of the transfer, superimposed on chronic stagnation, may contribute to problems at the time of the embryo transfer and reduce pregnancy rates. Fibroids and polyps are associated with Liver Qi Stagnation and Spleen Deficiency, although fibroids and polyps may also be associated with generalized Qi Stagnation and Blood Stasis or Yin Deficiency and Empty-Fire Blazing.[118] Table 12.1 lists the signs and symptoms and treatment of Liver pathology.

Heart pathology

Heart Qi or Blood Deficiency and Stagnation frequently arise from the psychological distress of repeated failed IVF cycles. This can impair the vitality, circulation, and quality of Blood and Qi in the Uterus and reduce the embryo's chances of implantation.

The embryo signals its existence to the mother. Signalling ensures that the embryo's existence is acknowledged, thereby averting luteal regression. Heart pathology compromises the embryo's vitality and ability to initiate, and therefore facilitate, implantation, and the mother is unable to respond. Table 12.1 lists signs and symptoms and treatment of Heart pathology.

Spleen pathology

Spleen Qi Deficiency weakens the Extraordinary Vessels and reduces the nourishment available for the survival of the embryo. Spleen Qi Sinking fails to hold the embryo in the Uterus. Table 12.1 lists signs and symptoms and the treatment of Spleen pathology.

Blood Stasis

Free flow of Blood is required for the embryo's development and implantation into the endometrium. Blood Stasis blocks the flow of Blood and Qi, thereby reducing the quality, composition, and regeneration of Blood.[112] Blood Stasis damages the Ren and Chong Mai (Conception and Penetrating Vessels) and the Uterus.[112] Qi Stagnation and Blood Stasis affect the receptivity of the endometrium to the blastocyst and early pregnancy loss may result. Table 12.1 lists the signs and symptoms and the treatment of Blood Stasis pathology.

INTERESTING FACTS

BLOOD STASIS AND INFERTILITY

In medieval China, women unable to conceive were treated with vaginal suppositories and Uterus rinsing decoctions to correct Blood dysfunction in the Uterus.[119]

Cold

Cold harms Blood.[120] Cold, combined with Damp, can block the Uterus, thereby damaging the Chong and Ren Mai (Penetrating and Conception Vessels). A Cold-Uterus pathology prevents the free flow of Blood and coagulates and blocks Blood and Jing (Essence). Table 12.1 lists the signs and symptoms and the treatment of Cold pathology.

Phlegm-Damp

Fluids can become overabundant and overwhelm the Uterus[112] and the embryo. Phlegm-Damp generates congestion and poor circulation of Jing (Essence), Qi, and Blood. Therefore, the embryo loses the essential nourishment required for its growth and implantation. Phlegm-Damp can also obstruct the Uterus, so that the blastocyst lacks a clear attachment site. Table 12.1 lists the signs and symptoms and the treatment of Phlegm-Damp pathology.

Table 12.1 Syndrome differentiation and treatment in RIF patients

	Signs and symptoms	Associated with	Acupuncture (any time before embryo transfer)	Acupuncture (after embryo transfer)
Kidney Jing (Essence) Deficiency	Fearful, weak constitution Pulse: fine, weak, deep Tongue: pale, short	Older age Poor sperm parameters Low number of eggs or embryos	REN4, ZIGONG, KID13, KID3, ST27, LIV3 +moxibustion	BL23, BL52, BL18, BL20, BL22, DU4 +moxibustion
Kidney Yin Deficiency	Restless, thin body Pulse: fine, deep, weak Tongue: red, cracks	Older age Poor sperm parameters Low number of eggs or embryos	LU7 + KID6, REN12, REN7, SP6, P6	REN4, HE6, ST25, ST36, SP6
Kidney Yang Deficiency	Bright pale complexion, lethargy, cold hands and feet Pulse: right rear position weak Tongue: pale, swollen, wet	Older age Fertilization issues Reproductive immunological diagnosis Preclinical pregnancy loss First-trimester miscarriage	ST28, REN6, ST36, BL23, BL52, DU4 +moxibustion	BL23, BL52, DU4, DU20 +moxibustion
Liver Blood Deficiency and Qi Stagnation	Dull complexion, upset, crying and/or moodiness, unhappy, suppressed emotion Pulse: thin, choppy, wiry Tongue: pale (especially sides), red or normal	Diminishing ovarian reserve Low number of eggs or embryos	ST29, REN4, LIV3, SP6, LIV8, P6, SP10, ST30 +moxibustion (if no Heat signs)	LIV3, P6, ST30, DU20
Heart Qi Stagnation	Very emotional and anxious Pulse: thready, choppy Tongue: red tip	Psychological stress Poor fertilization rate Low number of embryos	HE5, HE6, P5, P6, KID5, ST36	REN14, REN15, REN16, REN17
Shen (Spirit) Affected	Dull eyes, anxious, restless, and fearful Pulse: moving, weak, fine Tongue: red tip	Psychological stress Older maternal age Poor fertilization rate Low number of embryos	HE6, KID4, HE4, SP4, ST25, REN15, REN16, REN17	YINTANG, DU24, KID3
Spleen Qi Deficiency	Complexion sallow, tired, reduced appetite, poor digestion Pulse: empty, soft Tongue: pale	Poor embryo development	TITUO, SP3, ST36, LU7, REN12, REN4 +moxibustion	TITUO, REN12, LU7, ST36, REN4 + moxibustion
Cold-Uterus	Feeling of cold, likes warmth Pulse: wiry, deep-slow, tight Tongue: white coat, blue body	Poor fertilization rate Poor embryo development Hardening of the zona pellucida (embryo's shell) and therefore reduces the embryo's ability to hatch Reduced endometrial receptivity	ST28, ZIGONG, REN8, REN4, ST30, DU4 +moxibustion + ginger[114]	BL23, BL52, DU4 +moxibustion
Blood Stasis	Dark complexion and circles under the eyes, lower abdominal pain after egg collection Pulse: wiry, thin Tongue: purple, dark red	Thrombophilia	ST29, LIV3, SP10, SP6, LIV2, KID14, SP8, REN3 If Heat from Blood Stasis use KID8, LIV4, SJ5	ST29, SP10, P6, BL17, BL18, BL23 Assess risks vs. benefits when strongly moving Blood[115] If Heat from Blood Stasis use KID8, LIV4, SJ5

Continued

Table 12.1 Syndrome differentiation and treatment in RIF patients—cont'd

	Signs and symptoms	Associated with	Acupuncture (any time before embryo transfer)	Acupuncture (after embryo transfer)
Blood-Heat	Feeling hot and agitated, dry mouth or throat, red colour on face Pulse: rapid, overflowing, slippery or normal Tongue: red, heat spots	Thrombophilia Reproductive immunological problems Poor fertilization rate	P7, LIV2, SP10, KID27, SP6	LI11, BL17, BL18
Phlegm-Damp	Overweight, sensation of heaviness Pulse: wiry, fine, slippery Tongue: swollen, raised, thin/thick coating	Poor egg quality and low numbers Hydrosalpinges	ST29, ST40, ST36, SP6, GB26	LU7, BL20, BL23 + moxibustion

Blood-Heat

Heat harms Qi[120] and Blood. Blood-Heat negatively affects implantation.[117] Heat/Fire forces the flow of Blood, stimulates and heats Blood, and can in some cases create Blood Stasis or Phlegm. Maternal Heat 'parches' or 'scorches' the embryo.[121] Table 12.1 lists signs and symptoms and treatment of Blood-Heat pathology.

The acupuncturist's role in the management of RIF

When treating RIF patients, acupuncturists may need to:

- Review the Orthodox medical management of their patients and potentially make recommendations.
- Refer for RIF tests and investigations where appropriate.
- Provide or reinforce advice on pre-conceptual care to increase the chances of successful ART treatment.
- Help to manage patients' stress levels.

Figure 12.3 provides a detailed algorithm on RIF patients management, and Appendix I provides an IVF audit tool, which can be used to help review each case.

Case study

Repeated Implantation Failure

Louise had six failed cycles of IVF/ICSI. Each time she had two good grade embryos transferred. The Orthodox medical cause of subfertility was male factor. After three failed cycles, Louise underwent a range of RIF investigations, all of which came back as normal.

Case study—cont'd

On the seventh IVF cycle, Louise decided to try acupuncture treatment alongside IVF in order to increase the chances of her embryos implanting. (Her husband was reluctant to have acupuncture.) Louise's TCM diagnosis was Spleen Qi Deficiency. She conceived following this treatment cycle.

Two years later Louise and her husband decided to try for a sibling for their son. The original syndrome had now progressed. She was suffering with Damp alongside pre-existing Spleen Qi Deficiency as well as Liver Blood Deficiency and had minor signs of Kidney pathology, presumably in part caused by breastfeeding her baby for a year, being drained from looking after her baby and being 2 years older. Treatment now focused on treating these syndromes in addition to IVF acupuncture protocols. Louise became pregnant with her second child and now has two healthy children.

MISCARRIAGES AND PREGNANCY LOSS

Background and terminology

A clinical pregnancy is a pregnancy diagnosed by ultrasonographic visualization of one or more gestational sacs or definitive clinical signs of pregnancy. The definition of a clinical pregnancy also includes an ectopic pregnancy![122] Miscarriage is probably the most common complication of an early pregnancy. It is estimated that 15–25% of pregnancies will result in clinical miscarriages.[67] Miscarriages

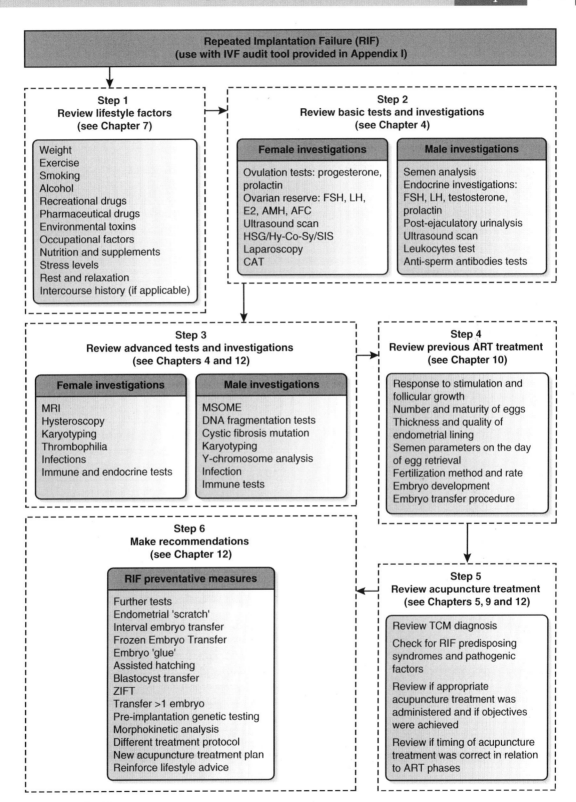

Figure 12.3 RIF algorithm.

are classified according to when they happen and the number of consecutive miscarriages:

- **Spontaneous clinical miscarriage** (also referred to as a spontaneous abortion): a clinical pregnancy loss before 24 weeks' gestation.[123]
- **Spontaneous preclinical miscarriage**: a pregnancy that is diagnosed by the detection of hCG in serum or urine, but that does not develop into a clinical pregnancy.[124]
- **Missed miscarriage** (also known as a blighted ovum): a clinical miscarriage where the pregnancy is nonviable but is not expelled spontaneously.[122]
- **Recurrent miscarriages (RMs)**: usually, two or more consecutive clinical pregnancy losses.[67,122] However, some experts feel that a diagnosis of RMs should only be made after three or more consecutive miscarriages.[123] Less than 5% of couples will experience two consecutive miscarriages and only 1% will experience three or more.[67]

Different expert bodies offer different recommendations regarding the timing of RM investigations. The ASRM recommends that clinical investigations should be undertaken following two first-trimester pregnancy losses.[67] In the United Kingdom, the Royal College of Obstetricians and Gynaecologists (RCOG) recommends investigations after three consecutive first-trimester miscarriages or after one second-trimester miscarriage.[123]

The rates of clinical miscarriages following IVF are higher compared to the rates of miscarriage in natural conceptions (a range of 21.7–23.5% vs. a range of 10–15%, respectively).[125,126] There are several hypotheses that attempt to explain these different rates. One hypothesis posits that women undergoing ART treatment tend to test earlier. If they miscarry shortly after testing positive, they will know that they were pregnant, whereas in a natural conception, pregnancy may have gone unnoticed and any bleeding would be perceived as a late period.[125] Another hypothesis is that women who get pregnant following IVF on average tend to be older. The risk of miscarriages is greater in older women. For example, a rate of 17.6% in women younger than 30 years old rising to a rate of 39.1% in women more than 40 years old.[125] The underlying pathology that causes subfertility is also implicated in miscarriages.[125]

Causes of miscarriages

Embryo genetic abnormalities and parental age

Age-related miscarriages are thought to be caused by the aneuploidy of embryos, where an embryo losses or gains one or more chromosome(s).[124] Pregnancies in older women, who are recipients of an egg donated by a younger woman, have similar rates of miscarriages to that of younger women.[67] This indicates that age has a detrimental effect on the quality of eggs and embryos and that women

who miscarry are less likely to have had their miscarriage caused by uterine issues. Up to 60% of first-trimester spontaneous miscarriages are believed to be due to embryonic chromosomal abnormalities.[67]

Both maternal and paternal ages are independent risk factors for miscarriages.[123] One study analysed 634,272 women and 1,221,546 pregnancy outcomes and found that the rate of spontaneous miscarriages was directly associated with maternal age (Figure 12.4).[127] In this study the rate of spontaneous miscarriages in women under 35 years old was around 7%, rising to 27% in women older than 45 years of age (Figure 12.4).[127] However, the risk of embryo aneuploidy is lower in women with RMs, irrespective of maternal age.[67,128] This is because chromosomal abnormalities are unlikely to cause three miscarriages in a row.

Paternal age is implicated in miscarriages.[123] In one study that retrospectively analysed outcomes of 3174 pregnancies, it was found that the risk of miscarriages was greatest in couples where a woman was aged ≥35 years and a man aged ≥40 years.[129]

Parental genetic abnormalities

Parental genetic abnormalities are observed in approximately 4% of couples with RM (compared to 0.2% in the general population).[130] It is recommended that both partners in a couple with a history of RM should undergo peripheral karyotyping in order to exclude a possibility of any balanced structural chromosomal abnormalities such as balanced reciprocal translocations and Robertsonian translocations.[67]

If a partner is found to have structural genetic abnormality, she may be offered PGT, amniocentesis, or chorionic villus sampling to detect genetic abnormalities in the offspring. Treatment options include PGD or use of donor gametes. Genetic counselling is also indicated. Routine pre-implantation embryo aneuploidy screening is not currently recommended.[67] Chapter 4 provides more information about parental genetic testing and embryo genetic testing is described later in this chapter.

Anatomical factors

Congenital uterine abnormalities are more common in women with a history of RMs, especially second-trimester pregnancy loss. Congenital uterine abnormalities are found in 12.6% of women with RM (compared to 4.3% of women with normal fertility).[67] Congenital uterine abnormalities are also associated with preterm labour, foetal malpresentation, and increased risk of caesarean delivery.[67]

The most common congenital uterine abnormalities associated with miscarriages are:[67]

- Uterine septum (risk of pregnancy loss 44.3%)
- Bicornuate uterus (risk of pregnancy loss 36.0%)
- Arcuate uterus (risk of pregnancy loss 25.7%)

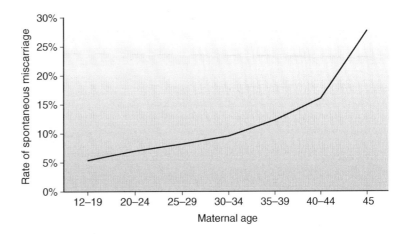

Figure 12.4 Rate of spontaneous miscarriages relative to maternal age.[127]

A uterine septum (where the uterine cavity is partitioned by a complete or incomplete wedge like longitudinal septum) is the most common uterine abnormality with the highest risk of pregnancy loss. A complete septum divides the cervix into two. Research shows that uterine septum is associated primarily with early (≤13 weeks) and less so with late (14–22 weeks) miscarriages, and with pregnancy losses of around 54% and 12%, respectively.[131] Patients who are found to have uterine septum prior to pregnancy would benefit from metroplasty, surgical resection of the septum.

Women with a bicornuate uterus (a 'heart shaped' uterus) have significantly higher rates of infertility, miscarriages, and combined infertility and miscarriages, compared to women in the general population, with a frequency of 0.4% (normal population) vs. 1.1% (infertility) vs. 2.1% (miscarriages) vs. 4.7% (infertility and miscarriages).[8]

An arcuate uterus is where the uterine fundus has a concave shape toward the uterine cavity and is mainly associated with second-trimester miscarriage.[123]

Congenital uterine abnormalities are usually picked up by HSG and can be evaluated more fully by 3D ultrasound imaging, hysteroscopy, or Magnetic Resonance Imaging scan. The RCOG recommends that all women with recurrent first-trimester miscarriages and all women with one or more second-trimester miscarriages should have their uterine cavity assessed using ultrasound.[123] Any suspected abnormalities should be evaluated further using hysteroscopy, laparoscopy, or a 3D ultrasound scan.[123]

Acquired uterine conditions, although the existing evidence is inconclusive, including such conditions as adhesions, Asherman syndrome, fibroids, and polyps, have been suggested to increase the risk of pregnancy loss.

Asherman's syndrome is where the uterine cavity is affected by post-traumatic adhesions,[130] for example, post-abortal or postpartum curettage.[132] These adhesions affect endometrial receptivity resulting in a foetal survivial rate estimated to be 30%.[132] Asherman syndrome usually presents as amenorrhoea or very scant menstruation. Diagnosis is confirmed by HSG or hysteroscopy.[132] Minor adhesions can be surgically corrected, but extensive dense fibrosis suggests a poor prognosis.[130]

In their extensive literature review Li *et al.* (2002) concluded that submucous fibroids significantly compromise reproductive outcome, whereas intramural and subserosal may possibly mildly compromise the reproduction outcomes. Removing submucous and intramural fibroids reduces the rate of miscarriages.[130]

The ASRM recommends that serious acquired uterine defects should be surgically corrected, if feasible. If surgical repair is not possible, ASRM recommend the use of a gestational carrier.[67]

Cervical weakness or insufficiency is a condition where the cervix shortens and dilates prematurely; this is strongly associated with second-trimester pregnancy losses.[123] Section 'Preterm birth and cervical insufficiency' discusses this in greater detail.

Infections

The ASRM acknowledges that *Ureaplasma urealyticum, Mycoplasma hominis, Chlamydia, Listeria monocytogenes, Toxoplasma gondii, Rubella virus, Cytomegalovirus,* and *herpes virus* are found more frequently in vaginal and cervical cultures and serum in women with a history of spontaneous miscarriages.[67] However, the ASRM does not recommend routine infection testing in RM or the use of empiric antibiotics due to lack of evidence that these infections actually cause RM.[67]

This ASRM approach is not supported by all experts. An alternative approach they suggest is that patients with RM should be screened for vaginal infections and daily vaginal pH measurements should be done.[133] More controversially, menstrual blood can be tested for presence of 'hidden' intra-uterine infections such as *Chlamydia*, which may be missed when using a standard vaginal swab. A course of microorganism specific antibiotics of high potency is prescribed for patients who test positive.

Bacterial vaginosis (BV) is one of the most common causes of abnormal vaginal discharge in women of child-bearing age.[134] It is associated with:

- Up to 40% of births before 32 weeks gestation[135]
- Early miscarriages (at or shortly after implantation) following IVF[134]
- Miscarriages of natural pregnancies before 16 weeks' gestation
- Urinary tract infections (UTIs)
- A history of infertility[136]

Some experts recommend that one BV screening in early pregnancy is sufficient to identify women at risk of preterm birth.[136] Others recommend another test shortly after embryo transfer, in the event of infection introduction during IVF procedures.[134]

CLINICAL TIPS

PREVENTION OF INFECTIONS DURING ROUTINE INVESTIGATIONS

Patients should always be prescribed prophylactic antibiotics when undergoing invasive investigations, such as HSG, just in case infection is introduced during the procedure.

Acquired and inherited thrombophilia

Thrombophilia is a group of different disorders that make blood clot abnormally.[39] These are subdivided into two types: acquired and inherited. The main type of acquired thrombophilia is Antiphospholipid Syndrome. Between 5% and up to as many as 42% of women with RM will test positive for antiphospholipid antibodies.[67] These antibodies affect the trophoblast and cause a maternal inflammatory response.[67]

There are many different discrete genetic clotting mutations, but not all have been linked to reproductive health issues. Protein S deficiency, activated protein C resistance, Factor V Leiden (homozygous and heterozygous), Prothrombin G20210A, and Hyperhomocysteinaemia have been strongly linked to either early or late pregnancy loss.[137] However, the ASRM recommends testing for inherited thrombophilia only in women with RM and *a personal history of venous thromboembolism in the setting of a non-recurrent risk factor (such as surgery) or a first-degree relative with a known or suspected high-risk thrombophilia*.[67]

Chapter 4 discusses thrombophilia testing in greater detail.

Endocrine factors

Endocrine disorders have been linked to recurrent pregnancy loss.[138] The most common ones are Polycystic Ovary Syndrome (PCOS), thyroid disease, and luteal phase deficiency.[138] Uncontrolled diabetes mellitus and hyperprolactinaemia have also been linked to pregnancy loss.[130,139]

Polycystic Ovary Syndrome

It is estimated that there is a threefold rise in the risk of miscarriage in PCOS patients.[140] However, not all studies support the link between PCOS and miscarriages.[141–143] The conflicting results may be in part due to different criteria and definitions of Polycystic Ovaries (PCO)/PCOS used in research studies.[144] It has been posited that PCOS may possibly cause miscarriages because of abnormal ovarian morphology, elevated Luteinizing Hormone levels, elevated androgen levels, hyperinsulinaemia, and insulin resistance and obesity.[144] Chapter 8 discusses PCOS in greater detail.

Hypothyroidism and thyroid autoimmunity

RM is significantly associated with thyroid disease and anti-thyroid antibodies.[138] Therefore, women with RM should be screened for thyroid disease. Chapter 8 discusses thyroid disease in greater detail.

Luteal phase insufficiency

The luteal phase requires adequate secretions of progesterone by the corpus luteum and adequate response to it by the endometrium (Chapter 2 described in detail luteal phase physiology).[138] In luteal phase deficiency this process is suboptimal, perhaps due to poor follicular development, poor corpus luteum function, or inadequate endometrial function.[138] Luteal phase insufficiency may be implicated in 20–60% of miscarriages.[132] Other diseases, such as thyroid and prolactin disorders, obesity, and ovarian aging may interfere with luteal function.[145]

There are no gold standard tests that can help to diagnose luteal phase deficiency. Measurements of progesterone levels are not helpful, because progesterone secretions are pulsatile, and the levels may vary up to sevenfold in a space of a few hours.[146,147] Basal Body Temperature (BBT) charting and endometrial biopsy are unreliable.[145] In its opinion paper, the ASRM states that luteal length of 11–13 days suggests normal luteal function, whereas a length of ≤8 days is considered evidence of abnormal luteal phase.[145]

Luteal phase deficiency treatment options include ovulation induction (for example, with Clomiphene Citrate (CC) or Clomid) or hCG or progesterone supplementation during the luteal phase.[138] The Cochrane review of progesterone supplementation for treating threatened miscarriages concluded that *'...the use of progesterone is effective in the treatment of threatened miscarriage...'* and is not harmful to the mother or foetus.[148]

Immunological factors

Immune factors, whereby the maternal immune system fails to adapt to the developing embryo, resulting in rejection, may be involved in some cases of RM.[130] See section 'Reproductive Immunology' for discussion on various immune conditions and their association with implantation failure and pregnancy loss.

Male factor

Two recent meta-analyses showed that the rate of miscarriages is significantly higher in patients with high sperm DNA fragmentation.[149,150] Therefore, sperm DNA fragmentation testing should be undertaken in patients with RM or even before undergoing ART.[150] Antioxidants may help to repair some DNA damage (see Chapter 7 for more details).

Environmental, lifestyle, and nutritional factors

Several environmental factors have been linked with miscarriages, including obesity, caffeine intake, alcohol intake, smoking, illicit drug use, medication, occupation factors, stress, and nutritional deficiencies. These are discussed in greater detail in Chapter 7.

Hyperhomocysteinaemia (elevated homocysteine levels) is linked to miscarriages. Hyperhomocysteinaemia is a common finding in patients with the methyl tetrahydrofolate reductase (MTHFR) gene mutation[151] and is associated with low folic acid and vitamin B12 levels.[130] Therefore, it is recommended that patients with elevated homocysteine levels should take high doses of folic acid and vitamin B6 and B12.[130]

Unexplained miscarriages

Even after patients have been thoroughly investigated, in approximately 50% of cases there are no medically identifiable causes for their miscarriages.[130]

Orthodox conventional medical management of patients presenting with suspected miscarriage

Presenting signs and symptoms

Early signs of a miscarriage are similar to the early signs of an ectopic pregnancy. These include irregular vaginal bleeding and/or abdominal pain. It is recommended that all patients reporting these symptoms should be referred to a doctor or an Early Pregnancy Unit (EPU) to exclude the possibility of an ectopic pregnancy, which can be fatal if not managed correctly. Ectopic pregnancy is discussed in more detail later in this chapter.

> **! Red flag**
>
> **Bleeding and/or abdominal pain in a woman of reproductive age**
>
> **Any woman of reproductive age** experiencing vaginal bleeding and/or abdominal pain should be referred to an EPU if known to be pregnant or to a doctor if not known to be pregnant.
>
> Urgent referral to an Accident and Emergency (A&E) department is indicated if the pain is severe and accompanied by:
> - Dizziness or fainting
> - Rapid pulse
> - Low blood pressure
> - Severe vaginal bleeding (more than 1 pad/h)
> - Severe pelvic pain
> - Temperature above 38°C (100.4°F)

Pregnancy viability assessment

The diagnostic classification of miscarriages depends on the clinical findings (see Table 12.2).

The initial assessment of the viability of a pregnancy should include a medical history, a bimanual examination, and a urinary hCG test. However, while this assessment may help physicians in their decision making, only ultrasound examination and blood serum beta-hCG test will help to confirm a diagnosis of a viable pregnancy or a miscarriage.

hCG is the hormone produced by the trophoblast when it implants. hCG can be detected in maternal urine and blood soon after implantation. Pregnancy is confirmed if beta-hCG levels are ≥5 IU/L.[152] An hCG level of ≥150 IU/L on day 15 after IVF embryo transfer is a good predictor of a viable pregnancy.[153] hCG levels between 25 and 50 IU/L 16 days after ovulation may indicate a low probability of continuation of the pregnancy (<35%), whereas levels of >500 IU/L were associated with high chance of ongoing pregnancy (>95%).[154]

Serum beta-hCG levels double every 48 h in most, but not all, healthy pregnancies. A rise of <53% is usually associated with an abnormal pregnancy.[155] Slow rising hCG may indicate an ectopic pregnancy. A high for gestational age hCG level may indicate a molar pregnancy. Declining levels of hCG suggests a failing pregnancy but may also indicate an ectopic pregnancy. Depending on the initial levels of hCG, in a failed pregnancy hCG levels decrease by 21–35% every 2 days.

CLINICAL TIPS

SLOW RISING OF HCG LEVELS AND ACUPUNCTURE

In our experience, acupuncture and moxa on REN4 and REN6 can help in cases where hCG is rising too slowly.

Table 12.2 Diagnostic classifications of miscarriages

Classifications of miscarriages	Signs and symptoms
Threatened	Vaginal bleeding and/or abdominal pain, but cervical os is closed and no tissue has been passed. 25% of all pregnancies have bleeding in the first two trimesters and around half of these will progress to a complete miscarriage
Inevitable	Progression from threatened, but now internal cervical os is opened and cervix dilated. Heavier bleeding and abdominal cramping
Incomplete	As per inevitable, but cervix may be open or closed and bleeding and pain are more intense. Retained product of conception may be seen on ultrasound scan
Complete	Bleeding and abdominal pain subsided. Pregnancy tissue has been passed. Diagnosis can be confirmed by ultrasonography or by beta-hCG tests
Missed	May or may not have history of vaginal bleeding and/or abdominal pain. No evidence of viable pregnancy on ultrasonography examination in previously confirmed pregnancy

A transvaginal ultrasound examination helps to visualize a pregnancy and helps to classify it. It is the most accurate diagnostic method in the first trimester of a pregnancy[156] and is superior to transabdominal ultrasound. It can help to ascertain the location and gestation of pregnancy and if a foetal heartbeat is seen. The following discriminatory findings apply in early pregnancy:[157]

- ∼4–5 weeks' gestation: a gestational sac should be seen on ultrasound examination.
- ∼5–6 weeks' gestation
  - yolk sac is visible when the diameter of gestational sac is >10 mm
  - embryo should be visible when the diameter of gestational sac is >18 mm
  - foetal heartbeat should be detected when embryonic crown-rump length is >5 mm

When beta-hCG levels rise above 1500 IU/L (known as the discriminatory level), there should, with the use of ultrasound examination, be evidence of pregnancy. If no gestational sac is seen on ultrasound in women with hCG levels above 1500 IU/L, it may indicate a complete miscarriage or an ectopic pregnancy.[155]

In twin pregnancies, the discriminatory level is set higher at 2300 IU/L, because beta-hCG levels are generally higher in multiple-gestation pregnancies. Multiple-gestation pregnancies are more common following ART treatment. Therefore, a gestational sac may not be seen on an ultrasound scan until beta-hCG levels are above 2300 IU/L.[158]

Other indications on ultrasound of a failing pregnancy are an abnormal gestational sac shape or size relative to gestation. If no foetal heartbeat is seen, an ultrasound scan should be repeated within 3–7 days. A slow foetal heartbeat (≤110 bpm) at 6–8 weeks' gestation is a poor prognostic sign.[159] The presence of a foetal heartbeat reduces the risk of miscarriage to 4.5% in women aged <36, 10% in women aged 36–39, and 29% in women ≥40 years of age.[160]

The medical management of a failed pregnancy depends on the diagnostic classification of a miscarriage. Expectant management (where women are expected to miscarry spontaneously) may be indicated in cases of inevitable miscarriage. These women must be closely monitored, in case they develop complications such as severe bleeding or infection. If women do not miscarry naturally or if there is incomplete or missed miscarriage, then surgical and pharmacological management is indicated. Second-trimester miscarriages may require induction of labour. In women who are Rh-negative, RhoGAM must be administered to prevent haemolytic disease in a newborn in this or future pregnancies. If available, foetal tissue may be sent for analysis.

TCM management of patients presenting with threatened miscarriage

Pathophysiology of miscarriages

There are many terms in TCM that indicate threatened miscarriage, for example, 'stirring foetus' or 'foetus displacement', where manifestations such as lower back pain, abdominal pain, and vaginal bleeding all suggest that the foetus is distressed.

Acupuncture and Chinese herbal medicine treatment and management can alter compromised physiology threatening a miscarriage and prevent a miscarriage from occurring. It does this by promoting the development of the embryo or foetus through optimizing maternal health to sustain and stabilize the pregnancy.[161]

In TCM, miscarriages are caused by a weakness of maternal Chong and Ren Mai (Penetrating and Directing Vessels),[162–164] through failure of gathering Blood and lack of nourishment of the foetus.[162] Dysfunction of the Chong and Ren Mai (Penetrating and Directing Vessels) is strongly related to maternal weakness of Kidney Jing (Essence),[165] Kidney Yin and/or Yang Deficiency, Qi and Blood Deficiency, and Blood-Heat.[163,165] Pathology of the Kidney,

Heart, Stomach,[165] and Spleen is also associated with threatened miscarriages.[161]

Pre- and Post-Natal Jing (Essence), Qi, Blood, and other vital substances influence maternal health, which in turn influences the embryo's health. ST36 with moxa is a classical treatment prescription for the prevention of threatened miscarriages.[166] Therefore, nourishing Qi and Blood enriches the mother, securing the Qi of the embryo or foetus.[161]

Blood flow enables pregnancy, and the general state of Qi and Blood directly affects the functions of the Extraordinary Vessels and the Uterus.[161] Blood Stagnation in the Uterus reduces the circulation of Qi, Blood, and Jing (Essence) to the embryo. This may halt its development and growth, leading to a miscarriage.[165] The treatment strategy in these cases is to warm and move Blood and regulate and circulate Qi of the mother and the embryo.[161]

A weak Uterus (from a varied TCM pathology) can lead to the opening of the Uterus, which can proceed to a threatened miscarriage.[161]

 Red flag

Frequent urination in pregnant patients

Frequent urination is a symptom Kidney Qi Deficiency. However, it is also a sign of a UTI. Because UTI can cause miscarriages, always check urine in pregnant patients who complain of frequent urination.

In contrast to Orthodox medicine, TCM places greater emphasis on prevention of miscarriage. When dealing with ART patients, it is important to remember that many of them are at higher risk of miscarrying, due to pre-existing medical conditions, extensive use of drugs during ART treatment, and emotional stress (see Chapter 7 for details on how stress affects fertility). Therefore, close monitoring of these patients in the first few weeks of pregnancy is essential for prevention of miscarriages.

Table 12.3 provides detailed miscarriage TCM diagnostic information, and Figure 12.5 provides an algorithm for the management of miscarriage patients.

TCM management of inevitable or missed miscarriages

If, following a scan or serial hCG tests, miscarriage is classed as inevitable, incomplete, or missed, acupuncture treatment may be attempted to help the patient to pass pregnancy tissue naturally. While treating these patients, they must be monitored very closely in case they develop infection or severe bleeding. Some of the acupuncture points that may be used include:

- LU7, LI4, SP6, BL32, REN4 (needled toward REN2)[164]

Treatment should be done daily until either pregnancy tissue is passed or it is no longer deemed safe to wait for a natural miscarriage and a patient is advised to undergo medical or surgical termination. In some countries, it may be illegal to assist patients in miscarrying pregnancy naturally in a non-hospital setting, even if the pregnancy is not viable. Acupuncturists must ensure that they follow the correct procedure for their country, for example, a written permission from a doctor may be needed.

Emotional support is also extremely important during this stage. Acupuncture points such as P6, KID27, and YINTANG are suitable for most patients. Other points may be chosen depending on patient's emotions and background history.

TCM management of patients with a history of RMs

RMs are usually a result of the same syndromes that cause spontaneous miscarriages, but much more advanced and serious. Acupuncture treatment principles are the same, but stronger Qi and Blood moving points can be used during the preventive phase of treatment. Other generic points for prevention of RMs are:

- ST36, KID7, DU20 to tonify and raise Qi and support the Kidneys
- SP4+P6, LI4*, SP6*, SP10 to move Qi and Blood

It may be helpful to use BBT charts in patients with a history of miscarriages. BBT often drops a day or two before the onset of bleeding. If such a pattern is observed, an emergency acupuncture treatment may help to rescue the pregnancy.

When to refer for miscarriage investigations

Acupuncture can address some causes of RMs, (but not all including, for example, serious genetic or anatomical abnormalities). Therefore, consideration should be given as to whether to refer a patient for advanced conventional medical investigations.

The decision when to refer patients will depend on the patient's individual set of circumstances and on local health policies. Investigations are always indicated in couples with three consecutive miscarriages or one miscarriage after 12 weeks' gestation.[123]

However, there may be instances when investigations could be recommended earlier. For example, if a young couple miscarry one pregnancy following IVF treatment, it may be seen as premature to refer them for investigations at this point in time, especially as such investigations may not be funded. But if a woman is over 40 years old and suffers a single spontaneous miscarriage following IVF treatment, it is justifiable to refer her for further

---

*These points may need to be avoided if a pregnancy is confirmed. See Chapter 14 for a discussion on forbidden points in pregnancy.

Table 12.3 Summary of common TCM syndromes in [121,162–164,167,168] miscarriages

	Blood Deficiency	Qi Deficiency and Qi Sinking	Kidney Deficiency	Blood-Heat	Blood Stasis
Explanation	Foetus fails to receive its nourishment from Blood in the Chong Mai (Penetrating Vessel)	Qi Deficiency leads to Qi sinking and therefore failure to hold foetus	Kidney Deficiency leads to deficiency in other channels, including the Chong and Ren Mai (Penetrating and Directing Vessels)	Heat dries Yin (which affects the endometrium). Heat also forces Blood out of Uterine vessels. Heat stops the development of the foetus ('scorches' and 'dries' it)	Blood stasis blocks Blood supply to foetus
Associated with	• End of first trimester or later miscarriages • Foetal growth issues after 2–3 months gestation, but may also be earlier • Low maternal iron levels	• Clinical or subclinical miscarriages • Also pregnancy loss during second trimester (e.g., cervical insufficiency)	• Very early miscarriages (pre-implantation or within the first few weeks of pregnancy) • Recurrent miscarriages • Reproductively older women	• Early miscarriages • Possibly recurrent miscarriages	• Pregnancy loss at any stage • Blood clotting disorders, such as antiphospholipid syndrome
Aetiology	• Diet low in Blood-building foods • History of bleeding (e.g., from previous miscarriages)	• Eating cold and raw foods • Worrying	• Working long hours • Heavy lifting • Over-exercising • Weak constitution	• Emotions such as worry, anger, resentment lead to Liver Qi Stagnation, which turns to Fire and as the Liver stores Blood, to Blood-Heat • Diet rich in hot and spicy foods, alcohol • Stimulating drugs (e.g., IVF downregulation medication) • Illnesses, such as infections	• Physical injuries (e.g., falls, trauma) injure Chong Mai and Ren Mai (Penetrating and Directing Vessels) • Excessive intercourse during pregnancy • Surgical procedures (e.g., IVF) • Pre-existing medical conditions related to Blood Stasis or Cold (e.g., endometriosis)
Pre-existing syndromes	Liver or Heart Blood Deficiency	Spleen Qi Deficiency	Kidney Yang or Yin or Jing (Essence) Deficiency	Liver Heat/Fire Heart Heat/Fire Empty-Heat from Yin Deficiency Blood Deficiency	Liver Qi and Blood Stasis Cold

Table 12.3 Summary of common TCM syndromes in[121,162–164,167,168] miscarriages—cont'd

	Blood Deficiency	Qi Deficiency and Qi Sinking	Kidney Deficiency	Blood-Heat	Blood Stasis
Vaginal bleeding[a]	**Pale** scanty (might be worse after exertion)	Spotting	Scanty	**Bright red**	**Dark or clotty**
Other symptoms[a]	**Pale face,** fatigue, possibly palpitations	**Bearing down sensation or dropping feeling in lower abdomen,** abdominal distension	**Back ache, frequent urination,** slight dizziness, feeling cold (if Yang Deficiency) or five palm heat and night sweats (if Yin Deficiency)	**Feeling hot, mental restlessness, dark urination, thirst,** red face, insomnia, dry stools	**Sharp stabbing abdominal pain**
Pulse	Weak	Fine (thready)	Weak and soft, especially in the Kidney positions	Rapid	Normal or choppy
Tongue	Pale	Swollen or pale	Pale and possibly swollen (if Yang Deficiency), red without coating (if Yin Deficiency)	Red, possibly with yellow coating Heat spots	Purple
Points	Generic points that can be used in all types of threatened miscarriage: SP1: apply moxa daily until bleeding has stopped; Qimen (extra point 3 cun lateral to REN4): to stop uterine contractions; YINTANG to calm Shen; DU20, HE5, REN12, REN6, ST36 to hold the foetus				
	BL17 (with moxa), ST36, BL20, LIV8	DU20, ST36, REN12, REN6	BL23, KID3, REN4 (moxa only)	SP10, LI11, KID8; plus HE5 (if HE-Fire), LIV2 (if LIV-Fire), KID2 (if Yin Deficiency)	ST29, SP10, P6, REN12 + DU20
Lifestyle advice	Bed rest is indicated for all types of threatened miscarriages. Chapter 7 provides details of foods beneficial in various syndromes				

[a] Bold signifies key differentiating signs and symptoms.

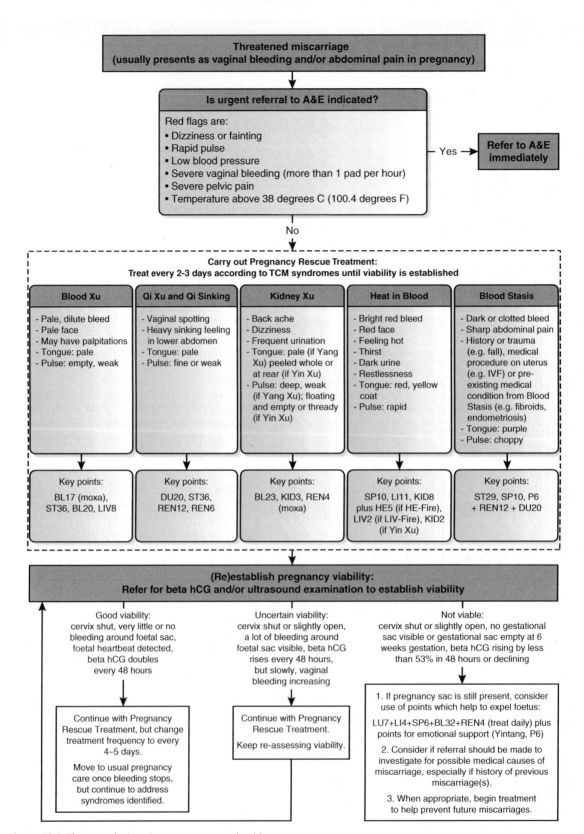

Figure 12.5 Threatened miscarriage management algorithm.

investigations. Even though it is likely that the miscarriage in this example was caused by age-related chromosomal abnormalities, it may be helpful to exclude other causes before further IVF is attempted. Otherwise, critically valuable time may be lost on several more failed IVF cycles or pregnancies.

CLINICAL TIPS

A MISCARRIAGE POST IVF AND SUBSEQUENT CHANCE OF SUCCESSFUL IVF

Women who experience an early pregnancy loss (biochemical pregnancy or clinical) after an IVF cycle were found to have a greater likelihood of success in a subsequent IVF cycle compared to patients who failed to conceive.[169]

TCM lifestyle advice in prevention of miscarriages

Physical activity

In order to help prevent a threatened miscarriage and as a way of preserving Qi if the miscarriage is inevitable, rest is advisable.[164] Physical overexertion and heavy lifting should be avoided.

Intercourse

From an Orthodox medical perspective, intercourse is not recommended if a woman is bleeding vaginally. Also, in couples with a history of miscarriage(s), it may be prudent to avoid intercourse until the pregnancy is well established (around 12 weeks' gestation).

From a TCM point of view, sexual intercourse during the first 3 months of pregnancy ought to be gentle or even avoided, because it may stir Ministerial Fire, which may damage Kidney Jing (Essence) and weaken Yin.[170] Intercourse in the middle stages of pregnancy is considered safe.[170]

Emotions

For women to see vaginal bleeding in pregnancy is extremely distressing and traumatic, especially so if the pregnancy was difficult to achieve. In all cases, acupuncture points that have a calming and tranquilizing effect on the mind must be used and are provided in Table 12.3. If the miscarriage could not be prevented and the pregnancy is lost, it is imperative that acupuncturists take great care with what they say to the patients. For example, saying *'At least you know you can get pregnant'* is insensitive and likely to make a woman even more annoyed and angry. Instead, it might be better to offer women hope by saying *'Most patients who miscarry subsequently achieve successful live birth'*.

Diet

TCM dietary advice is dependent on which TCM syndromes are diagnosed (see Chapter 7).

When to start trying for a baby again

In TCM, miscarriages are thought to be very damaging, similar in effect to labour. Miscarriages are very draining on a woman's body. However, a normal labour is followed by elation and happiness, whereas miscarriages are followed by grief, sadness, and often anger. This further stagnates and depletes Qi and Blood. Some TCM authors believe that it is vitally important that women do not try again for a baby for at least 6, preferably 12 months, so that they have time to fully recover, otherwise there is a risk of further miscarriages.[171,172]

While this advice is extremely important in younger patients, it may not be appropriate in subfertile or older patients. Many patients who consult fertility acupuncturists are older. In women 35 years or more in age, the chances for conception decline rapidly. A 6- to 12-month wait can be detrimental to their chances of conception through IVF. In some instances, women have no option but to retry IVF soon after a miscarriage. For example, if their treatment is funded by the state or by medical insurance, in order to qualify for funding, they need to start further treatment within a certain time frame. An appropriate time also needs to be allowed for the possible conception of any future pregnancies to add siblings to the family.

An interesting finding from one study that followed up 10,453 pregnancies that had ended in a miscarriage was that subsequent pregnancies that were conceived ≤3 months after a miscarriage were more likely to result in a live birth compared to pregnancies conceived 6–12 months after a miscarriage.[173]

For many women, a sense of loss following a miscarriage is so immense that the only way for them to heal is to replace what they lost. Thus advice to take a break from trying for a baby will be contra to their very deep instinctive need to try again as soon as possible. By discouraging them from trying again, we might inadvertently cause deterioration of their TCM syndromes. Women who miscarry often examine every detail of their lost pregnancy, just in case there was something they did wrong and therefore are to blame for losing the baby. We must be careful that we do not suggest that if they try too soon again, they will cause another miscarriage. To do so unhelpfully and wrongly attributes the blame for miscarriages to these vulnerable women. Therefore, in subfertile patients, the advice to take several months' break before trying for a baby again should be carefully balanced with the potential negative physiological, psychological, and age-related time-dependant impact it could have.

Management of patients experiencing anxiety about miscarrying

Tender loving care (TLC) is recommended as an established treatment for patients with a history of RMs.[151] TLC support (frequent contact with supporting clinicians, frequent scans, counselling, etc.) has been shown to significantly improve success of subsequent pregnancy. Regular acupuncture treatments during the first few weeks of pregnancy could benefit these patients as part of their TLC support.

Patients who have a history of miscarriage(s) benefit greatly psychologically from frequent 'reassurance' scans. Develop a working relationship with your local EPU or pregnancy scanning facility. Find out what their referral procedures are and refer patients when appropriate. Most EPUs are happy to scan patients from 6 weeks' gestation, when they are able to detect a foetal heartbeat.

Once patients reach 11–12 weeks' gestation, some may find it helpful to buy a foetal doppler to self-monitor a foetal heartbeat. Foetal dopplers are inexpensive to buy. However, while the use of foetal self-monitoring may help some patients, others may find the opposite to be true, especially if they find it difficult to locate the foetal heartbeat. If patients struggle to find the heartbeat, drinking a glass of cold water before attempting to locate the heartbeat can make it easier. Occasionally, patients confuse their own heartbeat with their baby's heartbeat. They need to be taught that foetal heartbeat is usually very fast, at least 120 beats/min. Some people benefit by being shown how to use the monitor correctly. Therefore, advice on doppler foetal self-monitoring should be given with extreme caution, and acupuncturists must use their knowledge of each patient when deciding who would benefit from using a foetal monitor.

Case study

Threatened Miscarriage

Sue, a 45-year-old nurse became pregnant following egg donation IVF treatment. She was diagnosed with a raised level of natural killer (NK) cells, but declined to have any medical treatment for this. Otherwise, Sue had good health.

Presentation at 4 Weeks' Gestation

- Two days of red blood alternating with brown spotting
    - Some cramping and a heavy feeling in the abdomen
    - Pulse: slippery
    - Tongue: red and very cracked

TCM Diagnosis

Threatened miscarriage due to Qi Sinking and Heat in the Blood

Case study—cont'd

Point Prescription and Rationale

KID3, KID7 to benefit the embryo, SP3, ST36 supporting Spleen Qi in holding the baby, KID9 to stop uterine cramping, LIV2 to clear Heat, and Shenmen to calm Shen.

Bleeding stopped 2 h after the treatment. There was no bleeding for the next four days, but Sue felt very tired. Point prescription was repeated.

Heavy bleeding and cramping restarted 5 days after the second treatment. Sue became distressed. During the emergency acupuncture session her pulse was very thin on all positions. Point prescription was repeated with the addition of LIV8 to boost Liver Blood. Her bleeding stopped soon after.

Two days later Sue passed a large clot. Her hCG levels were 8000 IU/L. Pulse was stronger. Points prescription was repeated with addition of REN6, DU20 to raise Qi, magnetic seeds were placed on Shenmen ear points.

Two days later ultrasound scan showed one foetal heartbeat, but it was slow. Sue's pulse remained strong, but her tongue was still red. Repeated point prescription.

Bleeding ceased soon after treatment, but restarted with cramping 5 days later. Her latest hCG results were 16,000 IU/L (doubled in 7 days, which was too slow a rate of increase for a viable pregnancy). Points prescription was once again repeated.

Two days later, there was only minor spotting, ultrasound scan showed a faster heartbeat. Sue's pulse was very slippery. But her tongue was less red. Repeated the same point prescription.

At 9 weeks Sue's spotting had resolved.

Sue had a healthy baby boy delivered by elective caesarean section at 38 weeks gestation.

Frequent (every 2–3 daily) acupuncture treatment helped to rescue this pregnancy, even though initially the prognostic signs were not good (slow foetal heartbeat, slow rising hCG).

Ectopic pregnancy

Ectopic pregnancy is defined as pregnancy that implants outside of the uterus. Ninety percent of ectopic pregnancies occur in the fallopian tubes.[155] The rest are found in the cervix, ovary, or abdomen. An analysis of 108,130 cycles of ART treatment showed that the rate of ectopic pregnancies following ART is between 0.6% and 1.8%, depending on the type of ART procedure used.[174]

Early diagnosis is very important, because an undiagnosed ectopic pregnancy can lead to internal bleeding from a ruptured fallopian tube, which can potentially be fatal. An ectopic pregnancy can lead to subsequent subfertility. Mortality rates from ectopic pregnancies are low at a rate of 0.5 per 100,000, but these rates have remained static since 1985.[175]

Risk factors for developing ectopic pregnancy are:[155]

- History of previous ectopic pregnancy
- History of tubal surgery (including tubal sterilization)
- History of sexually transmitted infection or tubal infection
- Pelvic adhesions
- Current use of intrauterine device
- Smoking
- Conception following ART
- *In utero* exposure to diethylstilboestrol

Early symptoms of ectopic pregnancy include vaginal bleeding and abdominal pain. **Any woman of reproductive age** presenting with these symptoms (even if not known to be pregnant) should be referred for further investigations.[155]

In more advanced ectopic pregnancies, a patient will complain of severe cramping, usually to one side, or stabbing pain. She may also show signs of hypovolemic shock, such as dizziness or fainting, her pulse will be rapid, and her blood pressure low.[125] These patients need immediate emergency medical services.

Red flag

Signs of possible ectopic pregnancy that require urgent referral to A&E

Any woman of reproductive age having vaginal bleeding with or without:

- Severe abdominal cramping, possibly to one side, or stabbing pain
- Dizziness or fainting
- Rapid pulse
- Low blood pressure

Case study

Ectopic Pregnancy

Kate had recently started acupuncture treatment to prepare her for her second IVF treatment cycle. She emailed me to find out if the mid-cycle bleeding she was experiencing was normal. I advised her to do a pregnancy test to exclude a possibility of pregnancy. The pregnancy test was positive.

I then advised her to see her medical practitioner urgently with a view to being referred for an ultrasound scan to assess viability of her pregnancy and to exclude the possibility of ectopic pregnancy. Unfortunately, it took several days before her scan was arranged and performed. The scan showed an ectopic pregnancy and substantial internal bleeding. Surgery was performed on the same day and Kate lost one of her fallopian tubes.

Preterm birth and cervical insufficiency

The risk of preterm birth (defined as birth before 37 weeks' gestation)[176] is greater in pregnancies conceived as a result of ART treatment, independent of maternal age or number of foetuses.[82] 75–95% of neonatal deaths occur as a result of preterm births.[176] Surviving preterm infants are at greater risk of severe handicap and long-term health problems.[176] Although great efforts are being made by researchers to identify causes of preterm births, the rates of preterm births have remained largely unchanged over the last 30 years.[176]

Risk factors for premature labour include:

- BMI <19.8 kg/m^2[135,177]
- Vaginal bleeding[135]
- Pulmonary disease[177]
- Hormonal fertility treatment (excluding CC)[178]
- BV infection[135,177]
- Pelvic infection[135]
- Uterine contractions (regular or irregular)[135,177]
- Black race[135]
- **Previous preterm birth**[†135,177]
- **Cervical length $\leq$25 mm**[†135,177]
- **A positive foetal fibronectin (fFN) test**[†135,177]

BV accounts for up to 40% of births before 32 weeks' gestation.[135] It is also associated with early miscarriages in IVF pregnancies.[134] Some experts recommend that one BV screen in early pregnancy is sufficient to identify women at risk for preterm birth.[136] However, while this will help to identify women at high risk of preterm birth, it will not help to prevent miscarriages associated with BV, because they happen very early, usually around the implantation stage or shortly after implantation.[134] Therefore, it might be advisable to screen all women undergoing ART for BV before ART treatment starts, and perhaps on one more occasion shortly after embryo transfer, to exclude the possibility of infection being introduced during the medical procedures.

Uterine contractions are subjective and may not be completely reliable as a diagnostic feature. Home Uterine Activity Monitoring may help to monitor contractions more objectively.[176]

Cervical length measurements taken during transvaginal ultrasound scans have proved to be highly predictive of preterm birth. Shortening of the cervix is known as cervical incompetence or insufficiency. Opinions vary about what the cervical length should be during various stages of pregnancy. However, measurement of $\leq$25 mm before 32[176] to 34[179] weeks' gestation is seen as a reliable significant risk

---

†The last three risk factors are the strongest predictors of preterm birth.[135] The presence of two or more risk factors significantly increases the probability of preterm birth,[135] especially if one of the risk factors is cervical length shorter than 25 mm or a positive fFN test.

factor. In one study that examined 2915 women with singleton pregnancies, average cervical lengths were as follows:[180]

- 24 weeks' gestation: 35.2 mm (±8.3 mm)
- 28 weeks' gestation: 33.7 mm (±8.5 mm)

Cervical funnelling (dilation of the internal cervical os) is also considered to be a sign of poor prognosis. Women with cervical shortening may be offered cervical cerclage ('stitch') done transvaginally or transabdominally. Transabdominal cerclage is more beneficial in multiple-gestation pregnancies, but this procedure must be carried out preconceptually or early in pregnancy (ideally by 10 weeks' gestation) if it is to be of benefit.[181] Progesterone supplementation has recently been shown to be of benefit.

fFN is a fibronectin protein produced by foetal cells that acts as glue that attaches the foetal sack to the uterine lining. It is normally present in higher quantities in cervicovaginal secretions before 20 weeks' gestation and also from 37 weeks' gestation, but should be almost undetectable between 22 and 37 weeks.[182] A value of >50 ng/mL between weeks 22 and 37 is considered to be positive and highly predictive of preterm birth.[182]

Fertility acupuncturists who continue to treat patients throughout a pregnancy must be aware of the risk factors for a premature birth and initiate a referral when appropriate. Care should be taken not to alarm patients unnecessarily. For example, just because a patient's BMI is <19.8 kg/m^2, it does not necessarily mean that she will have preterm labour. However, if the patient were to mention menstrual-like cramps, she should be referred for further investigations, such as cervical length measurement and/or fFN test.

Women at high risk of premature delivery may derive great benefit from acupuncture. They should be treated weekly or fortnightly throughout the pregnancy. Treatment will depend on the underlying pathology and syndromes. In the majority of cases, the focus should be on strengthening Spleen's holding function and raising Qi. The Kidneys may also need to be supported.

CLINICAL TIPS

RISK FACTORS FOR PREMATURE DELIVERY

- BMI <19.8 kg/m^2
- Vaginal bleeding
- Pulmonary disease
- Hormonal fertility treatment (excluding clomiphene)
- BV infection
- Pelvic infection
- Uterine contractions (regular or irregular)
- Black race
- Previous preterm birth

CLINICAL TIPS—cont'd

If a patient has one or more of these risk factors, consider a referral for serial ultrasound scans to monitor cervical length and possibly also for a fFN test. Vaginal bleeding and/or uterine contractions indicate an urgent referral to a maternity ward.

The risk of premature delivery is much greater if a patient has:

- **Cervical length ≤25 mm and/or**
- **A positive fFN test (>50 ng/mL) between 22 and 37 weeks' gestation**

These patients will need to be very carefully managed, possibly requiring some form of cervical cerclage ('stitch'), progesterone supplementation, and prophylactic antenatal corticosteroids. Acupuncture treatment is applicable if a patient is managed on outpatient basis.

 Case study

Cervical Shortening in Twin Gestation Pregnancy Following IVF

Oksana was pregnant with twins following a third round of IVF and gruelling immunological and anti-clotting treatments.

Following a routine scan at 10 weeks' gestation, Oksana contacted me with an update. Everything was looking good, her babies were 'wriggling', had healthy heartbeats, and measured perfectly for 10 weeks' gestation. However, her fertility specialist was concerned because Oksana's cervix measurement was 27.5 mm and advised Oksana to seek urgent referral to an obstetric specialist.

Oksana contacted her midwife and was told that it was nothing to worry about and that she will probably need to wait until her routine 16 weeks' monitoring appointment with her obstetric consultant.

I was concerned as Oksana had several risk factors for cervical insufficiency:

- Cervical biopsy a few years previously due to an abnormal smear
- Slight vaginal bleeding
- Twin pregnancy

I was also aware that a standard transvaginal 'stitch' was not effective in twin gestation pregnancies and possibly could cause even more issues. On the other hand, a transabdominally placed 'stitch' known as Transabdominal Cervicoisthmic Cerclage (TAC) was more likely to be effective, but it needed to be performed ideally before 12 weeks' gestation.

I explained to Oksana how urgent it was, and she arranged to see a consultant who specialized in this condition. She was scanned again and advised to undergo TAC as soon as possible. TAC was successfully performed at just before 12 weeks' gestation. Apart from a brief period of rest during the recovery from the procedure, Oksana

Case study—cont'd

could resume her normal activity levels. Oksana successfully carried the twins until 37.5 weeks' gestation, at which point she underwent elective caesarean section.

This is a case where acupuncture treatment alone would not offer this patient the best chance of live birth. Instead, my role was to facilitate a quick referral to ensure that the surgical procedure, which would give this patient the best chance of successful pregnancy, was carried out within the optimal timeframe.

REPRODUCTIVE IMMUNOLOGY

Introduction

The role of the immune system is to identify and destroy cells that are genetically different from ours. Because the foetus has 50% of paternal DNA, it is genetically different to its mother and therefore theoretically the maternal immune system would see it as foreign and destroy it. Yet, in a healthy pregnancy, a foetus is not rejected, because of protective mechanisms that are not well understood.[183,184]

The proponents of reproductive immunology believe that these mechanisms can become faulty, and the maternal immune system attacks and destroys the foetus. This is, then, a reason why some couples experience RIFs and/or miscarriages. Although there is some evidence to support this view, it is not a fully empirically established theory.[185] Therefore, reproductive immunology is a highly controversial topic, about which divergent opinions polarize reproductive medicine professionals.

A full review of this area of reproductive medicine is outside of the scope of this book. This section only briefly outlines the most common immune issues, tests, and treatments. Anyone wishing to explore this subject in greater depth is advised to read a book written by a prominent reproductive immunology proponent Dr Alan Beer, *Is Your Body Baby Friendly?* ISBN 0-9785078-0-0.

Reproductive immune pathology and tests

CD56+ natural killer

CD56+ NK cells are lymphocytes, which help to fight an infection.[186,187] They can be found in the peripheral blood supply (PBNK). Cells resembling PBNK called uterine natural killer (uNK) cells are present in large numbers in the uterine mucosa during implantation and in the early stages of pregnancy,[187] particularly in the first 12 days of pregnancy.[188] They are thought to help with implantation by

helping to establish a blood supply to the placenta, although it is not known exactly how.[187]

Controversially, some experts believe that uNK cells can become cytotoxic and cause implantation or pregnancy failure[189] by leading to production of other cells (for example, Th1 helper cells such as tumour necrosis factor, or TNF-alpha cells) that attack the placenta.[188] In turn, TNF-alpha cells can trigger migration into the uterus of other immune cells (CD3, CD4, and CD8 T cells).[188] Later in pregnancy, blood clotting can occur and lead to separation of the placenta and foetal death.[188] Therefore, suppressing these cytotoxic uNK cells is believed to help with implantation and early pregnancy failure and reduce the risks of pregnancy complications.

A test has been developed called NK Cell Assay, which tests the killing power of NK cells. It is based on the premise that the activity of the uNK cells can be measured by testing the activity of the PBNK cells in the lab.[190] The PBNK cells are placed in a test tube with cells similar to embryo cells in various dilutions. Then the number of cells that have been killed by the PBNK cells is calculated (expressed as a percentage of killed cells).[191] Table 12.4 lists reference ranges for killing powers.

Criticism of this test is that there is no evidence that measuring PBNK cells is indicative of the uNK cells' activity, there is no agreement on what constitutes a raised level and that a number of variables can affect the result (for example, the time of day a sample is taken and parity of the mother).[186]

An alternative way to check for activity of uNK is to do an endometrial biopsy.

Reproductive immunophenotype

An immunophenotype test is done to determine the concentrations of white blood cells, which, if elevated, are thought to cause infertility and/or pregnancy loss. Table 12.5 provides reference ranges.

Th1:Th2 assay

High levels of lymphocytes T helper 1 (TNF-alpha, IFNγ) compared to T helper 2 (IL-10) cytokines may be implicated in miscarriages and subfertility.[36,199] Th1:Th2 assay measures the ratio between these two types of lymphocytes. Th1 (TNF-alpha) should be <30.[192]

Table 12.4 NK cell assay reference values[192]		
Dilutions	**Reference range (%)**	**Notes**
50:1	10–40	Levels >15% are damaging to the embryo
25:1	5–20	
12:1	2.5–10	

Table 12.5 Immunophenotype reference ranges[192]

Cells	Reference range	Notes
CD3	63–86%	Elevated levels are associated with autoimmune disease such as thyroiditis, systemic lupus erythematosus (SLE) and rheumatoid arthritis
CD4	31–53%	Very low values are associated with severe immunodeficiency, for example, in patients with AIDS
CD8	17–35%	Low levels can lead to up-regulation of Th1 lymphocytes
CD19	3–8%	Levels of >12% may lead to infertility or recurrent pregnancy loss
CD56+/ CD16+	3–12%	Elevated levels can lead to infertility and recurrent miscarriages
CD56+	3–12%	Levels of >18% maybe predictive of a poor reproductive outcome
CD3/IL-2R+	0–5%	Women with autoimmune disease may have elevated levels
CD19+/ 5+	2–10% of B Cells	Women with raised levels may not respond well to ovarian stimulation and also suffer embryonic damage or loss

Leukocyte Antibody Detection test

The Lymphocyte Antibody Detection (LAD) test determines whether the mother is producing enough blocking antibodies to her partner's lymphocytes (T and B cells).[192]

Levels of IgG T cells or IgG B cells of <30% are associated with increased risk of implantation failure and pregnancy loss and are therefore abnormal.[200,201]

Lymphocyte Immune Therapy (LIT) may be recommended to boost the level of recognition of paternal proteins.

Human leukocyte antigen HLA-DQ alpha test

When a couple's genetic tissue type is closely matched, the woman's immune system may see the resulting embryo tissue as a distorted part of her own body. This may activate NK cells against the cells of the embryo. Human Leukocyte

Antigen HLA-DQ alpha test identifies if mother and her partner share a similar DQ alpha match.[192] LIT may be recommended if DQ alpha match is identified.

Immunotherapy

Several immune therapies have been proposed to help to overcome reproductive immune issues, but the evidence for most is very limited. Therefore, immunotherapy is controversial, and both the RCOG and the ASRM do not currently recommend it until more evidence emerges.[67,123]

However, many of our patients are prescribed these treatments. Perhaps it is because a large proportion of patients presenting for infertility acupuncture are complex cases, often with a history of failed IVFs and/or RMs. Therefore, they turn to more aggressive treatments with the hope of better future success. For this reason, the most commonly used immune therapies are outlined in this section.

Intravenous Immune Globulin

Intravenous Immune Globulin (IVIG) is the best-known immune therapy. Its mode of action is believed to be by suppressing circulating antibodies and cytotoxicity and modulating the release of cytokines from lymphocytes.[130] IVIG preparations such as Venoglobin-S, Gamimune-N, and Gammagard are infused at doses of 0.2 g to 0.4 g/kg of weight.[202] Typically, the first infusion is done at the end of the pre-treatment cycle and shortly before egg retrieval, soon after a positive pregnancy test, and 3–4 weekly frequency thereafter. However, different consultants recommend different timings and number of infusions.

The disadvantages of IVIG are that it is a donor blood product and therefore bloodborne infections such as hepatitis, HIV, and CJD may be introduced.[187] It contains antibodies, which may cross the placenta,[187] and it is also very expensive.[203]

A recent meta-analysis of RCTs and cohort studies on IVIG therapy in patients with a history of implantation failure concluded that IVIG therapy in this patient group significantly increases live birth rate.[204]

The evidence for IVIG therapy for prevention of miscarriages is weak. A Cochrane review did not find that IVIG significantly improves pregnancy outcomes.[185] A 2011 meta-analysis of six RCTs on IVIG therapy in women with unexplained RMs also did not find that IVIG was beneficial.[205] However, an earlier review found that IVIG therapy may be effective for prevention of secondary miscarriages.[206] The ASRM concluded that IVIG efficacy in prevention of miscarriages is unproven and ASRM views it as an experimental treatment.[203]

Intralipid therapy

Intralipid infusion is another type of immunotherapy.[202,207] It is administered intravenously at a dose of

2–3 mL in 250 mL of sterile saline at approximately 250 cm³/h.[202,208] Intralipid therapy appears to be as effective at immunosuppression as IVIG,[208,209] but does not have the disadvantages of IVIG. Therefore, IVIG is being phased out by some clinics in favour of intralipid therapy.

Glucocorticoids

Glucocorticoids may help to modulate the immune system. Glucocorticoid therapy involves one of the following medications:[202]

- Oral prednisone (5, 7.5, 10, 15, 30, and 60 mg/day)
- Oral methylprednisone (4 and 16 mg/day)
- Oral dexamethasone (0.5 and 1 mg/day), less commonly used
- Intravenous hydrocortisone (100 mg), less commonly used

A 2012 Cochrane review did not find clear evidence that routine use of glucocorticoids improves ART cycles outcomes, although there was some borderline evidence that IVF (as opposed to ICSI) outcomes were improved.[210] Because this review looked at routine use of glucocorticoids, it is not possible to say if targeted use (for example, in women diagnosed with autoantibodies or with a history of RIF) would produce a more significant therapeutic effect.

Lymphocyte Immunization Therapy

In active immunotherapy, either paternal or embryonic membrane infusion is injected into the mother in order to boost future maternal recognition of the developing embryo.[130] Paternal immunization (also known as Lymphocyte Immune Therapy or LIT) is highly controversial. In their review of evidence for LIT for RMs, Li *et al.* concluded that, although there are studies demonstrating beneficial effect of LIT, there are also studies that failed to show such effect.[130] They postulated that a reason for conflicting findings is the indiscriminate inclusion of participants in research studies.[130] Therefore, for now LIT is considered an experimental therapy, and it is suggested that it should only be used within the context of a carefully designed research.[130] However, there is some promising evidence for third-party donor leukocytes, although further research is necessary.[151]

TNF-alpha inhibitors (Th1:Th2)

Anti TNF-alpha therapy such as adalimumab (Humira®) together with IVIG has been shown to improve IVF outcome in women with raised Th1:Th2.[211]

Peripheral blood mononuclear cells

Intrauterine administration of maternal peripheral blood mononuclear cells (PBMCs) is suggested to positively enhance implantation. In this therapy, PBMCs are obtained on the day of egg retrieval, cultured with hCG, then on the day of embryo transfer cultured PBMCs are combined with freshly obtained PBMCs and then administered into the uterine cavity. This has been shown to significantly improve live birth rates in patients with RIF in a small controlled study.[212]

Granulocyte colony stimulating factor

Granulocyte colony stimulating factor (G-CSF) is a cytokine, which may help to reduce the risk of miscarriages.[213] In one RCT, G-CSF (1 µg/kg/day) was administered starting on day 6 post ovulation in women who suffered from RMs and in whom other immune therapies (for example, IVIG) had failed. The live birth rate was significantly higher in the active treatment group compared with placebo group.[213]

REPRODUCTIVE IMMUNOLOGY FROM A TCM POINT OF VIEW

Research on the effect of acupuncture on the immune system

Acupuncture and Th1:Th2 (TNF-alpha) cells

A small study on rats assessed implantation and Th1:Th2 ratio and showed that acupuncture can inhibit Th1 and increase Th2 secretions. The protocol used was stimulation for 25 min ('rolling needle' every 5 min) on ST36 and SP6 acupuncture points bilaterally, beginning on the day when male sperm was detected by vaginal smear. The treatment was administered daily for 5–8 days (day 8 was a test day). The implantation rate was also significantly higher in the acupuncture group.[214]

Other treatment protocols, which have been shown to have a downregulating effect on TNF-alpha (Th1) levels in non-reproductive population, include:

- Electroacupuncture (EA) and/or moxa on DU14 (1 Hz 500 µs or 50 µs)[215]
- EA on ST36 and extra point M-LE-13 Lanwei ('strings of dense-sparse frequencies 60 Hz for 1.05 s and 2 Hz for 2.85 s alternately'), intensity adjusted until slight muscle contraction of the hindlimb was induced (≤1.5 mA)[216]
- EA on ST36 daily for 10 days[217]

In their review paper Kim and Bae concluded that the effect of acupuncture on Th1:Th2 ratio is modulating or balancing.[218] This is similar to the effect in other studies where high Th2 levels contributed to a disease process, and acupuncture was shown to have an inhibitory effect on Th2 production.[218] Interestingly, in one study, acupuncture was shown to have no effect on TNF-alpha levels in healthy young individuals, thereby providing further support to the modulating effect theory.[219]

Acupuncture and NK cells

The potential benefit of acupuncture in patients with abnormal uNK cell expressions is less clear. We have not been able to find any research on acupuncture and NK cells in human or animal studies relating to reproduction. But the evidence from non-reproductive patient group studies suggests that acupuncture has a modulating effect on the immune system.[218,220,221]

INTERESTING FACTS

IMMUNOMODULATION: COMPARISON OF ACUPUNCTURE AND IVIG

Recent research suggests that acupuncture has an immunomodulating effect.[218,220,221] That means that in patients whose immune system is deficient, acupuncture boosts it, and in patients whose immune system is overactive, acupuncture suppresses it.

IVIG, one of the immunotherapy treatments used in reproductive immunology, is also immunomodulating in its action,[222] but it has a number of serious side effects.

More research is necessary to understand exactly how acupuncture works and which treatment regimens are best. But for now it is probably safe to say that acupuncture should be tried as first-line treatment in patients with suspected or diagnosed reproductive immune issues.

Acupuncture has been shown to increase the number of splenic NK cells.[220,221] If acupuncture was also able to increase the number of uNK cells, then this may possibly create a more favourable environment for implantation. The high numbers of uNK cells during the first 12 days of pregnancy may possibly assist with the formation of the blood supply to the baby. It is only when these cells become cytotoxic that they can lead to implantation or pregnancy failure.[189] NK cells do this by stimulating production of other cells (for example, Th1 helper cells such as tumour necrosis factor, or TNF-alpha cells), which attack the placenta.[188] In turn, TNF-alpha cells can trigger migration into the uterus of other immune cells (CD3, CD4, and CD8 T cells).[188]

Acupuncture points that modulate the immune system

In their review, Silverio-Lopes and da Mota found that ST36 and LI4 (either with manual or EA stimulation) are the most frequently used acupuncture points in acupuncture immunomodulation research. Other points that have been used in research studies include SP6, LI11, YINTANG, DU20, BL23, REN4, and LU6.[221]

Associations of reproductive immunology and TCM

Other TCM authors have previously identified several syndromes that may be involved in immune reproductive failure. These include:

- Liver and Kidney Yin Deficiency generating Toxic-Heat[117]
- Kidney Jing Deficiency[223]
- Kidney Yin Deficiency[224]
- Kidney Yin (Jing) Deficiency with Empty Fire, Liver Qi Stagnation, and Blood Deficiency[223]
- Damp-Heat and Blood Stasis[117,223]

In our opinion and experience, Blood Stasis is the most common syndrome associated with reproductive immunology issues. Blood Stasis may either lead to infertility or, if conception occurs, there is a danger of losing the foetus, which can happen as early as implantation stage. It is interesting that according to Orthodox medical thinking, most reproductive immune pathology leads to a blood clotting reaction, producing a vascular necrosis of the foetal blood supply.

However, in many cases Blood Stasis is a result of other underlying pathology, including:

- Kidney Yang Deficiency
- Spleen Qi Deficiency with Dampness
- Stomach Yin Deficiency Empty-Heat/Fire
- Lung and Spleen Qi Deficiency
- Internal Cold

Once Blood Stasis is formed, it can cause additional complications associated with reproductive failure. The severity level of reproductive failure depends on the extent of pathology. Figure 12.6 outlines the pathogenesis of Blood Stasis in relation to reproductive immunology patients.

As in Orthodox medicine, reproductive immunology is a very new concept in contemporary acupuncture practice. There are very few if any established treatment protocols or diagnostic criteria. The syndromes just listed are perhaps the more prevalent. However, it is important to 'treat what you find' when dealing with reproductive immunology cases.

IMPLICATIONS FOR ACUPUNCTURISTS: TO REFER OR NOT TO REFER?

As already stated, reproductive immunology is a highly controversial area of medicine. Reproductive tests and treatments are not fully proven or accepted, are expensive, and have associated adverse events. Yet, in the authors'

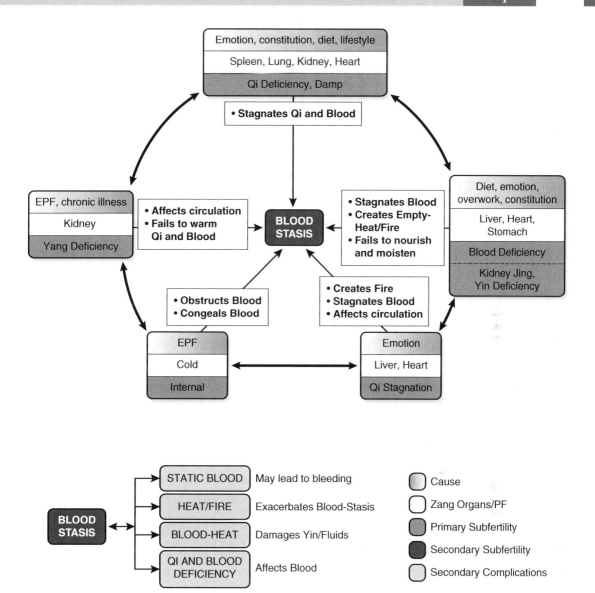

Figure 12.6 Pathogenesis of Blood Stasis in reproductive immunology patients.

experience, there are patients who seem to succeed with their ART and acupuncture interventions only with the addition of immune treatments.

Ethically, it is very difficult to make recommendations if and when we should refer our patients for reproductive immunology tests and treatments. In our opinion, the best recommendation that we can make is that acupuncturists should be aware of the threat that immunological risk factors may pose for a pregnancy to be initially conceived and then to be kept viable to term. Therefore,

those patients who may potentially benefit from immune investigations and interventions should be referred once they are aware of the risks and benefits of these approaches.

Box 12.1 outlines relevant diseases and facts of a patient's medical history that are associated with reproductive immune issues. If patients are diagnosed with these diseases and have a history of RIFs or RMs, it may be prudent to recommend reproductive immunology assessment.

Box 12.1 Diseases associated with reproductive autoimmune issues

Diseases/associations

Negative reproductive history/infertility:[188]

- ≥1 live child followed by secondary infertility or recurrent pregnancy loss
- ≥3 RIFs
- ≥3 pregnancy losses

Advancing maternal age[193]

Premature ovarian failure[194,195]

Premature ovarian aging[194]

Endometriosis[188,196,197]

Pelvic inflammatory disease and tubal blockage and abnormal APA test result[188]

Infections:[188]

- *Chlamydia*
- Gonorrhoea
- *Candida*
- Herpes (HSV-2)
- Dysplasia (Genital warts) due to Human Papilloma Virus (HPV)

DQ alpha genetic compatibility with partner[188]

Allergies and intolerances[188]

Bowel disease:

- Irritable bowel diseases (IBS), especially associated with very aggressive CD57 cells[188]
- Coeliac disease[194,198]
- Crohn's disease[188]

Other autoimmune diseases:

- Thyroid disease[194] (anti-thyroid antibodies, hypothyroidism, hyperthyroidism)[188]
- Systemic lupus erythematosus[194]
- Rheumatoid arthritis[194]
- Scleroderma[194]
- Mixed connective tissue disease[194]
- Phospholipid antibody syndrome[194]
- Coeliac disease[194]
- Multiple autoimmune endocrinopathies[194]
- Type I diabetes mellitus[194]
- Addison disease[194]
- Other autoimmune disease[194]

Stress[188]

CLINICAL TIPS

REPRODUCTIVE IMMUNOLOGY REFERRAL

In the authors' experience the following patients may also benefit from reproductive immunology investigations:

CLINICAL TIPS—cont'd

- ◆ Patients who have a history of vaginal bleeding during the luteal phase of an ART cycle and
- ◆ Patients who suffer from ≥2 implantation failures despite receiving specialist fertility acupuncture support during ART treatment

---

 ## Case study

RIF and Reproductive Immunology

Josie was 33 years old when she presented for acupuncture treatment support during her sixth IVF cycle.

Formal Orthodox Medical Diagnosis

Unexplained infertility

IVF History

- ◆ First cycle resulted in ectopic pregnancy and the loss of her right fallopian tube.
- ◆ Second cycle resulted in a biochemical miscarriage (positive pregnancy test and bleeding, both at 13 days post-egg collection).

- ◆ The last three IVF cycles resulted in negative pregnancy test results, but Josie experienced vaginal bleeding during the luteal phase in all three cycles.

Each time two good-quality blastocysts were transferred and the lining was 'well thickened'. Her reproductive consultant advised Josie to undergo immune investigations.

Immune Tests Results

- ◆ Th1 TNF-alpha ratio 34.3 (raised)
- ◆ NK cell assay 50:1 level 16.7% (slightly raised)

Case study—cont'd

- LAD levels of IgG T cells 23.3% and IgG B cells 2.8% (both low)
- Positive (heterozygote) for the MTHFR C677T mutation

She received a very basic immunotherapy (one intralipid infusion) with the last two IVF cycles, but they still failed.

Josie and her husband were frustrated. She wrote in her email to me, 'One of the hardest and most frustrating things about the whole process is that there are no answers and sometimes it doesn't seem that people are willing to try and find them. Just keep trying another cycle'.

I referred Josie to a reproductive immunologist with a view of possibly undergoing a more individualized immunotherapy. In preparation for her next IVF cycle, her reproductive immunologist provided several months of immunotherapy, including TNF-alpha inhibitors (Humira®), LIT, and IVIG. She was also prescribed glucocorticoids and Clexane to be used during IVF treatment.

In the meantime Josie received weekly acupuncture treatments.

TCM Diagnosis

- Blood Stasis: menstrual pain (dull or stabbing), large clots, wiry pulse.
- Full Heat: thirst for cold drinks, sleeping difficulties, can feel hot in the face especially, very heavy menstrual blood flow, headaches, constipation, red tongue body.

Basic Acupuncture Points Prescription

SP4 + P6, LU7 + KID6, LIV2, LI11, LI4, SP6, SP10, ST36, ST29, ZIGONG

After several months of preparation both with immunotherapy and acupuncture, Josie was ready to undergo her sixth cycle of IVF. She conceived and the pregnancy went well, although Josie needed regular immunotherapy and acupuncture treatment. She had a healthy baby boy.

Discussion

Combined Orthodox and TCM treatment approaches almost certainly made a difference in this case.

SUMMARY

Success rates of ART treatments are frustratingly low. In some cases, despite having good embryos transferred, patients still fail to conceive or miscarry soon after conception.

In some cases, the addition of a thorough preparation programme (including acupuncture treatment) is all that is needed for a successful outcome. In other cases, however, patients may require more advanced investigations and treatments.

For patients with a history of RIF, several additional options exist, including immunological testing and immunotherapy, but not all patients know about these. Not all ART clinics have the facilities to provide RIF investigations and/or treatments.

In the authors' experience, often the responsibility to refer patients for such investigations devolves to the fertility acupuncturist. Therefore, acupuncturists specializing in this field must be aware of what tests are available and the indications for each test.

REFERENCES

1. Thornhill AR, deDie-Smulders CE, Geraedts JP, et al. ESHRE PGD consortium 'best practice guidelines for clinical preimplantation genetic diagnosis (PGD) and preimplantation genetic screening (PGS)'. Hum Reprod 2005;20:35–48.

2. Rinehart J. Recurrent implantation failure: definition. J Assist Reprod Genet 2007;24:284–7.

3. Chard T. Frequency of implantation and early pregnancy loss in natural cycles. Baillieres Clin Obstet Gynaecol 1991;5:179–89.

4. Boomsma CM, Kavelaars A, Eijkemans MJ, et al. Endometrial secretion analysis identifies a cytokine profile predictive of pregnancy in IVF. Hum Reprod 2009;24:1427–35.

5. Macklon NS, Geraedts JP, Fauser BC. Conception to ongoing pregnancy: the 'black box' of early pregnancy loss. Hum Reprod Update 2002;8:333–43.

6. Nikas G, Makrigiannakis A, Hovatta O, et al. Surface morphology of the human endometrium. Basic and clinical aspects. Ann N Y Acad Sci 2000;900:316–24.

7. Achache H, Revel A. Endometrial receptivity markers, the journey to successful embryo implantation. Hum Reprod Update 2006;12:731–46.

8. Chan YY, Jayaprakasan K, Zamora J, et al. The prevalence of congenital uterine anomalies in unselected and high-risk populations: a systematic review. Hum Reprod Update 2011;17:761–71.

9. Taşkın EA, Berker B, Ozmen B, et al. Comparison of hysterosalpingography and hysteroscopy in the evaluation of the uterine cavity in patients undergoing

assisted reproductive techniques. Fertil Steril 2011;96:349–52.

10. Makrakis E, Hassiakos D, Stathis D, et al. Hysteroscopy in women with implantation failures after in vitro fertilization: findings and effect on subsequent pregnancy rates. J Minim Invasive Gynecol 2009;16:181–7.

11. Makrakis E, Pantos K. The outcomes of hysteroscopy in women with implantation failures after in-vitro fertilization: findings and effect on subsequent pregnancy rates. Curr Opin Obstet Gynecol 2010;22:339–43.

12. El-Mazny A, Abou-Salem N, El-Sherbiny W, et al. Outpatient hysteroscopy: a routine investigation before assisted reproductive techniques? Fertil Steril 2011;95:272–6.

13. Aletebi F. Hysteroscopy in women with implantation failures after in vitro fertilization: findings and effect on subsequent pregnancy rates. Middle East Fertil Soc J 2010;15:288–91.

14. Potdar N, Gelbaya T, Nardo LG. Endometrial injury to overcome recurrent embryo implantation failure: a systematic review and meta-analysis. Reprod Biomed Online 2012;25:561–71.

15. Machtinger R, Dor J, Margolin M, et al. Sequential transfer of day 3 embryos and blastocysts after previous IVF failures despite adequate ovarian response. Reprod Biomed Online 2006;13:376–9.

16. Loutradis D, Drakakis P, Dallianidis K, et al. A double embryo transfer on days 2 and 4 or 5 improves pregnancy outcome in patients with good embryos but repeated failures in IVF or ICSI. Clin Exp Obstet Gynecol 2004;31:63–6.

17. Fang C, Huang R, Li TT, et al. Day-2 and day-3 sequential transfer improves pregnancy rate in patients with repeated IVF-embryo transfer failure: a retrospective case–control study. Reprod Biomed Online 2013;26:30–5.

18. Abramovici H, Dirnfeld M, Weisman Z, et al. Pregnancies following the interval double-transfer technique in an in vitro fertilization-embryo transfer

program. J in vitro Fert Embryo Transf 1988;5:175–6.

19. Almog B, Levin I, Wagman I, et al. Interval double transfer improves treatment success in patients with repeated IVF/ET failures. J Assist Reprod Genet 2008;25:353–7.

20. Roque M, Lattes K, Serra S, et al. Fresh embryo transfer versus frozen embryo transfer in in vitro fertilization cycles: a systematic review and meta-analysis. Fertil Steril 2013;99:156–62.

21. Maheshwari A, Bhattacharya S. Elective frozen replacement cycles for all: ready for prime time? Hum Reprod 2013;28:6–9.

22. Revel A. Defective endometrial receptivity. Fertil Steril 2012;97:1028–32.

23. Bontekoe S, Blake D, Heineman MJ, et al. Adherence compounds in embryo transfer media for assisted reproductive technologies. Cochrane Database Syst Rev 2010;CD007421.

24. Barnhart K, Dunsmoor-Su R, Coutifaris C. Effect of endometriosis on in vitro fertilization. Fertil Steril 2002;77:1148–55.

25. Strandell A. The influence of hydrosalpinx on IVF and embryo transfer: a review. Hum Reprod Update 2000;6:387–95.

26. Al-Ghamdi A, Coskun S, Al-Hassan S, et al. The correlation between endometrial thickness and outcome of in vitro fertilization and embryo transfer (IVF-ET) outcome. Reprod Biol Endocrinol 2008;6:37.

27. El-Toukhy T, Coomarasamy A, Khairy M, et al. The relationship between endometrial thickness and outcome of medicated frozen embryo replacement cycles. Fertil Steril 2008;89:832–9.

28. Mains L, Van Voorhis BJ. Optimizing the technique of embryo transfer. Fertil Steril 2010;94:785–90.

29. Moore DE, Soules MR, Klein NA, et al. Bacteria in the transfer catheter tip influence the live-birth rate after in vitro fertilization. Fertil Steril 2000;74:1118–24.

30. Brook N, Khalaf Y, Coomarasamy A, et al. A randomized controlled trial of prophylactic antibiotics (co-amoxiclav) prior to embryo transfer. Hum Reprod 2006;21:2911–5.

31. Thum MY, Bhaskaran S, Abdalla HI, et al. An increase in the absolute count of CD56dim CD16+ CD69+ NK cells in the peripheral blood is associated with a poorer IVF treatment and pregnancy outcome. Hum Reprod 2004;19:2395–400.

32. Fukui A, Kwak-Kim J, Ntrivalas E, et al. Intracellular cytokine expression of peripheral blood natural killer cell subsets in women with recurrent spontaneous abortions and implantation failures. Fertil Steril 2008;89:157–65.

33. Chernyshov VP, Sudoma IO, Dons'koi BV, et al. Elevated NK cell cytotoxicity, CD158a expression in NK cells and activated T lymphocytes in peripheral blood of women with IVF failures. Am J Reprod Immunol 2010;64:58–67.

34. Tuckerman E, Mariee N, Prakash A, et al. Uterine natural killer cells in peri-implantation endometrium from women with repeated implantation failure after IVF. J Reprod Immunol 2010;87:60–6.

35. Miko E, Manfai Z, Meggyes M, et al. Possible role of natural killer and natural killer T-like cells in implantation failure after IVF. Reprod Biomed Online 2010;21:750–6.

36. Makrigiannakis A, Petsas G, Toth B, et al. Recent advances in understanding immunology of reproductive failure. J Reprod Immunol 2011;90:96–104.

37. Karami N, Boroujerdnia MG, Nikbakht R, et al. Enhancement of peripheral blood CD56(dim) cell and NK cell cytotoxicity in women with recurrent spontaneous abortion or in vitro fertilization failure. J Reprod Immunol 2012;95:87–92.

38. Sacks G, Yang Y, Gowen E, et al. Detailed analysis of peripheral blood natural killer cells in women with repeated IVF failure. Am J Reprod Immunol 2012;67:434–42.

39. Heit JA. Thrombophilia: common questions on laboratory assessment and management. Hematology Am Soc Hematol Educ Program 2007;(1):127–35.

40. Qublan HS, Eid SS, Ababneh HA, et al. Acquired and inherited thrombophilia: implication in recurrent IVF and embryo transfer

failure. Hum Reprod 2006;21:2694–8.

41. Bellver J, Soares SR, Alvarez C, et al. The role of thrombophilia and thyroid autoimmunity in unexplained infertility, implantation failure and recurrent spontaneous abortion. Hum Reprod 2008;23:278–84.

42. Sauer R, Roussev R, Jeyendran RS, et al. Prevalence of antiphospholipid antibodies among women experiencing unexplained infertility and recurrent implantation failure. Fertil Steril 2010;93:2441–3.

43. Azem F, Many A, Yovel I, et al. Increased rates of thrombophilia in women with repeated IVF failures. Hum Reprod 2004;19:368–70.

44. Simur A, Ozdemir S, Acar H, et al. Repeated in vitro fertilization failure and its relation with thrombophilia. Gynecol Obstet Invest 2009;67:109–12.

45. Buckingham KL, Stone PR, Smith JF, et al. Antiphospholipid antibodies in serum and follicular fluid – is there a correlation with IVF implantation failure? Hum Reprod 2006;21:728–34.

46. Practice Committee of American Society for Reproductive Medicine. Anti-phospholipid antibodies do not affect IVF success. Fertil Steril 2008;90:S172–3.

47. Lodigiani C, Di Micco P, Ferrazzi P, et al. Low-molecular-weight heparin in women with repeated implantation failure. Womens Health (Lond Engl) 2011;7:425–31.

48. Urman B, Ata B, Yakin K, et al. Luteal phase empirical low molecular weight heparin administration in patients with failed ICSI embryo transfer cycles: a randomized open-labeled pilot trial. Hum Reprod 2009;24:1640–7.

49. Qublan H, Amarin Z, Dabbas M, et al. Low-molecular-weight heparin in the treatment of recurrent IVF-ET failure and thrombophilia: a prospective randomized placebo-controlled trial. Hum Fertil (Camb) 2008;11:246–53.

50. Bohlmann MK. Effects and effectiveness of heparin in assisted reproduction. J Reprod Immunol 2011;90:82–90.

51. Berker B, Taşkin S, Kahraman K, et al. The role of low-molecular-weight heparin in recurrent implantation failure: a prospective, quasi-randomized, controlled study. Fertil Steril 2011;95:2499–502.

52. Thum MY, Abdalla HI, Taylor D. Relationship between women's age and basal follicle-stimulating hormone levels with aneuploidy risk in in vitro fertilization treatment. Fertil Steril 2008;90:315–21.

53. Wang YA, Healy D, Black D, et al. Age-specific success rate for women undertaking their first assisted reproduction technology treatment using their own oocytes in Australia, 2002–2005. Hum Reprod 2008;23:1633–8.

54. Klipstein S, Regan M, Ryley DA, et al. One last chance for pregnancy: a review of 2,705 in vitro fertilization cycles initiated in women age 40 years and above. Fertil Steril 2005;84:435–45.

55. Serour G, Mansour R, Serour A, et al. Analysis of 2,386 consecutive cycles of in vitro fertilization or intracytoplasmic sperm injection using autologous oocytes in women aged 40 years and above. Fertil Steril 2010;94:1707–12.

56. Sullivan E, Wang Y, Chapman M, et al. Success rates and cost of a live birth following fresh assisted reproduction treatment in women aged 45 years and older, Australia 2002–2004. Hum Reprod 2008;23:1639–43.

57. Tsafrir A, Simon A, Revel A, et al. Retrospective analysis of 1217 IVF cycles in women aged 40 years and older. Reprod Biomed Online 2007;14:348–55.

58. Brodin T, Bergh T, Berglund L, et al. Menstrual cycle length is an age-independent marker of female fertility: results from 6271 treatment cycles of in vitro fertilization. Fertil Steril 2008;90:1656–61.

59. Terriou P, Sapin C, Giorgetti C, et al. Embryo score is a better predictor of pregnancy than the number of transferred embryos or female age. Fertil Steril 2001;75:525–31.

60. Ruiz-Flores FJ, Garcia-Velasco JA. What strategies are the most effective in optimizing IVF outcome in patients with advanced maternal age? Expert Rev Obstet Gynecol 2011;6:591–8.

61. Orris JJ, Taylor TH, Gilchrist JW, et al. The utility of embryo banking in order to increase the number of embryos available for preimplantation genetic screening in advanced maternal age patients. J Assist Reprod Genet 2010;27:729–33.

62. Farhi J, Ben-Haroush A, Dresler H, et al. Male factor infertility, low fertilisation rate following ICSI and low number of high-quality embryos are associated with high order recurrent implantation failure in young IVF patients. Acta Obstet Gynecol Scand 2008;87:76–80.

63. Zini A. Are sperm chromatin and DNA defects relevant in the clinic? Syst Biol Reprod Med 2011;57:78–85.

64. Evenson D, Wixon R. Meta-analysis of sperm DNA fragmentation using the sperm chromatin structure assay. Reprod Biomed Online 2006;12:466–72.

65. Collins JA, Barnhart KT, Schlegel PN. Do sperm DNA integrity tests predict pregnancy with in vitro fertilization? Fertil Steril 2008;89:823–31.

66. Speyer BE, Pizzey AR, Ranieri M, et al. Fall in implantation rates following ICSI with sperm with high DNA fragmentation. Hum Reprod 2010;25:1609–18.

67. The Practice Committee of the American Society for Reproductive Medicine. Evaluation and treatment of recurrent pregnancy loss: a committee opinion. Fertil Steril 2012;98:1103–11.

68. Simon A, Laufer N. Repeated implantation failure: clinical approach. Fertil Steril 2012;97:1039–43.

69. The Practice Committee of the American Society for Reproductive Medicine. The clinical utility of sperm DNA integrity testing: a guideline. Fertil Steril 2013;99:673–7.

70. Klement AH, Koren-Morag N, Itsykson P, et al. Intracytoplasmic morphologically selected sperm injection versus intracytoplasmic sperm injection: a step toward a clinical algorithm. Fertil Steril 2013;99:1290–3.

71. Das M, Holzer HE. Recurrent implantation failure: gamete and

embryo factors. Fertil Steril 2012;97:1021–7.

72. Gianaroli L, Racowsky C, Geraedts J, et al. Best practices of ASRM and ESHRE: a journey through reproductive medicine. Fertil Steril 2012;98:1380–94.

73. Mantikou E, Youssef MA, van Wely M, et al. Embryo culture media and IVF/ICSI success rates: a systematic review. Hum Reprod Update 2013;19:210–20.

74. Glujovsky D, Blake D, Farquhar C, et al. Cleavage stage versus blastocyst stage embryo transfer in assisted reproductive technology. Cochrane Database Syst Rev 2012;7: CD002118.

75. Gunby J, Daya S, Olive D, et al. Day three versus day two embryo transfer following in vitro fertilization or intracytoplasmic sperm injection. Cochrane Database Syst Rev 2004; CD004378.

76. Kyrou D, Kolibianakis EM, Venetis CA, et al. How to improve the probability of pregnancy in poor responders undergoing in vitro fertilization: a systematic review and meta-analysis. Fertil Steril 2009;91:749–66.

77. Bahceci M, Ulug U, Ciray HN, et al. Efficiency of changing the embryo transfer time from day 3 to day 2 among women with poor ovarian response: a prospective randomized trial. Fertil Steril 2006;86:81–5.

78. Margalioth EJ, Ben-Chetrit A, Gal M, et al. Investigation and treatment of repeated implantation failure following IVF-ET. Hum Reprod 2006;21:3036–43.

79. Habana AE, Palter SF. Is tubal embryo transfer of any value? A meta-analysis and comparison with the Society for Assisted Reproductive Technology database. Fertil Steril 2001;76:286–93.

80. Research and evidence – facts and figures. Available from: http://www. oneatatime.org.uk/126.htm [accessed 23 September 2012].

81. Barnhart KT. Epidemiology of male and female reproductive disorders and impact on fertility regulation and population growth. Fertil Steril 2011;95:2200–3.

82. ASRM. Practice committee opinion: multiple pregnancy associated with infertility therapy. American Society for Reproductive Medicine. Continuing Medical Education for Physicians. Online course. Syllabus COM003; 2012.

83. Baruffi RL, Mauri AL, Petersen CG, et al. Single-embryo transfer reduces clinical pregnancy rates and live births in fresh IVF and intracytoplasmic sperm injection (ICSI) cycles: a meta-analysis. Reprod Biol Endocrinol 2009;7:36.

84. Pandian Z, Bhattacharya S, Ozturk O, et al. Number of embryos for transfer following in-vitro fertilisation or intra-cytoplasmic sperm injection. Cochrane Database Syst Rev 2009; CD003416.

85. Lawlor DA, Nelson SM. Effect of age on decisions about the numbers of embryos to transfer in assisted conception: a prospective study. Lancet 2012;379:521–7.

86. Schreurs A, Legius E, Meuleman C, et al. Increased frequency of chromosomal abnormalities in female partners of couples undergoing in vitro fertilization or intracytoplasmic sperm injection. Fertil Steril 2000;74:94–6.

87. Riccaboni A, Lalatta F, Caliari I, et al. Genetic screening in 2,710 infertile candidate couples for assisted reproductive techniques: results of application of Italian guidelines for the appropriate use of genetic tests. Fertil Steril 2008;89:800–8.

88. Stern C, Pertile M, Norris H, et al. Chromosome translocations in couples with in-vitro fertilization implantation failure. Hum Reprod 1999;14:2097–101.

89. Raziel A, Friedler S, Schachter M, et al. Increased frequency of female partner chromosomal abnormalities in patients with high-order implantation failure after in vitro fertilization. Fertil Steril 2002;78:515–9.

90. Practice Committee of American Society for Reproductive Medicine. Preimplantation genetic testing: a practice committee opinion. Fertil Steril 2008;90:S136–43.

91. Harton GL, De Rycke M, Fiorentino F, et al. ESHRE PGD consortium best practice guidelines for amplification-based PGD. Hum Reprod 2011;26:33–40.

92. Harton GL, Harper JC, Coonen E, et al. ESHRE PGD consortium best practice guidelines for fluorescence in situ hybridization-based PGD. Hum Reprod 2011;26:25–32.

93. Harper JC, Sengupta SB. Preimplantation genetic diagnosis: state of the art 2011. Hum Genet 2012;131:175–86.

94. Wong C, Chen AA, Behr B, et al. Time-lapse microscopy and image analysis in basic and clinical embryo development research. Reprod Biomed Online 2013;26:120–9.

95. Montag M. Morphokinetics and embryo aneuploidy: gas time come or not yet? Reprod Biomed Online 2013;26:528–30.

96. Herrero J, Meseguer M. Selection of high potential embryos using time-lapse imaging: the era of morphokinetics. Fertil Steril 2013;99:1030–4.

97. Campbell A, Fishel S, Bowman N, et al. Modelling a risk classification of aneuploidy in human embryos using non-invasive morphokinetics. Reprod Biomed Online 2013;26:477–85.

98. Prados FJ, Debrock S, Lemmen JG, et al. The cleavage stage embryo. Hum Reprod 2012;27(Suppl. 1): i50–i71.

99. Boomsma CM, Macklon NS. What can the clinician do to improve implantation? Reprod Biomed Online 2006;13:845–55.

100. Berin I, Stein DE, Keltz MD. A comparison of gonadotropin-releasing hormone (GnRH) antagonist and GnRH agonist flare protocols for poor responders undergoing in vitro fertilization. Fertil Steril 2010;93:360–3.

101. Takahashi K, Mukaida T, Tomiyama T, et al. GnRH antagonist improved blastocyst quality and pregnancy outcome after multiple failures of IVF/ICSI-ET with a GnRH agonist protocol. J Assist Reprod Genet 2004;21:317–22.

102. Al-Inany HG, Youssef MA, Aboulghar M, et al. Gonadotrophin-releasing hormone antagonists for assisted reproductive technology. Cochrane Database Syst Rev 2011; CD001750.

103. van der Linden M, Buckingham K, Farquhar C, et al. Luteal phase support for assisted reproduction

cycles. Cochrane Database Syst Rev 2011;CD009154.

104. Tomás C, Tikkinen K, Tuomivaara L, et al. The degree of difficulty of embryo transfer is an independent factor for predicting pregnancy. Hum Reprod 2002;17:2632–5.

105. Spitzer D, Haidbauer R, Corn C, et al. Effects of embryo transfer quality on pregnancy and live birth delivery rates. J Assist Reprod Genet 2012;29:131–5.

106. Spandorfer SD, Goldstein J, Navarro J, et al. Difficult embryo transfer has a negative impact on the outcome of in vitro fertilization. Fertil Steril 2003;79:654–5.

107. Mansour RT, Aboulghar MA. Optimizing the embryo transfer technique. Hum Reprod 2002;17:1149–53.

108. Matthiesen SM, Frederiksen Y, Ingerslev HJ, et al. Stress, distress and outcome of assisted reproductive technology (ART): a meta-analysis. Hum Reprod 2011;26:2763–76.

109. Domar AD, Rooney KL, Wiegand B, et al. Impact of a group mind/body intervention on pregnancy rates in IVF patients. Fertil Steril 2011;95:2269–73.

110. Tan BK, Vandekerckhove P, Kennedy R, et al. Investigation and current management of recurrent IVF treatment failure in the UK. BJOG 2005;112:773–80.

111. Isoyama Manca di Villahermosa D, Dos Santos LG, Nogueira MB, et al. Influence of acupuncture on the outcomes of in vitro fertilisation when embryo implantation has failed: a prospective randomised controlled clinical trial. Acupunct Med 2013;31:157–61.

112. Rochat de la Vallee E. Infertility. In: Root C, editor. The essential women, female health and fertility in Chinese classical texts. Norfolk: Monkey Press; 2007. p. 72–83.

113. Carman N. The treatment of recurrent implantation failure in Assisted Reproductive Technology. J Chin Med 2008;88:53–9.

114. Auteroche B, Kivity O. Reinforcing, reducing and balancing. In: Acupuncture and moxibustion: a guide to clinical practice. Edinburgh: Churchill Livingstone; 1992. p. 43–8, Section 1 [chapter 4].

115. Jiang J, Li G, Zang M. Clinical observation on 41 cases of threatened and habitual abortion treated by blood activation and stasis removal. J Tradit Chin Med 1997;17:259–65.

116. Rochat de la Vallee E. Zang and Fu. In: Root C, editor. The essential women, female health and fertility in Chinese classical texts. Norfolk: Monkey Press; 2007. p. 26–46.

117. Maughan TA, Zhai X. The acupuncture treatment of female infertility – with particular reference to egg quality and endometrial receptiveness. J Chin Med 2012;13–21.

118. Zhou J, Qu F. Treating gynaecological disorders with Traditional Chinese Medicine: a review. Afr J Tradit Complement Altern Med 2009;6:494–517.

119. Sun Si-Miao. Translation. In: Wilms S, translator. Bèi Jí Qian Jin Yào Fang. Essential prescriptions worth a thousand in gold for every emergency. 3 Volumes on gynecology, vol. 2. Portland: The Chinese Medicine Database; 2007. p. 52–216 [chapter 2].

120. Lu HC. Great treatise on Yin Yang classifications of natural phenomena. In: A complete translation of the Yellow Emperor's classics of internal medicine and the difficult classic (Nei-Jing and Nan-Jing). Vancouver: International College of Traditional Chinese Medicine; 2004. p. 86–98, Section two: Essential questions [Su Wen] [chapter 5].

121. Jin Y. Complications of pregnancy. In: Hakim C, editor. Handbook of obstetrics & gynecology in Chinese medicine: an integrated approach. Seattle, WA: Eastland Press; 1998. p. 95–120 [chapter 7].

122. Zegers-Hochschild F, Adamson GD, de Mouzon J, et al. The International Committee for Monitoring Assisted Reproductive Technology (ICMART) and the World Health Organization (WHO) revised glossary on ART terminology, 2009. Hum Reprod 2009;24:2683–7.

123. Royal College of Obstetricians and Gynaecologists. GTG17 the investigation and treatment of couples with recurrent first-trimester and second-trimester miscarriage. Report of the Royal College of Obstetricians and Gynaecologists; 2011.

124. Assisted Reproductive Technology (ART) – glossary. Available from: http://www.eshre.eu/ESHRE/ English/Guidelines-Legal/ART-glossary/page.aspx/1062 [accessed 26 January 2013].

125. Blok L, Kremer J. In vitro fertilisation and intracytoplasmic sperm injection. In: de Haan N, Spelt M, Gobel R, editors. Reproductive medicine: a textbook for paramedics. Amsterdam: Elsevier Gezondheidszorg; 2010. p. 105–26 [chapter 8].

126. Tummers P. Risk of spontaneous abortion in singleton and twin pregnancies after IVF/ICSI. Hum Reprod 2003;18:1720–3.

127. Nybo Andersen AM, Wohlfahrt J, Christens P, et al. Maternal age and fetal loss: population based register linkage study. BMJ 2000;320:1708–12.

128. Stephenson MD, Awartani KA, Robinson WP. Cytogenetic analysis of miscarriages from couples with recurrent miscarriage: a case–control study. Hum Reprod 2002;17:446–51.

129. de la Rochebrochard E, Thonneau P. Paternal age and maternal age are risk factors for miscarriage; results of a multicentre European study. Hum Reprod 2002;17:1649–56.

130. Li TC, Makris M, Tomsu M, et al. Recurrent miscarriage: aetiology, management and prognosis. Hum Reprod Update 2002;8:463–81.

131. Ghi T, De Musso F, Maroni E, et al. The pregnancy outcome in women with incidental diagnosis of septate uterus at first trimester scan. Hum Reprod 2012;27:2671–5.

132. García-Enguídanos A, Calle ME, Valero J, et al. Risk factors in miscarriage: a review. Eur J Obstet Gynecol Reprod Biol 2002;102:111–9.

133. Toth B, Jeschke U, Rogenhofer N, et al. Recurrent miscarriage: current concepts in diagnosis and treatment. J Reprod Immunol 2010;85:25–32.

134. Ralph SG, Rutherford AJ, Wilson JD. Influence of bacterial vaginosis on conception and miscarriage in the first trimester: cohort study. BMJ 1999;319:220–3.

135. Goldenberg RL, Iams JD, Mercer BM, et al. The preterm prediction study: the value of new vs standard risk factors in predicting early and all spontaneous preterm births. NICHD MFMU network. Am J Public Health 1998;88:233–8.

136. Larsson PG, Fåhraeus L, Carlsson B, et al. Predisposing factors for bacterial vaginosis, treatment efficacy and pregnancy outcome among term deliveries; results from a preterm delivery study. BMC Womens Health 2007;7:20–6.

137. Robertson L, Wu O, Langhorne P, et al. Thrombophilia in pregnancy: a systematic review. Br J Haematol 2006;132:171–96.

138. Smith ML, Schust DJ. Endocrinology and recurrent early pregnancy loss. Semin Reprod Med 2011;29:482–90.

139. Christiansen OB, Nybo Andersen AM, Bosch E, et al. Evidence-based investigations and treatments of recurrent pregnancy loss. Fertil Steril 2005;83:821–39.

140. Jakubowicz DJ, Iuorno MJ, Jakubowicz S, et al. Effects of metformin on early pregnancy loss in the polycystic ovary syndrome. J Clin Endocrinol Metab 2002;87:524–9.

141. Rai R, Backos M, Rushworth F, et al. Polycystic ovaries and recurrent miscarriage – a reappraisal. Hum Reprod 2000;15:612–5.

142. Amsterdam ESHRE/ASRM-Sponsored 3rd PCOS Consensus Workshop Group. Consensus on women's health aspects of polycystic ovary syndrome (PCOS). Hum Reprod 2012;27:14–24.

143. ESHRE Capri Workshop Group. Health and fertility in World Health Organization group 2 anovulatory women. Hum Reprod Update 2012;18:586–99.

144. Cocksedge KA, Li TC, Saravelos SH, et al. A reappraisal of the role of polycystic ovary syndrome in recurrent miscarriage. Reprod Biomed Online 2008;17:151–60.

145. The Practice Committee of the American Society for Reproductive Medicine. The clinical relevance of luteal phase deficiency. Fertil Steril 2012;98:1112–7.

146. Practice Committee of American Society for Reproductive Medicine. Diagnostic evaluation of the infertile female: a committee opinion. Fertil Steril 2012;98:302–7.

147. Filicori M, Butler JP, Crowley WF. Neuroendocrine regulation of the corpus luteum in the human. Evidence for pulsatile progesterone secretion. J Clin Invest 1984;73:1638–47.

148. Wahabi HA, Fayed AA, Esmaeil SA, et al. Progestogen for treating threatened miscarriage. Cochrane Database Syst Rev 2011;(12): CD005943.

149. Robinson L, Gallos ID, Conner SJ, et al. The effect of sperm DNA fragmentation on miscarriage rates: a systematic review and meta-analysis. Hum Reprod 2012;27:2908–17.

150. Zini A, Boman JM, Belzile E, et al. Sperm DNA damage is associated with an increased risk of pregnancy loss after IVF and ICSI: systematic review and meta-analysis. Hum Reprod 2008;23:2663–8.

151. Jauniaux E, Farquharson RG, Christiansen OB, et al. Evidence-based guidelines for the investigation and medical treatment of recurrent miscarriage. Hum Reprod 2006;21:2216–22.

152. Lawler CC, Budrys NM, Rodgers AK, et al. Serum beta human chorionic gonadotropin levels can inform outcome counseling after in vitro fertilization. Fertil Steril 2011;96:505–7.

153. Chen CD, Ho HN, Wu MY, et al. Paired human chorionic gonadotrophin determinations for the prediction of pregnancy outcome in assisted reproduction. Hum Reprod 1997;12:2538–41.

154. Homan G, Brown S, Moran J, et al. Human chorionic gonadotropin as a predictor of outcome in assisted reproductive technology pregnancies. Fertil Steril 2000;73:270–4.

155. Practice Committee of American Society for Reproductive Medicine. Medical treatment of ectopic pregnancy. Fertil Steril 2008;90: S206–12.

156. Tayal VS, Cohen H, Norton HJ. Outcome of patients with an indeterminate emergency department first-trimester pelvic ultrasound to rule out ectopic pregnancy. Acad Emerg Med 2004;11:912–7.

157. Deutchman M, Tubay AT, Turok D. First trimester bleeding. Am Fam Physician 2009;79:985–94.

158. Kadar N, Bohrer M, Kemmann E, et al. The discriminatory human chorionic gonadotropin zone for endovaginal sonography: a prospective, randomized study. Fertil Steril 1994;61:1016–20.

159. Rauch ER, Schattman GL, Christos PJ, et al. Embryonic heart rate as a predictor of first-trimester pregnancy loss in infertility patients after in vitro fertilization. Fertil Steril 2009;91:2451–4.

160. Deaton JL, Honoré GM, Huffman CS, et al. Early transvaginal ultrasound following an accurately dated pregnancy: the importance of finding a yolk sac or fetal heart motion. Hum Reprod 1997;12:2820–3.

161. Wu YL. An uncertain harvest, pregnancy and miscarriage. In: Reproducing women: medicine, metaphor, and childbirth in late imperial China. Berkeley: University of California Press; 2010. p. 120–46 [chapter 4].

162. Maciocia G. Threatened miscarriage. In: Obstetrics and gynecology in Chinese medicine. 2nd ed. Edinburgh: Elsevier Health Sciences; 2011. p. 477–90 [chapter 31].

163. Lyttleton J. Pregnancy loss, miscarriage and ectopic pregnancy. In: Treatment of infertility with Chinese medicine. London: Churchill Livingstone; 2004. p. 277–336 [chapter 8].

164. Betts D. Miscarriage. In: Deadman P, Heese I, editors. Essential guide to acupuncture in pregnancy and childbirth. Hove, UK: Journal Of Chinese Medicine; 2006. p. 8–18 [chapter 2].

165. Zhao LQ. TCM preventative treatment of recurrent spontaneous miscarriage. J Assoc Tradit Chin Med 2009;16:14–8.

166. Sun Si-Miao. Translation. In: Wilms S, translator. Bèi Jí Qian Jin Yào Fang, Essential prescriptions worth a thousand in gold for every emergency, 3 Volumes on gynecology, vol. 3. Portland: The Chinese Medicine Database; 2007. p. 232–362 [chapter 3].

167. Liang L. Prevention of miscarriages. In: Acupuncture & IVF. Boulder, CO: Blue Poppy Press; 2003. p. 69–77 [chapter 7].

168. West Z. High risk pregnancies. In: Acupuncture in pregnancy and childbirth. Edinburgh: Churchill Livingstone/Elsevier; 2001. p. 121–30 [chapter 8].

169. Bates GW, Ginsburg ES. Early pregnancy loss in in vitro fertilization (IVF) is a positive predictor of subsequent IVF success. Fertil Steril 2002;77:337–41.

170. Liu Z, Ma L. Common methods used in health preservation of TCM. In: Health preservation of Traditional Chinese Medicine. Beijing: People's Medical Publishing House; 2007. p. 294–442 [chapter 2].

171. Maciocia G. Habitual miscarriage. In: Obstetrics and gynecology in Chinese medicine. 2nd ed. Edinburgh: Elsevier Health Sciences; 2011. p. 545–54 [chapter 43].

172. Flaws B. Hua Tai slippery fetus. Shu Duo Tai repeated fallen fetus. Xi Guan Xing Liu Chan habitual miscarriage. In: Path of pregnancy. Volume 1. A handbook of traditional Chinese gestational & birthing disease. Boulder, CO: Blue Poppy Press; 1993. p. 69–73 [chapter 7].

173. Davanzo J, Hale L, Rahman M. How long after a miscarriage should women wait before becoming pregnant again? Multivariate analysis of cohort data from Matlab, Bangladesh. BMJ Open 2012;(12): doi:10.1136/bmjopen-2012-001591.

174. American Society for Reproductive Medicine. Assisted reproductive technology in the United States: 2001 results generated from the American Society for Reproductive Medicine/Society for Assisted Reproductive technology registry. Fertil Steril 2007;87:1253–66.

175. Mol F, van den Boogaard E, van Mello NM, et al. Guideline adherence in ectopic pregnancy management. Hum Reprod 2011;26:307–15.

176. Lee HJ, Park TC, Norwitz ER. Management of pregnancies with cervical shortening: a very short cervix is a very big problem. Rev Obstet Gynecol 2009;2:107–15.

177. Mercer B. The preterm prediction study: prediction of preterm premature rupture of membranes through clinical findings and ancillary testing. Am J Obstet Gynecol 2000;183:738–45.

178. Dekker GA, Lee SY, North RA, et al. Risk factors for preterm birth in an international prospective cohort of nulliparous women. PLoS One 2012;7:e39154.

179. Honest H, Bachmann LM, Coomarasamy A, et al. Accuracy of cervical transvaginal sonography in predicting preterm birth: a systematic review. Ultrasound Obstet Gynecol 2003;22:305–22.

180. Iams JD, Goldenberg RL, Meis PJ, et al. The length of the cervix and the risk of spontaneous premature delivery. N Engl J Med 1996;334:567–73.

181. Farquharson RG. Late pregnancy loss. In: Farquharson RG, Stephenson MD, editors. Early pregnancy. Cambridge: Cambridge University Press; 2010. p. 277–86.

182. Lockwood CJ, Senyei AE, Dische MR, et al. Fetal fibronectin in cervical and vaginal secretions as a predictor of preterm delivery. N Engl J Med 1991;325:669–74.

183. Chen SJ, Liu YL, Sytwu HK. Immunologic regulation in pregnancy: from mechanism to therapeutic strategy for immunomodulation. Clin Dev Immunol 2012;2012:258391.

184. Aagaard-Tillery KM, Silver R, Dalton J. Immunology of normal pregnancy. Semin Fetal Neonatal Med 2006;11:279–95.

185. Porter TF, LaCoursiere Y, Scott JR. Immunotherapy for recurrent miscarriage. Cochrane Database Syst Rev 2006;(2):CD000112 [review].

186. Royal College of Obstetricians and Gynaecologists Immunological Testing and Interventions for Reproductive Failure. Scientific advisory committee opinion paper 5. Report of the Royal College of Obstetricians and Gynaecologists. June, 2008.

187. Reproductive immunology – natural killer cells – fertility. Available from: http://www.hfea.gov.uk/fertility-treatment-options-reproductive-immunology.html [accessed 7 July 2013].

188. Beer AE, Kantecki J, Reed J. Category 5 immune problems – part one. In: Is your body baby-friendly: "unexplained" infertility, miscarriage and IVF failure explained. Houston, TX: AJR Pub.; 2006. p. 69–90

189. Quenby S, Farquharson R. Uterine natural killer cells, implantation failure and recurrent miscarriage. Reprod Biomed Online 2006;13:24–8.

190. A guide to interpreting the results of the reproductive immunophenotype. Available from: http://repro-med.net/repro-med-site2/index.php?option=com_content&view=article&id=6:immunophenotype&catid=2:pages-ett&Itemid=25 [accessed 7 July 2013].

191. Natural killer (NK) cell assay. Available from: http://www.repro-med.net/repro-med-site2/index.php?option=com_content&view=article&id=7:nk-assay-&catid=2:pages-ett&Itemid=70 [accessed 7 July 2013].

192. Beer AE, Kantecki J, Reed J. Comprehensive immune testing. In: Is your body baby-friendly: "unexplained" infertility, miscarriage and IVF failure explained. Houston, TX: AJR Pub.; 2006. p. 127–40.

193. Beaman KD, Ntrivalas E, Mallers TM, et al. Immune etiology of recurrent pregnancy loss and its diagnosis. Am J Reprod Immunol 2012;67:319–25.

194. Gleicher N, Weghofer A, Barad DH. Cutting edge assessment of the impact of autoimmunity on female reproductive success. J Autoimmun 2011;38:J74–80.

195. Carp HJ, Selmi C, Shoenfeld Y. The autoimmune bases of infertility and pregnancy loss. J Autoimmun 2012;38:J266–74.

196. Christodoulakos G, Augoulea A, Lambrinoudaki I, et al. Pathogenesis of endometriosis: the role of defective 'immunosurveillance'. Eur J Contracep Reprod Health Care 2007;12:194–202.

197. Eisenberg VH, Zolti M, Soriano D. Is there an association between autoimmunity and endometriosis? Autoimmun Rev 2012;11:806–14.

198. Ozgör B, Selimoğlu MA. Coeliac disease and reproductive disorders. Scand J Gastroenterol 2010;45:395–402.

199. Clark DA. Anti-TNFalpha therapy in immune-mediated subfertility: state of the art. J Reprod Immunol 2010;85:15–24.

200. Leukocyte antibody detection (LAD) test. Available from: http://www.repro-med.net/repro-med-site2/index.php?option=com_content&view=article&id=75%3Aleukocyte-antibody-detection-lad-test&catid=12%3Atests-and-testaments&Itemid=12 [accessed 26 July 2013].

201. Beer AE, Kantecki J, Reed J. Dr. beer's treatments. In: Is your body baby-friendly: "unexplained" infertility, miscarriage and IVF failure explained. Houston, TX: AJR Pub.; 2006. p. 141–57

202. Benschop L, Seshadri S, Toulis KA, et al. Immune therapies for women with history of failed implantation undergoing IVF treatment. Cochrane Database Syst Rev 2012; doi: 10.1002/14651858.CD009602.

203. Practice Committee of the American Society for Reproductive Medicine. Intravenous immunoglobulin (IVIG) and recurrent spontaneous pregnancy loss. Fertil Steril 2006;86:S226–7.

204. Clark DA, Coulam CB, Stricker RB. Is intravenous immunoglobulins (IVIG) efficacious in early pregnancy failure? A critical review and meta-analysis for patients who fail in vitro fertilization and embryo transfer (IVF). J Assist Reprod Genet 2006;23:1–13.

205. Ata B, Tan SL, Shehata F, et al. A systematic review of intravenous immunoglobulin for treatment of unexplained recurrent miscarriage. Fertil Steril 2011;95:1080–1085.e1-2.

206. Hutton B, Sharma R, Fergusson D, et al. Use of intravenous immunoglobulin for treatment of recurrent miscarriage: a systematic review. BJOG 2007;114:134–42.

207. Shreeve N, Sadek K. Intralipid therapy for recurrent implantation failure: new hope or false dawn? J Reprod Immunol 2012;93:38–40.

208. Roussev RG, Ng SC, Coulam CB. Natural killer cell functional activity suppression by intravenous immunoglobulin, intralipid and soluble human leukocyte antigen-g. Am J Reprod Immunol 2007;57:262–9.

209. Coulam CB, Acacio B. Does immunotherapy for treatment of reproductive failure enhance live births? Am J Reprod Immunol 2012;67:296–304.

210. Boomsma CM, Keay SD, Macklon NS. Peri-implantation glucocorticoid administration for assisted reproductive technology cycles. Cochrane Database Syst Rev 2012;6, CD005996.

211. Winger EE, Reed JL, Ashoush S, et al. Treatment with adalimumab (Humira) and intravenous immunoglobulin improves pregnancy rates in women undergoing IVF. Am J Reprod Immunol 2009;61:113–20.

212. Yoshioka S, Fujiwara H, Nakayama T, et al. Intrauterine administration of autologous peripheral blood mononuclear cells promotes implantation rates in patients with repeated failure of IVF-embryo transfer. Hum Reprod 2006;21:3290–4.

213. Scarpellini F, Sbracia M. Use of granulocyte colony-stimulating factor for the treatment of unexplained recurrent miscarriage: a randomised controlled trial. Hum Reprod 2009;24:2703–8.

214. Gui J, Xiong F, Li J, et al. Effects of acupuncture on th1, th2 cytokines in rats of implantation failure. Evid Based Complement Alternat Med 2012;2012:893023.

215. Aoki E, Kasahara T, Hagiwara H, et al. Electroacupuncture and moxibustion influence the lipopolysaccharide-induced TNF-alpha production by macrophages. In Vivo 2005;19:495–500.

216. Wang J, Zhao H, Mao-Ying QL, et al. Electroacupuncture downregulates TLR2/4 and pro-inflammatory cytokine expression after surgical trauma stress without adrenal glands involvement. Brain Res Bull 2009;80:89–94.

217. Tian L, Huang YX, Tian M, et al. Downregulation of electroacupuncture at ST36 on TNF-alpha in rats with ulcerative colitis. World J Gastroenterol 2003;9:1028–33.

218. Kim SK, Bae H. Acupuncture and immune modulation. Auton Neurosci 2010;157:38–41.

219. Karatay S, Akcay F, Yildirim K, et al. Effects of some acupoints (DU-14, LI-11, ST-36, and SP-6) on serum TNF-α and HSCRP levels in healthy young subjects. J Altern Complement Med 2011;17:347–50.

220. Takahashi T, Sumino S, Kanda K, et al. Acupuncture modifies immune cells. J Exp Clin Med 2009;1:17–22.

221. Silverio-Lopes S, da Mota MPG. Acupuncture in modulation of immunity. In: Chen J, Cheng T, editors. Acupuncture in modern medicine. Rijeka, Croatia: InTech; 2013. p. 51–76 [chapter 3].

222. Hartung HP, Mouthon L, Ahmed R, et al. Clinical applications of intravenous immunoglobulins (ivig) – beyond immunodeficiencies and neurology. Clin Exp Immunol 2009;158(Suppl. 1):23–33.

223. Zhao L. Treating infertility by the integration of Traditional Chinese Medicine and assisted conception therapy. J Assoc Tradit Chin Med 2011;28:9–14.

224. Xu X, Yin H, Tang D, et al. Application of traditional Chinese medicine in the treatment of infertility. Hum Fertil 2003;6:161–8.

Chapter 13

The therapeutic relationship in acupuncture practice

Practitioner and patient interaction is a fundamental attribute in the practical application of the philosophy of Traditional Chinese Medicine (TCM). The therapeutic relationship is formed through a series of actions that occur during the consultation, treatment, and management of the subfertile patient. Various methods of inquiry involve active participation between the patient and practitioner.

TCM philosophical concepts unify Mind, Body, Emotion, and Spirit, and recognize emotions as a cause and/or consequence of subfertility. Fertility acupuncturists need to ensure that the social and psychological consequences of subfertility are identified and are appropriately taken into consideration in patient management. This can help to put in context a patient's emotional disposition and allow appropriate and empathetic management.[1]

Fertility acupuncturists can positively influence patients' experience of subfertility and assisted reproductive technology (ART) treatment. At the same time, acupuncture supports their health and well-being and positively influences Qi, Shen (Spirit), and Jing (Essence). As shown in other healthcare contexts, a good therapeutic relationship psychologically supports a patient's treatment and management.[1,2] This is especially important in fertility-based acupuncture practice management of subfertility patients.

The synergy of TCM diagnosis, treatment, management, and the therapeutic relationship with the practitioner allows the patient to understand more about his or her subfertility and to be potentially more motivated to improve the factors associated with fertility. It may also help to reduce anxieties and fears about the treatment outcome. In this respect, subfertility patients may be comparable to dental patients, who also have concerns and anxieties about treatment that, when appropriately addressed in the therapeutic relationship, can be dispersed.[1]

Mitchell and Cormack suggest that there are five important aspects in the development of the therapeutic relationship in the practice of complementary medicine: mutuality, trust, care, challenge and performance, and return to mutuality.[3] Equally so, the evolution of the patient–practitioner therapeutic relationship in TCM involves a complexity of interactions.

MUTUALITY

The initial acupuncture fertility consultation provides the foundation for mutuality by means of active participation. A patient-centred approach to diagnosis[4] that is holistic in its theoretical foundation gives the patient the opportunity to identify with his or her health and subfertility. The acupuncturist's clinical skills such as enquiry, looking, and listening facilitate empathy, validation, and shared understanding.

An integrated approach to the acupuncture consultation combining TCM and Orthodox medical knowledge strengthens the subfertility review, identifying other causes, contributing factors, and methods of treatment. This approach to management and treatment enables the patient to conceptualize his or her health and illness in different and meaningful ways.

Patients' expectations of what they want from acupuncture are clear. In the authors' experience, subfertility patients seek acupuncture treatment to help them conceive, reduce their stress levels, and improve their health. Patients often comment that they obtain a sense of control over their fertility issues and aspects of their lifestyle through acupuncture treatment. They feel reassured that they are taking active steps to optimize their chances of success with IVF.

Discussing and analysing their main complaint highlights their individual needs, their specific points of concern, and their expectations of what acupuncture treatment and management can provide for them.

However, it is necessary for both patients and acupuncturists to appreciate the limits of what acupuncture can achieve in each individual case. A realistic and an integrated approach along with problem solving initiates shared understandings and agreement. Mitchell and Cormack proposed several key steps that demonstrate mutuality within the therapeutic relationship that can help complementary practitioners explain to patients how they can help them:[3,5]

- Explain what the treatment may involve, for example, the way you approach the treatment of fertility.
- Respond helpfully to questions raised by the patient.
- Discuss your plan of action to help the patient.
- Discuss the patient's views so he or she can consider the appropriateness of your approach to treatment in the context of what the patient believes he or she needs and wants from the acupuncture treatment.

TRUST

Patients place a lot of trust in the decisions that are made on their behalf, for example, in consultants who deem their suitability for IVF/ART intervention, the medication they are prescribed, the embryologists who look after their embryos and who make the choices about which embryos are suitable for transfer, and in their acupuncturist's skills and abilities.

Subfertile patients may at times be sensitive and vulnerable. Therefore, for them to have a feeling of safety, empathy[2] and trust is very important.[3] Patients often feel safer as a result of seeing practitioners who have the expertise in the treatment of subfertility and are well versed in understanding IVF and ART.[4,6] An acupuncturist can achieve the trust of a patient by demonstrating excellent knowledge of reproduction, subfertility, medical tests and investigations, and ART treatment. The fertility acupuncturists who can do this provide reassuring feelings of safety and added security for the patient.

The practitioner's sensitivity to the patient's need for information during the reproductive medicine consultation provides the foundation for trust, care, and patient satisfaction.[2] Information provision is important, but it should be delivered according to the individual patient's needs and requirements.[4] Some patients like to know everything about their treatment, medical tests, and procedures. Other patients would rather not know very much (which in itself may raise issues of obtaining appropriately informed patient consent).

Boundaries are also important,[3] especially so in subfertile patients. Maintaining appropriate boundaries can help patients feel and remain safe and comfortable during the clinical encounter.

Reassuring a patient that the information he or she divulges will be kept confidential is another essential element of trust.[3] It is not unusual for the practitioner to treat both partners or friends of the patient. Patients must feel that they can share all the nuances of their information with the practitioner, without worrying about confidentiality.

Explaining the TCM treatment plan, associated benefits and risks from treatment, and the associated costs enables the patient to give informed consent to treatment and facilitates trust and compliance.[3]

As Mitchel and Cormack have noted, behaving courteously and respectfully to patients is a cornerstone of clinical practice.[3] In subfertility patients this is especially important when discussing sensitive subjects such as age, interpretation of signs and symptoms, test results, treatment prognosis, and other parameters.

As a fertility acupuncturist, it is very important to understand the fertility patients' individual needs and special requirements and manage a range of emotions (which can alter very quickly, for example, following a test result) in order to gain their trust in your abilities and skills.[3] As a normal part of fertility acupuncture practice, you will need to support and manage each patient you see in each clinical encounter, because each one will present with a variety of emotions and reactions. Patients' emotions can be radically different from one consultation to the next.

TCM pulse and tongue diagnosis are tools that can facilitate both a spoken and unspoken dialogue between practitioner and patient, encourage the development of a therapeutic relationship, and provide the foundations for trust; methods that are able to positively influence the Shen (Spirit). This is because the patient can observe the approach, care, concern, importance, and knowledge obtained during the TCM diagnostic process. These factors also act as treatment quality controls for the patient and practitioner alike. For example, pulse taking involves holding or touching the patient's hand. For the acupuncturist, assessment of the pulse assists in the diagnosis process and acts as one of the outcome measures.

CARE

Care for and empathy with the patient is important, as it demonstrates a willingness to help the patient at one of the most important times of his or her life – creating a family. Empathy by the clinician shows understanding and acceptance of the patient's situation.[3] An empathic approach helps patients feel more at ease and satisfied. One example of this is illustrated in a study of 2146 patients who rated their satisfaction levels with their first consultation, at a private fertility clinic, significantly higher after physicians received training in empathic skills.[2]

A range of negative feelings and emotions may be expressed at different times by patients, for example, hopelessness, despair, depression, anxiety, jealousy, or suspicion. Patients may worry about the outcome of the various aspects of their fertility treatment. A very good therapeutic relationship helps to manage these concerns and emotions, and also reassure and safeguard the patient. The fertility acupuncturist becomes central to the patient's support network, with highly sensitive care being a fundamental aspect of treatment and management.

Caring for the patient also means caring for yourself.[3] Self-reflection is useful, especially after clinical encounters and the countertransference of emotions that may have affected the practitioner adversely.

The provision of acupuncture treatment at time-specific critical times during their IVF cycle is an important aspect of care for the patient, and it is expected and valued by patients. However, there are logistical limitations on your ability to be always available for treatments. Ensuring that the patient's acupuncture treatment can still be provided, even if you personally are unavailable to administer it, is very important. So, for example, a smooth transition between you and your locum helps to support the patient's experience and confidence in the locum and you.

Manage issues, which may affect the patient or influence the outcome, professionally. For example, you may need to emphasize the value of controlling alcohol intake. Show you can tolerate patients' feelings and understand their concerns and difficulties.[1,3] A patient may be annoyed and find it difficult to lose weight as suggested by a clinician, or, alternatively, the patient may be overweight, but thus far may have not received information regarding the benefits of weight loss. Therefore, explaining or reinforcing this to the patient becomes your task. A therapeutic relationship facilitates compliance and professional intervention that is accepted and acted upon by the patient.

Acknowledge any personal biases or ethical considerations that you may have.[3] You may have particular opinions about reproductive medicine interventions or biases about a patient's age, sexual orientation, IVF itself, sex selection, or the use of donor sperm or eggs. These personal biases may influence your treatment choices or the patient's experience. Consider whether any such biases limit your objectivity to truly help the patient. If so, refer to another practitioner.

Acknowledge there are limits to what acupuncture treatment can achieve.[3]

CHALLENGE AND PERFORMANCE

Summarizing the clinical encounter and data relevant to the challenge and devising treatment principles based upon an integrated approach is essential. Always maintain a respectful and collaborative approach.[3,4] Ensure that it is relevant to the patient's constructs of both IVF and acupuncture and takes into account his or her physical, cognitive, and psychosocial state.

At times it is difficult to deal with obstacles (for example, from events such as failed IVF cycles, miscarriages, pregnancy-related complications, and stillbirth) that may have already compromised or may compromise the patient's current IVF treatment. Managing fertility patients' experiences of disappointment of their fertility status can be challenging. The fertility acupuncturist needs to listen, acknowledge, accept, and work toward developing a range of possible pragmatic solutions, so that they may improve the future fertility outcomes of each patient that presents to him or her.

Managing successful IVF outcomes against a background of complications and/or co-morbidities can at times be difficult for the practitioner, especially if the practitioner lacks experience in this field of practice. Advice sought from experienced colleagues can be of help. Professional forums can sometimes offer assistance.

Reproductive healthcare is a rapidly evolving field of medicine. Thus, the good fertility acupuncturist needs to be able to identify and critically review relevant high-quality literature. It is imperative that fertility acupuncturists remain current with advances in the field in order to be optimally able to support patients at differing times and stages of the patients' treatment cycle.

Continual professional development enhances theoretical knowledge. From this educational process the practitioner derives encouragement and reflective self-confidence, which is mutually beneficial and supportive to both the patient and practitioner. The practical application of the most appropriate clinical methodology skills (such as looking and listening), interface bidirectionally with the acupuncturist's theoretical knowledge base and philosophical constructs.

The use of self-reflection tools such as regular audits of practice results can help to provide some objectivity to the measurement of a practitioner's performance and success rates.

RETURN TO MUTUALITY

Ending treatments provides the means to incorporate relevant advice and the next plan of action.[3]

Decide on the appropriate time to discharge a patient, for example, once the treatment objectives have been achieved and the patient is clinically stable.[3] Ensure that the patient is ready and be prepared for this as the patient may have become dependent and rely on your treatments for support and feel that you are keeping his or her pregnancy hopes achievable. Thus the patient may feel a sense of abandonment or fear that withdrawal of treatment may compromise the pregnancy. Provide any relevant resources to help[3] and reassure the patient. For example, explain and reinforce any lifestyle and dietary advice for pregnancy. You may need to explain why it is important that the patient continues to be aware of doing everything necessary to stay healthy.[3] You may need to provide positive reinforcement, so discuss and highlight the achievements gained by working together. Give the patient credit for his or her hard work.[3] Reassure the patient that he or she can initiate appointments for pregnancy care and for prebirth acupuncture treatments or for any additional help, advice, and support should it be required.

For patients where the treatment has not had a successful outcome and accepting that ART and acupuncture treatment have not helped them, analysing the possible reasons for this outcome and respecting the patient's decision to end fertility treatments and move on with his or her life is important and should be done in an appropriate self-reflective manner.

MEASURING THE SUCCESS OF ACUPUNCTURE TREATMENT

As fertility acupuncturists, we can feel under pressure to help our patients become pregnant. However, it is important to remember that we work as part of a team: with both of the partners, their fertility consultant, nursing team, embryologists, and sometimes other professionals. Factors such as ART clinics' expertise or patients' compliance with lifestyle advice are just two examples of how circumstances beyond our control can affect the treatment outcome. We may provide the best acupuncture treatment possible, but random events (for example, a faulty medication batch or a fertility consultant having a bad day on the day of embryo transfer) can reduce the chance of success.

Although a healthy live birth is the most important goal of the treatment that we provide, other measures of treatment success should not be underestimated. These include, for example, achieving a better response by the patient to ovarian stimulation, more and better quality eggs and embryos, a thicker uterine lining, better semen parameters, lower stress levels, and an improvement in the patients' general well-being while they are undergoing ART treatment.

THE EFFECT OF SUBFERTILITY ON PATIENTS

The result of reproduction, that is having healthy, happy children, is an important part of most marriages. Subfertility is a heart-breaking condition that causes significant emotional suffering for both partners. It affects marital relationships and sexual satisfaction.[7] Some of the feelings infertile couples experience include anxiety, depression,

loss of control, guilt, low self-esteem, distress, stigmatization, isolation, grief, shame, failure, and resentment.

Infertility takes over couples' lives, with women in particular putting their lives on hold until they conceive.[8] Fifty percent of women report that subfertility is the most upsetting experience of their lives.[9] Subfertility has been shown to cause the same distress as suffering a life-threatening disease. One study that compared psychological symptoms of subfertile women who were undergoing fertility treatment found that women had the same depression and anxiety scores as those women who were undergoing treatment for cancer.[10]

Men are affected by infertility too. A structured review of 73 studies concluded that both men as well as women experience desire for parenthood in equal measures. In the short term, infertile men experience infertility specific anxiety and, if their goal is never fulfilled, they experience lasting sadness.[11]

Childlessness causes persistent, prolonged anxiety and depression.[8] Failure to overcome subfertility increases depressive symptoms.[12] Infertility is also linked to a greater risk of suicide in women.[13]

LEGAL AND ETHICAL CONSIDERATIONS

Assisted reproduction ethics

Is fertility treatment ethical?

Technology advances more rapidly than cultural views. There is a lag between what is culturally acceptable and what is technologically possible. IVF has divided society into those who feel it should be offered to infertile couples and those who feel it is unethical.

Some of the arguments against treating infertility are that infertility is normal and natural; it is argued that it is nature's or God's will and that infertile couples should not think that they have a right to have a baby. As already mentioned, infertility causes significant levels of suffering to couples, which is comparable to that of other chronic illnesses and which has a lasting effect. Infertility is no more natural a state than it is to have a cancer or any other illness. Yet, a cancer sufferer would never be told to accept that cancer is a natural condition given by God or nature and therefore should not be treated.

Another argument against ART treatment is that it is very expensive to provide to infertile couples. Yet infertility treatments (including IVF and similar treatment) account for only 0.07% of US healthcare costs.[14]

Health of babies born as a result of ART

Approximately 1% of babies in developed countries are conceived through ART.[15] ART babies are at greater risk of premature birth, low birth weight; they are also at an increased risk of perinatal death.[16] These risks are greater for multiples, but even singletons are at risk. However, such increased perinatal morbidity is also common in subfertile women who have not undergone ART, but who experienced delayed conception or had ovulation-induction treatments, albeit that the risks are incrementally lower.[15,16] Therefore, it would be wrong to attribute these increased risks purely to ART treatment, and it is important to emphasize that the vast majority of ART children are healthy.[15,17]

Treatment of much older patients

In 1984 the first baby was born following a successful egg donor IVF treatment. The mother of the baby had secondary amenorrhoea and premature ovarian failure.[18] The treatment is now widely used in women of advanced reproductive age who delay parenthood to pursue education or career opportunities or simply do not meet the right partner until later in life. Treatment of older patients has galvanized strong opinions about the ethical aspects of third-party donor treatments, especially in older recipients. There are also many social and legal concerns. In treating older patients, should there, for example, be a cutoff age for recipients and if so, what should it be?

Medically, with appropriate hormonal support, the uterus is capable of sustaining the pregnancy even in women in their 60s and 70s. However, these women experience higher rates of complications, such as pregnancy-induced hypertension (16–40%), caesarean section (40–76%), and gestational diabetes (20%).[18–21]

Third-party reproduction

Campbell explored the issue of the ethical dilemmas potentially being faced by fertility acupuncturists, in particular donor conception.[22] He pointed out that individuals born as a result of donated eggs or sperm may suffer from identity problems, especially if the biological parents' identity is kept hidden. Some countries, for example, the UK, no longer give the right to anonymity for donors. This drives patients (who wish to keep their infertility treatment a secret) to travel to other countries where donor anonymity is still the norm. This is referred to as cross-border reproduction. It remains to be seen if in the UK the removal of anonymity status will result in a further exacerbation of donor shortage.

Regulation of ART treatments

Reproductive medicine is highly regulated in different countries. In the UK the Human Fertilisation and Embryology Act 2008 covers areas of reproductive medicine such as:[23]

- Definition and status of 'embryo,' 'gamete,' 'mother,' 'father,' 'intended female parent,' 'marriage,' and 'civil partnership'
- Prohibition of embryo and genetic material use
- Storage of gametes, embryos
- Surrogacy arrangements
- Consents
- Cloning
- Donor anonymity

The Human Fertilisation and Embryology Authority is an independent regulatory body that oversees the use of gametes and embryos, as prescribed by the 2008 Act.

In the United States reproductive medicine is one of the most regulated forms of medicine.[24] State regulation, among other things, covers areas such as licencing; federal regulation includes the Fertility Clinic Success Rate and Certification Act and self-regulation guidelines cover ethics and other practice-related matters.[24]

Other countries have similar regulatory and self-regulatory frameworks, based on local laws, religious beliefs, and cultural values. Regulation in different countries varies in areas such as donor anonymity, remuneration of donors, number of embryos transferred, freezing of embryos, treatment funding, and age limits.

Ethical fertility acupuncture practice

Fertility patients are a highly motivated group of patients and often will comply with anything they are asked to do. But this makes them very vulnerable. Therefore, ART and fertility acupuncturists face even more ethical dilemmas than when dealing with other less vulnerable patient groups. Some of the common ethical issues such as fees, professional boundaries, confidentiality, and continuity of care are explored in this section.

Fees structure

Fertility patients require a much higher level of "outside of the normal office hours" care. For example, fertility patients regularly send text or email messages that need to be responded to very quickly to avoid anxiety issues developing, but also to help ensure their care is optimized. They often require weekend and evening treatments made available to them at short notice and at great personal life sacrifice on behalf of their acupuncturists.

Since assisted reproduction is a rapidly evolving area of medicine, acupuncturists specializing in this field require a high level of commitment to continual professional development. That means that a greater level of investment in time and money is needed in order to keep learning and researching about the very latest TCM and Orthodox medical techniques.

Therefore, it could be argued that it is only fair that fertility acupuncturists charge higher fees for their services and expertise. However, is it ethical to charge more to a vulnerable patient group? On the other hand, is it ethical to charge other patients who do not require such a level of commitment from the acupuncturist, the same fees as patients who need a lot of extra time and care?

Ultimately, acupuncturists must decide for themselves of what they consider is an appropriate fee to charge their fertility patients based on the acupuncturist's personal and practice circumstances. For example, if an acupuncturist needs to rent premises 7 days a week to ensure availability for treatments for fertility patients or if he or she subscribes to expensive reproductive medicine journals in order to remain current with the literature, then these extra expenses may need to be included in his or her fee structure.

Professional boundaries

Sometimes professional boundaries are blurred when dealing with fertility patients. For example, fertility patients may need to be provided with a practitioner's personal contact details in order to update their acupuncturist with the latest scan details or to arrange an emergency treatment session. In the authors' experience, patients do not abuse this. However, some acupuncturists may feel uncomfortable about blurring the boundaries.

It is also very difficult to remain emotionally detached when dealing with fertility cases, and fertility acupuncturists may suffer emotionally with their patients. Therefore, it is imperative that fertility acupuncturists develop effective coping strategies.

Continuity of care

ART patients require time-critical treatments, for example, on the embryo transfer day. It is the authors' opinion that acupuncturists who take on fertility patients and treat them for prolonged periods of time in preparation for IVF must make themselves available or must make appropriate alternative arrangements to ensure that patients are treated whenever the treatment is required (including weekends and public holidays). Practitioners should have contingency plans in place in the event of not being available to provide treatment due to unexpected illnesses or holiday arrangements. Cover arrangements could be achieved by teaming up with another fertility acupuncturist and providing cover for each other.

Case study

Ethical Fertility Acupuncture Practice: Treatment Continuity

Sue contacted me to see if I would be willing to treat her on the day of her embryo transfer, which was in 2 days' time on

Case study—cont'd

a Sunday. She explained that her existing acupuncturist (who she had been seeing for over 9 months in preparation for this IVF cycle) could not see her as the acupuncturist 'does not work on Sundays'. I agreed to see her.

However, I felt that this patient was let down by her existing acupuncturist. It is unfair to take on a patient and charge her for 9 months' worth of treatment, only to then refuse to see her on Sunday and offer no alternative arrangements.

Unfortunately, that cycle of IVF did not result in conception. In preparation for her next IVF cycle, Sue did not go back to her existing acupuncturist despite my encouraging her to do so, as she felt let down by him.

Confidentiality

It is our responsibility to keep all information confidential, no matter what condition patients seek treatment for. However, when dealing with fertility patients, we are privy to very personal and at times compromising information. The difficulties can arise when treating both partners or a donor and the recipient. They may disclose information to us that they wish to keep private from each other. Difficulties may also arise when treating friends. While friends may be aware of the fact that they are each undergoing IVF, they may not know the full extent of each other's personal circumstances and we must respect and protect their right to confidentiality. In some cases it may be advisable to ask a colleague to see one of the patients to ensure total confidentiality.

Limit of competence

As fertility acupuncturists, our role has evolved. We are expected by patients to give an opinion on medical aspects of their treatment. We must do so within the limits of our professional competence and recognize when the advice we may wish to provide may be outside of our level of qualifications or professional responsibility.

Treating patients when the prognosis is very poor or futile

The American Society for Reproductive Medicine defines 'poor prognosis' as very low odds of achieving a live birth (>1% to ≤5% per cycle) and 'futility' as ≤1% chance of achieving a live birth.[25] The decision whether to treat patients with a poor or a futile prognosis should be made purely on the grounds of what is in the patient's best interests and should be done in consultation with the patient. It should not be guided by the prospect of financial gain or for reasons of protecting one's success rates.[25]

Refusing to treat a patient

There may be circumstances when we may feel unable to treat a patient on the basis of our own personal beliefs. For example, we may disagree on religious or other grounds about women having donor egg babies in their 50s or 60s or about a gay couple raising a child. While we are not obliged to take on a patient, we must be aware of legal ramifications of refusing to treat a particular subgroup of patients. Specialist legal advice should be sought in these circumstances.

SUMMARY

The therapeutic relationship between the practitioner and the patient is extremely important. It begins to develop from the very first consultation and continues developing through the treatment course. The therapeutic relationship is a fundamental part of the treatment and patient management and can make a significant difference in the patients' experience and perhaps even an outcome of ART.

Fertility acupuncturists need to be aware of patients' needs. They also need to be aware of their own feelings, especially with respect to emotionally challenging situations or when the treatment fails. Acupuncturists must realize that the success of acupuncture is not just about helping patients conceive, but also about enhancing and easing patients' experience of ART.

Fertility patients are considered a vulnerable patient group. Therefore it is essential that acupuncturists adhere to strict ethical principles.

REFERENCES

1. Aquilina L, Wilkinson C. The therapeutic relationship in the dental setting. In: Wilkinson C, editor. Professional perspectives in health care. Hampshire: Palgrave Macmillan; 2007. p. 205–301 [chapter 10].
2. García D, Bautista O, Venereo L, et al. Training in empathic skills improves the patient-physician relationship during the first consultation in a fertility clinic. Fertil Steril 2013;99:1413–1418.e1.
3. Mitchell A, Cormack MA. The process of treatment. In: The therapeutic relationship in complementary health care. Edinburgh: Elsevier; 1998. p. 107–28 [chapter 8].
4. Dancet EA, Nelen WL, Sermeus W, et al. The patients' perspective on fertility care: a systematic review. Hum Reprod Update 2010;16:467–87.
5. Leite RC, Makuch MY, Petta CA, et al. Women's satisfaction with physicians' communication skills during an infertility consultation. Patient Educ Couns 2005;59:38–45.
6. Van Voorhis BJ, Thomas M, Surrey ES, et al. What do consistently high-performing in vitro fertilization programs in the U.S. do? Fertil Steril 2010;94:1346–9.
7. Monga M, Alexandrescu B, Katz SE, et al. Impact of infertility on quality of life, marital adjustment, and sexual function. Urology 2004;63:126–30.
8. Beaurepaire J, Jones M, Thiering P, et al. Psychosocial adjustment to infertility and its treatment: male and female responses at different stages of IVF/ET treatment. J Psychosom Res 1994;38:229–40.
9. Freeman EW, Boxer AS, Rickels K, et al. Psychological evaluation and support in a program of in vitro fertilization and embryo transfer. Fertil Steril 1985;43:48–53.
10. Domar AD, Zuttermeister PC, Friedman R. The psychological impact of infertility: a comparison with patients with other medical conditions. J Psychosom Obstet Gynaecol 1993;14 (Suppl.):45–52.
11. Fisher JR, Hammarberg K. Psychological and social aspects of infertility in men: an overview of the evidence and implications for psychologically informed clinical care and future research. Asian J Androl 2012;14:121–9.
12. Salmela-Aro K, Suikkari AM. Letting go of your dreams–adjustment of child-related goal appraisals and depressive symptoms during infertility treatment. J Res Pers 2008;42:988–1003.
13. Kjaer TK, Jensen A, Dalton SO, et al. Suicide in Danish women evaluated for fertility problems. Hum Reprod 2011;26:2401–7.
14. ASRM infographic. Infertility treatments, including IVF and similar procedures, account for approx 0.07 percent of U.S. health care costs. Available from: http://www.asrm.org/awards/detail.aspx?id=9640 [accessed 13 April 2013].
15. Pinborg A, Henningsen AK, Malchau SS, et al. Congenital anomalies after assisted reproductive technology. Fertil Steril 2013;99:327–32.
16. Barnhart KT. Epidemiology of male and female reproductive disorders and impact on fertility regulation and population growth. Fertil Steril 2011;95:2200–3.
17. Hart R, Norman RJ. The longer-term health outcomes for children born as a result of IVF treatment. Part II: Mental health and development outcomes. Hum Reprod Update 2013;19:244–50.
18. Wang J, Sauer MV. In vitro fertilization (IVF): a review of 3 decades of clinical innovation and technological advancement. Ther Clin Risk Manag 2006;2:355–64.
19. Söderström-Anttila V. Pregnancy and child outcome after oocyte donation. Hum Reprod Update 2001;7:28–32.
20. Obasaju M, Kadam A, Biancardi T, et al. Pregnancies from single normal embryo transfer in women older than 40 years. Reprod Biomed Online 2001;2:98–101.
21. Paulson RJ, Boostanfar R, Saadat P, et al. Pregnancy in the sixth decade of life: obstetric outcomes in women of advanced reproductive age. JAMA 2002;288:2320–3.
22. Campbell R. Ethics in fertility medicine? EJOM 2008;6:4–8.

23. Human fertilisation and embryology act 2008. Available from: http://www.legislation.gov.uk/ukpga/2008/22/contents [accessed 1 June 2013].

24. ASRM patient resources: oversight of assisted reproductive technology. Available from: http://www.asrm.org/Oversight_of_ART/ [accessed 1 June 2013].

25. Ethics Committee of the American Society for Reproductive Medicine. Fertility treatment when the prognosis is very poor or futile. Fertil Steril 2009;92:1194–7.

Chapter | 14 |

Aftercare

Fertility acupuncturists play an important role in the weeks following a pregnancy test. If the test is negative, we can assist patients in their decision-making processes about all the considerations they may need to take into account when planning for any future attempts at conceiving. If the test is positive, we can help patients make a healthy transition from subfertility to pregnancy and parenthood.

NEGATIVE OUTCOME

On the day of a pregnancy test, silence from a patient often, but not always, means the result is negative. Patients are usually very quick to share good news, but it is typically absolutely heartbreaking for them to share the news about an unsuccessful outcome.

As acupuncturists, we have a responsibility to help these patients get through such devastating times. There are several ways in which we can help.

Immediate aftermath of a negative test

Most patients, in our experience, prefer to grieve in private. However, some may wish to come in for treatment to help them in their recovery process. Fertility acupuncturists can help with the immediate emotional and physical trauma. On an emotional level, these patients often feel sadness, loss, and sometimes anger and frustration. Emotional symptoms are frequently made worse by physical symptoms, such as heavy and often very painful withdrawal bleeding. Table 14.1 lists some of the acupuncture points that may be beneficial in treating patients immediately after a failed treatment cycle.

Guiding patients in their possible future steps

Initial disappointment with fertility treatment turns to questions being asked. Why did the treatment not work? What else can we try? Will the treatment ever work? What do we do next? These are difficult questions with no definitive answers. However, in almost all cases, Assisted Reproductive Technology (ART) treatment cycles can be improved upon, additional tests can be carried out, and different fertility treatment techniques can be tried.

Providing patients with some feedback on what went well, what could have gone better, and what else they can try in the next treatment cycle is often well received by patients and gives them both hope and knowledge. The feedback can be provided formally in the form of a report or less formally, for example, in person or as advice over the phone. Emails can work well in these circumstances.

In order to provide feedback and any recommendations, it is helpful to carry out an audit of the patients' current and past treatment cycles. Chapter 10 provides information on what to expect at different stages of the treatment cycle and what solutions exist for overcoming the obstacles. Chapter 12 discusses possible reasons for In Vitro Fertilization (IVF) failure and available solutions and provides an algorithm for auditing implantation failure cases. Appendix I provides an IVF Audit Tool, which can be used when reviewing each case.

When is the right time to stop the treatment?

There are several reasons why couples may decide to discontinue ART treatment, accept that they will never have a child, and instead consider the use of alternative options,

Table 14.1 Acupuncture points beneficial immediately after a failed treatment cycle

Acupuncture points	Indications
LIV14	Spiritual symptoms: give hope and strength[1]
DU13	Unhappiness and disorientation[2]
KID26	Stabilize the Kidney–Heart relationship to help cope with shock and disappointment[3]
BL10	Crying and sadness[4]

such as third party donor treatment, surrogacy, or adoption.

Some patients discontinue with ART due to an erroneous belief that they have a poor prognosis. Some discontinue due to erroneously believing that they have tried every available ART treatment option. But successful IVF is to an extent dependant on the roll of the dice, and some patients need to roll them more times than others. One study demonstrated that the chances of conception increase with each failed IVF cycle. This trend is even more evident in older women, who may need up to 14 cycles of IVF before they conceive.[5]

In our experience, very few couples who undertake ART and acupuncture management during the same time period discontinue their ART treatment. We would posit that this may possibly result from a reduction of the pressure on their coping abilities secondary to a reduction of their perception of the stress they associate with, and possibly expect to have, when undergoing ART treatment cycles.

It would be interesting to see how the discontinuation rates for acupuncture and ART patients compare with non-acupuncture patients. However, to the best of our knowledge, no such studies exist.

In Israel, IVF treatment is free of charge to couples until they have two children, and the IVF discontinuation rate is very low.[6] Although the research is inconclusive, the high financial burden of undertaking ART may lead some couples to stop their ART treatment. However, even when cost is not an issue, some couples still choose to discontinue their treatment, citing the emotional stress of undergoing ART as one of the most common reasons for their ART treatment cessation.[7]

While research identifies that the main reasons for discontinuing IVF treatment are psychological stress and poor prognosis,[8–10] assuming the stress aspect of the continued treatment can be managed and there are no financial constraints, so long as ART options exist that the patients have not yet explored, there is no reason why they should discontinue their treatment.

As fertility acupuncturists, we may also be able to influence patients' decisions whether to carry on with further IVF treatment. However, once all the most logical and potentially applicable options have been explored and there is still no successful pregnancy outcome, this would indicate that it would be appropriate to consider alternative routes to becoming parents.

INTERESTING FACTS

HOW LONG TO ALLOW BETWEEN IVF TREATMENT CYCLES

A recent study found that there is no advantage of waiting for two to three menstrual cycles before undergoing a further cycle of IVF, so couples can proceed with another treatment cycle after just one menstrual cycle, if their clinic supports this.[11]

However, there may be instances where waiting is advisable, for example, if new pathology is identified following a failed IVF treatment cycle and this pathology needs resolving before starting the next treatment cycle.

POSITIVE OUTCOME: HEALTHY TRANSITION FROM SUBFERTILITY TO PREGNANCY

Pregnancy following ART and the risk of complications

The best measure of success of ART treatment is a live birth resulting in a healthy mother and a healthy baby. While a positive pregnancy test is a good start, it is by no means a guarantee of a live baby.

Some acupuncturists can be fearful about treating patients during pregnancy, especially if the pregnancy was achieved as a result of ART treatment. However, acupuncture has a lot to offer during pregnancy, especially for such a clinically challenging group of patients.

As recent reviews have highlighted, ART pregnancies are associated with increased risks of obstetric complications, such as:

- Miscarriages[12,13]
- Preeclampsia[14]
- Gestational hypertension[14] (2-fold)[15]
- Gestational diabetes[14] (2-fold)[15]
- Placenta abruptio[14] (2-fold)[15]
- Placenta previan[14] (3–6-fold)[15]
- Preterm delivery (1–2-fold)[15]

Potentially, acupuncture may help to reduce the risks of developing some of these complications. Acupuncture can also help to manage minor complications, such as pregnancy-related aches and pains, headaches, anxiety, digestive complaints, tiredness, morning sickness, etc.

It is beyond the scope of this book to discuss each ART pregnancy complication. Chapter 12 provided information on prevention of miscarriages and pregnancy loss. The remainder of this chapter discusses how to support patients during the early stages of pregnancy.

It is recommended that any acupuncturist who works with pregnant patients should have advanced training in obstetric acupuncture. There are also a number of books written on the subject of acupuncture in pregnancy, including:

- *Acupuncture in Pregnancy and Childbirth* by Zita West
- *The Essential Guide to Acupuncture in Pregnancy and Childbirth* by Debra Betts
- *Medical Acupuncture in Pregnancy* by Ansgar Roemer
- *Pregnancy and Gestation in Classical Texts* by Elisabeth Rochat De La Vallee

Transition from subfertility to pregnancy

After a positive pregnancy test, many women remain worried and anxious about their pregnancy, especially those women who have a history of miscarriage(s).

These patients suffer from the consequences of emotional reactivity, sensitivity, and hypervigilance as a result of everything they had to go through in order to achieve a pregnancy. They may experience any number of the following:

- Inability to relax and enjoy the pregnancy
- Fear that something will go wrong
- Compulsion to repeatedly do pregnancy tests and visit the toilet to check they are not bleeding
- Feeling like they do not belong to either a pregnant or infertile 'category', therefore they are not easily able to access the emotional support they require
- Loss of friends they made while undergoing treatment, who may still be going through ART treatment
- Problems with the transition from reproductive to obstetric medical care
- Desire for more intensive antenatal care (more scans, more blood tests, more midwife appointments)
- Guilt, especially if they have a history of miscarriage(s) or pregnancy losses
- Fear of sharing the news with family and friends and anxiety about questions that they may be asked
- Worry that they are too old to be parents, if conception took place later in life
- Bonding issues
- 'Putting up' with negative pregnancy symptoms and not complaining, for fear of being seen as ungrateful

Patients should be reassured that to experience any of these feelings is not unusual. Encouragement to do the 'normal' things that all pregnant women do should be given. Acupuncture treatment in these patients should include points to support pregnancy as well as address any psychological–emotional symptomatology. Supporting patients emotionally and reducing their feeling of being stressed during pregnancy is important,[16] since maintaining negative emotions may adversely influence the mother's and embryo's Qi.[17]

Acupuncture treatment during early pregnancy

During the first month of pregnancy, the embryo develops via its own transformation and is influenced by the maternal environment (see Chapter 3 for more details on embryo development).[17] A range of factors (for example, parental age, emotions, overexertion) or Traditional Chinese Medicine (TCM) pathology (for example, Internal dysfunction, Heat,[17] Fire,[16] or Cold), may damage the embryo.[17]

Table 14.2 summarizes TCM understanding of the embryonic development.

Maternal age and/or constitutional weakness[16] may compromise the embryo's development due to a reduction of Qi, Blood, Yin, Yang, and Kidney Jing (Essence). These are the same syndromes that are associated with subfertility (see Chapter 5) and may affect the embryo's ability to develop. Therefore assessment and treatment of maternal Qi, Blood, and Jing (Essence) is essential during pregnancy, because it supports the embryo's development.

There are two main ways to support early pregnancy and reduce the risk of pregnancy loss:

- At initial diagnosis: identification of high-risk syndromes that may be implicated in preclinical pregnancy loss is essential. These potential syndromes include Liver Blood Stasis, Spleen Qi Deficiency, Kidney Yang Deficiency, Liver and/or Heart Blood Deficiency.
- The provision of continuous care: Careful monitoring and the early identification of abnormal manifestations developing in pregnancy enable the acupuncturist to provide timely intervention, thus reducing the risk of pathology progressing.

Pulse reading is one of the ways to assess the viability of pregnancy from a TCM perspective. Pulse readings that indicate Qi, Blood, Yin, or Yang Deficiency may identify a high-risk pregnancy. A healthy pregnancy is generally represented by a pulse with strength.[19]

During the first 3 months of pregnancy, the embryo develops into a foetus and transforms under a range of maternal influences, particularly Liver Blood, Jing (Essence), Shen (Spirit), and the Mind.

Several acupuncture points have been suggested as 'forbidden' in pregnancy, including LI4,[20] SP6,[21] GB21,[22] and BL60.[23] However, some authors argue that there is no physiological (medical) basis for this rule.[24,25]

Table 14.2 Pregnancy development and TCM supportive intervention

	2–4 weeks' gestation	4–8 weeks' gestation	8–12 weeks' gestation
Vital Substance and Shen (Spirit)	Blood[18]	Jing (Essences)	Shen (Spirit)
Embryo/foetus development	Beginning of embryo[18]	Beginning of the formation of 'paste'. This fertile paste takes a new 'form and hardens'.[18] Jing (Essences) condense and become concentrated[18]	Beginning of a foetus; foetus shape becomes stabilized[18]
Yin Yang	Yin and Yang combine, constituting the embryo[18]	Yin and Yang occupy the channels[18]	Yin and Yang undergo change, developing further until birth[18]
Meridian and Zangfu	Mother's Liver nourishes the embryo[18] and supports the functions of the Uterus	Mother's Gallbladder and Liver provide Jing (Essence), nourishing and forming the embryo in the Uterus[18]	Mother's Heart Shen (Spirit) and Mind nourish and influence the foetus[18]
Treatment principle and method	Assess maternal Qi, Blood, Jing (Essence), Shen (Spirit), Yin and Yang through pulse reading, observation, and manifestations Support the Liver if dysfunctional, for example if patient suffers from mood fluctuations Calm the Shen (Spirit), balance emotions (for example, fear of a miscarriage) with acupuncture and through psycho-education appropriately delivered via a good patient–practitioner therapeutic relationship Tonify Qi, enrich Blood, Jing (Essence), support Yin and/or Yang if deficient with acupuncture and dietary and lifestyle advice	Assess maternal Kidney Jing (Essence) and Heart Shen (Spirit) function through pulse reading and observation Enrich Yin and fortify Yang if deficient Tonify the Kidney, Stomach, and Spleen with acupuncture to support Qi and Jing (Essence) Relevant lifestyle and dietary advice should be provided to the patient	Assess maternal Shen (Spirit) Support and balance Qi, the Mind and the emotions. For example, balance the Heart to treat sadness, the Lung to treat grief, the Spleen to treat overthinking and worrying, and the Kidney to treat fear Prevent injury caused by emotions Balance the Heart if disordered
Additional patient advice	Advise avoiding strenuous exercise to preserve Liver function and support the Uterus in its reproductive functions. Especially so if Qi, Blood, or Kidney Jing (Essence) Deficiency is evident	Advise to ensure adequate clothing according to environment, to reduce the risk of invasion by EPFs	Advise patients to regulate their emotion and to avoid circumstances that cause emotional upset to prevent injury by negative emotion
Gestation-specific points	P6, REN4 BL18, BL20, BL23	KID9, REN4, LU9	DU23, YINTANG BL15
Other points	*Generic points throughout first trimester:* REN12, ST36, KID7, DU20, REN6, KID3, YINTANG *Modifications:* Liver Blood Deficiency: LIV8, YINTANG, P6 Spleen Qi Deficiency: SP3 with moxa Kidney Yang Deficiency: BL23, DU4 with moxa, moxa right area of lower back Heat/Fire: LI11, LIV2 Cold: REN4 with moxa Dampness: SP2, SP9 with moxa Severe Kidney weakness and aging: LU7+KID6, REN4, KID9 Blood Stagnation: SP4+P6, SP10		

Studies appear to show that there are no adverse consequences to the pregnancy from needling of the 'forbidden' points in pregnant rats.[26,27] To the contrary, needling LI4[28] and SP6[29] has been shown to reduce uterine contractions, which are associated with negative pregnancy outcomes.

Ultimately, each acupuncturist must make his or her own decision about whether to use these points in pregnant patients. For example, if a patient has a history of recurrent miscarriages due to Blood Stasis, SP6 may help to treat the underlying pathology and prevent another miscarriage. This example illustrates that patient's constitution and underlying pathology should also be taken into account when deciding on the points prescription.

When to discharge pregnant patients

For the majority of patients, acupuncture should be continued until at least 12 weeks' gestation. For high-risk pregnancies, it may be prudent to continue with acupuncture treatment until the baby is delivered. Table 14.3 provides detailed treatment frequency recommendations.

However, these are not prescriptive. They are proposed guidelines that should be adapted to the individual patient.

It is important to note that some women prefer to stop seeing their fertility acupuncturist as soon as they are pregnant. For some women the maintenance of acupuncture at this stage is psychologically discomforting. Acupuncture treatments act as a reminder to these patients of their infertility and they are keen to put their infertility history behind them and move on with their lives. However, such patients are a minority. Most women feel attached to their acupuncturist and develop a real strong sense of bond and trust.

ACUPUNCTURIST'S SELF-CARE: SAYING GOODBYE TO PATIENTS

As a result of the complex nature of their reproductive health, fertility patients are often treated over a long period of time. We get to know these patients very intimately and share in their extreme lows and highs. However, there comes a time when we need to say goodbye. In many cases, it is because they have conceived or have had their baby. Sometimes, it is because there is nothing else we can do to help them. It is surprising how emotional the discharge appointment can be.

Table 14.3 Recommended treatment frequency and discharge

Criteria	Treatment frequency and discharge recommendations
Low risk: • Patient ≤35 years old, in good health (from both Orthodox and TCM perspectives) • Single gestation pregnancy • No history of pregnancy loss • No complications in this or any previous pregnancies • If ART pregnancy with no complications following standard ART treatment	Treat weekly until 10–12 weeks' gestation. Then discharge or move to 2–3 monthly maintenance treatment. Optionally consider treating weekly from around 34 weeks' gestation in preparation for birth
Medium risk: • Patient >35 years of age • Very anxious • Complex pathology from TCM perspective • Some minor pregnancy symptomatology (for example, anaemia, abdominal pain, backache, tiredness, headaches/migraines)	Treat weekly until 12 weeks' gestation. Move to monthly treatment frequency until 34 weeks' gestation. Weekly treatments thereafter in preparation for birth
Very high risk: • Multiple gestation • History of previous late pregnancy loss or serious pregnancy complications • Patient suffers from a known or suspected condition, which may threaten pregnancy or affect foetus (for example, diabetes, thyroid disease, immune or clotting disorders, high blood pressure, frequent urinary tract infections, incompetent cervix) • Patient is managed by an obstetric consultant (rather than by midwife; suggests high-risk pregnancy)	Treat weekly until 20 weeks' gestation. Thereafter, 1–2 weekly until 34 weeks' gestation. Weekly treatments thereafter in preparation for birth

As fertility acupuncturists, we can also feel a range of different emotions, including sadness, happiness, loss, or even grief. In cases where we were unable to help our patients, we might feel frustration and guilt, and we may feel we have failed. Sometimes these feelings can get so strong that we may need to share them with a colleague. However, all of these feelings are normal and a reflection and a reminder of how much we care for our patients and how emotionally charged this field of medicine can be. The feeling of elation and jubilation when we 'crack' a challenging case and when we get to share in our patients' excitement and joy when they conceive and when they go onto have a baby is really special. Then the desire sets in to repeat it all over again with other patients.

SUMMARY

Although many of our patients succeed in having a baby, some do not. Fertility acupuncturists can help these patients to decide on what their next course of action should be, whether it be to try more ART and other treatments or make a decision to move on by accepting their infertility.

When a course of ART treatment succeeds in creating a pregnancy, fertility acupuncturists must be cognisant that things can and sometimes do go wrong. Fertility acupuncturists should carry out a risk assessment when planning to continue with any further acupuncture treatment or when deciding to discharge their patient. The risk of some pregnancy complications can be minimized with acupuncture, and where possible, an attempt should be made to reduce the possibility of complications.

For those patients who conceive, acupuncture treatment should be continued during the first trimester and in some cases throughout pregnancy to reduce the risks of complications that may ultimately threaten the viability of the pregnancy and the delivery of a healthy baby or the wellbeing of the mother.

REFERENCES

1. Jarrett LS. The Liver. In: The clinical practice of Chinese medicine. Stockbridge, MA: Spirit Path Press; 2003. p. 549–70 [chapter 31].

2. Deadman P, Al-Khafaji M, Baker K. The governing vessel. In: A manual of acupuncture. England: Journal of Chinese Medicine Publications; 1998. p. 527–62.

3. Jarrett LS. Kidney. In: The clinical practice of Chinese medicine. Stockbridge, MA: Spirit Path Press; 2003. p. 427–59 [chapter 27].

4. Lu HC. Verbal questions. In: A complete translation of the Yellow Emperor's classics of internal medicine and the difficult classic (Nei-Jing and Nan-Jing). Vancouver: International College of Traditional Chinese Medicine; 2004. p. 481–7, Section three: Spiritual pivot [Ling Shu] [chapter 28].

5. Verit FF, Verit A. How effective is in vitro fertilization, and how can it be improved? Fertil Steril 2011;95:1677–83.

6. Lande Y, Seidman DS, Maman E, et al. Couples offered free assisted reproduction treatment have a very high chance of achieving a live birth within 4 years. Fertil Steril 2011;95:568–72.

7. Domar AD. Impact of psychological factors on dropout rates in insured infertility patients. Fertil Steril 2004;81:271–3.

8. McDowell S, Murray A. Barriers to continuing in vitro fertilisation – why do patients exit fertility treatment? Aust N Z J Obstet Gynaecol 2011;51:84–90.

9. Olivius C, Friden B, Borg G, et al. Why do couples discontinue in vitro fertilization treatment? A cohort study. Fertil Steril 2004;81:258–61.

10. Domar AD, Smith K, Conboy L, et al. A prospective investigation into the reasons why insured United States patients drop out of in vitro fertilization treatment. Fertil Steril 2010;94:1457–9.

11. Reichman DE, Chung P, Meyer L, et al. Consecutive GnRH – antagonist IVF cycles: does the elapsed time interval between successive treatments affect outcomes? Fertil Steril 2013;99:1277–82.

12. Blok L, Kremer J. In vitro fertilisation and intracytoplasmic sperm injection. In: de Haan N, Spelt M, Gobel R, editors. Reproductive medicine: a textbook for paramedics. Amsterdam: Elsevier Gezondheidszorg; 2010. p. 105–26 [chapter 8].

13. Tummers P. Risk of spontaneous abortion in singleton and twin pregnancies after IVF/ICSI. Hum Reprod 2003;18:1720–3.

14. Mukhopadhaya N, Arulkumaran S. Reproductive outcomes after in-vitro fertilization. Curr Opin Obstet Gynecol 2007;19:113–9.

15. Allen VM, Wilson RD, Cheung A, et al. Pregnancy outcomes after assisted reproductive technology. J Obstet Gynaecol Can 2006;28:220–50.

16. Wu YL. An uncertain harvest, pregnancy and miscarriage. In: Reproducing women: medicine, metaphor, and childbirth in late imperial China. Berkeley: University of California Press; 2010. p. 120–46 [chapter 4].

17. Sun Si-Miao. Translation. In: Wilms S, editor. Bèi Jí Qian Jin Yào Fang. Essential prescriptions worth a thousand in gold for every emergency. 3 Volumes on gynecology, vol. 3. Portland: The Chinese Medicine Database; 2007. p. 232–362 [chapter 3].

18. Sun Si-Miao. Translation. In: Wilms S, translator. Bèi Jí Qian Jin Yào Fang. Essential prescriptions worth a thousand in gold for every emergency. 3 Volumes on gynecology, vol. 2. Portland: The Chinese Medicine Database; 2007. p. 52–216 [chapter 2].

19. Rochat de la Vallee E. Pulses in pregnancy. In: Root C, editor. Pregnancy and gestation: in Chinese classical texts. Norfolk: Monkey Press; 2007. p. 3–8.

20. Deadman P, Al-Khafaji M, Baker K. The Large Intestine channel. In: A manual of acupuncture. England: Journal of Chinese Medicine Publications; 1998. p. 93–122.

21. Deadman P, Al-Khafaji M, Baker K. The Spleen channel. In: A manual of acupuncture. England: Journal of Chinese Medicine Publications; 1998. p. 175–206.

22. Deadman P, Al-Khafaji M, Baker K. The Gallbladder channel. In: A manual of acupuncture. England: Journal of Chinese Medicine Publications; 1998. p. 415–66.

23. Deadman P, Al-Khafaji M, Baker K. The Bladder channel. In: A manual of acupuncture. England: Journal of Chinese Medicine Publications; 1998. p. 249–328.

24. da Silva AV, Nakamura MU, da Silva JB. 'Forbidden points' in pregnancy: do they exist? Acupunct Med 2011;29:135–6.

25. Cummings M. 'Forbidden points' in pregnancy: no plausible mechanism for risk. Acupunct Med 2011;29:140–2.

26. Guerreiro da Silva AV, Nakamura MU, Cordeiro JA, et al. The effects of so-called 'forbidden acupuncture points' on pregnancy outcome in wistar rats. Forsch Komplementmed 2011;18:10–4.

27. Guerreiro da Silva AV, Nakamura MU, Guerreiro da Silva JB, et al. Could acupuncture at the so-called forbidden points be harmful to the health of pregnant wistar rats? Acupunct Med 2013;31:202–6. Available from: http://dx.doi.org/10.1136/acupmed-2012-010246.

28. Kim J-S, Shin KH, Na CS. Effect of acupuncture treatment on uterine motility and cyclooxygenase-2 expression in pregnant rats. Gynecol Obstet Invest 2000;50:225–30.

29. Kim JS, Na CS, Hwang WJ, et al. Immunohistochemical localization of cyclooxygenase-2 in pregnant rat uterus by Sp-6 acupuncture. Am J Chin Med 2003;31:481–8.

Appendix

Templates

Medical and fertility history (female)	
Personal details	
Full name	**DOB and age**
Home address	**Contact details**
	Tel (H) Tel (M) Tel (W) Email
Family doctor's name and clinic contact details	**Fertility doctor's name and clinic contact details (if relevant)**
Occupation	**Hobbies**
Presentation	
Reason for presenting (natural conception/ART support (e.g. IVF)/miscarriage prevention/other)	
Date of planned ART/IVF, if applicable:_____ART/IVF protocol attached: yes/no	
Length of subfertility	**When stopped contraception and type**
_____ months/years _____ actual chances of conception	
Confirmed medical illnesses	**Confirmed infertility diagnosis**
Suspected Orthodox medical diagnosis (requiring further investigations)	
Patient's opinion why they cannot conceive	
Patient's treatment goal	

Figure A1.1 Medical and fertility history (female).

	Menstrual cycle										Notes (see Chapters 2, 5 and 8)
Age at menarche											
Cycle length and regularity	Range: from_____days to_____days Changes over time: shorter, longer, more irregular, less irregular										

Menses	**Days**										
	−3	−2	−1	1	2	3	4	5	6	7	
Colour											
Flow: spotting (S)/heavy (H)/ normal (N)/light (L)											
Consistency											
Clots and size											
Other remarks											

Menstrual pain	When Location Type Severity Medication What makes it better What makes it worse	
Premenstrual symptoms	When Breast tenderness Mood alteration Bloating Bowel habits Headaches Back pain Other	
Pelvic pain outside of period	When Location Type Severity Medication What makes it better What makes it worse	
Vaginal bleeding outside of period		

Continued

	Manifestations	Notes (see Chapter 5)
Temperature		
Sweating		
Thirst, drink preferences		
Mouth, throat		
Digestive problems		
Bowels		
Urination		
Sleep, dreaming		
Chest pain/palpitations		
Lungs and breathing		
Headaches		
Dizziness		
Memory, concentration		
Musculoskeletal pain		
Energy levels		
Skin, hair		
Ears and hearing		
Eyes and eyesight		
Vaginal discharges		
Emotional disposition		
Constitution		

	Observations		Notes (see Chapter 5)
Jing-Shen (overall complexion, eyes)			
Spirit/emotion/colour/odour			
Pulse	L	R	
Tongue			
Abdominal palpation			
Other (hair, complexion, skin, body build, etc.)			

Figure A1.1, cont'd

	Past medical history	Notes (see Chapter 5)
STDs		
Pelvic inflammatory disease or infections		
Pelvic surgery (e.g. appendicitis, ovarian cysts)		
Cervical conization		
Cancer		
Other		

	Past pregnancies (Childbirth, terminations, miscarriages)	Notes (see Chapters 5 and 12)
Past pregnancies and outcome of each (in this or previous relationship(s))		

	Family medical history	Notes (see Chapter 5)
Major illnesses (e.g., thyroid disease, diabetes, PCOS, early onset menopause, high blood pressure, etc.)		
Reproductive health (miscarriages, infertility, twins delivery, etc.)		

Continued

BBT diagnosis (see Chapter 5)	
Syndromes	**Signs and symptoms**

TCM diagnosis (see Chapter 5)		
Syndromes	**Signs and symptoms**	**Aetiology**

Pathology diagram	TCM treatment plan (Acupuncture point prescription/needle technique/moxa/cupping/electroacupuncture/other)

Figure A1.1, cont'd

Medical and fertility history (male)	
Personal details	
Full name	**DOB and age**
Home address	**Contact details**
	Tel (H) Tel (M) Tel (W) Email
Family doctor's name and clinic contact details	**ART doctor's name and clinic contact details (if relevant)**
Occupation	**Hobbies**

Presentation

Reason for presenting (natural conception/ART support (e.g. IVF)/miscarriage prevention)

Date of planned ART/IVF, if applicable:_____ART/IVF protocol attached: yes/no

Length of subfertility

_____ months/years

_____ actual chances of conception

Confirmed medical illnesses	**Confirmed infertility diagnosis**

Suspected Orthodox medical diagnosis (requiring further investigations)

Patient's opinion why he and his partner cannot conceive

Patient's treatment goal

Figure A1.2 Medical and fertility history (male).

	Manifestations	Notes (see Chapter 5)
Vasectomy		
Temperature		
Sweating		
Thirst, drink preference		
Mouth, throat		
Digestive problems		
Bowels		
Urination		
Sleep, dreaming		
Chest pain/palpitations		
Lungs and breathing		
Headaches		
Dizziness		
Memory, concentration		
Musculoskeletal pain		
Energy levels		
Skin, hair		
Ears and hearing		
Eyes and eyesight		
Emotional disposition		
Breast discharges		
Constitution		

	Observations		Notes (see Chapter 5)
Jing-Shen (overall complexion, eyes)			
Spirit/emotion/ colour/odour			
Pulse	L	R	
Tongue			
Other (hair, complexion, skin, body build, etc.)			

Figure A1.2, cont'd

	Past medical history	Notes (see Chapter 5)
STDs		
Testicular trauma or torsion		
Surgery (e.g., hernia, orchidopexy, vasectomy)		
Undescended testis		
Mumps		
Cancer		
Other		

	Past pregnancies (Childbirth, terminations, miscarriages)	Notes (see Chapter 5)
Past pregnancies and outcome of each (in this or previous relationship(s))		

	Family medical history	Notes (see Chapter 5)
Major illnesses (e.g., thyroid disease, blood pressure, diabetes, etc.)		
Reproductive health (miscarriages, infertility, twins delivery, etc.)		

Continued

	TCM diagnosis (see Chapter 5)	
Syndromes	Signs and symptoms	Aetiology

Pathology diagram	TCM treatment plan (Acupuncture point prescription/needle technique/moxa/cupping/electroacupuncture/other)

Figure A1.2, cont'd

Tests and investigations (female)

Patient's name: _____ DOB: _____

	Initial test	Retest	Notes (see Chapters 4 and 12)
Ovarian reserve			
Reproductive hormones: **FSH** **LH** **E2** **FSH:LH ratio** **FSH:E2 ratio**	Date _____ _____ IU/L / mIU/mL _____ IU/L / mIU/mL _____ pmol/L / pg/mL _____ _____	Date _____ _____ IU/L / mIU/mL _____ IU/L / mIU/mL _____ pmol/L / pg/mL _____ _____	
AMH	Date _____ _____ pmol/L / ng/mL	Date _____ _____ pmol/L / ng/mL	
Antral follicle count (AFC) scan	Date _____ Left _____ Right _____	Date _____ Left _____ Right _____	
Ovulation			
Progesterone	Date _____ _____ nmol/L / ng/mL day____of____days cycle	Date _____ _____ nmol/L / ng/mL day____of____days cycle	
Prolactin	Date _____ _____ mIU/L / µg/L	Date _____ _____ mIU/L / µg/L	
Thyroid screen: **TSH** **T3** **T4** **Thyroid antibodies**	Date _____ _____ _____ _____ _____ _____	Date _____ _____ _____ _____ _____ _____	
Utero-tubal investigations			
Ovaries assessment	Date _____ Details	Date _____ Details	
Tubal assessment	Date _____ Details	Date _____ Details	
Uterine assessment	Date _____ Details	Date _____ Details	

Figure A1.3 Tests and investigations (female).

Thrombophilia screen			
Inherited thrombophilia	Protein C Protein S Antithrombin III Factor V Leiden Prothrombin Gene Mutation (20210A) Protein Z Homocysteine Other FV mutations	Thrombomodulin gene variants PAI-1 activity levels PAI-1 4G/4G polymorphism MTHFR C677T Factor evaluation (VII, VIII, IX, XI) Platelet count Other	
APS: LA aCL IgG aCL IgM anti-b2 IgG anti-b2 IgM	Date_____ _____ _____ _____ _____ _____	Date_____ _____ _____ _____ _____ _____	
Clotting screen: Platelet count Bleeding time Prothrombin time (PT) APTT TCT or fibrinogen level	Date_____ _____ _____ sec _____ sec _____ _____	Date_____ _____ _____ sec _____ sec _____ _____	
Immune screen			
Date			
NK cell assay	50:1_____ 25:1_____ 12:1_____	50:1_____ 25:1_____ 12:1_____	
Immunophenotype	CD3_____ CD4_____ CD8_____ CD19_____ CD56$^+$/CD16$^+$_____ CD56$^+$_____ CD3/IL-2R$^+$_____ CD 19$^+$/5$^+$_____	CD3_____ CD4_____ CD8_____ CD19_____ CD56$^+$/CD16$^+$_____ CD56$^+$_____ CD3/IL-2R$^+$_____ CD 19$^+$/5$^+$_____	
Th1:Th2			
IgG T **IgG B**			
HLA-Dq alpha			
Other immune investigations			

Figure A1.3, cont'd

Infection screen			
Infection screen	Date _____ Details	Date _____ Details	

Genetic tests			
Karyotyping, fragile X syndrome, etc.	Date _____ Details		

Other			
Rubella status	Date _____ Details	Date _____ Details	
Other blood tests (e.g., testosterone, glucose, vitamin levels, etc.)	Date _____ Test _____ Result _____ Date _____ Test _____ Result _____ Date _____ Test _____ Result _____ Date _____ Test _____ Result _____	Date _____ Test _____ Result _____ Date _____ Test _____ Result _____ Date _____ Test _____ Result _____ Date _____ Test _____ Result _____	

Tests and investigations (male)			
Patient's name:_____ DOB:_____			
	Initial test	**Retest**	**Notes** (see Chapters 4 and 12)
Semen analysis			
	Date _____	Date _____	
Days of abstinence	_____	_____	
Exposure to heat/fever	yes/no	yes/no	
Influencing lifestyle factors	_____	_____	
Semen volume	_____mL	_____mL	
Sperm concentration	_____10^6 per mL	_____10^6 per mL	
Total sperm number	_____10^6 per ejaculate	_____10^6 per ejaculate	
Total motility (PR+NP)	_____%	_____%	
Progressive motility (PR)	_____%	_____%	
Vitality (live spermatozoa)	_____%	_____%	
Sperm morphology (normal forms)	_____%	_____%	
pH	_____	_____	
Peroxidase-positive leukocytes	_____10^6 per mL	_____10^6 per mL	
MAR test (motile spermatozoa with bound particles)	_____%	_____%	
Immunobead test (motile spermatozoa with bound beads)	_____%	_____%	
Seminal zinc	_____μmol/ejaculate	_____μmol/ejaculate	
Seminal fructose	_____μmol/ejaculate	_____μmol/ejaculate	
Seminal neutral glucosidase	_____mU/ejaculate	_____mU/ejaculate	
Semen leukocytes	Round cells_____mil/mL White blood cells_____mil/mL	Round cells_____mil/mL White blood cells_____mil/mL	
DNA fragmentation			
	Date _____	Date _____	
SCSA	_____%	_____%	
TUNEL	_____%	_____%	
COMET	_____%	_____%	
MSOME			
Findings	Date _____ Details	Date _____ Details	
Endocrine investigations			
	Date _____	Date _____	
FSH	low/normal/high	low/normal/high	
LH	low/normal/high	low/normal/high	
Testosterone	low/normal	low/normal	
Prolactin	normal/high	normal/high	

Figure A1.4 Tests and investigations (male).

Ultrasound			
Transrectal ultrasound (TRUS):	Date _____		
Dilated seminal vesicles	yes/no		
Dilated ejaculatory ducts	yes/no		
Midline cystic prostatic structures	yes/no		
Scrotal ultrasound:	Date _____		
Varicoceles	yes/no		
Spermatoceles	yes/no		
Absent vasa	yes/no		
Epididymal induration	yes/no		
Testicular masses	yes/no		
Infection screen			
Infection screen	Date _____ Details	Date _____ Details	
Genetic tests			
Karyotyping **Cystic fibrosis gene mutation** **Y-chromosome analysis**	Date _____ Details		
Other			
Anti-sperm antibodies (ASA)	Date _____ yes/no		
Post-ejaculatory urinalysis:	Date _____	Date _____	
Sperm found?	yes/low numbers/no	yes/low numbers/no	
Other tests	Date _____ Test _____ Result _____ Date _____ Test _____ Result _____ Date _____ Test _____ Result _____	Date _____ Test _____ Result _____ Date _____ Test _____ Result _____ Date _____ Test _____ Result _____	

Preconception care (female or male)

Patient's name:_____DOB:_____

	Initial details	Review	Notes (see Chapter 7)
Date			
Weight BMI	_____kg _____kg/m²	_____kg _____kg/m²	
Smoking Exposed to second-hand smoke?	_____cigarettes/day yes/no	_____cigarettes/day yes/no	
Recreation drugs use			
Exercise	_____hours/week Details	_____hours/week Details	
Rest and relaxation			
Stress levels Coping methods	_____out of 10	_____out of 10	
Environmental toxins exposure			
Occupational risk factors			
Medication (prescribed and over the counter)			
Supplements (details and dose)			
Alcohol	_____units/week	_____units/week	
Caffeine	_____cups/day (or equivalent)	_____cups/day (or equivalent)	
Water	_____L/day	_____L/day	

Figure A1.5 Preconception care (female or male).

Diet: Special diet followed (e.g., vegan, vegetarian, etc.)			
Diet on a typical day: Breakfast			
Snack			
Lunch			
Snack			
Dinner			
Snack			
Cravings			
Dislikes			

Coitus

(For couples where natural conception is possible)

Patient's name (female):_____ DOB:_____

Patient's name (male):_____ DOB:_____

	Initial details	Review	Notes (see Chapter 7)
Date			
Fertile window estimation	Shortest cycle length: ____ – 14 – 5 =____(a) Longest cycle length: ____ – 13 =____(b) Fertile window: from (a)____to (b)____	Shortest cycle length: ____ – 14 – 5 =____(a) Longest cycle length: ____ – 13 =____(b) Fertile window: from (a)____to (b)____	
Fertile mucus: when quantity	_____day(s) of cycle scanty/profuse	_____day(s) of cycle scanty/profuse	
Intercourse frequency: During fertile window Outside of fertile window	_____ _____	_____ _____	
Method of fertile window detection	None/fertile mucus/ ovulation detection kits (LH or oestrogen and LH)/ BBT charting/other	None/fertile mucus/ ovulation detection kits (LH or oestrogen and LH)/ BBT charting/other	
Use of lubricants	yes/no type_____	yes/no type_____	
Libido: Male partner Female partner	_____out of 10 _____out of 10	_____out of 10 _____out of 10	
Pain during intercourse	yes/no	yes/no	
Erection problems	yes/no	yes/no	
Ejaculation problems	yes/no	yes/no	
Arousal, enjoyment			
Other intercourse issues (being away a lot, relationship issues, inability to have intercourse for other health reasons, etc.)			

Figure A1.6 Coitus.

ART audit tool

Patient's name (female):_____ DOB:_____

Patient's name (male):_____ DOB:_____

	Treatment cycle 1	Treatment cycle 2	Notes (see Chapters 4 and 12)
Date treatment cycle started			
Age when treatment started	Female_____ Male_____	Female_____ Male_____	
ART clinic, consultant and contact details			
Stress levels, emotional imbalances			
Implantation failure – prevention steps taken			
Hysteroscopy/ endometrial scratch Embryo glue Vaginal Viagra Immune treatments Thrombophilia treatment IMSI fertilization method Assisted hatching Other			
Lifestyle modifications made in preparation for ART treatment and how long for			
What modifications were made?			
Preparation acupuncture (within 3 months of treatment cycle)			
Acupuncture treatment (female): TCM syndromes/ improvement rate	No. of sessions_____ _____/____% _____/____% _____/____% _____/____% _____/____%	No. of sessions_____ _____/____% _____/____% _____/____% _____/____% _____/____%	
Acupuncture treatment (male): TCM syndromes/ improvement rate	No. of sessions_____ _____/____% _____/____% _____/____% _____/____% _____/____%	No. of sessions_____ _____/____% _____/____% _____/____% _____/____% _____/____%	

Figure A1.7 ART audit tool.

Continued

Pretreatment phase up to 4 weeks before treatment cycle (downregulation, contraceptive pill, etc.)			
Acupuncture treatment (female)	Day____ Day____ Day____ Day____	Day____ Day____ Day____ Day____	
Acupuncture treatment (male)	Day____ Day____ Day____ Day____	Day____ Day____ Day____ Day____	
Medication, dose, length of administration			
Issues (e.g. side effects, problems with medication, etc.)			
Ovarian stimulation (or follicular preparation, if not a stimulated cycle)			

Baseline scan and blood tests	AFC: Left____Right____
	Endometrium____mm
	Oestrogen____pmol/L / pg/mL
	Cysts: Left____mm
	     Right____mm
		AFC: Left____Right____
		Endometrium____mm
		Oestrogen____pmol/L / pg/mL
		Cysts: Left____mm
		     Right____mm	

Acupuncture treatment (female): day of stimulation and observations	Day____ Day____ Day____ Day____ Day____ Day____	Day____ Day____ Day____ Day____ Day____ Day____	
Acupuncture treatment (male): day of stimulation and observations	Day____ Day____ Day____ Day____ Day____ Day____	Day____ Day____ Day____ Day____ Day____ Day____	
Medication, dose, length of administration			
Other medication (e.g. aspirin, clexane, steroids, intralipids, thyroid medication, etc.)			

Figure A1.7, cont'd

Last monitoring scan	Day of stimulation_____ Days before egg retrieval_____ Endometrium_____mm Oestrogen_____pmol/L / pg/mL		Day of stimulation_____ Days before egg retrieval_____ Endometrium_____mm Oestrogen_____pmol/L / pg/mL		
	Follicles:		**Follicles:**		
	Left	**Right**	**Left**	**Right**	
	1_____mm 2_____mm 3_____mm 4_____mm 5_____mm 6_____mm 7_____mm 8_____mm 9_____mm 10_____mm	1_____mm 2_____mm 3_____mm 4_____mm 5_____mm 6_____mm 7_____mm 8_____mm 9_____mm 10_____mm	1_____mm 2_____mm 3_____mm 4_____mm 5_____mm 6_____mm 7_____mm 8_____mm 9_____mm 10_____mm	1_____mm 2_____mm 3_____mm 4_____mm 5_____mm 6_____mm 7_____mm 8_____mm 9_____mm 10_____mm	
Hyperstimulation (OHSS) symptoms (bloating, diarrhoea, constipation, reduced urination, breathing difficulties, weight gain)					
Ovulation induction/final egg maturation (hCG trigger to egg retrieval)					
Trigger medication	Day of trigger Medication Dose		Day of trigger Medication Dose		
Acupuncture session between trigger and egg retrieval?	yes/no		yes/no		
Egg retrieval, if applicable (day 0)					
Day of egg retrieval					
Expected no. of eggs (most follicles ≥15 mm should have a mature egg)					
No. of eggs retrieved					
No. of eggs matured with IVM					
Anaesthetics	Local/sedation/general/ acupuncture		Local/sedation/general/ acupuncture		
Pain during retrieval **Pain after retrieval**	_____out of 10 _____out of 10		_____out of 10 _____out of 10		
Sperm parameters on the day					
Fertilization (day 0–1)					
Method of fertilization	IVF/ICSI/IMSI/other		IVF/ICSI/IMSI/other		
No. of eggs suitable for fertilization					
No. and % of eggs fertilized	_____eggs_____%		_____eggs_____%		
No. of eggs fertilized abnormally	No._____ Details		No._____ Details		

Continued

375

Embryo development (days 2 to 6 post-egg retrieval)			
No. of embryos and quality	Day 2 Day 3 Day 4 Day 5	Day 2 Day 3 Day 4 Day 5	
Was embryoscope/ EEVA used?			
Results of embryo genetic diagnosis, if done (e.g. CGH, PGD, etc.)			
Embryo transfer			
Embryos transferred	Grade_____ day____ Grade_____ day____ Grade_____ day____	Grade_____ day____ Grade_____ day____ Grade_____ day____	
No. of embryos frozen, their grades and day of development (e.g. day 1, 2, 3, 5, reached blastocysts stage)	Grade_____ day____ Grade_____ day____ Grade_____ day____ Grade_____ day____ Grade_____ day____ Grade_____ day____ Grade_____ day____ Grade_____ day____ Grade_____ day____ Grade_____ day____ Grade_____ day____	Grade_____ day____ Grade_____ day____ Grade_____ day____ Grade_____ day____ Grade_____ day____ Grade_____ day____ Grade_____ day____ Grade_____ day____ Grade_____ day____ Grade_____ day____ Grade_____ day____	
Pain during or after transfer?	_____out of 10	_____out of 10	
Any issues with ejecting the embryos from catheter?			
Acupuncture embryo transfer	Protocol _____hours before transfer _____hours after transfer	Protocol _____hours before transfer _____hours after transfer	
Luteal phase or 'two-week wait' (embryo transfer to pregnancy test)			
Acupuncture treatment (days of treatment, clinical findings)			
Early pregnancy symptoms			
Poor prognostic symptoms (bleeding, abdominal cramping, etc.)			
Stress levels Strong emotions	_____out of 10	_____out of 10	

Figure A1.7, cont'd

Early pregnancy (if applicable)			
Home pregnancy test (egg retrieval = day 0)	Day____result_____ Day____result_____ Day____result_____	Day____result_____ Day____result_____ Day____result_____	
hCG blood test (egg retrieval = day 0)	Day____result_____ Day____result_____ Day____result_____	Day____result_____ Day____result_____ Day____result_____	
Threatened miscarriage symptoms (bleeding, abdominal or back cramping)			
Acupuncture treatment			
Pregnancy outcome: Live birth Miscarriage Ectopic pregnancy Still birth	_____weeks' gestation _____weeks' gestation _____ _____weeks' gestation	_____weeks' gestation _____weeks' gestation _____ _____weeks' gestation	
Ultrasound scan 1: Heartbeat(s) Any bleeding visible?	_____weeks' gestation ____bpm ____bpm ____bpm yes/no	_____weeks' gestation ____bpm ____bpm ____bpm yes/no	
Ultrasound scan 2: Heartbeat(s) Any bleeding visible?	_____weeks' gestation ____bpm ____bpm ____bpm yes/no	_____weeks' gestation ____bpm ____bpm ____bpm yes/no	
Ultrasound scan 3: Heartbeat(s) Any bleeding visible?	_____weeks' gestation ____bpm ____bpm ____bpm yes/no	_____weeks' gestation ____bpm ____bpm ____bpm yes/no	

Appendix

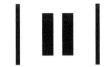

Basal body temperature (BBT) chart template and instructions

Basal Body Temperature (BBT) Charting Instructions

Taking the Temperature

- Use a special fertility thermometer (in °C). It should have two decimal places and is more sensitive than a standard thermometer.
- Keep the thermometer next to your bed ready to be used in the morning.
- Your temperature should be taken at the same time every morning after at least three consecutive hours of sleep and immediately when you wake up, before you get out of bed or do anything else (for example before you go to the toilet, feed a cat etc).
- Most people prefer to take their temperature orally. But it can also be taken vaginally, rectally or under your arm. Use the same method throughout.

Recording the Temperature

- Start taking your temperature on day one of your menstrual bleed. If you have spotting before proper bleeding starts, wait until the proper bleed and this will be classed as your menstrual cycle day 1.
- Record on the chart the date and the time on the relevant menstrual cycle day.
- Put a cross on the square with the temperature nearest to the one your thermometer is showing.

Intercourse

- It would also be helpful if you could mark the days when you have intercourse.

Cervical Fluid

- Observe what kind of vaginal secretions you have and log at the end of the day. Use the relevant keys provided at the bottom of the chart. For example, if you have fertile mucus, which looks like egg white and stretches without breaking, enter E on the relevant day, for blood enter B, if you have no secretions, enter D and if your secretions are moist or creamy, enter C.

Ovulation Test Results

- If you use an ovulation detection kit, mark the days on the chart when you get positive or peak reading on your ovulation test.

Other Notes

- The following factors are known to affect the temperature. Please make a note in the "special notes" section when any of these are applicable:
  - If you have alcohol the night before (even small amounts)
  - If you have an illness (for example cold, flu or other infections)
  - If you have bad night's sleep (especially if you slept for less than 3 hours before taking temperature)
  - If you had to take medication (especially temperature lowering medication, such as paracetamol or ibuprofen)
  - If the bedroom is unusually hot or cold
  - If you feel stressed
  - If you travel, especially air travel

Table A2.1 Basal body temperature chart

Cycle day	1	2	3	4	5	6	7	8	9	10	11	12	13	14	15	16	17	18	19
Date																			
Time																			
Waking basal temp.	37.60	37.60	37.60	37.60	37.60	37.60	37.60	37.60	37.60	37.60	37.60	37.60	37.60	37.60	37.60	37.60	37.60	37.60	37.60
	37.55	37.55	37.55	37.55	37.55	37.55	37.55	37.55	37.55	37.55	37.55	37.55	37.55	37.55	37.55	37.55	37.55	37.55	37.55
	37.50	37.50	37.50	37.50	37.50	37.50	37.50	37.50	37.50	37.50	37.50	37.50	37.50	37.50	37.50	37.50	37.50	37.50	37.50
	37.45	37.45	37.45	37.45	37.45	37.45	37.45	37.45	37.45	37.45	37.45	37.45	37.45	37.45	37.45	37.45	37.45	37.45	37.45
	37.40	37.40	37.40	37.40	37.40	37.40	37.40	37.40	37.40	37.40	37.40	37.40	37.40	37.40	37.40	37.40	37.40	37.40	37.40
	37.35	37.35	37.35	37.35	37.35	37.35	37.35	37.35	37.35	37.35	37.35	37.35	37.35	37.35	37.35	37.35	37.35	37.35	37.35
	37.30	37.30	37.30	37.30	37.30	37.30	37.30	37.30	37.30	37.30	37.30	37.30	37.30	37.30	37.30	37.30	37.30	37.30	37.30
	37.25	37.25	37.25	37.25	37.25	37.25	37.25	37.25	37.25	37.25	37.25	37.25	37.25	37.25	37.25	37.25	37.25	37.25	37.25
	37.20	37.20	37.20	37.20	37.20	37.20	37.20	37.20	37.20	37.20	37.20	37.20	37.20	37.20	37.20	37.20	37.20	37.20	37.20
	37.15	37.15	37.15	37.15	37.15	37.15	37.15	37.15	37.15	37.15	37.15	37.15	37.15	37.15	37.15	37.15	37.15	37.15	37.15
	37.10	37.10	37.10	37.10	37.10	37.10	37.10	37.10	37.10	37.10	37.10	37.10	37.10	37.10	37.10	37.10	37.10	37.10	37.10
	37.05	37.05	37.05	37.05	37.05	37.05	37.05	37.05	37.05	37.05	37.05	37.05	37.05	37.05	37.05	37.05	37.05	37.05	37.05
	37.00	37.00	37.00	37.00	37.00	37.00	37.00	37.00	37.00	37.00	37.00	37.00	37.00	37.00	37.00	37.00	37.00	37.00	37.00
	36.95	36.95	36.95	36.95	36.95	36.95	36.95	36.95	36.95	36.95	36.95	36.95	36.95	36.95	36.95	36.95	36.95	36.95	36.95
	36.90	36.90	36.90	36.90	36.90	36.90	36.90	36.90	36.90	36.90	36.90	36.90	36.90	36.90	36.90	36.90	36.90	36.90	36.90
	36.85	36.85	36.85	36.85	36.85	36.85	36.85	36.85	36.85	36.85	36.85	36.85	36.85	36.85	36.85	36.85	36.85	36.85	36.85
	36.80	36.80	36.80	36.80	36.80	36.80	36.80	36.80	36.80	36.80	36.80	36.80	36.80	36.80	36.80	36.80	36.80	36.80	36.80
	36.75	36.75	36.75	36.75	36.75	36.75	36.75	36.75	36.75	36.75	36.75	36.75	36.75	36.75	36.75	36.75	36.75	36.75	36.75
	36.70	36.70	36.70	36.70	36.70	36.70	36.70	36.70	36.70	36.70	36.70	36.70	36.70	36.70	36.70	36.70	36.70	36.70	36.70
	36.65	36.65	36.65	36.65	36.65	36.65	36.65	36.65	36.65	36.65	36.65	36.65	36.65	36.65	36.65	36.65	36.65	36.65	36.65
	36.60	36.60	36.60	36.60	36.60	36.60	36.60	36.60	36.60	36.60	36.60	36.60	36.60	36.60	36.60	36.60	36.60	36.60	36.60
	36.55	36.55	36.55	36.55	36.55	36.55	36.55	36.55	36.55	36.55	36.55	36.55	36.55	36.55	36.55	36.55	36.55	36.55	36.55
	36.50	36.50	36.50	36.50	36.50	36.50	36.50	36.50	36.50	36.50	36.50	36.50	36.50	36.50	36.50	36.50	36.50	36.50	36.50
	36.45	36.45	36.45	36.45	36.45	36.45	36.45	36.45	36.45	36.45	36.45	36.45	36.45	36.45	36.45	36.45	36.45	36.45	36.45
	36.40	36.40	36.40	36.40	36.40	36.40	36.40	36.40	36.40	36.40	36.40	36.40	36.40	36.40	36.40	36.40	36.40	36.40	36.40
	36.35	36.35	36.35	36.35	36.35	36.35	36.35	36.35	36.35	36.35	36.35	36.35	36.35	36.35	36.35	36.35	36.35	36.35	36.35
	36.30	36.30	36.30	36.30	36.30	36.30	36.30	36.30	36.30	36.30	36.30	36.30	36.30	36.30	36.30	36.30	36.30	36.30	36.30
	36.25	36.25	36.25	36.25	36.25	36.25	36.25	36.25	36.25	36.25	36.25	36.25	36.25	36.25	36.25	36.25	36.25	36.25	36.25
	36.20	36.20	36.20	36.20	36.20	36.20	36.20	36.20	36.20	36.20	36.20	36.20	36.20	36.20	36.20	36.20	36.20	36.20	36.20
	36.15	36.15	36.15	36.15	36.15	36.15	36.15	36.15	36.15	36.15	36.15	36.15	36.15	36.15	36.15	36.15	36.15	36.15	36.15
	36.10	36.10	36.10	36.10	36.10	36.10	36.10	36.10	36.10	36.10	36.10	36.10	36.10	36.10	36.10	36.10	36.10	36.10	36.10
	36.05	36.05	36.05	36.05	36.05	36.05	36.05	36.05	36.05	36.05	36.05	36.05	36.05	36.05	36.05	36.05	36.05	36.05	36.05
	36.00	36.00	36.00	36.00	36.00	36.00	36.00	36.00	36.00	36.00	36.00	36.00	36.00	36.00	36.00	36.00	36.00	36.00	36.00
	35.95	35.95	35.95	35.95	35.95	35.95	35.95	35.95	35.95	35.95	35.95	35.95	35.95	35.95	35.95	35.95	35.95	35.95	35.95
	35.90	35.90	35.90	35.90	35.90	35.90	35.90	35.90	35.90	35.90	35.90	35.90	35.90	35.90	35.90	35.90	35.90	35.90	35.90
	35.85	35.85	35.85	35.85	35.85	35.85	35.85	35.85	35.85	35.85	35.85	35.85	35.85	35.85	35.85	35.85	35.85	35.85	35.85
	35.80	35.80	35.80	35.80	35.80	35.80	35.80	35.80	35.80	35.80	35.80	35.80	35.80	35.80	35.80	35.80	35.80	35.80	35.80
	35.75	35.75	35.75	35.75	35.75	35.75	35.75	35.75	35.75	35.75	35.75	35.75	35.75	35.75	35.75	35.75	35.75	35.75	35.75
	35.70	35.70	35.70	35.70	35.70	35.70	35.70	35.70	35.70	35.70	35.70	35.70	35.70	35.70	35.70	35.70	35.70	35.70	35.70
Cycle day	1	2	3	4	5	6	7	8	9	10	11	12	13	14	15	16	17	18	19
Intercourse																			
Cervical fluid*																			
Ovulation test result																			
Pregnancy test result																			
Other notes:																			
Poor sleep																			
Alcohol																			
Illness																			
Additional information:																			

*Cervical fluid: E, Egg white; C, Creamy; D, Dry; B, Blood.

20	21	22	23	24	25	26	27	28	29	30	31	32	33	34	35	36	37	38	39	40
37.60	37.60	37.60	37.60	37.60	37.60	37.60	37.60	37.60	37.60	37.60	37.60	37.60	37.60	37.60	37.60	37.60	37.60	37.60	37.60	37.60
37.55	37.55	37.55	37.55	37.55	37.55	37.55	37.55	37.55	37.55	37.55	37.55	37.55	37.55	37.55	37.55	37.55	37.55	37.55	37.55	37.55
37.50	37.50	37.50	37.50	37.50	37.50	37.50	37.50	37.50	37.50	37.50	37.50	37.50	37.50	37.50	37.50	37.50	37.50	37.50	37.50	37.50
37.45	37.45	37.45	37.45	37.45	37.45	37.45	37.45	37.45	37.45	37.45	37.45	37.45	37.45	37.45	37.45	37.45	37.45	37.45	37.45	37.45
37.40	37.40	37.40	37.40	37.40	37.40	37.40	37.40	37.40	37.40	37.40	37.40	37.40	37.40	37.40	37.40	37.40	37.40	37.40	37.40	37.40
37.35	37.35	37.35	37.35	37.35	37.35	37.35	37.35	37.35	37.35	37.35	37.35	37.35	37.35	37.35	37.35	37.35	37.35	37.35	37.35	37.35
37.30	37.30	37.30	37.30	37.30	37.30	37.30	37.30	37.30	37.30	37.30	37.30	37.30	37.30	37.30	37.30	37.30	37.30	37.30	37.30	37.30
37.25	37.25	37.25	37.25	37.25	37.25	37.25	37.25	37.25	37.25	37.25	37.25	37.25	37.25	37.25	37.25	37.25	37.25	37.25	37.25	37.25
37.20	37.20	37.20	37.20	37.20	37.20	37.20	37.20	37.20	37.20	37.20	37.20	37.20	37.20	37.20	37.20	37.20	37.20	37.20	37.20	37.20
37.15	37.15	37.15	37.15	37.15	37.15	37.15	37.15	37.15	37.15	37.15	37.15	37.15	37.15	37.15	37.15	37.15	37.15	37.15	37.15	37.15
37.10	37.10	37.10	37.10	37.10	37.10	37.10	37.10	37.10	37.10	37.10	37.10	37.10	37.10	37.10	37.10	37.10	37.10	37.10	37.10	37.10
37.05	37.05	37.05	37.05	37.05	37.05	37.05	37.05	37.05	37.05	37.05	37.05	37.05	37.05	37.05	37.05	37.05	37.05	37.05	37.05	37.05
37.00	37.00	37.00	37.00	37.00	37.00	37.00	37.00	37.00	37.00	37.00	37.00	37.00	37.00	37.00	37.00	37.00	37.00	37.00	37.00	37.00
36.95	36.95	36.95	36.95	36.95	36.95	36.95	36.95	36.95	36.95	36.95	36.95	36.95	36.95	36.95	36.95	36.95	36.95	36.95	36.95	36.95
36.90	36.90	36.90	36.90	36.90	36.90	36.90	36.90	36.90	36.90	36.90	36.90	36.90	36.90	36.90	36.90	36.90	36.90	36.90	36.90	36.90
36.85	36.85	36.85	36.85	36.85	36.85	36.85	36.85	36.85	36.85	36.85	36.85	36.85	36.85	36.85	36.85	36.85	36.85	36.85	36.85	36.85
36.80	36.80	36.80	36.80	36.80	36.80	36.80	36.80	36.80	36.80	36.80	36.80	36.80	36.80	36.80	36.80	36.80	36.80	36.80	36.80	36.80
36.75	36.75	36.75	36.75	36.75	36.75	36.75	36.75	36.75	36.75	36.75	36.75	36.75	36.75	36.75	36.75	36.75	36.75	36.75	36.75	36.75
36.70	36.70	36.70	36.70	36.70	36.70	36.70	36.70	36.70	36.70	36.70	36.70	36.70	36.70	36.70	36.70	36.70	36.70	36.70	36.70	36.70
36.65	36.65	36.65	36.65	36.65	36.65	36.65	36.65	36.65	36.65	36.65	36.65	36.65	36.65	36.65	36.65	36.65	36.65	36.65	36.65	36.65
36.60	36.60	36.60	36.60	36.60	36.60	36.60	36.60	36.60	36.60	36.60	36.60	36.60	36.60	36.60	36.60	36.60	36.60	36.60	36.60	36.60
36.55	36.55	36.55	36.55	36.55	36.55	36.55	36.55	36.55	36.55	36.55	36.55	36.55	36.55	36.55	36.55	36.55	36.55	36.55	36.55	36.55
36.50	36.50	36.50	36.50	36.50	36.50	36.50	36.50	36.50	36.50	36.50	36.50	36.50	36.50	36.50	36.50	36.50	36.50	36.50	36.50	36.50
36.45	36.45	36.45	36.45	36.45	36.45	36.45	36.45	36.45	36.45	36.45	36.45	36.45	36.45	36.45	36.45	36.45	36.45	36.45	36.45	36.45
36.40	36.40	36.40	36.40	36.40	36.40	36.40	36.40	36.40	36.40	36.40	36.40	36.40	36.40	36.40	36.40	36.40	36.40	36.40	36.40	36.40
36.35	36.35	36.35	36.35	36.35	36.35	36.35	36.35	36.35	36.35	36.35	36.35	36.35	36.35	36.35	36.35	36.35	36.35	36.35	36.35	36.35
36.30	36.30	36.30	36.30	36.30	36.30	36.30	36.30	36.30	36.30	36.30	36.30	36.30	36.30	36.30	36.30	36.30	36.30	36.30	36.30	36.30
36.25	36.25	36.25	36.25	36.25	36.25	36.25	36.25	36.25	36.25	36.25	36.25	36.25	36.25	36.25	36.25	36.25	36.25	36.25	36.25	36.25
36.20	36.20	36.20	36.20	36.20	36.20	36.20	36.20	36.20	36.20	36.20	36.20	36.20	36.20	36.20	36.20	36.20	36.20	36.20	36.20	36.20
36.15	36.15	36.15	36.15	36.15	36.15	36.15	36.15	36.15	36.15	36.15	36.15	36.15	36.15	36.15	36.15	36.15	36.15	36.15	36.15	36.15
36.10	36.10	36.10	36.10	36.10	36.10	36.10	36.10	36.10	36.10	36.10	36.10	36.10	36.10	36.10	36.10	36.10	36.10	36.10	36.10	36.10
36.05	36.05	36.05	36.05	36.05	36.05	36.05	36.05	36.05	36.05	36.05	36.05	36.05	36.05	36.05	36.05	36.05	36.05	36.05	36.05	36.05
36.00	36.00	36.00	36.00	36.00	36.00	36.00	36.00	36.00	36.00	36.00	36.00	36.00	36.00	36.00	36.00	36.00	36.00	36.00	36.00	36.00
35.95	35.95	35.95	35.95	35.95	35.95	35.95	35.95	35.95	35.95	35.95	35.95	35.95	35.95	35.95	35.95	35.95	35.95	35.95	35.95	35.95
35.90	35.90	35.90	35.90	35.90	35.90	35.90	35.90	35.90	35.90	35.90	35.90	35.90	35.90	35.90	35.90	35.90	35.90	35.90	35.90	35.90
35.85	35.85	35.85	35.85	35.85	35.85	35.85	35.85	35.85	35.85	35.85	35.85	35.85	35.85	35.85	35.85	35.85	35.85	35.85	35.85	35.85
35.80	35.80	35.80	35.80	35.80	35.80	35.80	35.80	35.80	35.80	35.80	35.80	35.80	35.80	35.80	35.80	35.80	35.80	35.80	35.80	35.80
35.75	35.75	35.75	35.75	35.75	35.75	35.75	35.75	35.75	35.75	35.75	35.75	35.75	35.75	35.75	35.75	35.75	35.75	35.75	35.75	35.75
35.70	35.70	35.70	35.70	35.70	35.70	35.70	35.70	35.70	35.70	35.70	35.70	35.70	35.70	35.70	35.70	35.70	35.70	35.70	35.70	35.70
20	21	22	23	24	25	26	27	28	29	30	31	32	33	34	35	36	37	38	39	40

Appendix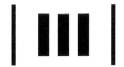

Investigation reference ranges at a glance

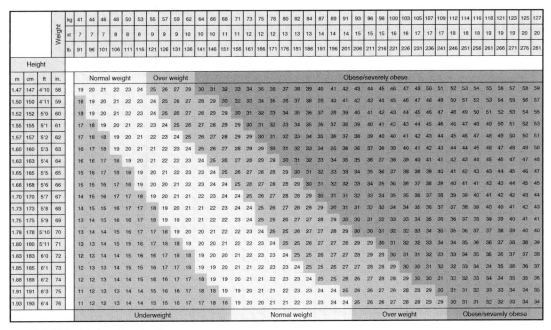

Figure A3.1 BMI table (see Chapter 7).
Source: WHO (2013). Available from: http://apps.who.int/bmi/index.jsp?introPage=intro_3.html (accessed 8 October 2013).

Table A3.1 Ovulation investigations: reference ranges for progesterone and prolactin (see Chapter 4)

Hormones	Timing relative to menstrual cycle	Reference range[a]	Notes
Progesterone	Seven days before expected start of next period. In women with irregular cycles the test may need to be repeated every 7 days until the next period starts[1]	>9.54 nmol/L (>3 ng/mL): ovulation has occurred[2] ≤3 ng/mL (≤9.54 nmol/L): ovulation has not occurred[2]	Some fertility clinics prefer to see higher levels, as levels of ≥31.8 nmol/L (≥10 ng/mL) may be suggestive of better quality luteal function[3]
Prolactin	Any cycle day	Values depend on assay used by the laboratory, ranging from[4]: 3.35–4.65 µg/L (71–98 mIU/L): lower limit to 16.4–23.2 µg/L (348–492 mIU/L): upper limit	Even mildly elevated prolactin may be a sign of central nervous system lesion. Therefore Magnetic Resonance Imaging (MRI) is indicated in all cases of raised prolactin[5] Other causes of raised prolactin include physical and emotional stress, high protein diet and intense breast stimulation,[6] kidney or thyroid disease, use of certain drugs, and hypersensitive prolactin releasing cells in the pituitary[7]

[a] Reference values may vary between different laboratories and assays used. Therefore, laboratory reports should be checked for reference ranges applicable to the individual patient's results profile.

Table A3.2 Ovarian reserve reference ranges: FSH, LH, and E2 (see Chapter 4)

Hormones	Timing relative to menstrual cycle	Reference ranges[a]	Notes
FSH[a]	Cycle days 2–5	*ASRM*[2]: <10 IU/L (<10 mIU/mL): normal ovarian reserve[a] 10–20 IU/L (10–20 mIU/mL): poor ovarian reserve >20 IU/L (>20 mIU/mL): may signify menopause *National Institute for Health and Care Excellence (NICE)*[1]: <4 IU/L (<4 mIU/mL): likely high ovarian response[a] >8.9 IU/L (>8.9 mIU/mL): likely low ovarian response	An imperfect measure, as FSH fluctuates from cycle to cycle Should be tested and interpreted together with E2. High E2 may suppress FSH, resulting in false normal FSH reading.[8,9] This is usually seen in premenopausal women[a]
LH	Days 2–5 together with FSH	1.4–7.8 IU/L (1.4–7.8 mIU/mL): normal range[10]	High LH + normal FSH suggests Polycystic Ovarian Syndrome (PCOS),[11] although this is not a diagnostic test and specific PCOS tests need to be carried out (see Chapter 8 for further details on PCOS) High LH + high FSH suggest diminished ovarian reserve (DOR)
E2	Days 2–5 together with FSH	>188–210 pmol/L (51–57 pg/mL): high levels[10]	Helps to interpret FSH correctly. If FSH is within normal range, raised E2 may be artificially suppressing FSH, thus giving a false normal FSH level. E2 levels during IVF may be much higher E2 also helps to distinguish between different types of amenorrhoea[2]: • High FSH + low E2 = ovarian failure requiring egg donation • Normal FSH + low E2 = hypothalamic amenorrhoea requiring exogenous gonadotrophin stimulation for ovulation induction

[a] Reference values may vary between different laboratories and assays used. Therefore, laboratory reports should be checked for reference ranges applicable to the individual patient's results profile.

Table A3.3 Ovarian reserve reference ranges: AMH (see Chapter 4)

Hormones	Timing relative to menstrual cycle	Reference ranges[a]			Notes
AMH	Any cycle day	*ASRM*[9]: <1.4–5 pmol/L (<0.2–0.7 ng/mL DSL ELISA): likely low ovarian response, poor embryo quality, and low chance of achieving pregnancy *NICE*[1]: ≤5.3 pmol/L (≤0.7 ng/mL): likely low ovarian response ≥25.0 pmol/L (≥3.5 ng/mL): likely high ovarian response >48 pmol/L (>6.7 ng/mL): likely PCOS[12]			Very good predictive value of ovarian response[9]
		Age	pmol/L	ng/mL[13]	Age-specific AMH values may be better for assessing ovarian reserve on an individual basis[14]
		24	29.3	4.1	
		25	29.3	4.1	
		26	30.0	4.2	
		27	26.4	3.7	
		28	27.1	3.8	
		29	25.0	3.5	
		30	22.8	3.2	
		31	22.1	3.1	
		32	17.9	2.5	
		33	18.6	2.6	
		34	16.4	2.3	
		35	15.0	2.1	
		36	12.9	1.8	
		37	11.4	1.6	
		38	10.0	1.4	
		39	9.3	1.3	
		40	7.9	1.1	
		41	7.1	1.0	
		42	6.4	0.9	
		43	5.0	0.7	
		44	4.3	0.6	
		45	3.6	0.5	

Table A3.3 Ovarian reserve reference ranges: AMH—cont'd

Hormones	Timing relative to menstrual cycle	Reference ranges[a]		Notes
		46	2.9	0.4
		47	2.9	0.4
		48	1.4	0.2
		49	0.7	0.1
		50	0	0

[a] Reference values may vary between different laboratories and assays used. Therefore, laboratory reports should be checked for reference ranges applicable to the individual patient's results profile.

Table A3.4 Ovarian reserve reference ranges: AFC (see Chapter 4)

Scan	Timing relative to menstrual cycle	Reference ranges	Notes
AFC	Usually performed during the early follicular phase (but can be done at any point)[15]	*ASRM*[2,9]: >10 total antral follicles: good ovarian reserve 3–10 total antral follicles: poor ovarian reserve, likely to have poor response to stimulation, and low chance of achieving pregnancy *NICE*[1]: ≤4 total antral follicles: likely low ovarian response >16 total antral follicles: likely high ovarian response ≥12 follicles on each ovary measuring 2–9 mm indicates Polycystic Ovarian (PCO)[16]	Very good predictive value of ovarian response[9]

Table A3.5 Criteria for diagnosing APS (see Chapter 4)

Clinical criteria	Laboratory criteria[a]

• Vascular thrombosis (one or more clinical episodes of arterial, venous, or small vessel thrombosis, in any tissue or organ. Thrombosis must be confirmed by objective validated criteria (i.e., unequivocal findings of appropriate imaging studies or histopathology). For histopathologic confirmation, thrombosis should be present without significant evidence of inflammation in the vessel wall
  ■ Pregnancy morbidity:
    a) One or more unexplained deaths of a morphologically normal foetus at or beyond the 10th week of gestation, with normal foetal morphology documented by ultrasound or by direct examination of the foetus, or
	• Lupus anticoagulant (LA) present in plasma, on two or more occasions at least 12 weeks apart, detected according to the guidelines of the International Society on Thrombosis and Haemostasis (Scientific Subcommittee on LAs/phospholipid-dependent antibodies)
	• Anticardiolipin (aCL) antibody of IgG and/or IgM isotype in serum or plasma, present in medium or high titre (i.e. >40 GPL or MPL, or >the 99th percentile), on two or more occasions, at least 12 weeks apart, measured by a standardized ELISA
	• Anti-b2 glycoprotein-I antibody of IgG and/or IgM isotype in serum or plasma (in titre >the 99th percentile), present on two or more occasions, at least 12 weeks apart,

Continued

Table A3.5 Criteria for diagnosing APS—cont'd	
Clinical criteria	**Laboratory criteria[a]**

b) One or more premature births of a morphologically normal neonate before the 34th week of gestation because of:
   ○ Eclampsia or severe pre-eclampsia defined according to standard definitions, or
   ○ Recognized features of placental insufficiency, or
c) Three or more unexplained consecutive spontaneous abortions before the 10th week of gestation, with maternal anatomic or hormonal abnormalities and paternal and maternal chromosomal causes excluded. In studies of populations of patients who have more than one type of pregnancy morbidity, investigators are strongly encouraged to stratify groups of subjects according to a, b, or c above.
	measured by a standardized ELISA, according to recommended procedures

Reprinted with permission from Ref. 17.
[a] Other antibodies may be linked to APS. However, they are not included in the diagnostic criteria due to non-standardized testing.

Table A3.6 WHO interpretation of semen analysis (2010) (see Chapter 4)[18]

Parameter	Reference range[a]	Terminology relating to abnormal findings
Semen volume (mL)	≥ 1.5	*Aspermia*: no semen (or retrograde ejaculation)
Total sperm number (10^6 per ejaculate)	≥ 39	
Sperm concentration (10^6 per mL)	≥ 15	*Azoospermia*: absence of sperm in semen *Oligospermia*: total number of sperm below lower reference limit *Severe oligospermia*: sperm concentrations of <5 millions/mL
Total motility (PR + NP, %)	≥ 40	*Astheno-zoospermia*: sperm motility below reference limit *Astheno-terato-zoospermia*: low percentage of progressive motile (PR) and normal sperm
Progressive motility (PR, %)	≥ 32	*Oligo-astheno zoospermia*: low concentration and low percentage of progressively motile (PR) sperm
Vitality (live spermatozoa, %)	≥ 58	*Necro-zoospermia*: low percentage of live and high percentage of immotile sperm
Sperm morphology (normal forms, %)	≥ 4	*Terato-zoospermia*: percentage of normal sperm below reference limit *Oligo-terato-zoospermia*: low concentration and low normal forms *Oligo-astheno-terato-zoospermia*: low concentration, low percentage of progressively motile (PR) sperm and low normal forms
pH	≥ 7.2	
Peroxidase-positive leukocytes (10^6 per mL)	<1.0	*Leukospermia (leukocyto-spermia, pyospermia)*: presence of leukocytes in the ejaculate above reference limit
MAR test (motile spermatozoa with bound particles, %)	<50	

Table A3.6   WHO interpretation of semen analysis (2010)—cont'd

Parameter	Reference range[a]	Terminology relating to abnormal findings
Immunobead test (motile spermatozoa with bound beads, %)	<50	
Seminal zinc (μmol/ejaculate)	≥2.4	
Seminal fructose (μmol/ejaculate)	≥13	
Seminal neutral glucosidase (mU/ejaculate)	≥20	

[a] Men with semen parameters outside the reference range may still be fertile and equally men with semen parameters within normal range may be subfertile.[19]

Table A3.7 Interpretation of male factor hormone assessment (see Chapter 4)[19]

Parameter	FSH	LH	Testosterone	Prolactin
Normal spermatogenesis	Normal	Normal	Normal	Normal
Hypogonadotropic hypogonadism	Low	Low	Low	Normal
Abnormal spermatogenesis[a]	High/normal	Normal	Normal	Normal
Complete testicular failure/hypergonadotropic hypogonadism	High	High	Normal/low	Normal
Prolactin-secreting pituitary tumour	Normal/low	Normal/low	Low	High

Reprinted from Ref. 19, with permission from Elsevier.
[a] Elevated FSH always indicates abnormal spermatogenesis, but normal FSH levels may indicate abnormal spermatogenesis in some men.

Table A3.8 ASRM interpretation of post-ejaculatory urinalysis (see Chapter 4)[19]

Men with	Findings and interpretation
Azoospermia (no sperm) or aspermia (no semen)	• Any sperm: confirmed retrograde ejaculation • No sperm: consider ejaculatory duct obstruction, hypogonadism, or CBAVD (exclude incomplete semen collection)
Low ejaculate volume and oligospermia (low sperm concentration)	• Significant numbers of sperm: confirm retrograde ejaculation (significant is not defined) • No sperm or small numbers of sperm: consider ejaculatory duct obstruction, hypogonadism, or CBAVD (exclude incomplete semen collection)

Table A3.9 ASRM interpretation of ultrasound examination of male factor subfertility (see Chapter 4)[19]

Type of ultrasound	Findings	Interpretation and comments

Transrectal (TRUS)	• Dilated seminal vesicles or
	• Dilated ejaculatory ducts and/or
	• Midline cystic prostatic structures
		• Indicates (but not in itself establishes) complete or partial ejaculatory duct obstruction:
		  ▪ Complete obstruction typically presents as low semen volume, acidic ejaculate with no sperm or fructose
		  ▪ Partial obstruction may present as low semen volume, oligoasthenospermia (low sperm concentration and low motility), and poor progressive motility
		  ▪ Can also indicate CBAVD (due to absent or atrophic seminal vesicles)

Scrotal ultrasound	• Varicoceles • Spermatoceles • Absent vasa • Epididymal induration • Testicular masses	Ultrasound results help to confirm findings of physical examination

Table A3.10 Interpretation of sperm DNA tests (see Chapter 4)

Type of test	Findings	Interpretation and comments
SCSA	≥27% DNA damage[20]	Unlikely to result in pregnancy
TUNEL	>36.5% DNA damage[21]	Significantly lower pregnancy rates
COMET	>50% DNA damage[22]	Significantly lower live-birth rates
	25–50% DNA damage[22]	Reduced live-birth rates

Table A3.11 Vitamin D reference ranges[23,24]

Serum 25-OHD concentrations	Status
<25 nmol/L or <10 ng/mL	Severely deficient
25–50 nmol/L or 10–20 ng/mL	Deficient
50–75 nmol/L or 20–30 ng/mL	Adequate[23] or insufficient[24]
>75 nmol/L or >30 ng/mL	Optimal

Table A3.12 Thyroid test reference ranges (see Chapter 8)

Hormones	Normal reference ranges[a]	Notes
Thyroid Stimulating Hormone (TSH)	0.4–4.5 mU/L[25]	New emerging consensus 0.4–2.5 mIU/L[26]
		The American Thyroid Association guidelines recommend that women with a history of infertility or miscarriages should have a TSH <2.5 mU/L[27]
Free thyroxine (FT4)	9.0–25 picomol/L[25]	
Total thyroxine (TT4)	60–160 nanomol/L[25]	
Free triiodothyronine (FT3)	3.5–7.8 picomol/L[25]	
Total triiodothyronine (TT3)	1.2–2.6 nanomol/L[25]	
Thyroid peroxidase antibody (TPOAb)	0–35 IU/mL[28,29]	
Thyroglobulin antibody (TgAb)	0–40 IU/mL[28,29]	

[a] For exact values check laboratory report because reference ranges vary between different laboratories.

Table A3.13 NK cell assay reference values (see Chapter 12)[30]

Dilutions	Reference range (%)	Notes
50:1	10–40	Levels >15% are damaging to the embryo
25:1	5–20	
12:1	2.5–10	

Table A3.14 Immunophenotype reference ranges (see Chapter 12)[30]

Cells	Reference range	Notes
CD3	63–86%	Elevated levels are associated with autoimmune disease such as thyroiditis, systemic lupus erythematosus (SLE), and rheumatoid arthritis
CD4	31–53%	Very low values are associated with severe immunodeficiency, for example in patients with AIDS
CD8	17–35%	Low levels can lead to up-regulation of Th1 lymphocytes
CD19	3–8%	Levels of >12% may lead to infertility or recurrent pregnancy loss
CD56+/CD16+	3–12%	Elevated levels can lead to infertility and recurrent miscarriages
CD56+	3–12%	Levels of >18% may be predictive of a poor reproductive outcome
CD3/IL-2R+	0–5%	Women with autoimmune disease may have elevated levels
CD19+/5+	2–10% of B Cells	Women with raised levels may not respond well to ovarian stimulation and also suffer embryonic damage or loss

---

Table A3.15 Th1:Th2 ratio reference ranges (see Chapter 12)[30]

Reference range and explanation

Th1 (TNF-α) levels >30 are associated with miscarriages and subfertility

---

Table A3.16 Leukocyte Antibody Detection (LAD) test reference ranges (see Chapter 12)

Reference range and explanation

Levels of IgG T cells or IgG B cells <30% are associated with increased risk of implantation failure and pregnancy loss[31,32]

REFERENCES

1. National Collaborating Centre for Women's and Children's Health, Commissioned by the National Institute for Health and Clinical Excellence. Guideline summary. In: Fertility: assessment and treatment for people with fertility problems. NICE clinical guideline. 2nd ed. London: The Royal College of Obstetricians and Gynaecologists; 2013. p. 1–46 [chapter 1].

2. Practice Committee of American Society for Reproductive Medicine. Diagnostic evaluation of the infertile female: a committee opinion. Fertil Steril 2012;98:302–7.

3. Jordan J, Craig K, Clifton DK, et al. Luteal phase defect: the sensitivity and specificity of diagnostic methods in common clinical use. Fertil Steril 1994;62:54–62.

4. Beltran L, Fahie-Wilson MN, McKenna TJ, et al. Serum total prolactin and monomeric prolactin reference intervals determined by precipitation with polyethylene glycol: evaluation and validation on common immunoassay platforms. Clin Chem 2008;54:1673–81.

5. Collins JA. Evidence-based infertility: evaluation of the female partner. Int Congr Ser 2004; 1266:57–62.

6. Prolactin: MedlinePlus medical encyclopedia. Available from: http://www.nlm.nih.gov/medlineplus/ency/article/003718.htm [accessed 19 April 2013].

7. ASRM. Medication for inducing ovulation. A guide for patients. Report of the ASRM, ASRM, Birmingham, AL; 2012.

8. Montoya JM, Bernal A, Borrero C. Diagnostics in assisted human reproduction. Reprod Biomed Online 2002;5:198–210.

9. Practice Committee of the American Society for Reproductive Medicine. Testing and interpreting measures of ovarian reserve: a committee opinion. Fertil Steril 2012;98:1407–15.

10. Stricker R, Eberhart R, Chevailler MC, et al. Establishment of detailed reference values for luteinizing hormone, follicle stimulating hormone, estradiol, and progesterone during different phases of the menstrual cycle on the Abbott ARCHITECT analyzer. Clin Chem Lab Med 2006;44:883–7.

11. Cahill DJ, Wardle PG. Management of infertility. BMJ 2002;325:28–32.

12. Homburg R, Ray A, Bhide P, et al. The relationship of serum anti-Mullerian hormone with polycystic ovarian morphology and polycystic ovary syndrome: a prospective cohort study. Hum Reprod 2013;28:1077–83.

13. Seifer DB, Baker VL, Leader B. Age-specific serum anti-Müllerian hormone values for 17,120 women presenting to fertility centers within the United States. Fertil Steril 2011;95:747–50.

14. Lee JY, Jee BC, Lee JR, et al. Age-related distributions of anti-Müllerian hormone level and anti-müllerian hormone models. Acta Obstet Gynecol Scand 2012;91:970–5.

15. National Collaborating Centre for Women's and Children's Health, Commissioned by the National Institute for Health and Clinical Excellence. Investigation of fertility problems and management strategies. In: Fertility: assessment and treatment for people with fertility problems. NICE clinical guideline. 2nd ed. London: The Royal College of Obstetricians and Gynaecologists; 2013. p. 80–132 [chapter 6].

16. The Rotterdam ESHRE/ASRM-sponsored PCOS consensus workshop group. Revised 2003 consensus on diagnostic criteria and long-term health risks related to polycystic ovary syndrome (PCOS). Hum Reprod 2004;19:41–7.

17. Miyakis S, Lockshin MD, Atsumi T, et al. International consensus statement on an update of the classification criteria for definite antiphospholipid syndrome (APS). J Thromb Haemost 2006;4: 295–306.

18. WHO. Reference values and semen nomenclature. In: Cooper TG, editor-in-chief. WHO laboratory manual for the examination and processing of human semen. 5th ed. Geneva:

World Health Organization; 2010. p. 223–6 [Appendix 1].

19. Practice Committee of American Society for Reproductive Medicine. Diagnostic evaluation of the infertile male: a committee opinion. Fertil Steril 2012;98(2):294–301.

20. Larson-Cook KL, Brannian JD, Hansen KA, et al. Relationship between the outcomes of assisted reproductive techniques and sperm DNA fragmentation as measured by the sperm chromatin structure assay. Fertil Steril 2003;80:895–902.

21. Henkel R, Hajimohammad M, Stalf T, et al. Influence of deoxyribonucleic acid damage on fertilization and pregnancy. Fertil Steril 2004;81:965–72.

22. Simon L, Proutski I, Stevenson M, et al. Sperm DNA damage has a negative association with live-birth rates after IVF. Reprod Biomed Online 2013;26:68–78.

23. Pearce H, Cheetham D. Diagnosis and management of vitamin D deficiency. BMJ 2010;340:142–7.

24. Holick MF, Binkley NC, Bischoff-Ferrari HA, et al. Evaluation, treatment, and prevention of vitamin D deficiency:

an Endocrine Society clinical practice guideline. J Clin Endocrinol Metab 2011;96:1911–30.

25. The Association for Clinical Biochemistry (ACB), The British Thyroid Association (BTA) and The British Thyroid Foundation (BTF). UK guidelines for the use of thyroid function tests. Report of the The Association for Clinical Biochemistry (ACB), The British Thyroid Association (BTA) and The British Thyroid Foundation (BTF), British Thyroid Association, London; 2006.

26. The Practice Committee of the American Society for Reproductive Medicine. Evaluation and treatment of recurrent pregnancy loss: a committee opinion. Fertil Steril 2012;98:1103–11.

27. De Groot L, Abalovich M, Alexander EK, et al. Management of thyroid dysfunction during pregnancy and postpartum: an Endocrine Society clinical practice guideline. J Clin Endocrinol Metab 2012;97:2543–65.

28. Reh A, Chaudhry S, Mendelsohn F, et al. Effect of autoimmune thyroid disease in older euthyroid infertile woman during the first 35 days of an

IVF cycle. Fertil Steril 2011;95:1178–81.

29. Revelli A, Casano S, Piane LD, et al. A retrospective study on IVF outcome in euthyroid patients with anti-thyroid antibodies: effects of levothyroxine, acetyl-salicylic acid and prednisolone adjuvant treatments. Reprod Biol Endocrinol 2009;7:137.

30. Beer AE, Kantecki J, Reed J. Comprehensive immune testing. In: Is your body baby-friendly: "unexplained" infertility, miscarriage and IVF failure explained. Houston, TX: AJR Pub.; 2006. p. 127–40.

31. Leukocyte antibody detection (LAD) test. Available from: http://www.repro-med.net/repro-med-site2/index.php?option=com_content&view=article&id=75%3Aleukocyte-antibody-detection-lad-test&catid=12%3Atests-and-testaments&Itemid=12 [accessed 26 July 2013].

32. Beer AE, Kantecki J, Reed J. Dr. beer's treatments. In: Is your body baby-friendly: "unexplained" infertility, miscarriage and IVF failure explained. Houston, TX: AJR Pub.; 2006. p. 141–57.

393

Appendix | IV |

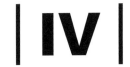

Fertility factsheets

OPTIMIZING FEMALE FERTILITY

Patient's factsheet

Weight

Ideally, aim to keep your weight between a BMI of 19 and 24 kg/m^2 because a BMI outside these limits has been linked to subfertility, poor IVF outcomes, and miscarriages.

If you need to lose weight, regular exercise (minimum 30 min of moderately intense exercise at least three times a week) and low calorie diet (1000–1200 kcal/day) is recommended. However, losing weight while undergoing reproductive treatment is not recommended.

Smoking

Smoking or inhalation of second-hand smoke is detrimental to fertility, it increases the risk of ectopic pregnancies and miscarriages, it reduces IVF success rates, it affects the menstrual cycle, and it reduces the reproductive lifespan by 1–4 years. Smoking is also linked to birth defects in the children of parents who smoke. Therefore, it is essential that you give up smoking and avoid exposure to second-hand smoke. Speak to your acupuncturist and/or family doctor if you need help with smoking cessation.

Alcohol

The research evidence on the effects of moderate alcohol intake and subfertility is at present mixed. Some studies suggest a detrimental effect with just one unit of alcohol a week, other studies have found a detrimental link with intakes of 7–14 units, and some have found no detrimental association. One large study found that women who consumed half to two units of alcohol a week conceived a little sooner compared with women who drank no alcohol. Therefore, it is probably not detrimental to have the occasional glass of wine. However, avoid binge drinking. Avoid alcohol completely in pregnancy. Speak to your acupuncturist and/or family doctor if you need help with reducing your alcohol intake.

Caffeine

Drinking caffeinated drinks (for example, coffee, tea, cola drinks) may reduce fertility and may also be linked to miscarriages. In the United Kingdom, the National Institute of Clinical Excellence guidelines recommend that women who are trying to conceive should ideally avoid all caffeinated drinks. In the United States, the American Society for Reproductive Medicine advises that the equivalent of 1–2 cups of caffeinated beverages are not detrimental to fertility or pregnancy.

Recreational drugs

The use of recreational drugs is strongly linked to subfertility. If using drugs, speak to your family doctor or your acupuncturist who may be able to advise you on how to give up. The information will be treated in a highly confidential manner.

Prescription or over-the-counter medication

Prescription or over-the-counter medication may affect your chances of conception and cause miscarriages or birth defects. Always check with your doctor or pharmacist if your medication is safe to take when trying to conceive or during pregnancy. Non-aspirin nonsteroidal anti-inflammatory medication such as diclofenac, naproxen, celecoxib, ibuprofen, or rofecoxib has been linked to increased risk of miscarriages, even in small dosages. Therefore, avoid taking this medication. **Never discontinue taking your medication without first checking with the doctor who prescribed it for you.**

Environmental toxins

Exposure to environmental toxins may affect reproductive health, although more research is needed to know exactly what types of chemicals are detrimental. In the meantime, minimize your exposure to as many toxins as possible. For example:

- Delay house decoration and renovations until after reproductive treatment is completed.
- Minimize the use of plastic containers, plastic food wrapping, and canned foods.
- Ideally, organic food should be eaten and fruits and vegetables thoroughly washed to reduce exposure to pesticides.
- Whenever possible, natural cosmetics and cleaning products should be used.
- When preparing fish, trimming the fat, removing or puncturing the skin, and not frying it may help to reduce exposure to chemicals and metals.
- Reduce exposure to chemicals at work. Consider changing your job if exposure is unavoidable.

Nutrition

A Mediterranean-type diet (with a high intake of vegetable oil, vegetables, fish, and legumes) has been shown to reduce the risk of subfertility and improve conception rates following IVF. Consuming a high-carbohydrate diet increases the risk of subfertility because it interferes with ovulation. Eating full-fat dairy products helps to reduce the risk of not ovulating. Seek specialist nutrition advice if you feel you need help with your nutrition. Your acupuncturist may also suggest other foods beneficial in your case, based on your acupuncture diagnosis.

Supplements

Advice in this section is provided for general information only. **Always seek specialist advice from a nutritionist regarding specific micronutrients.**

The following micronutrients are important for optimal reproductive health:

- Folic acid: take 0.4 mg/day for 3 months before conception and up to 3 months post conception. A higher dose of 5 mg/day is recommended for women who have previously had a baby with a neural tube defect, women who take anti-epileptic medication, and

diabetic women. Women with hyperhomocysteinaemia (elevated homocysteine) should also take a higher dose of folic acid together with vitamins B6 and B12. Good sources of folic acid include dark green leafy vegetables, fruits, nuts, beans, peas, dairy, poultry, eggs, seafood, and grains. The best sources of vitamin B12 are beef liver and clams, fish, meat, poultry, and dairy.

- Vitamin D: women who are pregnant or lactating should take a minimum of 600 IU (15 µg) of vitamin D per day, but may require an even higher dose of 1500–2000 IU (37.5–50 µg) per day. Do not take more than 4000 IU (100 µg) without medical supervision. Spend as much time in the sun as possible because sunlight helps the body to make vitamin D. Food sources of vitamin D include fish-liver oil, oily fish, egg yolks, and mushrooms.
- Iodine: it is recommended that all women who are trying to conceive should take 250 µg of iodine supplement in addition to eating foods rich in iodine (cow's milk, yoghurt, eggs, cheese, white fish, oily fish, shellfish, meat, poultry). Ideally, iodine should be taken a few hours apart from iron supplements. **If you have a diagnosed thyroid disease or take thyroid medication, you must check with your doctor regarding iodine supplementation.**
- Vitamin A: too much vitamin A may be harmful in pregnancy. Avoid taking supplements high in vitamin A or foods rich in vitamin A (e.g., crustaceans and liver) from ovulation (egg retrieval) to the beginning of your next menstrual cycle and throughout pregnancy.
- Vitamin E: doses 400–500 IU/day have been shown to improve the endometrial lining. Foods naturally rich in vitamin E include nuts, seeds, and vegetable oils.
- Omega-3: DHA and EPA are two types of omega-3 that have been shown to have a beneficial effect on reproductive health. Ensure that you consume at least 200–300 mg of DHA plus EPA per day. The best source of omega-3 is oily fish (salmon, sardines, herring, catfish, halibut, canned tuna). Avoid fish high in mercury (tilefish, shark, swordfish, king mackerel, fresh or frozen tuna steaks (not canned), orange roughy, marlin, Spanish mackerel). Alternatively, purified fish oil supplements with sufficiently high EPA and DHA levels can be taken. Avoid supplements made of cod livers because they are high in vitamin A. If you follow a vegan diet, you can take algal oil supplements. Fish feed on algae, which is what makes fish a rich source of omega-3. **Omega-3 can thin your blood. If you take blood thinning medication (for example, low molecular weight heparin (Clexane) or aspirin), speak to your doctor or nutritionist before increasing your omega-3 intake.**
- Selenium: if you have a history of recurrent miscarriages, selenium supplements may help to

reduce the risk of further pregnancy loss, especially if you have high thyroid antibody levels. Speak to a nutritionist to see if you are deficient in selenium.

- Iron: women of reproductive age are at high risk of iron deficiency anaemia. Ensure that you eat iron-rich foods (good-quality organic lean red meat, canned oysters, turkey, lentils, kidney beans) and take an iron supplement.

Exercise

If you are overweight (BMI ≥ 25 kg/m^2), intensive exercise is likely to significantly improve your fertility. If your BMI is normal (<25 kg/m^2 but ≥ 19 kg/m^2), moderate exercise is adequate. If you are underweight (BMI <19 kg/m^2), ensure you do not over-exercise because this may lead to subfertility.

Stress

If possible, reduce your stress levels. Engage in stress-reducing activities such as hobbies, positive visualization, meditation, and exercise. If you find it difficult to manage your stress levels, speak to your acupuncturist, who may be able to help.

Sexual intercourse

If you and your partner have not been diagnosed with complete sterility (for example, absence of fallopian tubes or an early onset menopause, very poor sperm parameters), you should carry on trying to conceive naturally.

Daily or every other day intercourse is most likely to result in conception. Timing intercourse to the fertile window is necessary. The most reliable methods of ovulation detection are fertile mucus days or E3G-based ovulation detection kits. Speak to your acupuncturist for more advice on this. Intercourse should be fun with emphasis on foreplay, visual stimulation, and high and prolonged arousal.

OPTIMIZING MALE FERTILITY

Patient's factsheet

Weight

Ideally, aim to keep your weight between a BMI of 19 and 24 kg/m^2 because a BMI outside these limits has been linked to subfertility, poor IVF outcomes, and miscarriages.

If you need to lose weight, regular exercise (minimum 30 min of moderately intense exercise at least three times a week) and a low calorie diet (1000–1200 kcal/day) is recommended. However, losing weight while undergoing reproductive treatment is not recommended.

Smoking

Semen parameters in smokers are poorer. Smoking reduces the fertilization rate when undergoing IVF or ICSI treatment. Smoking is also linked to birth defects in the children of parents who smoke. Therefore, it is essential that you give up smoking and avoid exposure to second-hand smoke. Speak to your acupuncturist and/or your family doctor if you need help with smoking cessation.

Alcohol

The research evidence on the effects of moderate alcohol intake and subfertility is at present mixed. There is no strong evidence to suggest that low to moderate alcohol intake (40–80 g or 4–8 units/week) in a man harms his fertility. Excessive alcohol intake (≥ 20 units/week) by a man has been shown to significantly increase how long it takes to conceive. Therefore, limit your alcohol intake and avoid binge drinking. Speak to your acupuncturist and/or your family doctor if you need help with reducing your alcohol intake.

Caffeine

There is no strong evidence that moderate caffeine intake reduces fertility in men. However, you may choose to limit your caffeine intake for general health reasons or as a way of supporting your female partner, who may be asked to stop drinking all caffeinated drinks.

Recreational drugs

The use of recreational drugs is strongly linked to subfertility. If using drugs, speak to your family doctor and/or your acupuncturist who will advise you on how to give up. The information will be treated in a highly confidential manner.

Prescription or over-the-counter medication

Prescription or over-the-counter medication may negatively affect your sperm production and ejaculation, cause erectile difficulties, produce changes in hormone levels, and affect libido. Always check with your doctor or pharmacist if your medication is safe to take when trying to conceive. **Never discontinue taking your medication without first checking with the doctor who prescribed it for you.**

Environmental toxins

Exposure to environmental toxins may affect reproductive health, although more research is needed to know exactly what types of chemicals should be avoided. In the meantime, minimize your exposure to as many toxins as possible. For example:

- Delay house decoration and renovations until after reproductive treatment is finished.
- Minimize the use of plastic containers, plastic food wrapping, and canned foods.
- Ideally, organic food should be eaten and fruits and vegetables thoroughly washed to reduce exposure to pesticides.
- Whenever possible, use only natural cleaning products.
- When preparing fish, trimming the fat, removing or puncturing the skin, and not frying it may help to reduce exposure to chemicals and metals.
- Reduce exposure to chemicals or heat when at work. Consider changing your job if exposure is unavoidable.

Heat in the scrotal area may be damaging to sperm. Therefore, avoid situations that would cause an increase in scrotal temperature (for example, sauna use, sitting down for prolonged periods of time, hot baths, use of electric blankets or heated car seats, use of a laptop on your lap).

Nutrition

To improve your fertility:

- Eat a diet rich in vegetables, fruits, grains, poultry, and seafood.
- Reduce processed meats, reduce high sugar foods, and avoid a high amount of carbohydrate foods.
- Replace full-fat dairy with low-fat dairy.

Seek specialist nutritionist advice if you feel you need help with your nutrition. Your acupuncturist may also suggest other foods beneficial in your case, based on your acupuncture diagnosis.

Supplements

Advice in this section is provided for general information only. **Always seek specialist advice from a nutritionist regarding specific micronutrients.**

The following micronutrients are important for optimal reproductive health:

- Vitamin D: take a minimum of 600 IU (15 µg) vitamin D per day, but you may require an even higher dose 1500–2000 IU (37.5–50 µg) per day if you are deficient in vitamin D. Do not take more than 4000 IU (100 µg) without medical supervision. Spend as much time in the sun as possible because sunlight helps the body to make vitamin D. Food sources of vitamin D include fish-liver oil, oily fish, egg yolks, mushrooms, and liver.
- Omega-3: DHA and EPA are two types of omega-3 that have been shown to have beneficial effect on reproductive health. Ensure you consume at least 200–300 mg of DHA plus EPA per day. The best source of omega-3 is oily fish (salmon, sardines, herring, catfish, halibut, canned tuna). Avoid fish high in mercury (tilefish, shark, swordfish, king mackerel, fresh or frozen tuna steaks (not canned), orange roughy,

marlin, Spanish mackerel). Alternatively, purified fish oil supplement with sufficiently high EPA and DHA levels can be taken. If you follow a vegan diet, you can take algal oil supplements. Fish feed on algae, which is what makes fish a rich source of omega-3. **Omega-3 can thin your blood. If you take blood-thinning medication (for example, low molecular weight heparin (Clexane) or aspirin), speak to your doctor or nutritionist before increasing your omega-3 intake.**

- Zinc: is important for testosterone and sperm production and sperm motility. In one study, taking 200 mg zinc twice daily improved sperm motility and reduced sperm DNA damage. Food sources of zinc are oysters (the richest source of zinc), red meat, poultry, seafood (crab, lobster).
- Vitamin B12: dosages between 1000 and up to 6000 µg/day taken for 2–3 months have been shown to improve sperm count. The best sources of vitamin B12 are beef liver and clams, fish, meat, poultry, and dairy.
- Antioxidants: help to repair sperm DNA damage. More research needs to be done to establish exactly which antioxidants and at what dosages are beneficial. However, there is some evidence that vitamin C and E are important. In one study it was found that taking 1 g vitamin C and 1 g vitamin E daily for 2 months significantly reduced sperm DNA damage. Selenium is another important antioxidant. Foods naturally rich in vitamin E include nuts, seeds, and vegetable oils. Vitamin C-rich foods are citrus fruits, red and green peppers, kiwifruit, broccoli, strawberries, cantaloupe, baked potatoes, and tomatoes.

Exercise

Exercise is important for general health and fertility. In one study it was found that men who exercised for ≥15 h a week had 73% higher sperm concentrations compared to men who exercised <5 h a week. However, bicycling ≥5 h/week is associated with low sperm concentrations and therefore must be avoided.

Stress

If possible, keep your stress levels down. Engage in stress-reducing activities such as hobbies, positive visualization, meditation, and exercise. If you find it difficult to manage your stress levels, speak to your acupuncturist, who may be able to help.

Sexual intercourse

If you and your partner have not been diagnosed with complete sterility (for example, absence of fallopian tubes or an early onset menopause in your partner, or if you have very poor sperm parameters), you should carry on trying to conceive naturally.

Daily or every other day intercourse is most likely to result in conception. Timing intercourse to the fertile window is necessary. Your female partner may need to use ovulation detection methods such as tracking fertile mucus days or using E3G-based ovulation detection kits. Speak to your acupuncturist for more advice on this. Intercourse should be fun with emphasis on foreplay, visual stimulation, and high and prolonged arousal. Ensure that you ejaculate regularly (that is, have an ejaculation every 2–5 days) outside of the fertile window because this has been shown to improve sperm, especially in men with suboptimal sperm parameters.

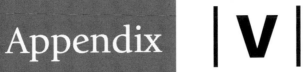

Appendix | V |

Commonly used medications in ART

Table A5.1 Commonly used medications in ART

Uses	Class	Active ingredient	Description	Trade names	Dose	Route	Common side effects
Ovarian suppression; Prevention of premature ovulation	Gonadorelin analogues (GnRH agonist)	Buserelin	Man-made gonadorelin, acts on LHRH receptors initially causing increase in FSH and LH, but after 10 days desensitizes the pituitary gland and leads to reduction in FSH and LH production, which inhibits androgen and oestrogen production	Suprefact	200–500 µg daily injection from cycle day 21 of suppression phase or cycle day 1 of stimulation phase until hCG administration	SC	Menopausal symptoms, such as hot flushes, increased sweating, vaginal dryness, dyspareunia, loss of libido, headaches
		Nafarelin		Synarel	200 µg/spray in each nostril daily from cycle day 21 of suppression phase or cycle day 2 of stimulation phase until hCG administration	Nasal spray	
	GnRH antagonist	Cetrorelix	Stops LH production by blocking LHRH action	Cetrotide	250 µg from cycle day 5 of stimulation phase until hCG administration	SC	Nausea, headaches
		Ganirelix		Orgalutran		SC	
Ovulation induction; Ovarian stimulation	Pulsed LHRH/GnRH	Gonadorelin acetate	Synthetic gonadotropin-releasing hormone (GnRH), which stimulates the production and release of LH and to lesser degree FSH	Factrel	5 µg every 90 min. If ineffective, can be increased incrementally up to 20 µg per 90 min pulse interval	IV	Rarely nausea, headaches, abdominal pain, increased menstrual bleeding
				Lutrepulse			
	Anti-oestrogen	Clomiphene citrate	Blocks oestrogen receptors in the hypothalamus, thus allowing for continued FSH/LH production and follicular development	Clomid	50–150 mg/day, days 1–5 of menstrual cycle	T	Hot flushes, abdominal discomfort
				Clomifene (generic)			
				Serophene			
	Gonadotrophin (Human Menopausal Gonadotrophin hMG)	Menotrophin FSH/LH	Purified extract of human post-menopausal urine containing FSH and LH (ratio 1:1) used to stimulate follicular development	Menopur	*Ovulation induction:* 150–450 IU/day for ~12 days *ART:* 150–450 IU/day for ~12 days	IM/SC	Gastrointestinal disturbances, headache, joint pain, fever
				Merional		IM/SC	
				Repronex		IM/SC	
		Urofollitropin FSH	Purified extract of human post-menopausal urine containing FSH used to stimulate follicular development	Bravelle		IM/SC	
				Fertinorm HP		IM/SC	
				Fostimon		IM/SC	
	Gonadotrophin (Recombinant LH)	Lutropin alfa	Recombinant (man-made) LH used with recombinant human FSH to stimulate follicular development	Luveris	*Ovulation induction:* 75–300 IU/day for up to 30 days *ART:* 150–450 IU/day for ~10 days	SC	Nausea, vomiting, abdominal and pelvic pain, headaches, somnolence
	Gonadotrophin (Recombinant FSH)	Follitropin alfa	Recombinant (man-made) FSH used to stimulate follicular development	Gonal-F		IM/SC	Gastrointestinal disturbances, headache, joint pain, fever

Indication	Drug class	Generic name	Description	Brand	Dose	Route	Side effects
Oocyte maturation	Chorionic gonadotrophin	Chorionic gonadotrophin	Urinary hCG obtained from the urine of pregnant women used in oocyte maturation	Pregnyl	5000–10,000 IU injection day after last dose of gonadotrophin	IM/SC	Oedema, headache, tiredness, mood changes, gynaecomastia
		Choriogonadotrophin alfa	Recombinant (man-made) hCG used in oocyte maturation	Ovitrelle	250 µg injection day after last dose of gonadotrophin	SC	Nausea, vomiting, abdominal pain, headache, tiredness
Luteal/endometrial support	Progestogen	Progesterone	Used for luteal phase and early pregnancy support	Crinone	90 mg (8% gel)/day from ovulation/egg retrieval for up to 12 weeks of pregnancy or discontinue on negative pregnancy test	VG	Menstrual disturbance, PMT (bloating, fluid retention, breast tenderness), weight change, nausea, headache, dizziness, insomnia, drowsiness, depression, change in libido. Pain, diarrhoea and flatulence (with rectal administration)
				Cyclogest	200 mg daily to 400 mg twice daily from ovulation/egg retrieval for up to 10 weeks of pregnancy or discontinue on negative pregnancy test	PE	
				Gestone	25–200 mg daily from embryo transfer for up to 8–16 weeks of pregnancy or discontinue on negative pregnancy test	IM	
Endometrial lining growth	Oestradiol	Estradiol valerate	Oestrogen used to promote endometrial lining growth	Progynova	2–8 mg/day from cycle day 1 for up to 12 weeks of pregnancy or discontinue on negative pregnancy test	T/P	Nausea, vomiting, abdominal cramps and bloating, weight changes, breast enlargement and tenderness, PMT, changes in libido, depression, mood changes, headache, migraine, dizziness, leg cramps, vaginal candidiasis, eye dryness
WHO grade II ovulatory disorders	Insulin sensitizer	Metformin hydrochloride	Used in PCO/PCOS patients to lower insulin levels, which leads to lower androgen levels and makes ovaries more responsive to own FSH	Metformin (generic)	500–2000 mg split into 2–3 doses/day	T	Anorexia, nausea, vomiting, diarrhoea, abdominal pain, taste disturbance
Ovulation induction (in patients with high prolactin levels)	Dopamine agonists	Bromocriptine	Reduces the amount of prolactin released by the pituitary	Parlodel	1.25 mg/evening for min 7–14 days. Dose can be increased by 1.25 every 2 weeks if no effect. Discontinued on positive pregnancy test	T	Nausea, constipation, headaches, hypotension, drowsiness, dyskinesia, pathological gambling, increased libido,
		Cabergoline		Dostinex	1–2 mg/week until pregnant	T	hypersexuality, leg cramps, alopecia, peripheral oedema

Continued

Table A5.1 Commonly used medications in ART—cont'd

Uses	Class	Active ingredient	Description	Trade names	Dose	Route	Common side effects
Blood thinners	Antiplatelet	Acetylsalicylic acid	Decreases platelet aggregation and inhibits thrombus formation	Aspirin	75–100 mg daily starting usually on day 5 of stimulated cycle. Stop for 1–2 days at egg retrieval. Continue until 12 weeks gestation, possibly longer. Discontinue on negative pregnancy test	T	Bronchospasm, gastrointestinal irritation, haemorrhage
	Parenteral anticoagulant – low molecular weight heparin	Enoxaparin sodium		Clexane / Lovenox	20–100 mg twice daily starting usually on day 5 of stimulated cycle. Stop for 1–2 days at egg retrieval. Continue until 12 weeks' gestation, possibly longer. Discontinue on negative pregnancy test	SC	Haemorrhage, thrombocytopenia, bruising

Sources: BNF.Org. Available from: http://bnf.org/bnf/index.htm [accessed 29 January 2012]. European medicines agency – find medicine. Available from: http://www.ema.europa.eu/ema/index.jsp?curl=/pages/medicines/landing/epar_search.jsp&mid=WC0b01ac058001d124 [accessed 29 January 2012]. Approved drugs. Available from: http://www.fda.gov/Drugs/InformationOnDrugs/ApprovedDrugs/default.htm [accessed 29 January 2012]. Drug, otcs & herbals l medscape reference. Available from: http://reference.medscape.com/drugs [accessed 29 January 2012].
Keys: IM, intramuscular injection; IV, intravenous injections; SC, subcutaneous injections; VG, vaginal gel; T, tablets; P, patches; PE, pessaries.

Appendix 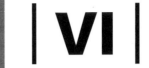 | VI |

Medications known to adversely affect fertility

Table A6.1

Drugs	Effect on male reproductive function	Effect on female reproductive function
Antibiotics Penicillin G, ampicillin, cephalotin, spiramycin, gentamicin, neomycin, nitrofurantoin, cotrimoxazole	Reversible impairment of spermatogenesis	
Dicloxacillin, tylosin, lincomycin, tetracycline, erythromycin, quinolones, neomycin, nitrofurantoin, cotrimoxazole	Reversible impairment of sperm motility	
Antimalarials: quinine and its derivatives	Reversible impairment of sperm motility	
Antischistosomal: niridazole	Reversible impairment of spermatogenesis and sperm motility	
Antimetabolites/antimitotics: colchicines, cyclophosphamide	Irreversible arrest of spermatogenesis and azoospermia	
Non-steroidal anti-inflammatory drugs, Cox-2 inhibitors		Reversible impairment of follicle rupture and ovulation, impairment of tubal function
Anti-inflammatory 5-ASA and derivatives: mesalazine, sulphasalazine	Reversible impairment of spermatogenesis and sperm motility	
Corticosteroids	Reversible impairment of sperm concentration and motility	
Antiandrogens: cyproterone acetate, danazol, finasteride, ketoconazole, spironolactone	Reversible impairment of spermatogenesis and erectile dysfunction	
Exogenous testosterone, GnRH analogues	Reversible impairment of spermatogenesis	

Continued

Table A6.1 —cont'd

Drugs	Effect on male reproductive function	Effect on female reproductive function
Anabolic steroids	Reversible impairment of spermatogenesis (up to 1 year recovery), may induce hypogonadism by affecting pituitary–gonadal axis	
Anti-oestrogens, e.g., clomiphene citrate		Reversible impairment of endometrial development
Anti-progestins, emergency contraceptive pills, progesterone-only pills		Impairment of implantation and tubal function
Local anaesthetics, halothane	Impair sperm motility	
Antiepileptics: phenytoin	Reversible impairment of sperm motility	
Antipsychotics Phenothiazine, antidepressants (particularly SSRIs), α blockers Butyrophenones	Raise prolactin concentrations and lead to sexual dysfunction Reversible impairment of spermatogenesis and sperm motility	Raise prolactin concentrations and lead to sexual dysfunction
Antihypertensives Calcium channel blockers (nifedipine) Beta blockers, α blockers (prazosin), α agonists (clonidine), thiazide diuretics, hydralazine, methyldopa	Fertilization failure Erectile dysfunction	Fertilization failure
H2 blockers: cimetidine, ranitidine	Raise prolactin concentrations and lead to loss of libido and erectile dysfunction	Raise prolactin concentrations and lead to impairment of luteal function and loss of libido
Metoclopramide	Erectile dysfunction	
Methadone	Depress spermatogenesis and sperm motility	

Reproduced with permission from Anderson K, Nisenblat V, Norman R. Lifestyle factors in people seeking infertility treatment – a review. Aust N Z J Obstet Gynaecol 2010;50(1):8–20. doi:10.1111/j.1479-828X.2009.01119.x.

Glossary of Orthodox medical terms

AH See Assisted Hatching

Aneuploidy The loss or gain of one or more chromosomes

ART See assisted reproductive technology

Assisted hatching (AH) An *in vitro* procedure in which the zona pellucida of an embryo is either thinned or perforated by chemical, mechanical, or laser methods to assist separation of the blastocyst

Assisted Reproductive Technology (ART) All treatments or procedures that include the *in vitro* handling of both human oocytes and sperm, or embryos, for the purpose of establishing a pregnancy. This includes, but is not limited to, *in vitro* fertilization and embryo transfer, gamete intra-fallopian transfer, zygote intra-fallopian transfer, tubal embryo transfer, gamete and embryo cryopreservation, oocyte and embryo donation, and gestational surrogacy

Biochemical pregnancy (preclinical spontaneous abortion/ miscarriage) A pregnancy diagnosed only by the detection of hCG in serum or urine and that does not develop into a clinical pregnancy

Blastocyst An embryo, 5 or 6 days after fertilization, with an inner cell mass, outer layer of trophectoderm, and a fluid-filled blastocoele cavity

Cancelled cycle An ART cycle in which ovarian stimulation or monitoring has been carried out with the intention to treat, but did not proceed to follicular aspiration or, in the case of a thawed embryo, to embryo transfer

Capacitation Changes that happen to sperm inside the female reproductive tract that allow the sperm to become capable of fertilizing the egg

Clinical pregnancy A pregnancy diagnosed by ultrasonographic visualization of one or more gestational sacs or definitive clinical signs of pregnancy. It includes ectopic pregnancy. *Note*: Multiple gestational sacs are counted as one clinical pregnancy

Clinical pregnancy rate The number of clinical pregnancies expressed per 100 initiated cycles, aspiration cycles or embryo transfer cycles. *Note*: When clinical pregnancy rates are given, the denominator (initiated, aspirated, or embryo transfer cycles) must be specified

Clinical pregnancy with foetal heart beat Pregnancy diagnosed by ultrasonographic or clinical documentation of at least one foetus with a heart beat. It includes ectopic pregnancy

Clone A copy of a (DNA) molecule, a (stem) cell or an individual. Cloning of an individual is done by replacing the nucleus of an egg cell with the genetic material from a somatic (non-germ) cell. Cloning can also be done to produce stem cells, the undifferentiated early cells from which all types of cells develop. This technique may in future enable people to access life-saving treatments tailor made from their own DNA

Congenital anomalies All structural, functional and genetic anomalies diagnosed in aborted foetuses, at birth or in the neonatal period

Controlled Ovarian Stimulation (COS) for ART Pharmacological treatment in which women are stimulated to induce the development of multiple ovarian follicles to obtain multiple oocytes at follicular aspiration

Controlled Ovarian Stimulation (COS) for non-ART cycles Pharmacological treatment for women in which the ovaries are stimulated to ovulate more than one oocyte

COS See Controlled Ovarian Stimulation (COS) for ART and Controlled Ovarian Stimulation (COS) for non-ART cycles

Cryopreservation Frozen storage of sperm, eggs, embryos, or ovarian and testicular tissues

Cumulative delivery rate with at least one live born baby The estimated number of deliveries with at least one live born baby resulting from one initiated or aspirated ART cycle including the cycle when fresh embryos are transferred and subsequent frozen/thawed ART cycles. This rate is used when less than the total number of embryos fresh and/or frozen/thawed have been utilized from one ART cycle. *Note*: The delivery of a singleton, twin, or other multiple pregnancy is registered as one delivery

Delivery The expulsion or extraction of one or more foetuses from the mother after 20 completed weeks of gestational age

Delivery rate The number of deliveries expressed per 100 initiated cycles, aspiration cycles, or embryo transfer cycles. When delivery rates are given, the denominator (initiated, aspirated, or embryo transfer cycles) must be specified. It includes deliveries that resulted in the birth of one or more live babies and/or stillborn babies. *Note*: The delivery of a singleton, twin, or other multiple pregnancy is registered as one delivery

Early neonatal death Death of a live born baby within 7 days of birth

Ectopic pregnancy Implantation of the embryo outside the uterus

Elective embryo transfer The transfer of one or more embryos, selected from a larger cohort of available embryos

Embryo The product up to 8 weeks after fertilization, later it is called a foetus

Embryo donation cycle Transfer of an embryo that did not originate from the recipient and her partner

Embryo/foetus reduction A procedure to reduce the number of viable embryos or foetuses in a multiple pregnancy

Embryo recipient cycle (See embryo donation cycle)

Embryo Transfer (ET) The procedure in which one or more embryos are placed in the uterus or fallopian tube

Embryo transfer cycle An ART cycle in which one or more embryos are transferred into the uterus or fallopian tube

Endometriosis Condition where endometrial tissue grows in areas other than the uterine cavity

ET See Embryo Transfer

ESHRE European Society of Human Reproduction and Embryology

Extremely low birth weight Birth weight less than 1000 g

Extremely preterm birth A live birth or stillbirth that takes place after at least 20 but less than 28 completed weeks of gestational age

FER See Frozen/thawed Embryo Transfer cycle

FET See Frozen/thawed Embryo Transfer cycle

Frozen Embryo Replacement (FER) See Frozen/thawed Embryo Transfer

Frozen/thawed Embryo Transfer (FET) cycle An ART procedure in which cycle monitoring is carried out with the intention of transferring a frozen/thawed embryo or frozen/thawed embryos. *Note*: An FET cycle is initiated when specific medication is provided or cycle monitoring is started with the intention to treat

Frozen/thawed oocyte cycle An ART procedure in which cycle monitoring is carried out with the intention of fertilizing thawed oocytes and performing embryo transfer

Fertilization A sperm penetrates the egg leading to a combination of genetic material resulting in a fertilized egg

Foetal death (stillbirth) Death prior to the complete expulsion or extraction from its mother of a product of fertilization, at or after 20 completed weeks of gestational age. The death is indicated by the fact that, after such separation, the foetus does not breathe or show any other evidence of life such as heart beat, umbilical cord pulsation, or definite movement of voluntary muscles

Foetus The product of fertilization from completion of embryonic development, at 8 completed weeks after fertilization, until abortion or birth

Follicle A fluid filled sac that contains an immature egg. Located in the ovaries, follicles develop each cycle, one ovulates into an egg

Full-term birth A live birth or stillbirth that takes place between 37 completed and 42 completed weeks of gestational age

Gamete A reproductive cell, egg in females and sperm in males

Gamete Intra-Fallopian Transfer (GIFT) An ART procedure in which both gametes (oocytes and spermatozoa) are transferred to the fallopian tubes

Gestational age Age of an embryo or foetus calculated by adding 2 weeks (14 days) to the number of completed weeks since fertilization. *Note*: For frozen/thawed embryo transfers, an estimated date of fertilization is computed by subtracting the embryo age at freezing from the transfer date of the FET cycle

Gestational carrier (surrogate) A woman who carries a pregnancy with an agreement that she will give the offspring to the intended parent(s). Gametes can originate from the intended parent(s) and/or a third party (or parties)

Gestational sac A fluid-filled structure associated with early pregnancy, which may be located inside or outside the uterus (in case of an ectopic pregnancy)

GIFT See Gamete Intra-Fallopian Transfer

Hatching The process by which an embryo at the blastocyst stage separates from the zona pellucida

High-order multiple A pregnancy or delivery with three or more foetuses or neonates

ICSI See Intra-Cytoplasmic Sperm Injection

Implantation The attachment and subsequent penetration by the zona-free blastocyst (usually in the endometrium) that starts 5–7 days after fertilization

Implantation rate The number of gestational sacs observed, divided by the number of embryos transferred

IMSI See Intra-Cytoplasmic Morphologically selected Sperm Injection

***In Vitro* Fertilization (IVF)** Fertilization of an egg by sperm in a laboratory dish

Induced abortion The termination of a clinical pregnancy, by deliberate interference that takes place before 20 completed weeks of gestational age (18 weeks' post fertilization) or, if gestational age is unknown, of an embryo/foetus of less than 400 g

Infertility A disease of the reproductive system defined by the failure to conceive after 12 months of regular unprotected sexual intercourse. Different reproductive health bodies may use a different definitions(s) for infertility

Initiated cycle An ART cycle in which the woman receives specific medication for ovarian stimulation, or monitoring in the case of natural cycles, with the intention to treat, irrespective of whether follicular aspiration is attempted

Intra-Cytoplasmic Morphologically Selected Sperm Injection (IMSI) Fertilization method in which spermatozoa are inspected and selected under ultra-magnification (6300×) and then injected into the egg

Intra-Cytoplasmic Sperm Injection (ICSI) Procedure in which an egg is fertilized by injecting a single sperm into the egg

Intra-Uterine Insemination (IUI) The insemination of washed semen directly into the uterus

IUI See Intra-Uterine Insemination

IVF See *In Vitro* Fertilization

Live birth The complete expulsion or extraction from its mother of a product of fertilization, irrespective of the duration of the pregnancy, which, after such separation, breathes or shows any other evidence of life such as heart beat, umbilical cord pulsation, or definite movement of voluntary muscles, irrespective of whether the umbilical cord has been cut or the placenta is attached

Live birth delivery rate The number of deliveries that resulted in at least one live born baby expressed per 100 initiated cycles, aspiration cycles or embryo transfer cycles. When delivery rates are given, the denominator (initiated, aspirated, or embryo transfer cycles) must be specified

Low birth weight Birth weight less than 2500 g

MESA See Micro-Epididymal Sperm Aspiration

MESE See Micro-Epididymal Sperm Extraction

Micro-Epididymal Sperm Aspiration (MESA) Surgical collection of sperm direct from the epididymis (tube that carries sperm out of the testis). Used when a blockage in the epididymis leads to absence of sperm in the semen

Mild ovarian stimulation for IVF A procedure in which the ovaries are stimulated with either gonadotropins and/or other

compounds, with the intent to limit the number of oocytes obtained for IVF to fewer than seven

Miscarriage/preclinical spontaneous abortion Pregnancy diagnosed by the detection of hCG in serum or urine that does not develop into a clinical pregnancy

Missed abortion/miscarriage A clinical abortion where the embryo(s) or foetus(es) is/are nonviable and is/are not expelled spontaneously from the uterus

Modified natural cycle An IVF procedure in which one or more oocytes are collected from the ovaries during a spontaneous menstrual cycle. Drugs are administered with the sole purpose of blocking the spontaneous LH surge and/or inducing final oocyte maturation

Motile Sperm Organelles Morphology Examination (MSOME) Is a method of sperm examination under high magnification (6000–8000×), which can detect morphological sperm abnormalities, which standard semen analysis could miss

MSOME See Motile Sperm Organelles Morphology Examination

Multiple gestation/birth A pregnancy/delivery with more than one foetus/neonate

Natural cycle IVF An IVF procedure in which one or more oocytes are collected from the ovaries during a spontaneous menstrual cycle without any drug use

Neonatal death Death of a live born baby within 28 days of birth

Neonatal period The time interval that commences at birth and ends 28 completed days after birth

OHSS See Ovarian Hyper Stimulation Syndrome

Oocyte donation cycle A cycle in which oocytes are collected from a donor for clinical application or research

Oocyte recipient cycle An ART cycle in which a woman receives oocytes from a donor

Ovarian Hyper Stimulation Syndrome (OHSS) An exaggerated

systemic response to ovarian stimulation characterized by a wide spectrum of clinical and laboratory manifestations. It is classified as mild, moderate, or severe according to the degree of abdominal distention, ovarian enlargement, and respiratory, haemodynamic, and metabolic complications

Ovarian torsion The partial or complete rotation of the ovarian vascular pedicle that causes obstruction to ovarian blood flow, potentially leading to necrosis of ovarian tissue

Ovulation Induction (OI) Pharmacological treatment of women with anovulation or oligo-ovulation with the intention of inducing normal ovulatory cycle

Percutaneous Epididymal Sperm Aspiration (PESA) Collection of sperm under local anaesthesia by needle aspiration of the epididymis

Perinatal mortality Foetal or neonatal death occurring during late pregnancy (at 20 completed weeks of gestational age and later), during childbirth and up to 7 completed days after birth

PESA See Percutaneous Epididymal Sperm Aspiration

PGD See Pre-implantation Genetic Diagnosis

PGS See Pre-implantation Genetic Screening

Polycystic Ovarian Syndrome (PCOS) A condition characterized by irregular or absent menstruation, acne, obesity, and excess hair growth

Post-term birth A live birth or stillbirth that takes place after 42 completed weeks of gestational age

Pre-implantation Genetic Diagnosis (PGD) Diagnostic technique involving genetic tests on an embryo or a polar body (a cell structure inside the egg). Usually done when the embryo is at the 6–8 cell stage. One cell is removed for analysis of its DNA or chromosomes to determine if the embryo is likely to develop a genetic disease

Pre-implantation Genetic Screening (PGS) Technique to check if an embryo has the correct number of chromosomes. Used particularly for older women (at increased risk of chromosomal abnormalities) and for women who have had recurrent miscarriages (often due to chromosomal abnormalities). It is still in the experimental phase, since it is not yet evidence based

Preterm birth A live birth or stillbirth that takes place after at least 20 but before 37 completed weeks of gestational age

Recurrent spontaneous abortion/miscarriage The spontaneous loss of two or more clinical pregnancies

Reproductive surgery Surgical procedures performed to diagnose, conserve, correct, and/or improve reproductive function

SET See Single Embryo Transfer

Severe Ovarian Hyper Stimulation Syndrome (severe OHSS) Severe OHSS is defined to occur when hospitalization is indicated. (See definition of Ovarian Hyper Stimulation Syndrome)

Single Embryo Transfer (SET) Method of selecting one embryo for transfer to lower the risk of multiple pregnancies

Small for gestational age Birth weight less than 2 standard deviations below the mean or less than the 10th centile

according to local intra-uterine growth charts

Sperm donation cycle See sperm recipient cycle

Sperm recipient cycle An ART cycle in which a woman receives spermatozoa from a donor who is someone other than her partner

SPOM See Simulated Physiological Oocyte Maturation

Spontaneous abortion/miscarriage The spontaneous loss of a clinical pregnancy that occurs before 20 completed weeks of gestational age (18 weeks post fertilization) or, if gestational age is unknown, the loss of an embryo/foetus of less than 400 g

STDs Sexually Transmitted Diseases

STIs Sexually Transmitted Infections

Stillbirth See Foetal death

TCM Traditional Chinese Medicine

TESA See Testicular Sperm Aspiration

TESE See Testicular Sperm Extraction

Testicular Sperm Aspiration (TESA) Needle aspiration of the testis to collect sperm, usually carried out in cases where PESA has been unsuccessful

Testicular Sperm Extraction (TESE) Done when other [sperm] extraction methods were unsuccessful

Total delivery rate with at least one live birth The estimated total number of deliveries with at least one live born baby resulting from one initiated or aspirated ART cycle

including all fresh cycles and all frozen/thawed ART cycles. This rate is used when all of the embryos fresh and/or frozen/thawed have been utilized from one ART cycles. *Note*: The delivery of a singleton, twin or other multiple pregnancy is registered as one delivery

TTC Time To Conception

Vanishing sac(s) or embryo(s) Spontaneous disappearance of one or more gestational sacs or embryos in an ongoing pregnancy, documented by ultrasound

Very low birth weight Birth weight less than 1500 g

Very preterm birth A live birth or stillbirth that takes place after at least 20 but less than 32 completed weeks of gestational age

Vitrification An ultra-rapid freezing method for eggs and embryos. It avoids the damage usually caused in freezing from ice crystals

ZIFT See Zygote Intra-Fallopian Transfer

Zygote A diploid cell resulting from the fertilization of an oocyte by a spermatozoon, which subsequently divides to form an embryo

Zygote Intra-Fallopian Transfer (ZIFT) A procedure in which zygote(s) is/are transferred into the fallopian tube

REFERENCES

1. Assisted Reproductive Technology (ART) – glossary. Available from: http://www.eshre.eu/ESHRE/English/Guidelines-Legal/ART-glossary/page.aspx/1062 [accessed 26 January 2013].
2. Zegers-Hochschild F, Adamson GD, de Mouzon J, et al. The International Committee for Monitoring Assisted Reproductive Technology (ICMART) and the World Health Organization (WHO) revised glossary on ART terminology, 2009. Hum Reprod 2009;24:2683–87.
3. Klement AH, Koren-Morag N, Itsykson P, et al. Intracytoplasmic morphologically selected sperm injection versus intracytoplasmic sperm injection: a step toward a clinical algorithm. Fertil Steril 2013;99:1290–3.

Glossary of Traditional Chinese Medicine (TCM) terms

Acupuncture (Zhen Jiu) TCM treatment modality characterized by the insertion of solid acupuncture needles into specific locations (acupuncture points) on the surface of the body for therapeutic purposes

Acupuncture point (Xue Wei) Specific locations on the surface of the body that are linked to meridians and network vessels. An acupuncture point has an anatomical location, needling specification, action and indication. A therapeutic change can be induced through stimulating these points by, for example, inserting into them fine needles (acupuncture), heating them (moxibustion) or by applying pressure to them

Blood (Xue) A TCM concept, which is different to the Orthodox medical understanding of blood. It is a vital substance derived from Gu Qi (food Qi) by the Stomach and Spleen. The Heart governs Blood, Blood circulates through the Vessels (Mai) and nourishes all of the body. Blood brings and offers life to the Body, Mind and Spirit. For example, it is responsible for sensation and perception. Blood is interrelated with Qi. It has a close relationship with the Liver, Spleen and Kidney

Blood Deficiency/Vacuity (Xue Xu) Pathology determined by signs of insufficient Blood

Blood-Heat (Xue Re) A pathological condition characterized by signs of Heat in the Blood

Blood Stasis (Xue Yu) Impaired flow of Blood

Brain (Nao) An Extraordinary Fu. Its growth and function is associated with Kidney Jing (Essence)

Cold (Han) One of the Six Evils or disease causing Qi. Cold can be either due to external environmental Cold or internally generated, for example from Yang deficiency

Conception Vessel (Ren Mai) One of the eight Extraordinary Vessels

Dampness (Shi) One of the Six Evils or disease causing Qi. Dampness can be either due to external environmental Dampness or Internal Dampness resulting from, for example, Spleen failing to transform and transport fluids

Damp-Heat (Shi Re) A combination of Dampness and Heat

Dietary irregularities (Yin Shi Shi Tiao) A miscellaneous cause of disease due to irregularities in a person's diet. For example, eating excessively or irregularly, eating an excessive quantity of raw, cold, hot, sweet or fatty foods, consuming too much alcohol

Eight Principles (Ba Gang) A TCM diagnostic system of the classification of disease, which helps to identify syndromes and formulate a treatment plan. The Eight Principles are Interior/Exterior, Hot/Cold, Full/Empty, Yin/Yang

Essence (Jing) The essential substance of the body. It determines and maintains life processes, including the constitution of a person. It is responsible for growth, development and reproduction. It is a combination of Pre-Natal (congenital) and Post-Natal (acquired) Jing (Essences)

Extraordinary Organ (Qi Heng Zhi Fu) Organs, which store Yin Essence (in the same way as Zang organs) and they also resemble the structure of the Fu organs. The Extraordinary Organs are the Brain, Uterus, Marrow, Bones, Vessels and the Gall Bladder

Fire (Huo) (1) A term that represents the motive force of life, a type of physiological fire which is transformed through Yang Qi. For example, the Ming Men (Fire of Life). (2) One of the Six Evils, disease causing Qi. Pathological Fire can also be caused by internal disharmony, for example Liver pathology

Five Phases (Wu Xing) A TCM diagnostic system of associated correspondences. The Five Phases are Wood, Fire, Earth, Metal, and Water

Food Qi (Gu Qi) Qi derived from food and water

Fu Yang organs. The Fu organs include the Stomach, Small Intestine, Large Intestine, Gall Bladder, Bladder, Triple Burner. They are paired with their Zang organs. Fu organs 'decompose' food and process 'matter', and eliminate waste products from the body

Girdle Vessel (Dai Mai) One of the eight Extraordinary Vessels

Governing Vessel (Du Mai) One of the eight Extraordinary Vessels

Gu Qi See Food Qi

Heart (Xin) One of the five Zang organs. The Heart governs Blood, controls Blood vessels, stores the Mind and Spirit

Heat (Re) One of the Six Evils or disease causing Qi. Heat is a manifestation of Fire, a pathological and lesser form. Heat can be either due to external environmental Heat or Internal Heat resulting from, for example, Yin Deficiency

Heavenly Gui/Heavenly Water/ Heavenly Tenth (Tian Gui) A TCM concept, which represents a person's reproductive potential. It is said to 'arrive' in girls at the age of 14 and in boys at the age of 16, peaks in the early /20s and declines as women and men age. Tian Gui also refers to 'original Yin' and 'menstruation'

Jing See Essence

Kidney (Shen) One of the five Zang organs. The Kidney is the basis for Pre-Natal Jing (Essence), it stores Jing (Essence) and governs reproduction

Liver (Gan) One of the five Zang organs. The Liver stores and regulates Blood and governs the flow of Qi

Lung (Fei) One of the five Zang organs. The Lungs govern Qi and respiration and significantly influence other Zang organs

Menstrual irregularities (Yue Jing Bu Tiao) Irregular menstrual cycles and abnormalities of the flow of menstruation such as the colour, amount and consistency of menstruation

Moxibustion (Jiu Fa) A TCM treatment technique involving heating acupuncture points and/or individual areas of the body by burning a herb called mugwort close to these areas

Original Qi or Source Qi (Yuan Qi) The original supply of Yin and Yang

Pathogenic Factor or Evil Qi (Xie Qi) Disease causing Qi, which affects the health of a person. Pathogenic Factors can be either external or internal. External Pathogenic Factors include: Wind, Cold, Fire,

Summer Heat, Dampness, Dryness (also known as the Six Excesses or Six Evil Qi). Internal Pathogenic Factors include: Dryness, Wind, Cold, Dampness, Fire. Pathogenic Factors can also be disease causing agents such as Phlegm or Blood Stasis

Penetrating Vessel (Chong Mai) One of the Eight Extraordinary Vessels

Phlegm (Tan) A thick and sticky substance which can be either a cause of a disease or a product of a disease. Phlegm may originate from internal disharmony of the Lung, Spleen and Kidney or through Fire condensing fluids. Dietary irregularities may also cause Phlegm. Dampness over time may lead to Phlegm

Post-Natal Jing (Essence), Post-Heaven Qi or later Heaven (Hou Tian) The constitution of a person, which is acquired after their birth under the influence of the Stomach and Spleen

Pre-Natal Jing (Essence)/Pre-Heaven Qi or Earlier Heaven (Xian Tian) The constitution of the person (or embryo) passed to them by their parents at the time of conception. Pre-Natal Jing (Essence) is under the influence of the Kidney

Qi The life force present in all living things. It is formed by the interaction between Yin and Yang. Qi flows in the body and provides vital energy to the organs and tissues

Source Qi See Original Qi

Spleen (Pi) The Spleen is one of the five Zang organs and is connected with the functions of the Stomach. The Spleen has an important role in the formation of Qi and Blood

Stagnation (Zhi) Slow or static movement of Qi and/or Blood

Stomach (Wei) A Fu organ connected with the functions of Spleen. It is involved in the formation of Blood by receiving and digesting Gu Qi (Food Qi)

and then sends this to the Heart and Spleen

Syndrome or Pattern Identification (Bian Zheng) A TCM classification and staging of a disease, derived through careful examination of clinical signs and symptoms

Tian Gui See Heavenly Gui

Uterus (Zi Gong) An Extraordinary Organ. It is interrelated with the Extraordinary Vessels and has a close association with the Kidney, Liver, Heart and Spleen. The Uterus controls menstruation, conception and pregnancy

Uterus Channel (Bao Luo) A Channel that joins the Kidney and Uterus together

Uterus Vessel (Bao Mai) A Vessel that joins the Heart and Uterus together

Wind (Feng) One of the Six Evils or disease causing Qi. Wind can be either due to external environmental Wind or internally generated, for example from Liver pathology. Wind easily combines with other Pathogenic Factors

Yang A concept opposite to Yin. Yang represents for example day, brightness, activity; whereas Yin represents night, darkness and rest

Yin A concept opposite to Yang. Yin represents for example night, darkness, and rest; whereas Yang represents day, brightness and activity

Yin Yang An ancient TCM concept that represents two opposing, yet mutually dependent forces. Yin Yang is a fundamental concept associated with TCM theoretical constructs, anatomy, physiology, diagnosis and clinical practice

Zang A Yin organ. The Zang organs include the Heart, Liver, Lung, Spleen, Kidney. Zang organs produce and store Jing (Essence)

Zangfu Zang and Fu internal organs. The Zangfu is an organ system that consists of functional interrelationships between the Zang and Fu

REFERENCES

1. Wiseman N, Feng Y. A practical dictionary of Chinese medicine. 2nd ed. Brookline, MA: Paradigm Publications; 1998. p. 14–52.

2. Larre C, Rochat de la Vallee E. Xue Blood. In: Root C, editor. Essence, Spirit, Blood and Qi. Norfolk: Monkey Press; 1999. p. 68–75 [chapter 4].

3. Wiseman N, Feng Y. A practical dictionary of Chinese medicine. 2nd ed. Brookline, MA: Paradigm Publications; 1998. p. 53–107.

4. Lu H. Causes of diseases. In: Terminology of traditional Chinese medicine. Milton Keynes: Lightening Source UK Ltd.; 2013. p. 99–112 [chapter 4].

5. Wiseman N, Feng Y. A practical dictionary of Chinese medicine. 2nd ed. Brookline, MA: Paradigm Publications; 1998. p. 108–65.

6. Wiseman N, Feng Y. A practical dictionary of Chinese medicine. 2nd ed. Brookline, MA: Paradigm Publications; 1998. p. 166–92.

7. Maciocia G. Identification of patterns. In: The foundations of Chinese medicine: a comprehensive text for acupuncturists and herbalists. Edinburgh, NY: Churchill Livingstone; 1989. p. 175–8 [chapter 17].

8. Wiseman N, Feng Y. A practical dictionary of Chinese medicine. 2nd ed. Brookline, MA: Paradigm Publications; 1998. p. 322–3.

9. Wiseman N, Feng Y. A practical dictionary of Chinese medicine. 2nd ed. Brookline, MA: Paradigm Publications; 1998. p. 251–94.

10. Lu H. Five elements. In: Terminology of traditional Chinese medicine. Milton Keynes: Lightening Source UK Ltd.; 2013. p. 18–34 [chapter 2].

11. Maciocia G. The functions of the Heart. In: The foundations of Chinese medicine: a comprehensive text for acupuncturists and herbalists. Edinburgh, NY: Churchill Livingstone; 1989. p. 71–87 [chapter 6].

12. Lu H. Physiology and pathology. In: Terminology of traditional Chinese medicine. Milton Keynes: Lightening Source UK Ltd.; 2013. p. 34–99 [chapter 3].

13. Wiseman N, Feng Y. A practical dictionary of Chinese medicine. 2nd ed. Brookline, MA: Paradigm Publications; 1998. p. 602–35.

14. Wiseman N, Feng Y. A practical dictionary of Chinese medicine. 2nd ed. Brookline, MA: Paradigm Publications; 1998. p. 324–37.

15. Maciocia G. The functions of the Liver. In: The foundations of Chinese medicine: a comprehensive text for acupuncturists and herbalists. Edinburgh, NY: Churchill Livingstone; 1989. p. 77–82 [chapter 7].

16. Maciocia G. The functions of the Lungs. In: The foundations of Chinese medicine: a comprehensive text for acupuncturists and herbalists. Edinburgh, NY:

ed. Brookline, MA: Paradigm Publications; 1998.

17. Wiseman N, Feng Y. A practical dictionary of Chinese medicine. 2nd ed. Brookline, MA: Paradigm Publications; 1998. p. 382–404.

18. Schatz J, Larre C, Rochat de la Vallée E, et al. The differential energies. In: Stang SE, translator. Survey of traditional Chinese medicine. 1st ed. Columbia, MD: Institut Ricci; 1986. p. 111–39. Part 2 [chapter 3].

19. Maciocia G. Identification according to Pathogenic Factors. In: The foundations of Chinese medicine: a comprehensive text for acupuncturists and herbalists. Edinburgh, NY: Churchill Livingstone; 1989. p. 293–302 [chapter 32].

20. Wiseman N, Feng Y. A practical dictionary of Chinese medicine. 2nd ed. Brookline, MA: Paradigm Publications; 1998. p. 423–74.

21. Wiseman N, Feng Y. A practical dictionary of Chinese medicine. 2nd ed. Brookline, MA: Paradigm Publications; 1998. p. 511–601.

22. Lu H. Yin and Yang. In: Terminology of traditional Chinese medicine. Milton Keynes: Lightening Source UK Ltd.; 2013. p. 6–18 [chapter 1].

23. Maciocia G. Yin and Yang. In: The foundations of Chinese medicine: a comprehensive text for acupuncturists and herbalists. Edinburgh, NY: Churchill Livingstone; 1989. p. 1–14 [chapter 1].

Churchill Livingstone; 1989. p. 83–7 [chapter 8].

Index

charting, 126
   advantages and disadvantages of,
      126, 127t
   analysing, 126–134
   in ART acupuncture practice, 127f
   as diagnostic aid, 126–134
   ovulation detection method,
      176–177
   working with, 126
BBT. *see* Basal body temperature (BBT)
Bicornuate uterus, 26, 313
Biochemical tests, for thyroid disease,
   197
Biopsy, endometrial, 82
Biphasic pattern, BBT chart, 128
Blastocysts
   versus day 2 *versus* day 3 transfer,
      Repeated Implantation Failure
      and, 305
   stage in embryogenesis, 62
Blastocyst scoring systems, 151, 152t
Blastomeres, 62
Blocked fallopian tubes, 186
Blood
   conjectural overview of production of,
      40f
   menstrual, conjectural composition
      from TCM point of view, 43f
   relationships between Qi, Jing
      (Essence), Body Fluids, and, 40f
   in reproductive physiology from TCM
      perspective, 39
Blood Deficiency syndromes
   foods beneficial in, 169
   in miscarriages, 318t
Blood-Heat
   in miscarriages, 318t
   Repeated Implantation Failure and,
      310
Blood Stasis syndromes, 309t
   foods beneficial in, 170
   and infertility, 308b
   in miscarriages, 318t
   Phlegm-Damp-Cold and, 122b
   and polycystic ovary syndrome, 194t
   Repeated Implantation Failure and,
      308
   in reproductive immunology, 328
   pathogenesis of, 329f
Blood-thinning medication
   in ART, 150
   and female fertility, 167b
BMI. *see* Body mass index (BMI)
Body Fluids, relationships between
      Blood, Qi, Jing (Essence),
      and, 40f
Body mass index (BMI), 161
Bravelle, in ART, 402t

British Acupuncture Council (BAcC), in
      medical causes of subfertility, 4
Buserelin (Suprefact®), 237
BV. *see* Bacterial vaginosis (BV)

C

Caffeine, 164
   effect on female fertility, 164
   effect on male fertility, 164
   in optimizing female fertility, 395
   in optimizing male fertility, 397
CAM. *see* Complementary and
      Alternative Medicine (CAM)
Canalization defect, in congenital
      uterine anomalies, 26
Capacitation, 12, 60
Care
   continuity of, 344
   for patients, 340–341
Case intake stage (review stage), in
      Assisted Reproductive
      Technology (ART) treatment,
      224–226
   lifestyle factors of, 224
   medical history and diagnosis of, 224
   previous ART treatment history of,
      224–225
   TCM history of, 226
CAT. *see* Chlamydia Antibody Test (CAT)
Cavitation, 62
CCCT. *see* Clomiphene Citrate Challenge
      Test (CCCT)
CD56+ natural killer cells, 325, 325t
Cervical assessment, in ovarian reserve
      screening, 80
Cervical funnelling, 324
Cervical insufficiency, 313, 323–325
Cervical length measurements,
      323–324
Cervical mucus, 60
   in ovulation detection methods, 176,
      176f
Cervical shortening, 325b
Cervical weakness, 313
Cervix, 25
Cetrorelix (Cetrotide®), 238
Cetrotide, in ART, 402t
Chinese medicine physicians, works of,
      reproductive history, 13–16
Chlamydia Antibody Test (CAT), 82
   in tubal pathology, 185
'Chocolate cysts.'. *see* Endometriomas
Chong Mai (Penetrating Vessel), 51
   functions of, 51
   vs. Ren Mai and Du Mai, 52t
Choragon, in ART, 402t
Circumcision, female, and subfertility, 6

Classical Chinese literature, conception
      and, 67–68
Cleavage, 62
Cleavage-stage embryo scoring systems,
      150–151, 151f, 151t, 152f
Clexane, in ART, 402t
Clomid. *see* Clomiphene citrate (CC)
Clomifene, in ART, 402t
Clomiphene citrate (CC), 12, 149, 149b
   in ART, 402t
   for ovulation disorders, 188–189
   ovulation induction with, 262
   for PCOS, 192
Clomiphene Citrate Challenge Test
      (CCCT), 80
Coital practices, 174–175
Coitus. *see* Sexual intercourse
Cold/coolness, 123–124, 124b
   acupuncture treatment of, 123–124,
      123t
   aetiology of, 123
   foods beneficial in, 170
   pathology of, 123
   possible consequences for
      reproduction and ART, 123
   Repeated Implantation Failure and,
      308
   signs and symptoms of, 123
Cold-Uterus, 309t
Compaction, 62
Competence, limit of, for acupuncture
      practice, 344
Complaint, presenting, for medical and
      fertility history taking, 97–98
Complementary and Alternative
      Medicine (CAM), 3
Conception, 59–72
   effect of male factor subfertility on,
      214
   female reproductive tract
      sperm transportation in, 60, 61b
      transportation of embryo down,
         62, 65f
   natural
      before IVF, 175b
      from TCM point of view, 67–68
   prerequirements for, 23–58
   from TCM point of view, 67–69
   in *In Vitro* Fertilization (IVF), 68, 68f
Conceptus stage, 63–66
Confidentiality, in acupuncture practice,
      344
Congenital uterine anomalies/
      abnormalities, 312
   American Fertility Society
      classification of, 26, 26f
   Repeated Implantation Failure and,
      302